John Charnley

Low Friction Arthroplasty of the Hip

Theory and Practice

With 440 Figures, 205 in Colour

Springer-Verlag Berlin Heidelberg New York 1979

Professor Sir John Charnley, C.B.E., F.R.S., F.R.C.S., F.A.C.S
Emeritus Professor of Orthopaedic Surgery, University of Manchester
Honorary Orthopaedic Surgeon, Centre for Hip Surgery, Wrightington Hospital
Consultant Orthopaedic Surgeon, King Edward VII Hospital, Midhurst, Sussex

Centre for Hip Surgery, Wrightington Hospital,
Wigan, Lancashire WN6 9EP, England

ISBN 978-3-642-67015-2
ISBN 978-3-642-67013-8 (eBook)
DOI 10.1007/978-3-642-67013-8

Library of Congress Cataloging in Publication Data. Charnley, John. Low friction arthroplasty of the hip. Bibliography: p. . Includes index. 1. Hip joint–Surgery. 2. Artificial hip joints. 3. Arthroplasty. 4. Friction. I. Title. RD549.C43 617'.58 78-22078

Softcover reprint of the hardcover 1st edition 1979

2125/3140-543210

To my wife Jill

and to the

Members of the Low Friction Society

all of whom have been personally associated with some part of this work during their period of Residency at Wrightington.

Contents

Preface

The theme of this work is the application of the engineering theory of frictional torque to total hip replacement.

The author adhered tenaciously to this theory, involving the use of a small-diameter femoral head, throughout the epoch when the large-diameter, metal-to-metal design dominated the field. During that considerable period general satisfaction with the early results rendered criticisms of the large-diameter head unwelcome. There was a formidable array of counter-criticism: the small head would pierce a film of synovial fluid; the small head would wear the socket too rapidly; the small head would always have a high risk of dislocation; detachment of the trochanter, to achieve precise orientation for the small head, was unacceptable.

But all these objections have now been largely overcome. Lubrication of high molecular weight polyethylene (HMWP) on metal is now accepted as being mainly by the boundary regime with thick fluid films playing no part. We now know that HMWP can indeed tolerate the very high stresses imposed by the small head and in tribological theory there may even be some advantage in high stress. Dislocation is now known not to be an automatic sequel to the small head.

There remains only the trochanter. Dissatisfaction with reattachment has been the cause of the many years of delay in writing this book. A method which satisfies the author has at last been found. This is important because it is now possible to view Chap. 21 (Biomechanics) for its practical application in attempting to reduce stress in total hips. It is quite possible that from this quarter will come the next phase of development, which is to prolong the survival of total hips in young patients, and to eliminate fatigue fractures in heavy men, by reducing stress, and doing so by engineering design.

Wrightington, September 1978 John Charnley

Acknowledgements

It is a pleasure to acknowledge help from colleagues who have not been named in the text; and especially pupils whose papers, published from Wrightington, have had to be excluded because not cogent to this work. There are a number of such papers to be found in *Clinical Orthopaedics and Related Research,* and my practice has been to add my name as the last of the authors for the purpose of aiding retrieval. I owe a debt of gratitude to Dr. Marshall Urist, Editor-in-Chief of *C.O.R.R.*, who has done so much to make that journal a true scientific archive; the publication of our papers from Wrightington in *C.O.R.R.* has been a vital encouragement to us over the years.

I am indebted to Mr. K.L. Barnes, F.R.C.S., Surgeon Superintendent of Wrightington Hospital, for casting a shrewd eye over the manuscript. Also, if in the course of time hydroxychloroquine should justify our hopes as a prophylactic agent against fatal pulmonary embolism, it is interesting to put on record that this potential in relation to total hip replacement was first spotted by Barnes, by clinical judgement, on a remarkably small series of patients and prompted the full-scale trials reported here. In a separate trial group, at King Edward VII Hospital, Midhurst, I am specially grateful to Dr. P.J. Doyle for his careful recording of data in relation to the prophylaxis of pulmonary embolism.

Mrs. A. Proffitt, Nursing Officer, Wrightington Hospital, and Sister Pring of King Edward VII Hospital, Midhurst, have kindly prepared for me the lists of instruments used in Chap. 14. I am greatly indebted to Mrs. Rosamunde Cock, M.C.S.P., Superintendent Physiotherapist, King Edward VII Hospital, for her most important help and advice in writing the chapter on post-operative rehabilitation.

Dr. Heinz Götze has taken the responsible step (for a publishing house so dedicated to perfection as Springer-Verlag) of permitting my own drawings to be used to illustrate the steps of the operation, (professionally 'touched up' where necessary) in order not to lose those surgeon's details which professional artists sometimes can miss. For this, and for the beautiful art work of his staff, I am very grateful.

I am also indebted to: Mr. Peter Kilshaw of the Department of Medical Illustration, Ribbleton Hospital; Mrs. E.M. Stringfellow for histological preparations; Mrs. S. Houghton and Mrs. D. Moss for work on many aspects of the clerical records; Mr. Ken Marsh and Mr. Frank Brown for the development of instruments and other researches in the Bioengineering Laboratory; Mr. Frank Dandy, Senior Laboratory Technician, for the immense amount of bacteriological work he carried out over a period of 10 years in the development of clean air operating; and above all Miss Margaret Green who has cheerfully undertaken the vast amount of typing and re-typing which was involved, at the same time pursuing her onerous clerical duties as my personal secretary.

In Britain it is not considered good form to acknowledge commercial undertakings in too glowing terms, even though the work would not have been possible without their collaboration; therefore I must satisfy myself merely by mentioning them by name: Messrs. Chas. F. Thackray Ltd. of Leeds; Codmann & Shurtleff Inc. of Randolph, Massachusetts, U.S.A.; Howorth Air Engineering of Farnworth; C.M.W. Laboratories of Blackpool.

Introduction

Many varieties of total hip replacement can give good results in the hands of surgeons who do not specialise in this field of surgery; but papers on complications, delivered to surgical societies even currently in 1978, make one wonder how consistently good are the good results in small groups of experience. The failure of most surgeons to stick to one type of operation, or to one surgical exposure, also implies underlying discontent.

The challenge comes when patients between 45 and 50 years of age are to be considered for the operation, because then every advance in technical detail must be used if there is to be a reasonable chance of 20 and more years of trouble-free activity. It is not in a young patient's interest for a surgeon to count on a successful 'revision' should mechanical failure ensue earlier than was expected. The best time to use acrylic cement is the first time; this is when the gritty surface of fresh cancellous bone can best accept cement. For this reason the author restricts this book to the primary intervention, in order to emphasize that only by performing easy operations very well shall we avoid an appalling accumulation of untreatable failures in the next two decades.

The longest duration of follow-up after this operation, in patients still alive and still successful, is 15 years. It is therefore a serious responsibility to extrapolate to another 50% for follow-up, and for age at operation to patients 10 years younger from the start. Therefore for vigorous patients of 45 years of age and over, it is emphasized that total hip replacement can be justified only when all the technical advances evolved during the last 5 years are adopted, some of which are described for the first time in this text.

Strictly speaking the procedure described in this book should not be regarded as a surgical operation at all. It should be seen as an exercise in practical mechanical engineering. Seen in this way the rate of mechanical failure ought to be as low as after any well-tried engineering routine. Practical engineering fortunately is easier than surgery, because in the traditional attitude to surgery the quality of a surgeon is revealed in the way he adapts himself to unforeseen difficulties in the course of an operation. But in practical engineering every job is first of all reduced to the same set of elements, by being 'taken to pieces', and the new components are then inserted without impediment and every time in exactly the same way. Therefore there should be no unforeseen difficulties. The fact that reassembly might take as long as the rest of the procedure is no matter if by this means we might some day aspire in hip surgery to a mechanical success rate of 99%.

Undoubtedly some who glance through these pages will be dismayed by what might appear to be the complexity of the operation, to judge from the number of steps needed to describe it and by the considerable armamentarium. But when an operative technique can be broken down into precise steps, each of which can be illustrated and facilitated by a special tool, the only difficulty facing the surgeon is to remember the sequence of the many easy steps. Keeping familiar with the sequence of the steps is the main problem, rather than their mere performance, and this is enormously helped by being able to perform three or four of these operations per week. This is the aspect of specialization which 'pays off' in the end-product.

Surgeons who are diffident about embarking on new and apparently complicated procedures can take heart in the knowledge that mechanical aptitude is a cerebral process. Aptitude which resides only in the fingers is a dangerous talent, though some hours of instruction at a fitter's bench can work wonders in boosting any postgraduate's self-confidence. This is an important aspect of the post-graduate training programme at Wrightington.

Finally the author thinks it important that he should state his belief that **in the case of osteoarthrosis** some type of artifical replacement of the hip is here to stay and that it could make a surgical specialty in itself. This might not apply to total replacement of the knee, and research into the pathology of rheumatoid arthritis may some day make joint replacement in that condition unnecessary. But in degenerative osteoarthrosis of the hip, total replacement must not be viewed as one of many passing phases in the evolution of surgery to be displaced in time by preventive measures. For the overwhelming majority of patients with osteoarthrosis of the hip, total replacement will always be the treatment of choice. It is most unlikely than anything will ever compete with it for speed of recovery and quality of the early result. Osteoarthrosis of the hip probably has its origin in a racial gene, as indicated in the remarkable differences in distribution throughout the world. There cannot therefore exist any prophylactic treatment for that strange, idiopathic condition of the hip correctly called **osteoarthrosis**.

Chapter 1

Low Friction Principle

The term low friction arthroplasty (or more correctly low frictional torque arthroplasty) was coined to emphasize the small diameter of the prosthetic head (22 mm) essential to the underlying theory. Low friction arthroplasty (LFA) is characterised even more particularly by the combination of a small prosthetic femoral head with a socket of maximum external diameter. Consequently the socket has maximum wall thickness.

The theory of low frictional torque arthroplasty is summarized in Fig. 1.1 reproduced from the Lancet 1961 under the title 'Arthroplasty of the hip—a new operation'.[1]

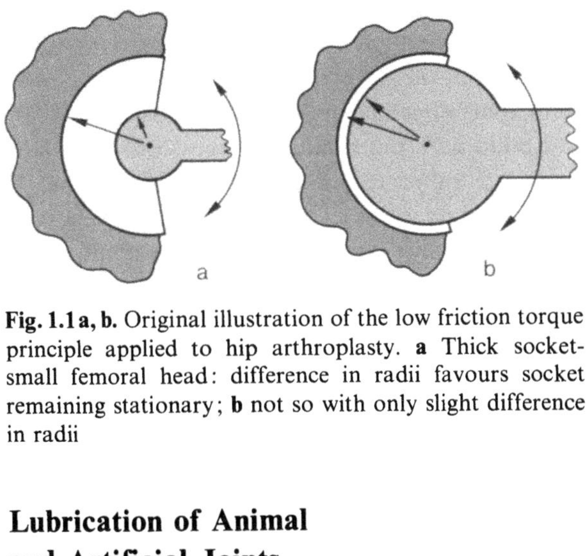

Fig. 1.1 a, b. Original illustration of the low friction torque principle applied to hip arthroplasty. **a** Thick socket-small femoral head: difference in radii favours socket remaining stationary; **b** not so with only slight difference in radii

Lubrication of Animal and Artificial Joints

The author's approach to total hip replacement from the point of view of lubrication started as a result of a chance encounter with a patient who had a Judet femoral head replacement for osteoarthrosis 1 or 2 years previously and whose hip in certain positions emitted an audible squeak. Enquiries established that colleagues had also had similar experiences. In the X-rays the stem of the prosthesis was seen to be lying in a grossly enlarged track in the femur, and this suggested that under load high friction between the head and the arthrosic socket was resisting movement and that the movement was now taking place between the loose stem and the femur.

This incident served to emphasize the ignorance of basic principles of lubrication, as applied to artificial animal joints, which existed at that time. The mere fact that a polished sphere of a plastics material, or of metal, felt 'slippery' when wetted with tissue fluids and handled in surgical rubber gloves, was no proof that this slippery behaviour would persist in an arthrosic acetabulum under heavy loads.

Lubrication of Animal Joints

At that time the universally accepted theory of lubrication in animal joints gave a dominant role to the action of synovial fluid. Maconnaill (1950)[2] was impressed by the incongruity existing between joint surfaces in the range of movement used when moving under load, compared with what he called the 'close-packed' situation adopted by some joints, as part of a muscle-sparing mechanism, when 'standing at ease'. Maconnaill saw in the incongruity of joint surfaces Nature adopting the principle of hydrodynamic lubrication, demonstrated par excellence in the Michel bearing, where convergent wedges of fluid generate pressure under the action of rotation and separate the surfaces moving under load.

Applied to animal joints however this concept was not convincing, because slow motion, and especially slow oscillating motion, is not ideally suited to the persistence of full-thickness fluid films between sliding surfaces.

Up to that time the only experimental work which had been published on the lubrication of animal joints was that of E. Shirley Jones (1936)[3], and of a number of experiments the one of greatest interest was that in which he made a freshly amputated human finger joint function as the pivot of a pendulum. This was an elegant experiment because it explored the resistance to movement of a loaded joint with the surfaces sliding at different speeds. This is because of the well-known fact of a pendulum that the time for each swing is the same whether the amplitude be large or small; therefore at the start of the experiment the speed of sliding will be high when the amplitude is great and will get progressively less as the amplitude decays. In his experiments with the amputated finger joint Jones found that when plotted against time the decrement of each swing behaved in an exponential fashion, which meant that frictional resistance was disproportionately high at high speeds of sliding. This was consistent with the viscous behaviour of a fluid and from this it was concluded that lubrication of the finger joint must incorporate a hydrodynamic mechanism (Fig. 1.2).

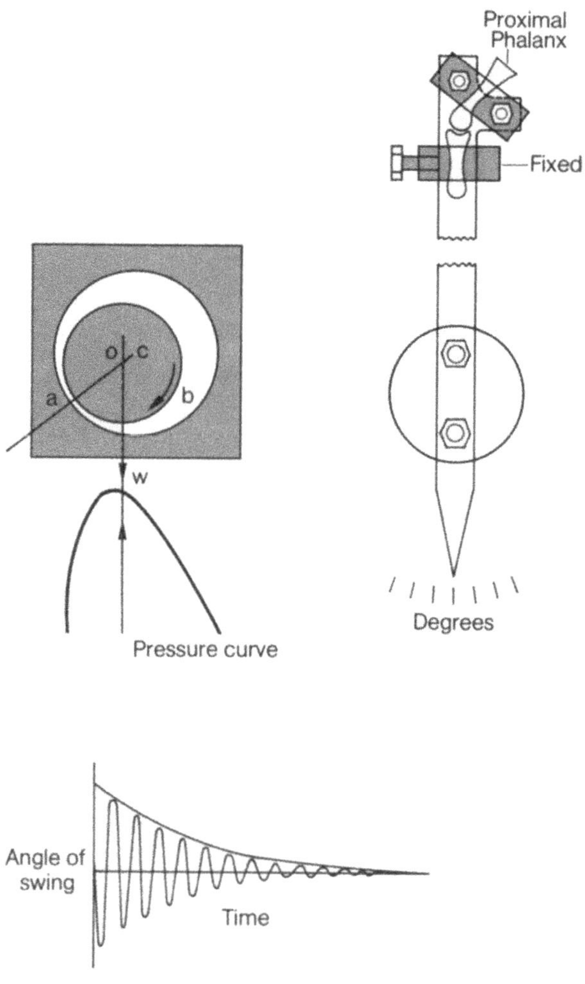

Fig. 1.2. Original experiment of E. Shirley Jones reproduced from his paper

The regime of lubrication which is the diametric opposite of hydrodynamic lubrication is known as 'boundary' lubrication. This mode of lubrication is equivalent to the sliding of dry surfaces which possess intrinsically slippery qualities; the extreme examples being graphite or molybdenum sulphide or polytetrafluorethylene. Also in this category is the lubricating action of substances which react chemically with the sliding surfaces and thereafter function as molecular films too thin to show viscosity in accordance with the laws of fluid mechanics. A good example of this is the lubricating action of fatty acids such as the oleic, stearic, palmitic acids, etc., which form soaps in combination with the metal surfaces of plain bearings. The intriguing feature of this mode of lubrication is that though extremely thin, as a result of being bound chemically to the sliding surfaces, the lubricating films are more resistant to rupture than thick films of grease or oil unable to make a chemical bond with the sliding surfaces. In these latter cases a film of oil or grease would be able to remain intact only as a result of the (relatively small) molecular forces acting between the molecules of the oil itself.

The boundary mode of lubrication seemed to the author ideally suited to the lubrication of slow-moving, heavily loaded animal joints and especially since these were exposed to oscillating motion and capable of remaining stationary under load for several seconds without exhibiting 'stiction' at the moment of resuming movement. It seemed possible that Jones had made an error in choosing a finger joint for the pivot of his pendulum because a finger joint is unstable in the absence of the collateral ligaments and to retain the ligaments would offer greater resistance at large amplitudes of swing than at small ones; this could explain an exponential pattern of decay of amplitude without postulating a viscous fluid mechanism.

The author repeated the pendulum experiment, this time choosing a human ankle joint (Fig. 1.3).

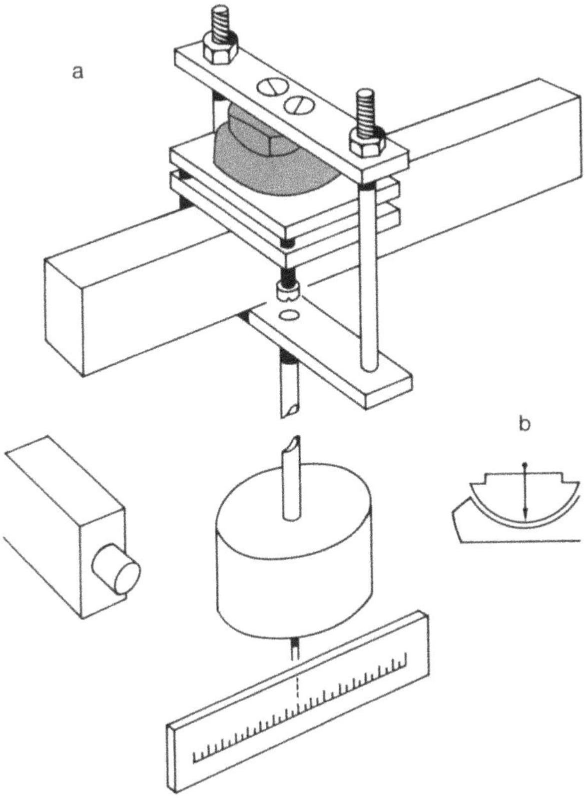

Fig. 1.3. Pendulum experiment using human ankle-joint

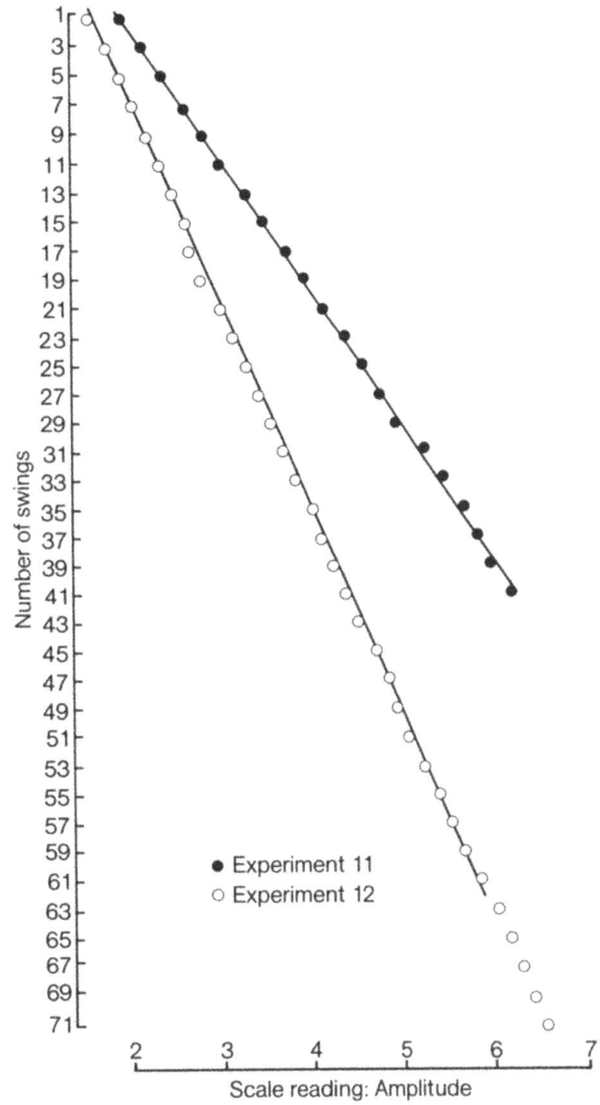

Fig. 1.4. Graphs of decay of amplitude with number of swings. Increase in number of swings when visible synovial fluid was not wiped away with dry cloth (Expt. 12 compared with Expt. 11) did not change straight line performance

Because of the deep curvature of the components of the ankle joint this biological pivot was self-locating in the absence of collateral ligaments. In these experiments the decay of amplitude followed a straight line (Fig. 1.4) indicating that the coefficient of friction in the joint remained the same despite changes in the rate of sliding. This is a recognised feature of boundary friction within certain fairly wide limits of speed. It was interesting also to note that the straight-line behaviour of the decrement of amplitude was not greatly changed whether the ankle joint was visibly wetted with synovial fluid or had been wiped clean of visible liquid with a dry cloth. This suggested that a smear of lubricant was as effective as a large volume, a state of affairs more in accordance with the theory of boundary lubrication than hydrodynamic lubrication.

Against the theory of boundary lubrication as the sole explanation of lubrication in animal joints is often advanced the fact that the coefficient of friction of an animal joint is so astonishingly low (in the region of 0.01 or even less) and in ordinary engineering practice most examples of boundary lubrication have coefficients of friction in the region of 0.10 or higher.

However, it is still possible that the last word has not yet been said on the ultimate nature of lubrication in animal joints and, as is commonly the case in matters of lubrication, a mixed regime of fluid film and boundary lubrication probably exists, with Nature having discovered a unique means of making a mixed regime.

Synovial Fluid as a Lubricant

In the designing of a total joint replacement the practical importance of the foregoing remarks is that when these experiments were extended to the substances likely to be used in the construction of artificial joints [before the introduction of high molecular weight polyethylene (HMWP)] it was found that synovial fluid was incapable of acting as a lubricant. Thus a chrome-cobalt surface sliding on chrome-cobalt; stainless steel sliding on bare bone; and Perspex (Lucite or polymethylmethacrylate) sliding on bare bone; when lubricated with bovine synovial fluid all presented coefficients of friction in the region of 0.5 and squeaked under load. On the other hand stainless steel sliding on normal articular cartilage was well lubricated with synovial fluid (coefficient of friction in region of 0.05) and this combination therefore was not greatly inferior to articular cartilage sliding on articular cartilage (Fig. 1.5).

These observations therefore seemed to indicate that synovial fluid was a specific lubricant for articular cartilage and for nothing else. The specificity of a lubricant for the material of a surface is characteristic of boundary lubrication because it involves that quality known as 'oiliness'. This does not apply in hydrodynamic lubrication where oiliness in a lubricant is unnecessary: water or air can be used to lubricate hydrodynamically, provided that the geometry of the rotating surfaces, the area of the surfaces, the load to be carried and the speed of rotation are all known.

From these considerations the author decided in 1958 that the only chance of success in lubricating an artificial animal joint would be by using surfaces which were intrinsically slippery on each other; in other words, self-lubricating irrespective of whether tissue fluid were present or not. This led to trials of polytetrafluorethylene (Teflon, PTFE), with spectacular early results. Unfortunately the poor wearing properties of pure PTFE, and the disastrous complications with PTFE 'filled' with material designed to enhance wear resistance, ended in PTFE being abandoned in 1961, after some 300 total hip operations had been performed with a number of different mechanical modifications. The PTFE era taught a number of very important lessons which might still have warnings for future development in this field and for this reason a brief review of selected experiences is cogent.

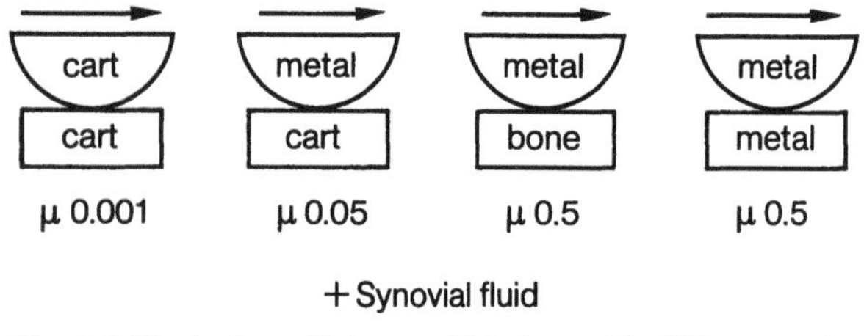

Fig. 1.5. Typical coefficients of friction with different pairs of substances in hip arthroplasty

a) Particle Size and Tissue Reaction

It is now well known that PTFE in the hip joint produced voluminous masses of amorphous caseous material. This presumably is the proteinaceous material resulting from vast numbers of dead foreign-body giant cells. Particle size might be very important in the production of granulomatous material because PTFE particles were very large (often 300 μm) and their large size could prevent transport away from the site of production. The high rate of production of PTFE particles (rapidity of wear) in addition to the large size of the particles, might have been responsible for defeating the available transport system for removing the particles and the caseous debris. Therefore slow production (high wear resistance) and small size of abraded particles might be important features in reducing local accumulations of caseous material even if the production of wear particles may never be avoided.

Therefore it would seem possible, if wear has to be accepted as inevitable, that the ideal implant will produce very small particles. The factors which control the size of abraded particles of HMWP as yet are unknown but the particles produced in the (LFA) hip in the author's experience seem to be smaller than those produced in knee arthroplasties. This might suggest that the high loading of a small-diameter ball can prevent 'third body' abrasion, perhaps by burnishing the particles into the surface, perhaps by the tendency of the small-diameter head to 'bore' into the plastic and remain close fitting, rather than combining elements of rolling and sliding encouraged by the large-diameter spherical surfaces of the knee.

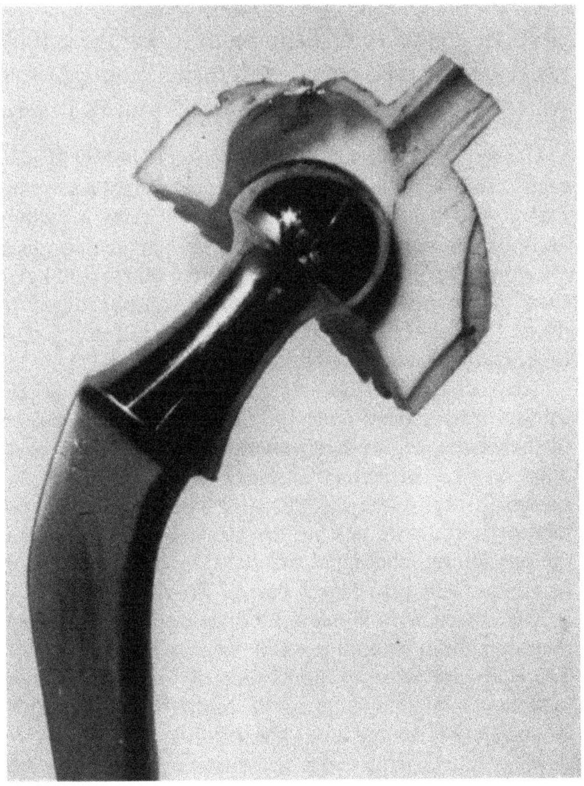

Fig. 1.6. Total wear-out of Teflon socket after 3 years. Note vertical direction of wear track

b) Direction of Socket Wear

The rapidity of wear of Teflon hip sockets enabled the direction of wear to be recognised in periods as short as 2 or 3 years (Fig. 1.6). When wear is very slight, as with HMWP, it is difficult to be sure of the precise direction of wear.

The frequency with which the direction of wear was vertically upwards, or even upwards and laterally, made Elson and Charnley (1968)[(4)] recommend that in designing total hip replacements we should not count on the joint force being advantageously inclined at 10° medially but we should assume that the joint force acts as though it were directed vertically. This emphasizes, among many other matters, the importance of designing the hip socket to be totally enclosed inside the acetabulum.

c) Fillers to Enhance Wear Resistance

PTFE filled with glass fibre, or with a synthetic proprietary substance (Fluorosint-Polypenco) showed enhanced wear resistance by a factor of 20 when lubricated with water in the laboratory. The surfaces of the plastics specimens also became highly polished in these laboratory experiments and the stainless steel counterface also remained in a high state of polish. In the human body however this type of filled PTFE behaved very badly. PTFE filled with glass fibre even after 1 year in the body developed a 'pasty' surface which could be scraped away with a blunt instrument. Fluorosint wore in the body just as rapidly as ordinary PTFE but the result was even worse, because the filler acted abrasively and lapped metal from the prosthetic head. The sockets retained a matt surface and never acquired the glazed surface that they did in the laboratory.

Ultra-High Molecular Weight Polyethylene

The introduction of HMWP by the author in 1962 as a material for socket surfaces in joint replacement necessitated a change of emphasis in lubrication theory as applied to artificial joints. The unique low coefficient of friction of PTFE could no longer be deployed and emphasis now had to be turned towards materials offering high resistance to wear and producing therefore a minimum of abraded detritus.

The coefficient of friction of HMWP is at least five times higher than that of PTFE, but its wear resistance in laboratory tests is 500–1000 times better. The very high wear resistance of HMWP now made acceptable the very high stresses on the plastics material produced by the small-diameter femoral head inseparable from concepts of low frictional torque. It thus became feasible to compensate for increased frictional resistance by designing for low frictional torque.

In this change of policy two unpredicted factors came to light which helped to offset the inferior coefficient of friction of HMWP compared with Teflon. In the first place HMWP is one of the plastics materials whose coefficient of friction becomes less under high stress; in the second place HMWP proved to be capable of a modest degree of boundary lubrication by synovial fluid. This latter property therefore made it an exception to the author's statement in the early stages of this work that there were no substances available for joint replacement which could avail themselves of synovial fluid as a lubricant.

Pendulum Comparator

A method of attempting to compare the frictional torque of different designs of total hip implant is the pendulum 'comparator' illustrated in Fig. 1.7. This device, developed by the author at Wrightington, is not intended to measure absolute values of friction but merely to make broad, even qualitative, comparisons of the frictional torque offered by different designs of total hip replacement when compared against a 22-mm-diameter stainless steel sphere in a socket of HMWP. Like all methods of measuring frictional resistance these tests are prone to erratic behaviour and it is impossible to make fine distinctions over the middle range of observed results; but for its main purpose, which is to reveal extremes of behaviour, it is valid.

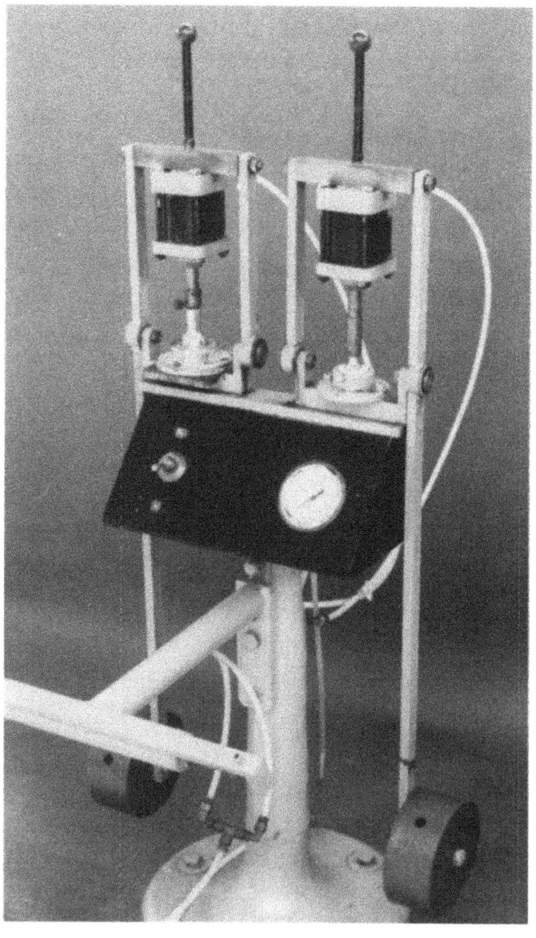

Fig. 1.7. Pendulum comparator

The device consists of two separate pendulum systems each with a heavy metal bob of identical weight and swinging on ball bearings. Each pendulum carries a cylinder and piston connected by a flexible tube to a compressed air source to deliver a force of about 200 lb (90 kg) at each piston rod. The femoral head component of the device to be tested must be cut from its stem and attached, by brazing, to a stub to fit the piston rod.

The sockets to be tested are mounted in metal holders using acrylic cement (Fig. 1.8). The point corresponding to the centre of the hemispherical cavity of the socket must be at a prescribed distance above the base plate on which the holder lies. This distance is the height of the horizontal axis passing through the ball bearings of the pendulum. The metal mounts taking the hip sockets locate on three pins on the base of the comparator.

The comparison is made by drawing both pendula to their maximum amplitude where they are held by a trigger. The bobs are released simultaneously without applying load to the hip implants to be compared. The number of swings is counted until the pendula start to be out of phase but of course are still swinging vigorously (this will usually be about 8–10 half-cycles). This demonstrates that in the unloaded state there is no gross difference between the two sides. The bobs are again brought back to the starting triggers and air pressure is applied to the two implants to be compared. The bobs are released and the number of half-cycles on each side are counted until each pendulum stops.

The tests are performed with bovine synovial fluid as a lubricant. It is important that the implants should be freshly washed in soapy water which is then eliminated by an adequate period under a running tap. Thereafter care should be taken not to get grease from the fingers on to the test surfaces.

The apparatus can be criticised as being unphysiological in that a constant load is maintained on the to and the fro half-cycles. It is not possible to design otherwise because slight errors of centring, inevitable when parts of the instrument deflect under the load, could produce serious errors if the load were applied repeatedly in one direction and removed in the other. By maintaining a constant load the errors caused by the load assisting the swing in one direction are neutralised by the load impeding the swing in the other direction.

Another criticism is that the state of any fluid film which might exist must be best at the start and that any contribution of fluid lubrication must decline throughout a test. Against this it is main-

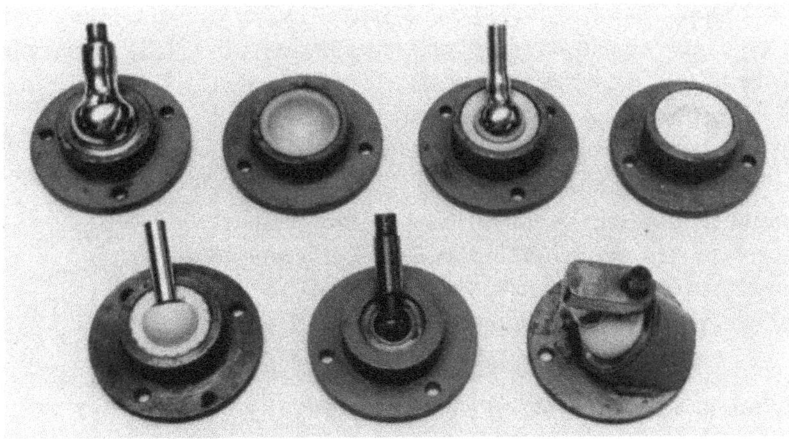

Fig. 1.8. Sockets mounted in holders to locate centre of rotation as near as possible to axis of the pendulum comparator

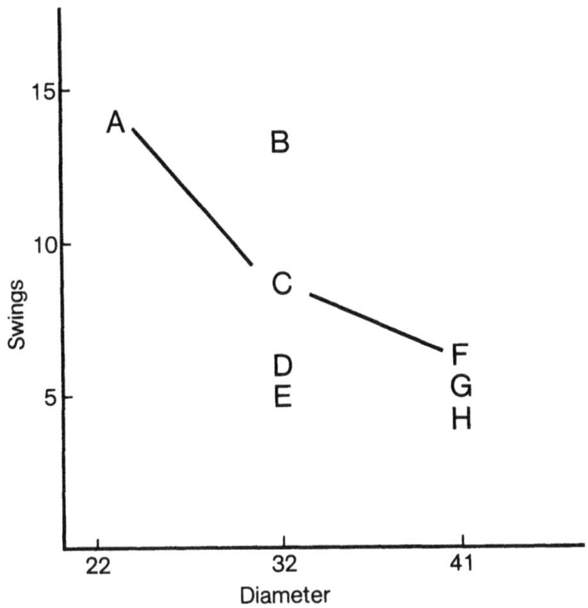

Fig. 1.9. *A, C, F,* represent different diameters of metal (stainless steel) ball on HMWP. The number of swings to stopping decreases as diameter increases: the opposite of what would be expected with fluid lubrication. Load 250 lb in all cases
D, polyester socket with 32-mm diameter chrome-cobalt head
E, ceramic (Al_3O_3) head 31-mm diamter on socket of same ceramic (Boutin)
B, ceramic (Biolox) head on HWMP socket
G, trunnion design (Weber) 42-mm polyester sphere
H, McKee–Farrar 41-mm chrome-cobalt head on socket of same

tained that, whatever may be the mechanism of lubrication, the comparison starts with all the joints being offered the same circumstances and the test reveals how different artificial joints react under these same starting conditions.

An important feature of the design is that the plane in which the ball oscillates is not unlike that during the weight-bearing phase of walking in the human body: the axis of rotation of the ball is at an angle to the central axis of the socket. To rotate the ball on the same axis as that of the socket would incur great variations in frictional torque depending on the fit of the ball in the socket: a large socket would give point contact with the head in the depth of the socket and therefore a very low frictional moment; a too-small socket would cause a 'cone-clutch' effect with binding of the head at the rim of the socket with very high frictional torque. An annular zone of contact halfway down the socket (as was recommended for the McKee-Farrar metal-to-metal implant) would give intermediate frictional torque. By oscillating in a plane perpendicular to the central axis of the socket, sensitivity to errors of fit of the ball in the socket is minimised because the length of the friction moment arm is the radius of the ball and is therefore constant.

Some typical results, the averages of many tests, all using lubrication with synovial fluid, are shown in Fig. 1.9. Points of special interest are as follows:

1. Metal/HMWP

The relationship between the number of swings and the diameter of the metal ball is well demonstrated in the sequence A (22 mm) – C (32 mm) – F (41 mm). If an important element of fluid-film lubrication were to be present one would expect that spheres with large diameters would make more swings than those with small diameters under the same load because large-diameter spheres would generate lower fluid pressures than small spheres and large-diameter sockets would present a longer distance through which a viscous fluid would have to extrude under low pressures.

In practical tests the opposite is the case. The number of swings becomes fewer as the diameter increases (14 swings falling to 7 as the diameter increases from 22 mm to 41 mm) which is in favour of boundary lubrication theory.

2. Metal 32 mm/HMWP (C) compared with metal 32 mm/polyester (D)

The inferior performance of the polyester socket could be explained in several ways: (a) on boundary theory as indicating that the friction between metal and polyester was greater than with HMWP or (b) again on boundary theory that very thin (boundary) films of synovial fluid are not encouraged by polyester but are by HMWP. On hydrodynamic theory the inferior performance might be explained by the greater hardness of the polyester causing any fluid film that might be present to be immediately ruptured, whereas the compliance of the HMWP socket could permit a fluid film to spread and so reach a thinner layer before finally rupturing (elasto-hydrodynamic lubrication).

These explanations also apply to the behaviour of metal-to-metal prostheses (41-mm McKee chrome-cobalt) where three or four swings when dry is not improved at all (or only marginally) by adding synovial fluid.

3. Ceramic Spheres and Ceramic Socket [31-mm diameter (E) Boutin]

When first tested this combination performed well, being equal to a 35-mm metal sphere on HMWP i.e. C (7 swings). At this time the sphere and the socket both had a matt surface finish. After about 30 demonstrations in the pendulum comparator (perhaps 200 swings) the performance deteriorated to the present state (E) of only 4 swings. But worse than this, it now emits a high-pitched audible squeak. The appearance of the squeak and the deterioration of performance coincided with the rubbing surfaces acquiring some degree of polish.

4. Ceramic Sphere and HMWP Socket [(B) 30-mm diameter Biolox (Muller)]

This combination performs better than any other in the range equalling the performance of the 22-mm metal head. Because the Biolox head is 30 mm in diameter compared with the 22-mm metal head the coefficient of friction between this ceramic and HMWP must be less than that between metal and HMWP (The 30-mm Biolox head was an experimental head—the one used clinically is 32 mm in diameter.)

5. Trunnion Hip. Polyester sphere (42-mm diameter (G) Weber)

This unit performs badly in the pendulum comparator and is only slightly better than the 41-mm metal-to-metal McKee. It appears that very high frictional resistance between the large-diameter polyester sphere and metal socket prevents the small-diameter trunnion revealing its potential. It would seem that for a better performance the axis of the trunnion would have to be more horizontal if it is to share more of the flexion range of the hip joint.

Coefficients of Friction in the Literature

The precise value of the coefficient of friction between any two sliding substances depends very much on the method used to make the measurement; for this reason the literature contains different values for the various combinations of materials which have been used in artificial joints.

An interesting feature of the pendulum comparator is how the performance has changed when giving monthly demonstrations with the same specimens over the years, though the relative values have been fairly constant. This would suggest that changes, possibly oxidative, can affect the rubbing surfaces over 10 years. When polished again the original values were restored.

Generally speaking a coefficient of friction between 0.05 and 0.10 would appear to the accepted value for metal on HMWP lubricated with synovial fluid (Simon and Radin) [5]. Compared with

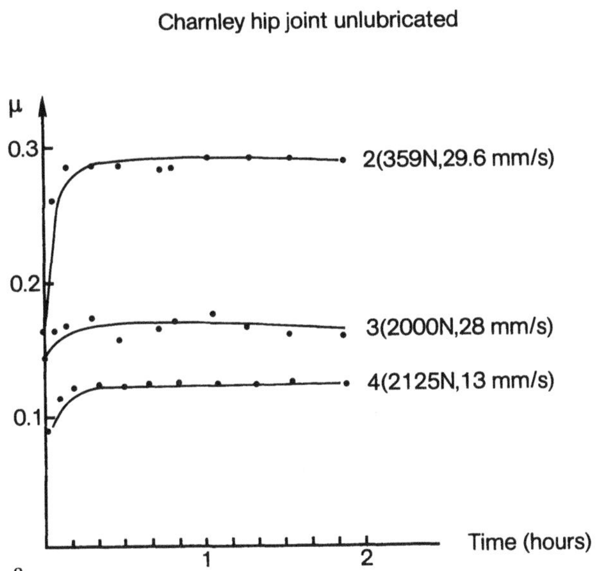

a

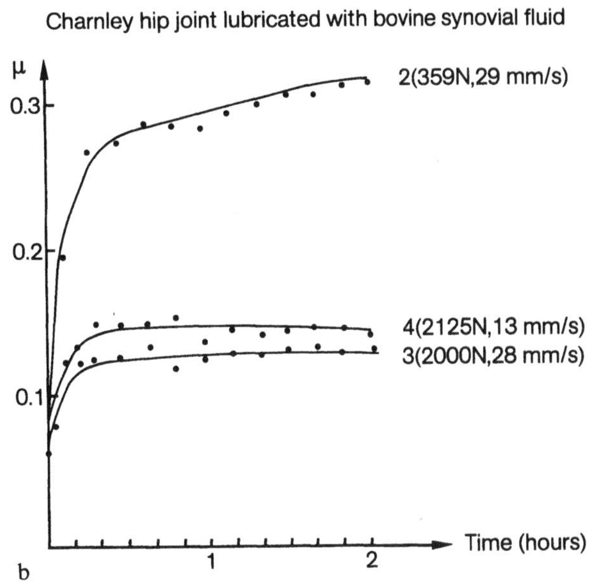

b

Fig. 1.10 a, b. Leeds pendulum experiment with load varied throughout each cycle, by hydraulic mechanism, to simulate human gait. **a** Lubricated with bovine synovial fluid and **b** unlubricated. Note decrease in coefficient of friction as load increases. Fact that performance is not different, lubricated or not lubricated with synovial fluid, despite loaded and unloaded half-cycles, strongly favours boundary lubrication mechanism as major contribution to lubrication

the coefficient of friction in normal animal joints, an order of magnitude lower, these are not particularly low values.

In a series of experiments carried out by the Bioengineering Group in Leeds [(6)], using a different type of test, even higher frictional resistance was recorded with the 22-mm Charnley prosthesis on HMWP and the results were not materially reduced when lubricated with synovial fluid. This test was a pendulum experiment but the amplitude was maintained by an external power source. The load on the joint was varied by a hydraulically operated system which applied peak loads at the extremes of motion corresponding to 'heel-strike' and 'toe-off' in human gait. This physiological method of loading therefore would encourage fluid lubrication in the non-weight-bearing half-cycle, not possible in the author's very simple comparator. The frictional resistance was monitored at each swing. Fig. 1.10 a, b reproduce their findings. It will be seen that within 10 min of starting a test, with or without synovial fluid, there was a rise in frictional resistance to 0.15 under a load of about 450 lb (2000 N). In this pendulum experiment it was notable that the coefficient of friction of the 22-mm head on HMWP, with or without synovial fluid, was less under high loads than when lightly loaded. Thus under 80 lb (359 N) $\mu = 0.3$ whereas at 450 lb approx. (2000 N) the coefficient of friction was half this value ($\mu = 0.15$).

Is Low Frictional Torque Essential?

High frictional torque in a total hip under the full load of joint force in theory will help to loosen cement bonds. In theory also high frictional torque will reduce the amount of external work which the muscles can do by energy lost as heat in the bearing. Energy lost cannot be demonstrated in clinical practice, though in metal-to-metal bearings in laboratory conditions it can always be demonstrated that they offer frictional resistance to movement under heavy load and become warm.

On four or five occasions the author has performed bilateral total hip replacement comparing the 22-mm metal-to-plastic LFA in one hip with a 41-mm-diameter metal-to-metal McKee in the other and, with technically sound implants on both sides, no subjective difference between the two sides was volunteered by the patient nor was admitted on questioning. These patients did not notice any feeling of weakness on the side of the metal-to-metal hip when ascending stairs compared with their sensations on the low-friction side.

The author suggests as one possible explanation that in the load-bearing phase of ascending stairs the metal-to-metal bearing might 'lock' and function as an arthrodesis. The same theory could conceivably apply even in bilateral metal-to-metal arthroplasties when ascending stairs: in this case the unloaded metal-to-metal hip will flex freely to reach the upper step, then it will progressively lock as load is transferred to it; the locked opposite hip which is taking load then progressively unlocks as load is removed. A considerable experience of arthrodesis of the hip indicates that in a unilateral arthrodesis the only defective phase in mounting stairs is that of reaching the upper step with the foot of the arthrodesed side. The act of putting weight on the arthrodesed hip and raising the body offers no problem and the sensation is indistinguishable from that of normal hip. In offering this explanation the locking is visualised as a gradual process, the change from free movement to seizure occupying perhaps 10°. Another 10° could easily be contributed by movement of pelvis and spine.

Another curious phenomenon, in the light of bad performance in the laboratory, when considering the behaviour of metal-to-metal total hip joints in clinical practice is that patients do not feel 'stick-slip' (which is the basis of a squeak) yet this is invariably detected when attempting to move a metal-to-metal total hip lubricated with synovial fluid under heavy load in the laboratory. In an experiment which the author has demonstrated many hundreds of times to visitors, a 41-mm McKee arthroplasty is wetted liberally with bovine synovial fluid and while the visitor is moving it slowly to and fro, manually through the medium of a lever, air pressure is suddenly applied to deliver 200 lb force. The metal-to-metal total hip locks instantaneously without a detectable period even as short as 0.5 s which might be occupied by the extrusion of the synovial fluid. Thereafter to move the metal-to-metal joint demands very considerable force, a grinding sound is audible and vibrations are detected through the lever.

One explanation could be that patients might not have a sensory mechanism in the bones of the hip capable of transmitting this type of vibration to consciousness. It is always surprising to observe how patients with unoperated arthrosic hips which emit loud grating sounds seem to detect this by their ears just as do others in the same room; they do not seem to associate it with a special sensation coinciding with the grating sound.

Yet another explanation might be that in the living body, metal-to-metal joints might be lubricated with a type of synovial fluid which cannot be imitated by bovine synovial fluid in the laboratory. In other words, a proteinaceous substance in the living environment might become conjugated with the metallic elements in the sliding surfaces in a way not reproducible in the non-living circumstances of the laboratory.

As regards the question whether low frictional torque in a total hip replacement plays a significant role in preventing loosening of the cemented components, an argument cited against this is derived from experimental work on sockets cemented into the cadaveric acetabulum (Anderson et al) [(7)]. In this study it was found that torsional moments needed to loosen cemented sockets were from 4 to more than 20 times greater than any frictional moment capable of being transmitted from a prosthetic femoral head. While there can be no disputing these laboratory findings this type of experiment overlooks the fact that if demarcation of a cemented socket from the adjacent cancellous bone is present (from the biological reaction of bone to microscopic movement of cement in contact with it over a period of years) the avoidance of high frictional torque might permit such a socket to function for many more years than would be the case if high frictional torque were present. The loading of a cemented socket in the relatively constant direction of the joint force is almost certainly the main cause of socket loosening; but add to this high frictional torque in the later stages of this process and then clinical failure is accelerated.

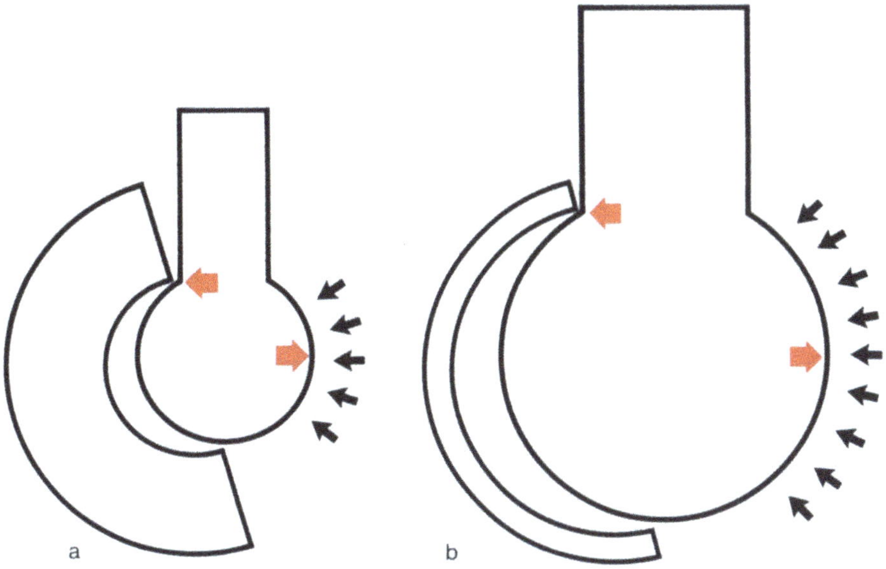

Fig. 1.11 a, b. Demonstrating magnitude of forces reacting on cement bonds, both of socket and of femoral prosthesis, at moment of traumatically exceeding designed range. **a** In case of small-diameter head, force resisting dilation of capsule is small; consequently equal and opposite force reacting against socket also is small; but thick-walled socket preserves maximum external surface area to resist shearing force imposed on it. **b** In case of large-diameter head, force resisting dilation of capsule is great; consequently equal and opposite force reacting against socket also is great; but external surface area of socket resisting shearing forces is identical with that in case **a**

Size of Femoral Head and the 'Safety Valve' of the Hip

The small-diameter femoral head demanded by the theory of low frictional torque originally caused some anxiety because obviously it could be prone to post-operative dislocation. Once the factors controlling stability had been clearly defined (Chap. 19) an advantageous side-effect was recognized in the possibility that transient subluxation could occur during severe trauma. By transient subluxation we mean momentary and incomplete escape of the femoral head from the socket when the joint is forcibly and traumatically made to exceed the designed range. Incomplete escape of the head is then followed instantaneously by return of the head to its normal position when the overstretched limb returns within its proper range.

In the case of the 41-mm McKee prosthesis a common observation at secondary interventions is a bright spot on the neck corresponding with a point of impingement on the rim of the socket. McKee himself frequently attributed loosening of one or other of the components to the patient sustaining trauma as the result of a fall. In our experience with the 22-mm head we cannot recall a single case where loosening of cement clearly followed trauma. On the contrary it is a common experience to have elderly patients reporting back to hospital after falls, proved by demonstrating cuts or bruises on their knees.

The author's explanation is that if a 41-mm-diameter McKee head is at the critical point of starting to be levered out of the socket, as the range is being forced beyond the point of impingement of the neck, the large head will have to stretch the capsule (or the fibrous reconstruction of the excised capsule) to produce a much greater volumetric distension of the capsule than would be the case with a small head (Fig. 1.11). The force needed to do this would react on the stem of the femoral prosthesis and possibly also on the socket.

Thickness of Socket Wall

The concept of low frictional torque in total hip replacement using a prosthetic head of minimum diameter and a socket of maximum external diameter, was prompted originally by the idea that a major difference in diameters would render cement in the acetabulum unnecessary. It was also recognized that a plastics socket with a thick wall would diffuse the load from a small ball more evenly over the socket-cement-bone interface than would a large ball acting through a thin-walled socket. The more uniformly loaded is the cement layer in the acetabulum the less likely is it to produce 'high spots' on the cement-bone interface which might precipitate minute, localised movement between cement and bone eventually producing a histiocyte reaction and bone cavitation with the start of loosening (Chap. 4).

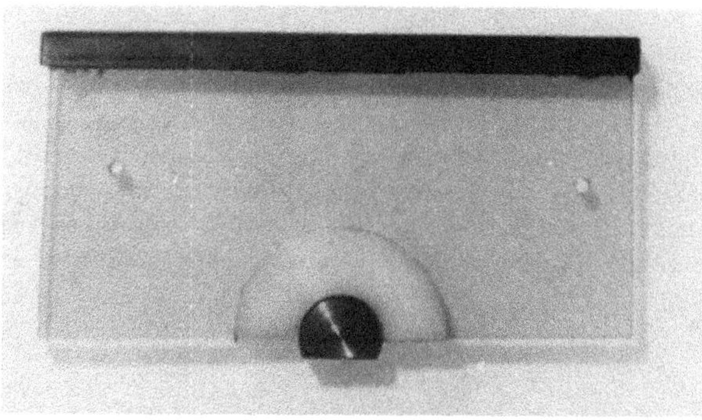

a

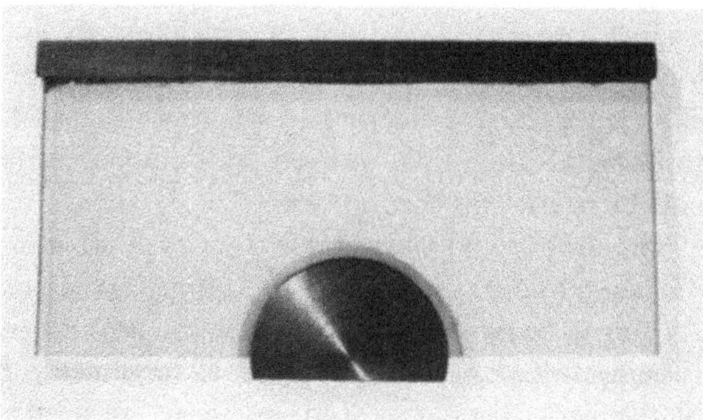

b

Fig. 1.12 a, b. Photoelastic models to illustrate effect of thickness of socket on distribution of load. Sheet of photosensitive plastics material represents the bone of the acetabulum. It is important that the external surface of HMWP socket should be *adherent* to substance representing bone (simulating the socket-cement-bone entity). Grooved metal bar cemented to top of sheet of photoelastic material helps to diffuse load from test apparatus equally over the specimen, so reducing 'high spots' to a minimum.
a 22.25 mm diameter metal cylinder – 56 mm external diameter HMWP 'socket'; **b** 50 mm diameter metal cylinder – 56 mm external diameter HMWP 'socket'

With the general trend (by 1977) for designs of metal-to-plastics total hip to be moving towards the smaller ranges of femoral head (32, 28 and 25 mm) it seemed unlikely to be profitable to examine further the effects of small differences in diameter, but in 1978 the 'double-cup' design of hip arthroplasty has emerged, using a metal sphere up to 50 mm in external diameter with a socket only about 3 mm thick (Appendix B). Because the 14-year studies of the LFA (Chap. 6) have shown that socket loosening is going to be the most likely cause of very late failure, even with a small-diameter head and a thick socket, there is a possibility that a very large head and a very thin socket could be a retrograde step. This prompted the author with engineering colleagues [1]) to undertake photo-elastic studies to illustrate load distribution at socket-cement-bone interfaces in relation to the thickness of the wall of a socket.

The photo-elastic demonstration used two models where the bone of the pelvis was represented by a sheet of Araldite CT 200 and the metal spheres by cylindrical steel discs (Fig. 1.12). The large metal disc measured 50 mm in external diameter and the small disc, 22.25 mm. The HMWP sockets were represented by semicircular discs both 56 mm in external diameter cemented into semicircular concavities of the same diameter in the Araldite. It was imperative to have a cemented joint between the polyethylene and the Araldite just as in the living situation.

The concavities of the polyethylene discs originally corresponded to the diameters of the metal cylinders but after cementing in position were too tight, and scraping was necessary to achieve a fit which gave the same sensation of free movement present in the hemispherical specimens used in surgery.

When viewed through a circular polariscope the resulting fringe patterns for an applied load of 325 lb are given in Fig. 1.13 for the small ball and for the large ball. The fringe orders are proportional to the principal stress in the Araldite. For the small ball the maximum fringe order is estimated to be 2.5 and stresses are more or less evenly distributed over the 180° interface between the socket and the Araldite. For the large ball the maximum fringe order is estimated to be 3.5 and stresses are concentrated over the central 90° of the interface between the socket and the Araldite.

[1]) Dr. R. Kitching and Dr. R.D. McLeish, Department of Mechanical Engineering, University of Manchester Institute of Science and Technology.

The maximum stresses in the plastic representing the bone of the acetabulum are (3.5/2.5) (1.4 times) higher with the thin socket than with the thick socket and these higher stresses are distributed over only about one-half of the area of cement-bone interface. The lower stresses produced by the thick socket are distributed more or less evenly over the whole area of the cement-bone interface. If the fit between the large ball and the thin socket were to be less good than in this experiment the zone of high stress would be more localised and higher in magnitude. With the thick socket on the other hand the stress will continue to be more evenly distributed on the cement-bone interfaces even if the ball were to be considerably smaller than a perfect fit.

From the point of view of the surgical manufacturer it is always difficult to be sure to what extent a socket of a plastics material made to close tolerances will hold these dimensions when internal stresses, etc. are relieved. It would be disastrous to use a socket which is too tight on a large head, because this could act as a powerful 'brake' and never have an opportunity to wear loose. Also to make different sockets and heads interchangeable, there will always be a tendency to deliver sockets erring on the side of looseness on a large head.

To this must also be added the fact that plastics materials have a much higher coefficient of thermal expansion than metal. Ideally a manufacturer should supply a socket which is too tight at room temperature so that it will be a perfect fit when at body temperature, but it is preferable to err on the side of a loose fit and hope that the head will adapt perfectly by a combination of wear and plastic flow.

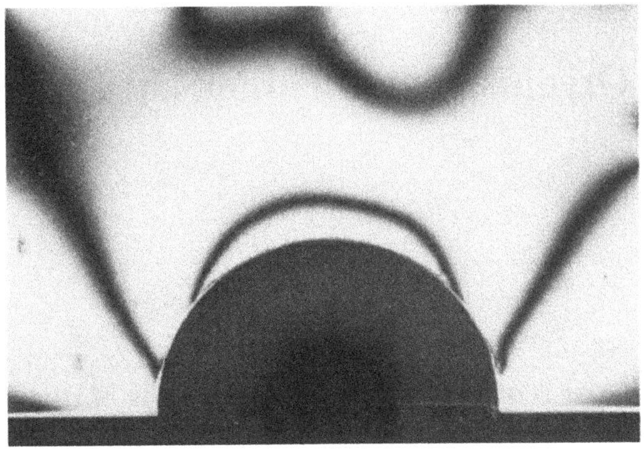

a

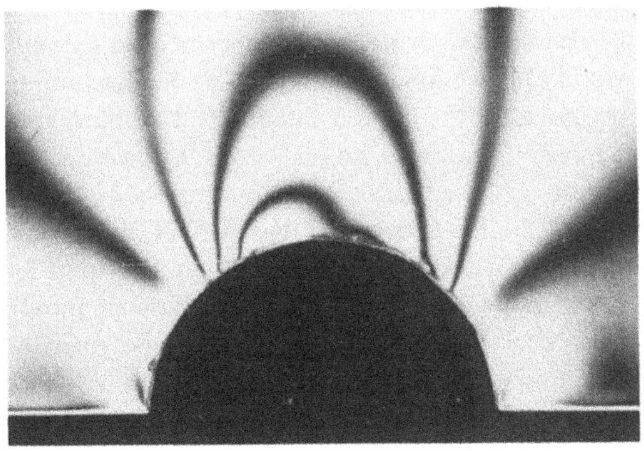

b

Fig. 1.13 a, b. *Top illustration* shows the thick socket under load from small-diameter metal prosthetic head. Fringes are distributed evenly over whole surface of socket. *Bottom illustration* shows thin socket and large-diameter metal prosthetic head under same load as above. Stresses are now concentrated over only a 90° quadrant of socket surface and are nearly 1.5 × higher than in case above. Under polarised light and both under load of 325 lb: **a** Two fringes on specimen (a) of Fig. 1.12; **b** three fringes on specimen (b) of Fig. 1.12

Chapter 2

Organisation of Follow-Up

There is only one really satisfactory way of studying the behaviour of acrylic cement in animal tissues under load-bearing conditions and that is by long-term surveillance in the human body. In this field of research animal experiments have been singularly unhelpful. The published work of almost all observations made on acrylic cement in animals would for ever dissuade surgeons from entertaining any hope for the human subject. It is ironical that the only favourable animal work known to the author was the first ever to be published: Wiltse et al.[8] in 1957 demonstrated perfect acceptance of acrylic cement after 3.5 years in the shaft of a long bone in a monkey but, because of purely theoretical objections to the heat of polymerisation, this work was not pursued.

During the 4 years from 1958 to 1962 the author introduced acrylic cement as a means of anchoring femoral prostheses and PTFE as a self-lubricating material for hip sockets in total hip replacement. In 1962 laboratory tests revealed the enormously improved wear resistance of HMWP compared with PTFE and for the first time it seemed possible that total hip replacement using a 'self-lubricating' socket of plastics material might well become a practical reality. The break with previous work by the introduction of HMWP was so clear-cut that the author decided that future work must form a prospective study and that a records system must be designed to follow up patients subjected to the new procedure by annual review for as many years as possible. It is important to describe how this system was organised and how it is still functioning 15 years later.

Long-Term Surveillance at Wrightington

The first requirement was a system of making clinical records. Proformata specially concentrating on brevity were designed for pre- and post-operative clinical examinations and for the operation notes. The number of essential data was kept to a minimum. It was considered that brevity would improve quality by avoiding the human tendency for surgeons to become lax when faced with documentation of computer type, a labour more properly done by clerks though, of course, clerks could never acquire the judgement necessary to make the original records.

Any system of numerical grading demands that all members of staff should acquire the same standards for estimating each grade and also that these standards should be maintained over the years. Written definitions of criteria for numerical grades were soon found to offer only a very rough guide and could be seriously misinterpreted by the resident surgical staff if left to work by themselves. Because the Hip Unit is organised so that all new patients are presented by the residents at a weekly clinical conference, it was possible to establish the criteria for numerical grading as part of the weekly teaching system.

Obviously the ideal prospective follow-up study would encompass all patients operated on; but by the end of 1965 it became obvious that the numbers of new patients applying for treatment was a chain-reaction and it would soon become impossible to make *annual* post-operative examinations of all patients when 1000 new patients were being added each year. It was therefore decided to make a prospective study of those patients operated on between November 1962 and the end of December 1965 and to continue this annually until they could no longer attend. This would produce truly long-term studies and this was considered likely to be better than to have many thousands of studies, none longer than about 5 years. This decision produced a group (referred to as the

'First 500') which returned annually, in batches of 8 or 10 every Wednesday afternoon. As the years have passed this number has fallen, by death from natural causes, by moves to distances too far to travel, and by the frailty of old age preventing attendance. But even so at the moment of writing (October 1977) we still have over 100 of this original group (Chaps. 5 and 6) able to attend or keep in communication by questionnaires sent out annually from the hospital, returning an annual radiograph taken near where they live.

For the patients who have been operated on since the First 500, now of the order of 12,000, the system is as follows: they return for their first post-operative attendance after 3 months and for their second, and final, attendance at 12 months when a full recording of the clinical condition and a final X-ray is made. If abnormalities are encountered, or if any case presents features of special interest, these patients are asked to return annually over an indefinite future period. This applies specially to the young patients and these are transferred for perpetual annual or bi-annual attendance to the diminishing group of the original prospective study.

The large group of patients operated on after the end of 1965 thus forms a source from which retrospective studies can be made and for this purpose every discharged patient is represented in the records department by:

1) Pre-operative clinical proforma
2) Pre-operative X-ray of pelvis and both hips
3) Operation proforma
4) Complications proformata (see below)
5) Portable post-operative X-ray
6) X-ray of pelvis and both hips at discharge from hospital
7) X-ray of pelvis and both hips 3 months after operation (clinical proforma only if progress not satisfactory)
8) Clinical record proforma 1 year after operation at discharge from follow-up
9) X-ray of pelvis and both hips 1 year after operation at discharge from follow-up

A significant proportion of patients return for operation on the opposite hip (perhaps 25%) so that there are frequent opportunities for clinical and radiographic studies of the first hip several years after the first operation even though these are not part of a prospective study.

X-Rays

Because the cement-bone interface is one of the subjects of prime importance in long-term follow-up, a consistently high quality of X-ray is of paramount importance. We are lucky in working in a hospital without an emergency surgical service and also with cordial relations with, and full co-operation of, the X-ray Department, which has been under the charge of the same Consultant Radiologist (Dr. David Mitchell) throughout the 15 years of this study.

All hip radiographs, with the exception of the immediate post-operative portable X-ray, are taken on 17 × 14 in. (42.5 × 35 cm) film to include both hips. The **pre-operative** film is centred on the fifth lumbar vertebra (to include some of the lumbar spine for assistance in diagnosis) but all **post-operative films** are centred on the symphysis pubis, in order to reach to a lower level on the femur and therefore include the whole length of the stem of a femoral prosthesis. A standard tube–film distance of 1 m is used throughout. **The most important post-operative film is that taken on discharge from hospital**, because this is on a mobile patient and is therefore comparable with those which will be taken at the subsequent follow-up attendances.

For studies of the cement-bone interface the importance of using radio-opaque acrylic cement was soon recognized and became routine early in 1963. In the same way a circumferential, radio-opaque wire in the coronal plane of the socket was introduced in 1963 to permit estimates of socket wear to be made.

Post-operative follow-up (both of the diminishing prospective study and the accumulating store of new patients available for retrospective study) has been made a precise subject by having this under the charge of one part-time secretary (Mrs. Margaret Weald), who has no other duties and has been with us since 1967. At discharge from hospital; after the 3 months visit; and after the final clinic at 1 year when the patient is discharged from further attendance, this secretary transfers comments made by residents in the clinical notes to a punch-card which covers all essential data including post-operative complications. This enormously facilitates the retrieval of original documents of cases pertinent to retrospective studies.

The original documents and X-rays of the First 500 are stored in our own research department, separately from the main hospital records, the latter being responsible only for storing the records of work done after 1965.

Complications

The recording and study of complications has always been of great interest and a special system of proformata was introduced for this purpose. The system functions in the following way.

If a complication of one of the several types specified on the proforma arises while the patient is still in hospital, it is the duty of the ward nurse and the resident doctor between them to send a 'current complication proforma' to the Director's office. This merely notifies the occurrence so that the Director thus has the opportunity to see the complication early, if he so wishes. When the patient is ready to be discharged from hospital a second type of complication proforma is completed (even if merely to state 'no complications') but this is permanently retained in the patient's records. After leaving hospital the patient's records pass through the Hip Centre, on their way to being stored in the main Records Office, and the two complication proformata are compared by Hip Centre staff. There are therefore two chances against the record of a complication being overlooked. The early record of a complication may be confirmed or negated by the second. In this way the system avoids the curse of most retrospective studies in which a single entry in the clinical records may state (for instance) '? pulmonary embolism?' without any further reference to it. It is possible to follow complications as a separate study and retrieve the original records only on those patients in whom a complication truly did exist.

A special duty of residents running the out-patient clinics is to return proformata for complications found after discharge from hospital, at the 3-month and 12-month post-operative attendances. These are returned directly to the Director's office. By this means late complications, or even only suspected complications, are not temporarily lost in the records, but can be the subject of an immediate study rather than be found, perhaps years later, in the course of a retrospective study.

The completion of these complication proformata requires no more than half-a-dozen words and is therefore no burden to the resident; the resident's main duty is not to forget his responsibility for initiating a proforma. Over several post-operative attendances the same patient may cause several proformata to be initiated and returned to the Director's office reporting the same condition but this is a 'fail-safe' error and causes no extra labour.

The data which the proformata record are:

While in hospital

1) Imperfect wound healing
2) Pulmonary embolus
3) Swollen leg (=DVT)
4) Trochanter detachment
5) Dislocation
6) Death
7) Positive bacterial cultures after second-hand surgery

At follow-up out-patient attendance

1) Clinical or radiological suspicion of infection
2) Defective union of trochanter
3) Persistence of fixed deformity
4) Other defects

Final Comment on Long-Term Surveillance

This account emphasizes how extreme specialisation facilitates the preservation of continuity of key personnel, vital to accurate long-term records, and that this can be done at modest cost. Only by concentrating this type of work in special centres can a consistent standard of high-quality work be performed and studied. Without a quick-acting feedback from surveillance of post-operative complications, the continuous performance of thousands of these operations every year cannot be justified, especially if small modifications of technique are always in progress.

Future Recommendations

The 12–15-year study of total hip replacement, concentrating particularly on the behaviour of the cement-bone interface, has shown that 5-year results can be of very great importance. Complications evident at 10 years in most cases (but certainly not in all) will be detectable at 5 years if one knows where to look for them, and their significance. Therefore a good research policy in the future could be to review all results radiographically after 5 years. In the first place this could be done locally and the X-rays sent to the hospital without the patient's personal attendance at the clinic being required.

Chapter 3

Numerical Grading of Clinical Results

The long-term study of clinical results at Wrightington has been greatly facilitated by the numerical system of grading the quality of results originally devised by d'Aubigné and Postel[9]; indeed, without this numerical system the long-term study would have been impossible.

The importance of a weekly teaching system so that the resident surgical staff can learn to use constant standards of grading has already been emphasized. Definitions of different grades are always difficult to make all-embracing and 'reading between the lines' is frequently necessary, but residents acquire a unified sense for the numbers indicating clear-cut categories when working continuously in this atmosphere.

Grading of Hips

Grading for **pain** and for the **function of walking** on a scale of 6 digits, is seen in Fig. 3.1, taken from our clinical proforma. In practice the appropriate compartments are merely ringed on the proforma without making written entries. Figure 3.1 indicates how a resident will do this using a red felt pen. The transfer of the digits from the proforma to a punch card or computer card is easily carried out by a clerk.

Grading of **range of motion** is performed on the proforma by drawing on the appropriate quadrants, using a red felt pen as indicated in Fig. 3.2. This visible way of demonstrating the range of

Bedridden	Chair Life	Two Crutches	Two Sticks	One Stick Always	One Stick Outside	No Sticks
PAIN	1 Severe Spontaneous R L	2 Severe on attempting to walk. Prevents all activity R L	3 Pain tolerable permitting limited activity R L	4 Pain only after some activity, disappears quickly with rest R L	5 Slight or intermittent Pain on starting to walk but getting less with normal activity R L	6 No pain R L
WALK	1 Bedridden or few yards; two sticks or crutches R L	2 Time and distance very limited with or without sticks. R L	3 Limited with one stick (less than one hour). Difficult without stick. Able to stand long periods R L	4 Long distances with one stick; limited without a stick R L	5 No stick but a limp R L	6 Normal R L
GAIT WITHOUT STICKS	Cannot walk	Just able to walk	Walks but with gross limp	Walks with moderate limp	Slight limp	Normal gait

Bizarre Gait (Describe)

Fig. 3.1. Method of 'ringing' appropriate data by resident using red felt pen. Transfer of digits to computer made by clerk

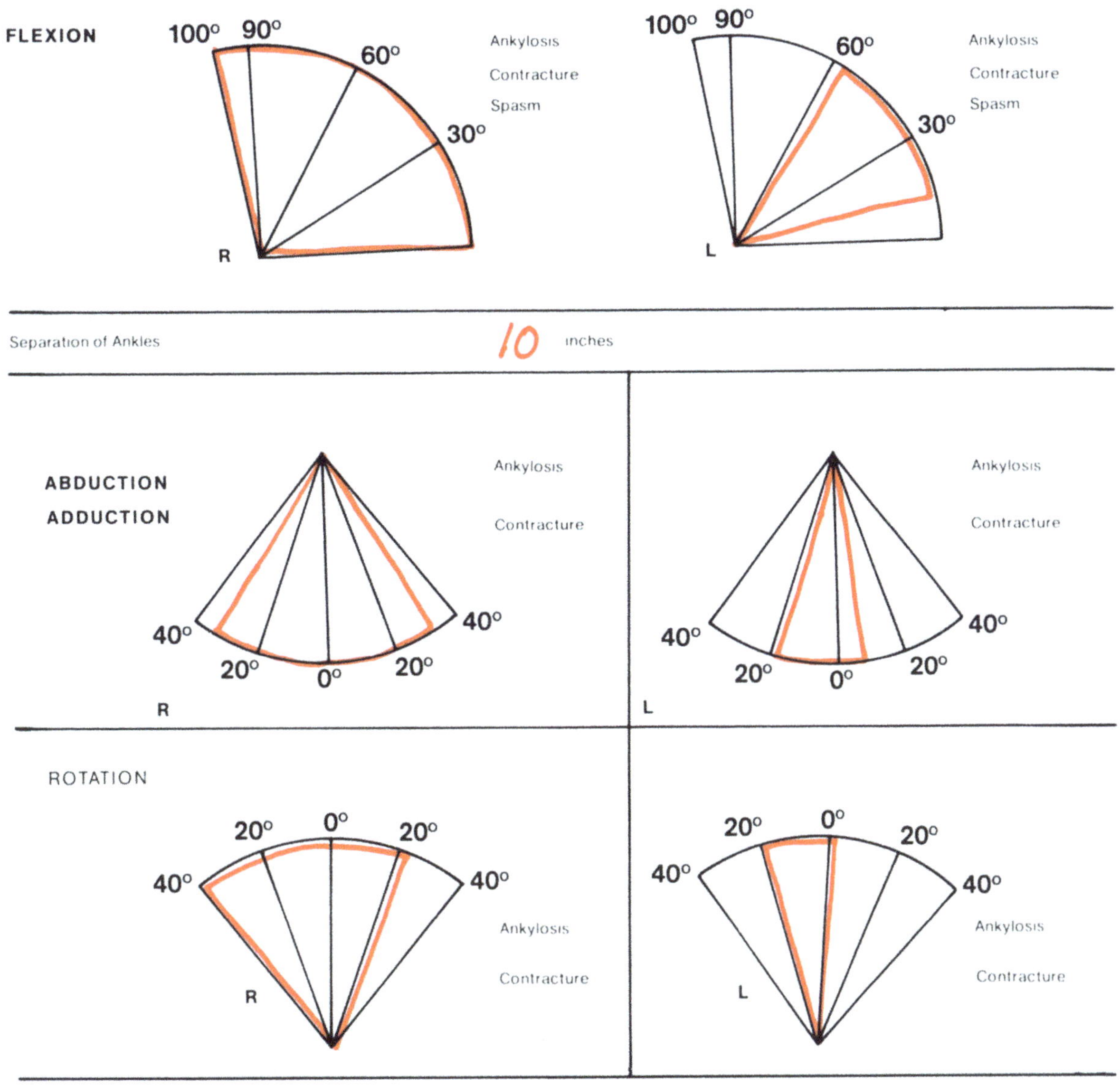

Fig. 3.2. Method of visibly recording range of motion by resident using red felt pen

movement conveys information visually and more easily than mere lists of numerical values. The method also makes it easy to demonstrate changes in the range of movement (as well as fixed contractures) to a seminar without reading out long lists of angles which are difficult for listeners to absorb.

Grades of motion are classified from the sum total of all the ranges of movement (flexion, abduction-adduction and rotation) according to the table:

Total	0–30°	30°–60°	60°–100°	100°–160°	160°–210°	over 210°
Grade	1	2	3	4	5	6

Because extreme accuracy is impossible and unnecessary, we approximate the total range to the nearest group.

Special Examples of Numerical Grading in Practice

Experience which adds to an understanding of numerical criteria has emerged since making the original definitions and because these cannot be condensed very briefly into a table the following expanded description may be of help.

Pain

Grade 4 pain is the lowest level of pain commonly encountered in osteoarthrosis when total hip replacement is indicated for pain.

Grade 5 pain in itself is not sufficient to warrant surgery. Grade 5 pain is merely discomfort; it is compatible with a 'fair' or 'satisfactory' result of surgery. Compared with the original state of disability, grade 5 pain should be a 'satisfactory' and even a 'good' post-operative result.

Grade 3 pain is a more painful hip than grade 4 because it is also a sensitive hip. Grade 3 pain is often associated with spontaneous pain at night. Night pain to be significant **must be volunteered** with unmistakable emphasis; it is not necessarily significant in reply to a leading question because in this case a positive reply will be obtained in 75%.

The most important sign of a sensitive or 'irritable' hip is the physical sign of **spasm** elicited on moving the hip towards its extremes of range. Grade 4 pain is not associated with spasm. Spasm is revealed by the patient exerting muscular resistance against further movement or by nothing more than a sudden expression of discomfort on the patient's face. (It is futile ever to ask the patient 'Does that hurt?'). Resting in hospital for 1 or 2 days before examination often will abolish spasm present in active daily life.

Grade 2 pain is the most severe pain encountered in chronic arthritis. In grade 2 pain scvcrc spasm always will be present and the patient will object to the surgeon touching or moving the limb. Drugs may be needed continuously for pain of grade 2.

Grade 1 pain is not encountered in chronic arthritis because this grade of pain is so severe that it would be equivalent to a suppurative arthritis, to a fresh fracture or to severe gout.

Function of Walking

Grade 3 function is the commonest grade demanding total hip replacement in chronic arthritis. In grade 3 function the patient can walk short distances in the clinic without disability being grossly obvious. Over short distances the patient may not use a stick or a cane. A female patient with grade 3 function could not go shopping for 1 hour without a walking aid.

Grade 2 function is most easily decided by observing the manner and speed with which the patient enters the consulting room. Whereas a patient with grade 3 function will enter the consulting room at normal speed and often without a cane, though perhaps with a distinct limp, a patient with grade 2 function will take a perceptible time to enter the consulting room and sit down. One or two sticks or crutches will always be needed. Sometimes a patient with grade 2 function may need a wheel-chair to reach the consulting room.

Grade 1 function signifies a patient who is bedridden or chair-bound.

Grade 4 function represents the patient, often a male, who has used a stick for many years almost as a habit. A good example is a hale and hearty farmer with an arthrosic hip who can walk long distances over rough ground. In these cases operation may be elective because pain may not be severe. Sometimes operation may be indicated mainly to correct adduction deformity and shortening and in order to dispense with the stick or cane.

Grade 5 function does not warrant total hip replacement. It is comparable with an acceptable or 'fair' post-operative result after total hip replacement.

Range of Movement

Range of motion is recorded as the sum of all the ranges of movement in flexion, abduction, internal and external rotation. No 'loading' factors are used, to give greater values to the most commonly used arcs, because arthroplasty purports to restore a near-normal hip; loading of certain useful ranges is only of value if the operation (such as osteotomy) does not purport to restore motion. Full range, grade 6, is anything over a total of 210° and this is less than the full anatomical range of a normal hip. **Grade 3** is the commonest grade for movement in the average patient with an established osteoarthrosis. It implies about 90° of flexion of the hip plus little else (i.e. very restricted abduction and rotation).

Grading of Both Hips

When, for instance, a patient is graded as:

Right 6.4.5. **Left** 5.4.2.

the numbers represent in sequence: pain; function of walking; total range of motion. It is important to realize that the middle number (function of walking) **always relates to the whole person** and not merely to the left or right hip. **The middle number of each group of three numbers therefore must always be the same for both hips.**

Example: A patient with an extremely painful hip on the right side and a normal hip on the left, could **not** be recorded as:

Right 2.**2**.5 **Left** 6.**6**.6

it would have to be:

Right 2.**2**.5 **Left** 6.**2**.6

even though the left hip (considered by itself) would be perfect i.e. 6.6.6.

Perhaps this system would be more logical if the function of walking were to be graded separately and this number used as a prefix: thus in the above example the prefix could be 2 and the right hip would then be 2.5, and the left 6.6. But we have become accustomed to the three-digit system invented by d'Aubigné and Postel and have not changed it.

Patient Categories

The use of categories A, B and C (as prefixes to the numerical grading for pain, function and range of movement) is a special development at Wrightington and has proved of great value.

The primary object of the categories is to make it possible to extract records of category A patients, **especially when study of the quality of function** is the primary object. Clinical material for the study of the function of walking on the artificial hip joint must not be impaired by other factors affecting the ability to walk. **A category A patient is therefore physically fit in all respects relating to function, with allowances for age, and without any defect other than the one hip affected by arthritis.** In category A the ability to walk means that the quality of the artificial hip can be compared with a normal hip in a patient of the same age. If **pain** or **range of movement** is being studied (i.e. comparisons before and after operation, or maintenance over the years) **all categories** can be examined and compared.

Category B patients have both hips affected but otherwise they are physically fit for their age and no other factor exists to interfere with function.

There is one special circumstance in defining category B which might be improved. A patient in category B **before operation** will have bilateral hip pathology but **post-operatively** category B could be a single-sided arthoplasty with an unoperated arthritis on the other side, or could be a bilateral arthroplasty. The bilateral operation could be distinguished from the pre-operative state as category B.B.

A bilateral arthritis which will be category B before a bilateral operation cannot be raised to category A even if the patient is functioning as well as a patient with two normal hips.

Whilst we cannot raise the category of a patient as a result of the operation, all categories can be lowered if the function of walking is impaired by factors which have developed since the operation. Thus a category A patient could be downgraded to B if the second hip became arthrosic; or could be downgraded to C with the onset of cardiac insufficiency, arthritis of the knees, or gross senility, etc.

If deterioration of the function of walking were to be solely from **deterioration of the arthroplasty** the patient would not become category C but the degeneration would be revealed in the change of the number related to that hip. Thus, if a patient changed from:

B Right 6.6.6. Left 6.6.6. (i.e. perfect bilateral arthroplasty) to
B Right 4.**3**.2. Left 6.**3**.6

this would show that the failure in function must come from deterioration of the right hip alone: by the onset of pain (6 down to 4), failure of walking function (6 to 3) and loss of motion (6 down to 2), **the left hip remaining normal**. (Remember that the middle number must always remain the same for both hips because it is function of the whole patient; therefore in this case the perfect left hip will be 6.3.6.)

When surveying columns of numbers representing the annual gradings of a patient, a life history can often be deduced almost at a glance, as in the case illustrated below: the patient was physically normal for his age before the operation, the only handicap being two arthrosic hips (i.e. category B). Bilateral arthroplasty was performed in 1966.

		R	L
1966	B	4 3 2	4 3 3
1967	B	6 6 5	6 6 5
1968	B	6 6 5	6 6 5
1969	B	6 5 5	5 5 5
1970	C	6 3 5	5 3 5

The annual gradings show that an excellent result was obtained from bilateral arthroplasty (range of motion being only slightly below perfect, i.e. 5) and this was maintained until 1969. The left hip then started to become slightly painful (grade 5) and this caused function to be slightly impaired (grade 5 for whole patient). The next year (1970) the left hip remained slightly uncomfortable (grade 5) but function had fallen to grade 3 (whole patient). There was no further deterioration in pain or range of motion in either hip. The patient had now been downgraded to C. Category C therefore explains the deterioration of walking function to 3 because the gradings for pain and motion indicate that both hips are still good, the right better than the left because of some discomfort in the left hip. Category C therefore could be the result of heart failure, cerebral thrombosis, etc.

When grading a patient category B, because the second hip is radiologically affected by arthritis though painless and clinically normal, there may be doubt whether or not it should be category A. There is no real problem because if the patient were graded A and some years later the second hip were to become painful it could always be reduced to category B without affecting the system.

Category C must be reserved for conditions **directly impairing the act of walking**. One can assess category C by asking whether the patient's function would be limited **if the hips were normal**; if the answer is 'yes' then the patient is category C. Obesity for instance would have to be pathologically gross to make a patient category C.

When age and sex are taken into account a guess at a diagnosis often can be made when scrutinising a patient's category and grading as illustrated in the following examples:

♀ 28	Cat. C	4 3 4	4 3 4	Rheumatoid arthritis
♂ 22	Cat. A	4 4 5	6 4 6	Road traffic accident, right hip
♀ 22	Cat. B	4 3 6	5 3 6	Bilateral congenital dislocation of the hip (CDH)
♀ 66	Cat. A	4 3 6	6 3 6	Unilateral osteoarthrosis
♂ 35	Cat. C	6 2 1	6 2 1	Ankylosing spondylitis
♂ 35	Cat. A	6 5 1	6 5 6	Surgical arthrodesis, one hip

The above list emphasizes again how the middle numbers, indicating the function of the whole patient, are always the same.

Pre-operative Assessment

An example of how valuable this numerical system of grading can be relates to a surgical consultation when the final decision is about to be made whether to advise a total hip replacement or not. After a long discussion, perhaps a harangue with a difficult patient who cannot give a consistent description of his or her troubles, on reassessing the evidence it may be found that during the early part of the interview pain had been recorded as 5 and the range of movement as 5. These numerical values show that serious re-thinking will be needed if the argument was leading towards the patient persuading the surgeon to operate, because sometimes an emotional aura from the patient can temporarily upset a surgeon's judgement. This is the type of case where, as delaying tactics, second or even third consultations may be valuable.

Chapter 4

Cement-Bone Interface*

If we are to contemplate total hip replacement in adults as young as 45 years of age with the idea of 25 years of trouble-free life ahead, it is necessary to hold definite opinions on the histological nature of the bone-cement interface. With the exception of some published observations of the author[10, 11] the literature so far contains very little histological work which justifies optimism for the late results of total hip replacement, except in the old and decrepit.

Most published histological studies of tissue derived from total hip replacements are concerned with reactions to the abraded particles derived from the wearing surfaces of different types of implant materials. Thus Willert and Semlitsch[12] studied tissue reactions to particles of HMWP, polyethylene terephthalate (polyester), polymethylmethacrylate (PMMA) and metallic particles from different types of chrome-cobalt alloys. Their results from 123 specimens of capsular tissue over a period of 5 years from the point of view of long-term results are disquieting. The conclusions from this well-illustrated paper are non-committal: the best these writers are prepared to say is that if foreign-body particles are generated in small amounts (which is almost the same as very slowly) it is possible that the particles may be eliminated via perivascular lymph channels, so avoiding the local accumulations which cause foreign-body granulomata. In their opinion it is the granulomatous material which invades the cement-bone interfaces which ultimately loosens the implants.

A recent general review of this subject is that of Vernon-Roberts and Freeman[13] but this presentation also tends to be dominated by the reaction of the tissues to particles of implanted materials. The opening section on the morphology of the 'normal' bone-cement interface offers little hope for success on a 25-year basis in vigorous male patients operated on at 45 years of age. In their introduction these writers say: 'The very good results which are generally observed in the period immediately following total joint replacement are, regrettably, no guarantee of permanent success in the long term since, even if a prosthesis is firmly fixed in place for a short or long period after the implantation, various factors can eventually lead to loosening at a late date.' There is little optimism here that good results may be permanent.

In addition to loosening caused by the invasion of the cement-bone interface by foreign-body granulomatous tissue these authors suggest that late loosening of cement may be the result of an excessive amount of bone death. They believe that dead bone is prone to fatigue and put forward the idea that when dead bone is fractured by fatigue it might be replaced by fibrous tissue. They suspect mechanical trauma as being more likely to cause extensive bone death than the thermal or chemical trauma of cement. This presumably would apply also when using expanded surfaces without acrylic cement.

The histological state of a bone-cement interface which is of most concern to patient and surgeon is that in the phase starting about 6 months after the operation. According to Vernon-Roberts and Freeman the typical appearance of a stabilised interface is: '.. a thin layer of acellular fibrin-like tissue in immediate contact with the main cement, with or without an outer layer of collagenised fibrous tissue up to 1.5 mm thick'. They present an illustration showing a thick layer of fibrous tissue, 2 years after implantation, which could be described as areolar tissue (i.e. a delicate stroma containing spaces or interstices) and certainly not

* This chapter incorporates material presented by the author in the Robert Jones Lecture of the British Orthopaedic Association, September 1976.

dense and collagenised. Another illustration is that of a transverse section of the femur of a patient who died 2 years after the operation. The cemented implant was stable in the medulla. The site occupied by the cement in the centre of the medulla is revealed as a thin shell of cancellous trabeculae orientated parallel to the cement surface. Between the external surface of the thin shell of bone surrounding the cement and the internal surface of the femoral cortex, there are only two trabeculae of any significant strength. The whole picture is one of gross osteoporosis as indicated by the uniformly thin cortex of the femur and the sparsity of cancellous trabeculae. Appearances such as this are common in advanced senility but it is only fair to the operation to say that even in cases such as this it is always surprising how firm the cemented metal implant can still be in the femur, giving a 100% clinical result for the diminished stresses to which it is exposed in advanced senility.

But these appearances are not cogent to the teaching of a surgical technique proposing 25 years of success in vigorous patients operated on at 45 years of age. Surgeons would be acting with irresponsibility if they offered this type of surgery to young and active persons with nothing more than these histological appearances as typical of the normal cement-bone interface. Fortunately the appearances described by Vernon-Roberts and Freeman are not typical of those found in the author's collection of post-mortem material representing the appearances between 5 and 12 years after implantation.

Long-Term Post-Mortem Material

It is necessary first to explain how the author's collection of post-mortem material was obtained, because the discouraging histology illustrated in the literature probably results from the specimens having been derived from secondary operations on replacements already in failure, or from cadaveric material from senile patients with sparse clinical and radiological records to supplement the study.

At Wrightington by about 1965 it became obvious that it was imperative as soon as possible to obtain post-mortem material **from highly successful cases.** The prospective long-term clinical study of the First 500 (p. 16) had already been organised, and the author devised a letter which he sent to patients who were **successful 3 years after their operation** explaining how it would benefit humanity, and especially young sufferers from hip arthritis, if elderly patients with excellent results would consider bequeathing their operated hips to medical science. The essential thing was that only patients showing

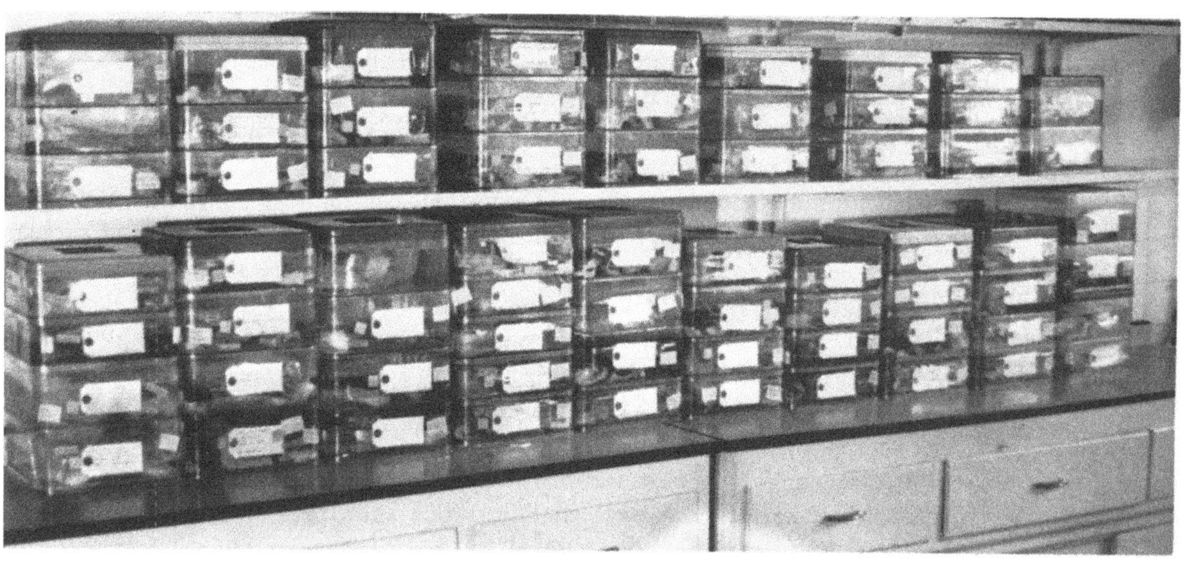

Fig. 4.1. Collection of 62 hips donated to medical research by patients operated on at Wrightington 1.5–13 years after surgery

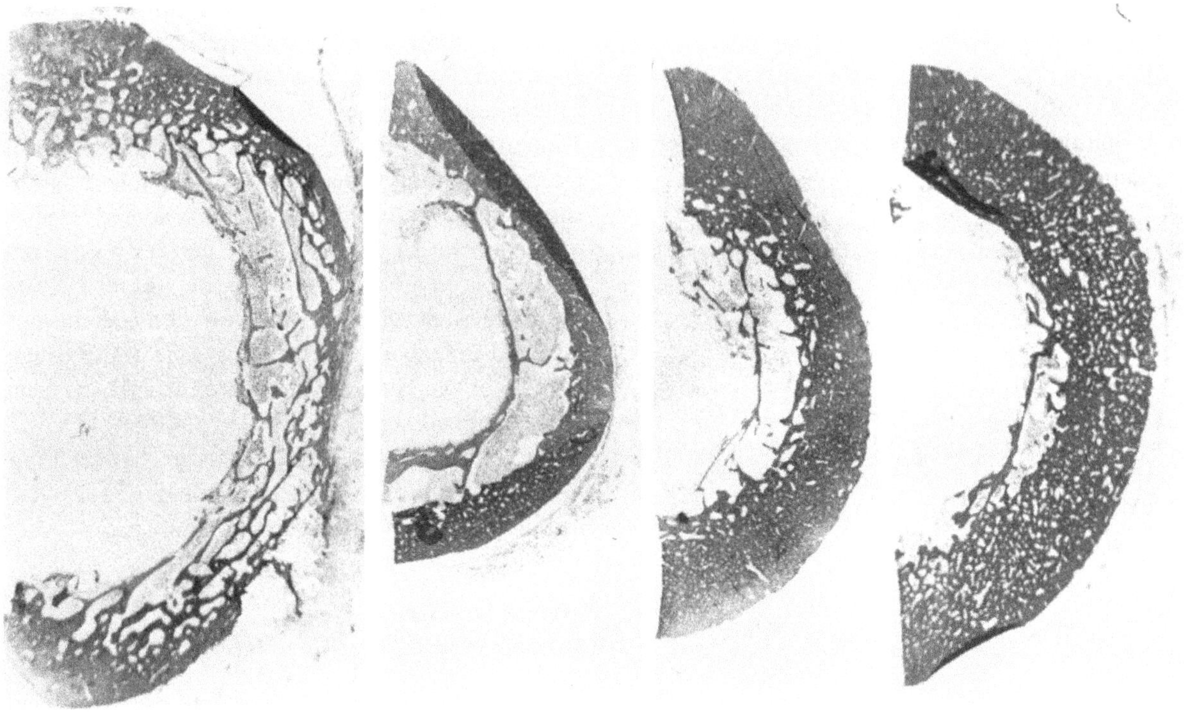

a b c d

Fig. 4.2 a–d. Selection of decalcified sections of shafts of femur, cement dissolved out, showing range of density of cortices, thickness of fibrous tissue intervening between cement surface and endosteal cancellous bone, and density of endosteal cencellous bone. **a** 10 years, **b** 8 years, **c** 7 years, **d** 8.5 years

very good results were approached. These were just those who in the normal course of events would be lost to science, whereas patients with clinical or radiological defects 3 years after the operation in all probability eventually would have to be explored; but these would not be typical of the excellent results. No patient with suspected deep infection was approached.

In this way all the specimens eventually obtained were from patients who had been operated on at Wrightington with clinical and radiographic records available. Many of these were patients of the prospective First 500 and these had records and X-rays made annually. A first survey of this post-mortem material was the subject of the author's Robert Jones Lecture to the British Orthopaedic Association in September 1976 and in due course it is hoped to complete the study and publish in full. Out of 62 hip specimens acquired at that time (Fig. 4.1), the histology of 41 had been completed and the lecture was based on the histology of 41 femoral shafts, 37 medial femoral necks and 26 acetabula. The average period between operation and death was 7.3 years; the longest period between operation and death was 11.75 years and 13 specimens were over 9 years. On macroscopic examination of the specimens the femoral prostheses were firm in the bone in every instance but the bond between the acetabulum and the cement was easily ruptured in 50% of cases and was frankly loose in two.

Femur

A typical selection of transverse sections of the femur at about the middle of the prosthetic stem, at low magnification, is shown in Fig. 4.2a, b, c, d. The selection is made to show (a) the range of thickness of the femoral cortex, (b) the range of thickness of soft tissues intervening between the cement surface and the endosteal cancellous bone and (c) the range of quality of cancellous bone intervening between the 'internal cortex' surrounding the cement and the cortex of the femur.

The density of the cortex in Fig. 4.2d is impressive as is also the thinness of the endosteal layer of fibrous tissue. These appearances are consistent with the X-ray of the longitudinal hemi-section of this specimen (Fig. 4.3): the cortical bone is of good density and no gap is visible between the radio-opaque cement and the endosteal surface of the femur.

This patient, 66 years of age at time of operation (April 1968) was a vigorous, extroverted male weighing 168 lb (75.6 kg). He had a perfect clinical result for 8.5 years and played golf regularly.

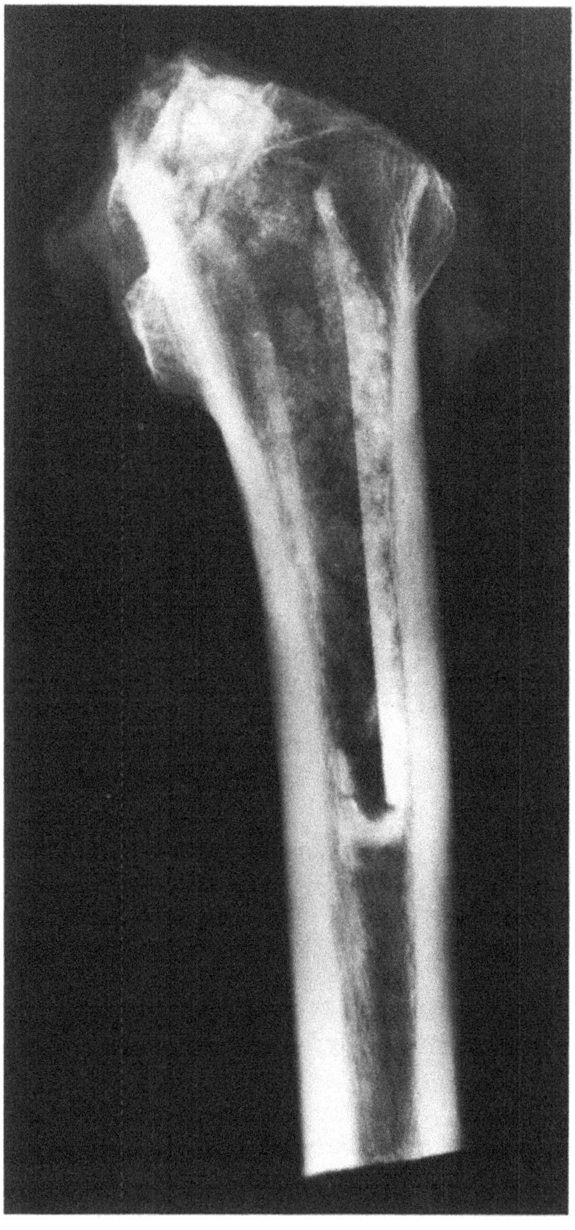

Fig. 4.3. X-ray of specimen corresponding to 4.2d above. Note density of femoral cortex. 8.5 years

A selection of transverse sections of undecalcified femora with acrylic cement in situ are shown in Fig. 4.4a, b, c (the author is indebted to Professor Rannie of the School of Dentistry, Newcastle-upon-Tyne, for making these sections from the author's specimens). These low-magnification transverse sections are considered typical of cement in the femur. There certainly does **not** exist '... a layer of fibrous tissue about 1.5 mm in thickness at all points between the cement surface and the adjacent cancellous bone'. Any osteoporosis of the cortex in these sections was present in the original state.

The thickness and density of the cortical bone in these sections is consistent with the 12–15-year radiological studies reported in Chap. 6.

Minute Structure of the Load-Bearing Cement-Bone Interface

Whereas the foregoing sections of the femur at low magnification prove that a **thick** layer of fibrous tissue does not exist as a **continuous layer** separating all the cement surface from the cancellous bone, the interpretation of the histology of the interface at high magnification demands some imagination. The technical problem is that very thin sections to permit high magnification cannot be made with cement in situ; therefore the cement must be dissolved out and decalcified sections made in wax in the usual way and then the tissues which have been in direct contact with cement must be deduced indirectly.

A striking feature of the sections of human femora from patients known to have had successful results, is that any fibrous tissue lining the medullary cavity, far from being thick, dense and collagenised, is so fine and delicate that it is often difficult to keep it adherent to the slide during staining. In some parts (especially where there are collections of broken, necrotic trabeculae; relics of the original trauma of insertion) no layer of any kind, organised or acellular, exists to indicate where the surface of the cement had been. Some of these disorganised zones probably do represent loss of the surface layer by artefact during the histological process, but the author thinks that many of these disorganised zones represent fluid-filled cavities between the cement and the endosteal surface of

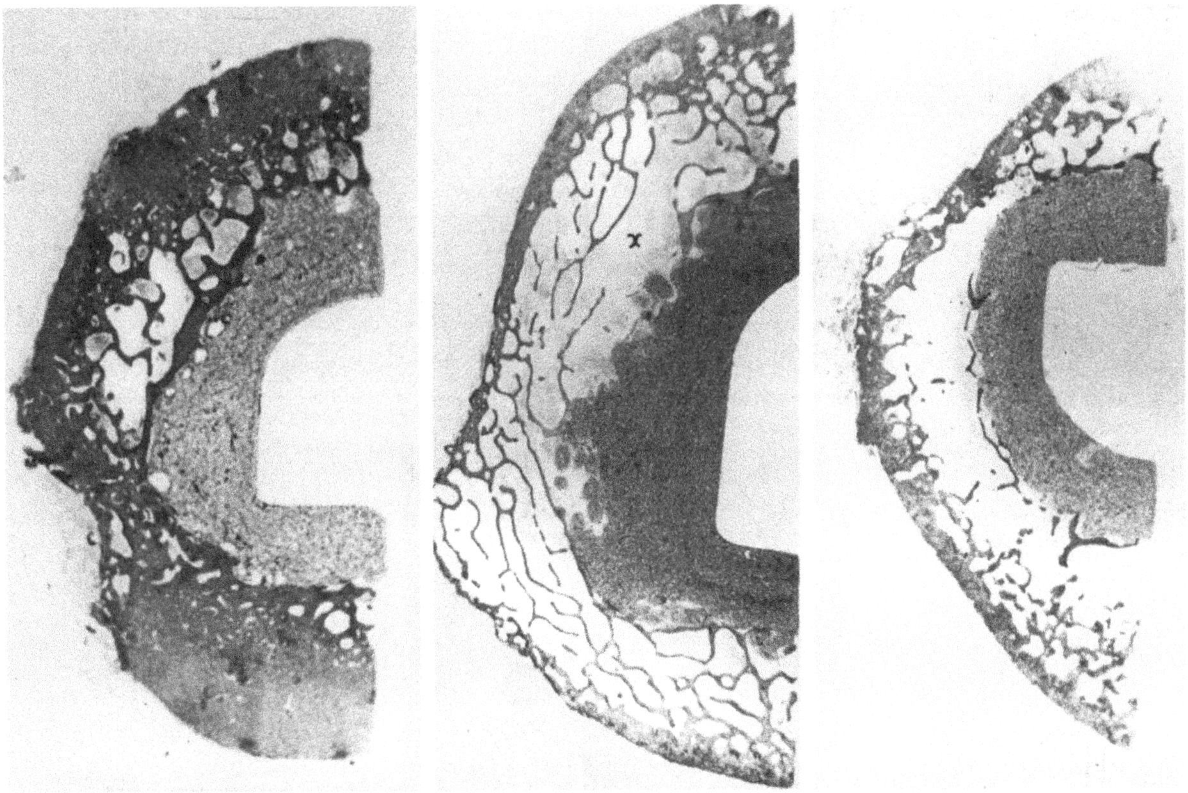

a b c

Fig. 4.4 a–c. Selection of undecalcified sections of shafts of femur with acrylic cement in position. Note variations in density of cortex and intervening cancellous bone. All clinically successful. In 4.4 b, *X* marks cavity without bone trabeculae on adjacent surface of cement (? fluid-filled cavity). (Courtesy of Prof. Rannie, School of Dentistry, Newcastle-on-Tyne, author's material.) **a** 8 years, **b** 7 years, **c** 7 years

the cancellous bone where no cellular layer ever formed on the cement surface. The area marked X in Fig. 4.4 b could represent such a space. Zones such as this obviously are incapable of load transmission between cement and the endosteal surface of the femoral cortex.

To recognize zones which have been in contact with a cement surface **and through which load could have been transmitted to bone**, it is necessary to describe the characteristic profile which a cement surface imposes on an organised tissue in contact with it. Acrylic cement is an aggregate of spherules of polymer, ranging in diameter from about 30 μm to about 80 μm, bonded together by the polymerised liquid phase. These spherules give the surface of the cement a mammillated appearance caused by spheres protruding from the surface to about a third or a quarter of their diameter. When a tissue receives such an impression, and when the histological section passes perpendicular to the surface, the section presents a characteristic scalloped outline (Fig. 4.5), and the curvatures of the scallops are, strikingly, parts of a true circle (unlike fat cells of approximately the same size). The curvatures are consistent with 30–80 μm-diameter spheres at the particular magnification in use. Less commonly a cement sphere may be revealed as a complete circular defect in the middle of a sheet of tissue, rather than as a scalloped outline seen on the margin of a section (Fig. 4.6). The circularity of these complete defects is quite perfect when compared with the shape of a fat cell. Sometimes (as in Fig. 4.6) these circular defects occur in clusters of two or three of different size and can be mistaken for isolated cement spheres (which of course they could be, through this is most unlikely considering the technique of using cement). The most likely explanation of this appearance, and of its rarity compared with the scalloped outline, is that the histological section must have passed

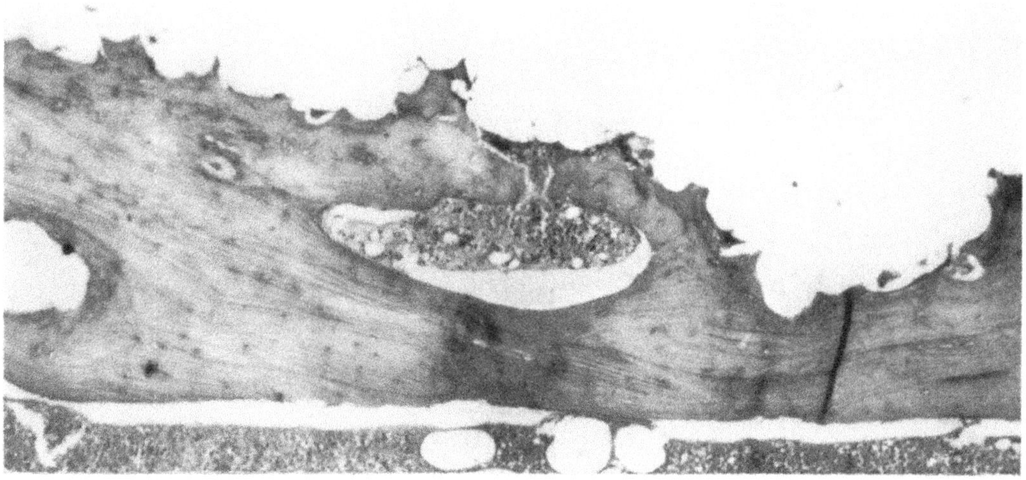

Fig. 4.5. Scalloped outline of bone on endosteal surface of femur with curvatures corresponding to sizes of cement spherules. Low-power H.E.

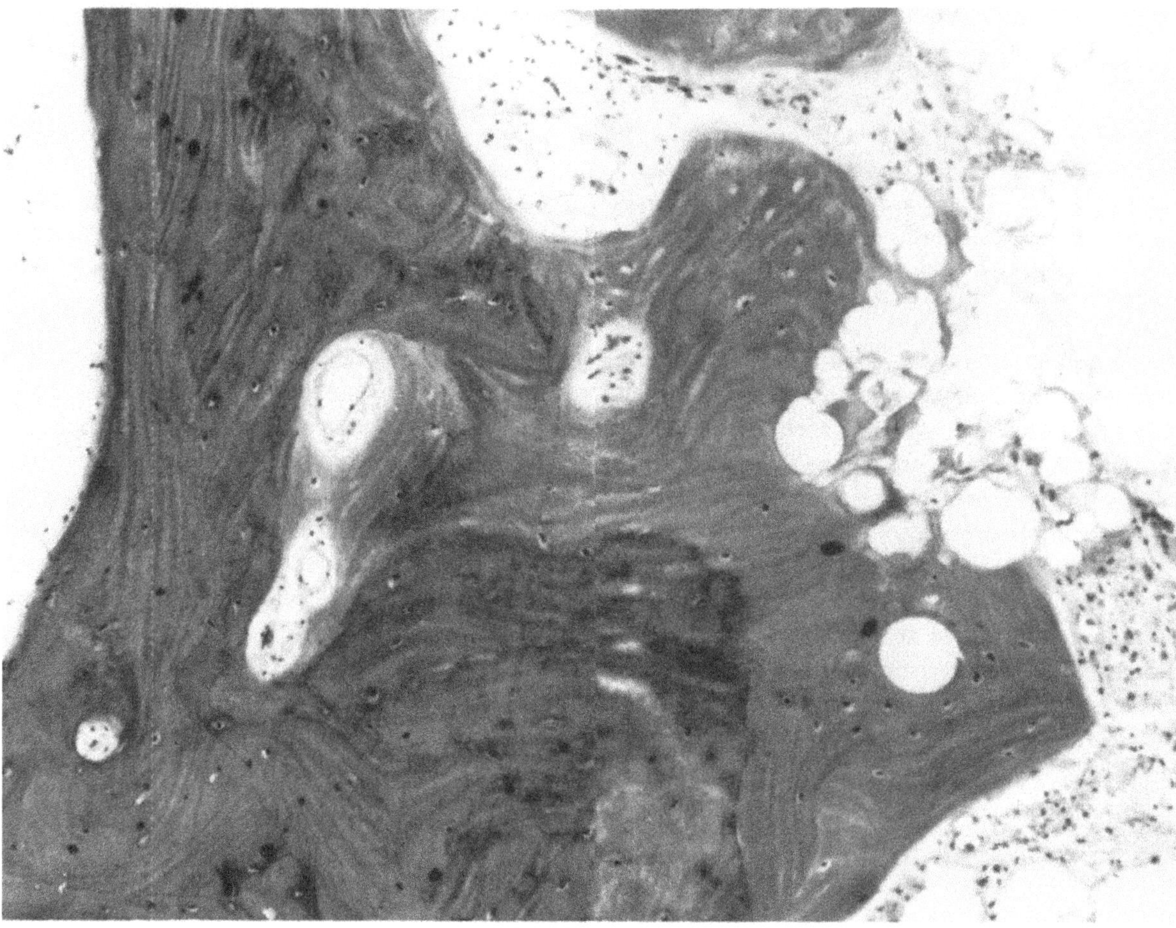

Fig. 4.6. Complete circular defects corresponding to cement spherules. Section tangential to surface. Living nuclei in tissue adjacent to spheres. 11 years in situ. No fibrous tissue between surface of spherules and tissue of trabecula. H.E.

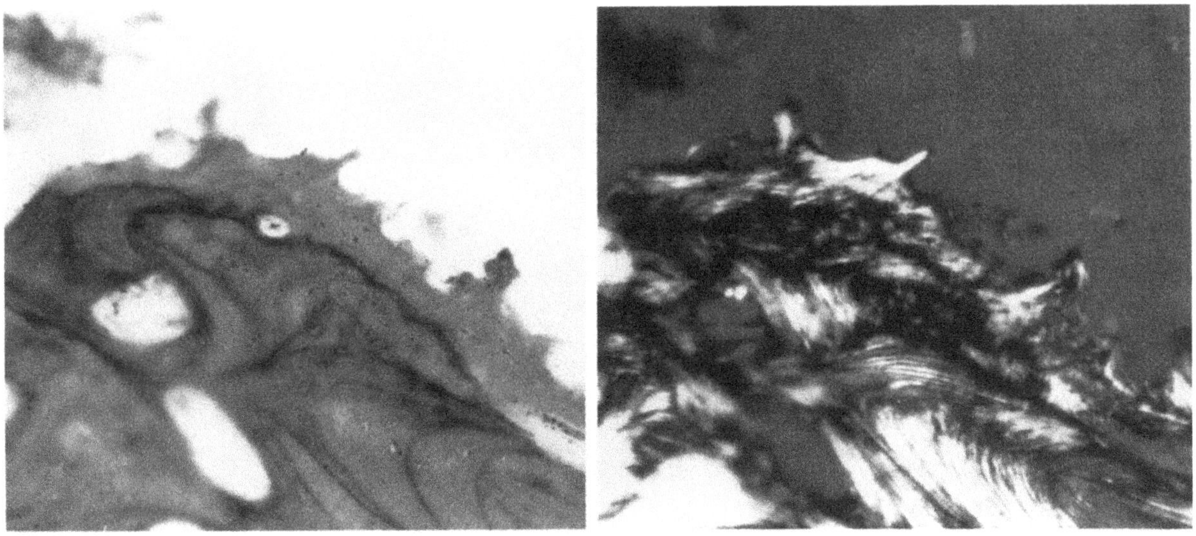

a b

Fig. 4.7. a Bone trabecula (with living osteocytes) 'capped' with tissue resembling fibro-cartilage. The cap bears hemispherical impressions of cement spherules. Living nuclei. H.E. **b** Same section under polarised light showing dense collagen in the cap with birefringent fibres (at *top left*) passing continuously from bone into the substance of the cap

tangentially to the cement surface, and not perpendicularly, as would give the commoner appearance of a scalloped outline.

When scalloped impressions are seen on a bony trabecula, close inspection will show that the impression is not usually in the lamellar bone of the trabecula but in a 'cap' of tissue on the end of the trabecula (Fig. 4.7a). That the cap is structurally continuous with the underlying bone is revealed by polarised light, in which case birefringent lamellae of the bone often will be seen to pass into the cap in direct continuity (Fig. 4.7b). The author thought at one time that these caps represented newly formed fibrocartilage and that this had grown from the bone surface towards the cement surface to receive the characteristic scalloped impression. Now however it seems more likely that these caps represent demineralised bone matrix and that the cement spheres have been impressed mechanically into it during load transmission.

The staining reactions of the caps differ from the underlying lamellar bone of the trabecula. Stained with haematoxylin and eosin the caps are less basophilic than the bone and present as pale pink zones almost devoid of texture. Compared with the bone they contain fewer cells and the cells are more spherical than osteocytes, being reminiscent of chondrocytes in shape and distribution (Figs. 4.8 and 4.9). With Masson's Tricolour stain the caps take a green colour against the red of the adjacent bone (Fig. 4.10). In this particular section, taken under partially polarised light, lamellae of collagen can be seen passing in continuity from the underlying bone into the cap of changed material.

An important feature of these caps of changed bone on the bony trabeculae is the absence of any tissue between the semicircular impressions and the cement. In Fig. 4.11 a hemispherical impression is seen in what would appear to be bone with living osteocytes. No soft tissue intervenes. The cement spheres causing these impressions therefore would appear perfectly accepted by the living tissue ('living' as judged by the presence of living nuclei).

A surprising feature of the cement impressions considered to be sites of load transmission to underlying bone trabeculae, is how sparsely they are distributed and what a small fraction they represent of the total length of the endosteal circumference. In any one complete section across the shaft of the femur only some 6–20 such capped trabeculae may be found. From the known excellence and duration of the clinical results one deduces that

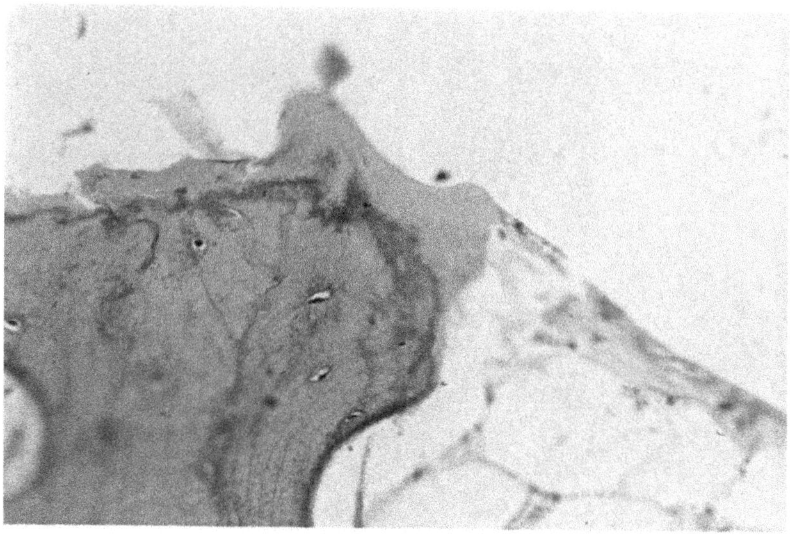

Fig. 4.8. Cap of pale-staining material on living bony trabecula

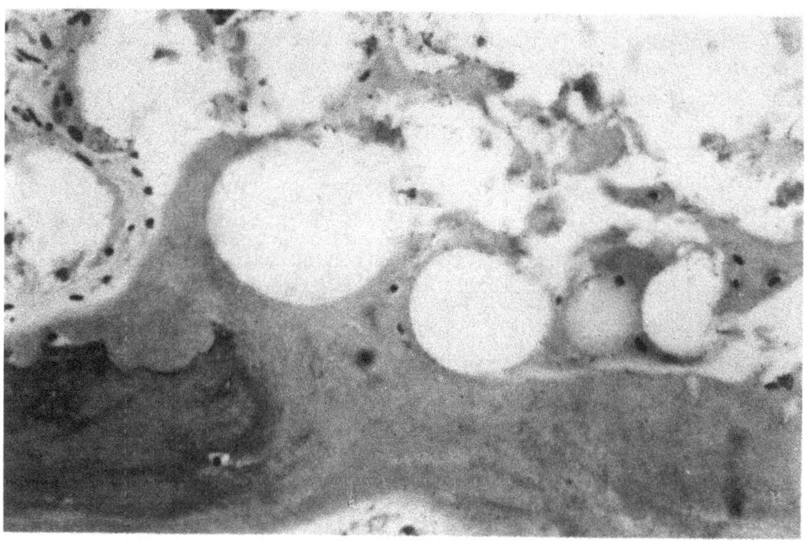

Fig. 4.9. Spherical impressions in 'cartilage-like' material (with living 'chondrocytes') in continuity with living bone

the total surface area of all the caps applied to the cement mass must be sufficient to carry the load required.

Histology of Non-Load-Bearing Soft Tissue Lining Femur

It has already been stated that where a fibrous layer intervenes between the cement surface and the endosteum in the **femoral** cavity, in human specimens with good clinical results this is never continuous, is never thick, and is often so delicate that it is best described as areolar tissue. It is suggested that the delicacy of this tissue indicates effective fixation of the cement in relation to the bone of the femur, because if fixation were not perfect (as is not infrequently the case in the acetabulum) a thick, densely collagenised layer of fibrous tissue would be expected between cement and bone.

Macrophage Layer

Where soft tissue in contact with cement bridges marrow spaces between trabeculae it is obvious from the anatomy that load transmission is not possible. Frequently the layer of tissue in contact with the cement at such a point is so thin that

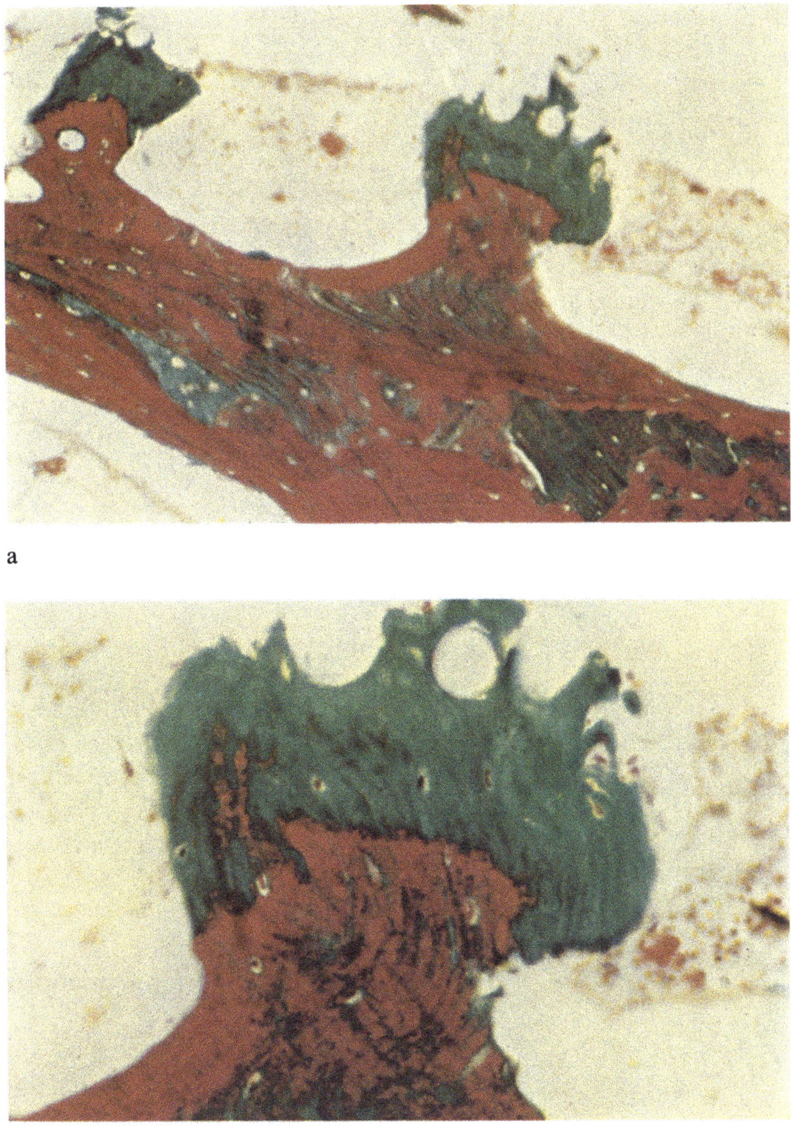

a

b

Fig. 4.10 a, b. Masson stain. Low and high power. Note changed staining reaction of caps bearing hemispherical impressions of cement spherules. In high power, under partially polarised light, note continuity of collagen lamellae with adjacent bone. **a** Low power, **b** High power

it is barely more than a membrane separating the cement surface from haemopoietic marrow and fat. Where a layer of fibrocytes can be distinguished in this membrane it may be only two or three cells thick (Fig. 4.12). In other sites a thicker layer of fibrocytes may be seen, as in Fig. 4.13, which shows very clearly the impressions of cement spheres.

Figure 4.14, at low magnification, shows a central trabecula of bone (A) with fatty haemopoietic marrow separated from cement in the medullary cavity by a thin layer of fibrous tissue (D). Figure 4.15, at higher magnification, shows that the central bony trabecula (A) carries a cap of changed bone tissue, with cells and living nuclei possessing some of the features of chondrocytes. It is to be noted that no tissue, fibrous or otherwise, intervenes between the cement and the load-bearing trabecula in the centre of this histological field. The scalloped outline indicates that cement spherules were in direct contact with the cap of changed bone. Figure 4.16 shows fibrous tissue in the non-load-bearing zone; the layer is about four fibrocytes thick, at D, and a layer of macrophages lines the surface in contact with cement. In several sites the macrophage layer is thicker and is forming foreign-body giant cells (E). Note how the fat cells, and haemopoietic cells, are healthy within a very

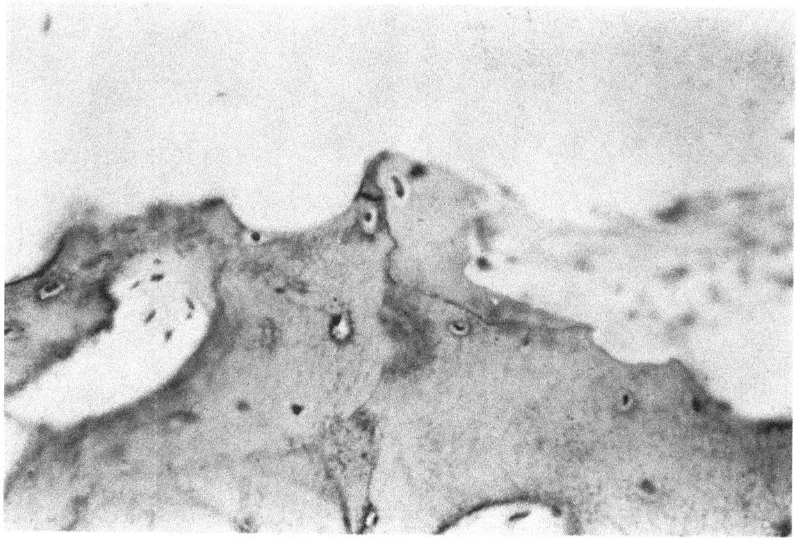

Fig. 4.11. Hemispherical impression in what appears to be bone. Living osteocytes. No fibrous tissue intervenes between bone, or changed bone, and cement surface

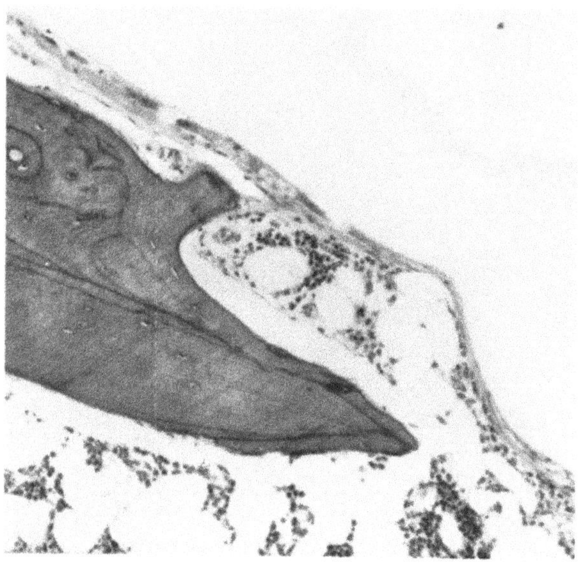

Fig. 4.12. Thin layer of fibrocytes separating cement surface from fatty and haemopoietic marrow. Non-weight-bearing zone

short distance of the cement surface. There is no caseous debris (the sequel to death of macrophages and giant cells).

Histiocytes (macrophages) and foreign-body giant cells represent a tissue reaction which no implant surgeon can lightly dismiss. Histiocytes are the root and origin of foreign-body granulomata. The caseating material derived from the death of histiocytes is the space-occupying material which invades cement-bone interfaces (probably by the mechanical effect of its increasing volume and the pumping action of slight relative movement) and causes destruction of cancellous bone with loosening of cement bonds.

Conclusions on Cement in the Femur

The clinical and radiological background of these post-mortem specimens representing an average period of 7 years, makes it possible to correlate certain facts relating to the macrophage tissue:

1) A surface of acrylic cement (in common with many other plastics materials) always tends to evoke a macrophage or histiocyte reaction. Metals, vitreous materials and ceramics evoke a fibroblastic reaction.

2) Acrylic cement evokes histiocytes in non-weight-bearing areas, as for instance where soft tissues bridge intertrabecular spaces.

3) In load-bearing areas no tissue of any kind intervenes between the cement surface and the caps of changed bone on the ends of the load-bearing trabeculae. At these sites acrylic cement appears to be completely accepted, and accepted for 10–12 years in the specimens of this duration available.

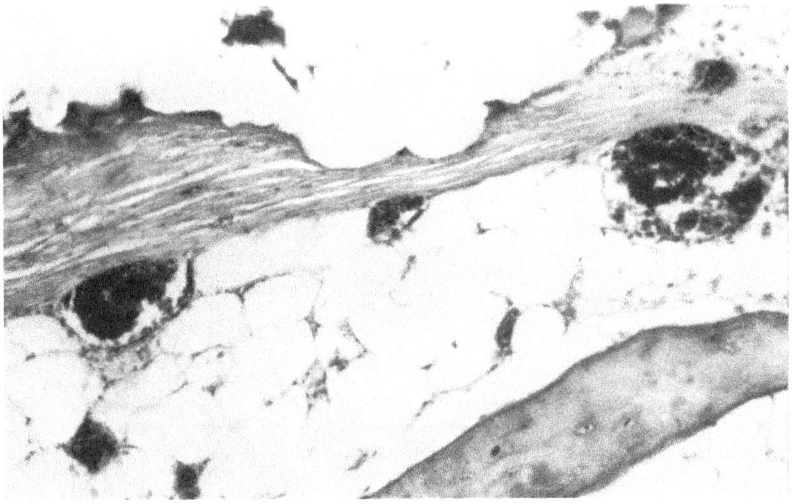

Fig. 4.13. Thicker layer of fibrocytes and collagen fibres separating cement (note hemispherical impressions) from fatty marrow. Non-weight-bearing zone

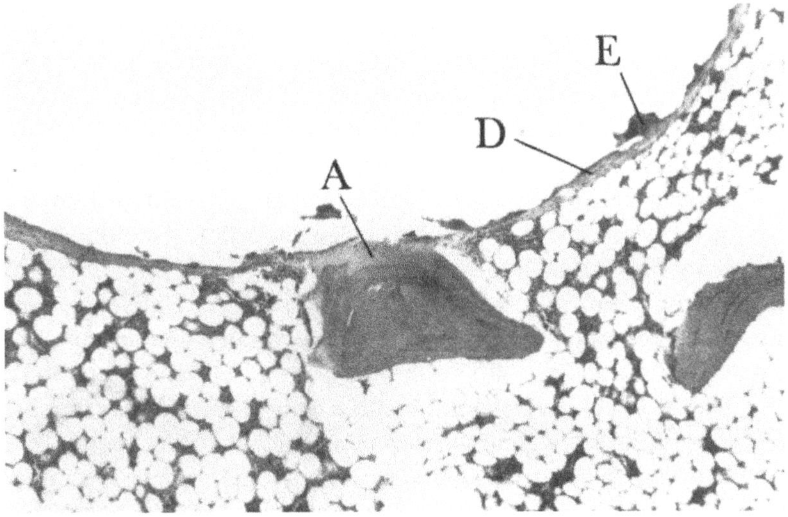

Fig. 4.14. Lining of medullary cavity of femur showing soft tissue in contact with cement except for central trabecula of bone (*A*). In contact with cement soft tissue lined with histiocytes (*D*); giant-cell collection of histiocytes (*E*)

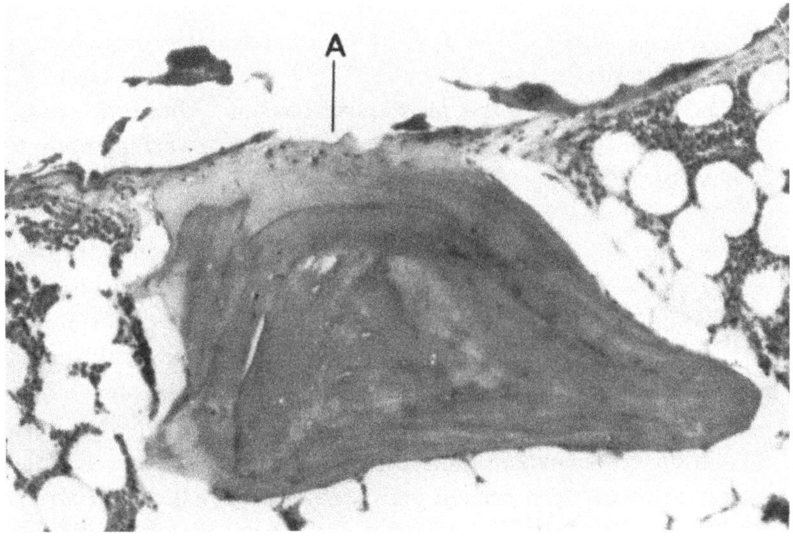

Fig. 4.15. Note cap of changed bone with cells resembling chondrocytes (*A*) and impressions of cement spherules. Higher mangification of Fig. 4.14

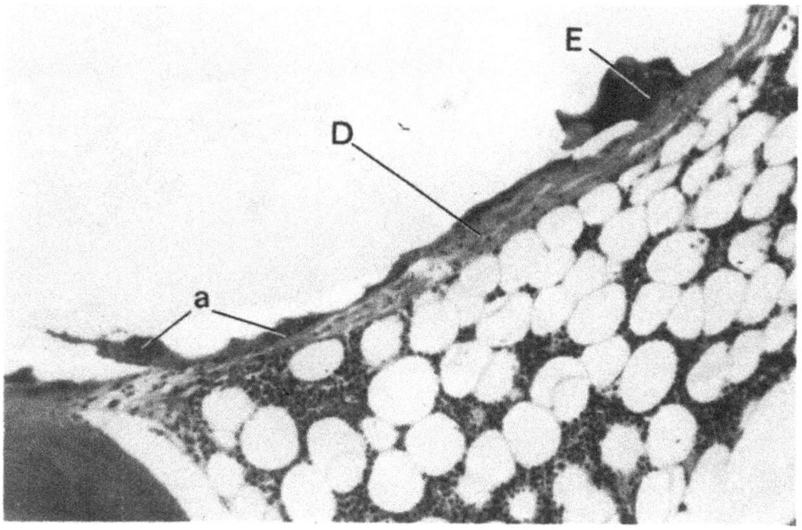

Fig. 4.16. Fibrous layer about four cells thick, lined with macrophages on cement side, and separating cement from normal fatty-haemopoietic marrow. Same specimen as Fig. 4.14. (*a*) Thick layer of histiocytes; (*D*) fibrocytes about four cells thick under the histiocytes and separating them from fatty marrow; (*E*) giant cell (nuclei not visible)

4) The clearly defined scalloped impressions produced by cement at load-bearing points is proof that no relative motion is taking place between cement and tissue; the impressions would not be clear cut and would be abraded away if movement were present.

5) In these specimens histiocytes and giant-cell collections have remained dormant, without any signs of granuloma formation (at least in the femur) for the longest period of observation (12 years).

6) The histiocyte layer on the surface of the cement can be isolated from haemopoietic marrow and fat by the thinnest of membranes. This indicates that histiocytes are not aggressive cells. Therefore, when granulomata arise and start to invade a cement-bone interface some additional factor must be at work which is not represented in these specimens.

It is postulated that sound mechanical fixation (resulting from a good cement technique) is responsible for the absence of thick layers of collagenised fibrous tissue intervening between cement and bone.

The Acetabulum

Unlike in the femur, where radiological suspicion of demarcation between cement and bone is very rare in our experience at Wrightington, in the acetabulum cement demarcates radiologically from the bone in about 60% of clinically successful cases (Chap. 6).

It will be shown that the histological nature of the cement-bone bond in the acetabulum is quite different from that in the femur and explains why some degree of demarcation in the acetabulum is compatible with good and long-lasting function. Unlike the femur the histological appearances in the acetabulum give no grounds for complacency and these studies urge the use of more sophisticated methods of handling cement in the acetabulum than was the case in the era which produced these specimens.

In none of the 26 sockets so far examined in the author's collection has direct contact between cement and bone of the acetabulum been observed. In most cases fibrous tissue, from 0.5 to 1.5 mm thick, intervenes between the cement and bone. In some cases, however, quite highly developed cartilaginous tissue, with good mechanical properties for load transmission, and often closely resembling hyaline cartilage, is present. Rather frequently the tissue lining the acetabulum is covered, on the surface applied to the cement, with a layer of amorphous material (Fig. 4.17). Almost certainly this is produced by cement, because it contains few birefringent particles of abraded HMWP and, when birefringent particles are present, they do not seem to be sufficiently numerous to be the main cause of the granulomatous material. Histiocytes are sometimes seen 'sandwiched' as mono-

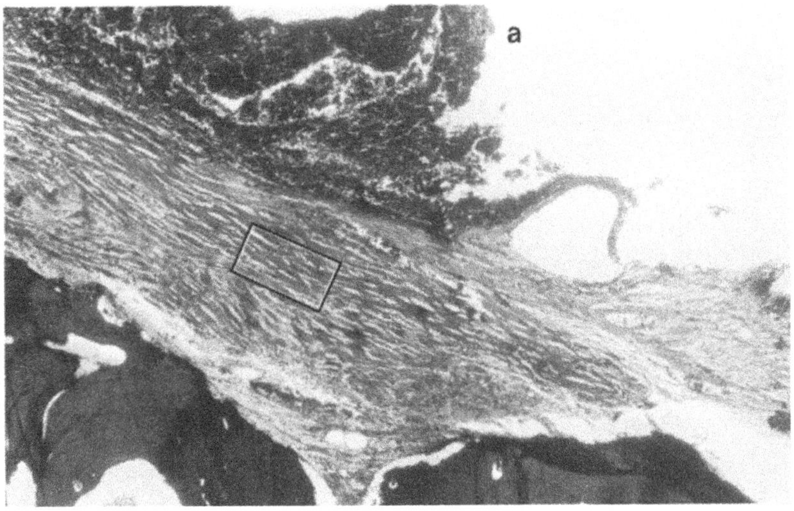

Fig. 4.17. Thick layer of fibrous tissue and collagen fibres lining acetabulum. Amorphous, caseous material (*a*)

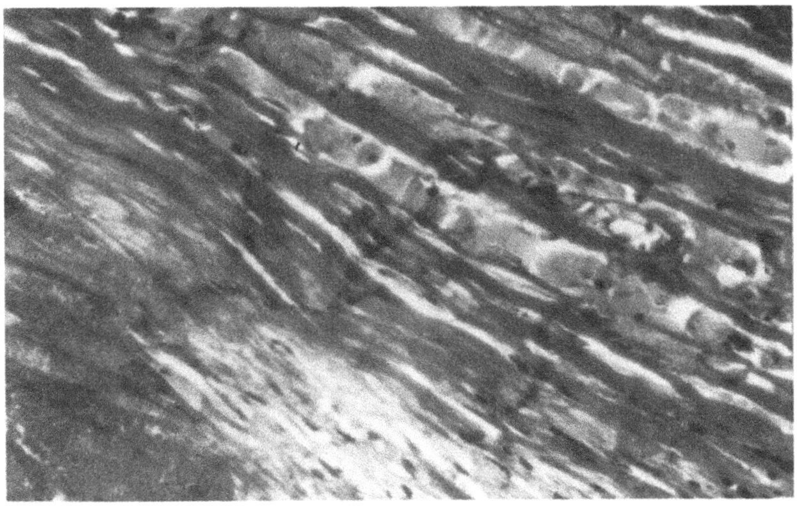

Fig. 4.18. Histiocytes in monocellular layers sandwiched between collagen fibres and fibrocytes (as from rectangle outlined in Fig. 4.17)

cellular layers between parallel laminae of collagenous material and fibrocytes (Fig. 4.18).

On the other hand and in marked contrast to this disappointing histological picture there are optimistic observations to be made. Thus the fibrous layer separating cement from the bone of the acetabulum is not infrequently interrupted by collections of cartilage through which there is clear evidence of load bearing from cement to bone (Fig. 4.19). The scalloped outline of the cartilaginous zone indicates direct contact with cement, and the underlying bone of the acetabulum clearly indicates a sound load-bearing arrangement (Fig. 4.20). A similar appearance of soft tissue, unfit for weight bearing, passing in continuity into cartilage at a load-bearing zone is seen in Fig. 4.21. At higher magnification transition of fibrous tissue into cartilaginous material is clearly seen (Fig. 4.22).

Sometimes the cartilage resembles the hyaline cartilage of a normal acetabulum, taking a basophilic stain, as is common in the deep layers of articular cartilage. It is possible that some of this type of cartilage might have started as remnants of articular cartilage left behind at the operation. On the other hand cartilage can often be demonstrated interrupting and in direct continuity with the fibrous lining of the acetabulum. The appearances suggest that ground substance, cartilaginous matrix, appears between the fibres of the fibro-

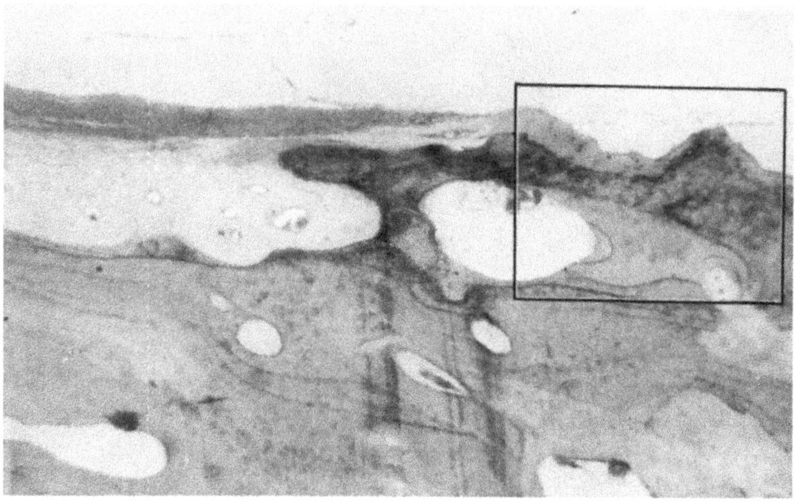

Fig. 4.19. Fibrous layer on left of picture, clearly unsuitable for load transmission, passing on right into cartilaginous material with scalloped outline indicating load transmission to bone. Acetabulum

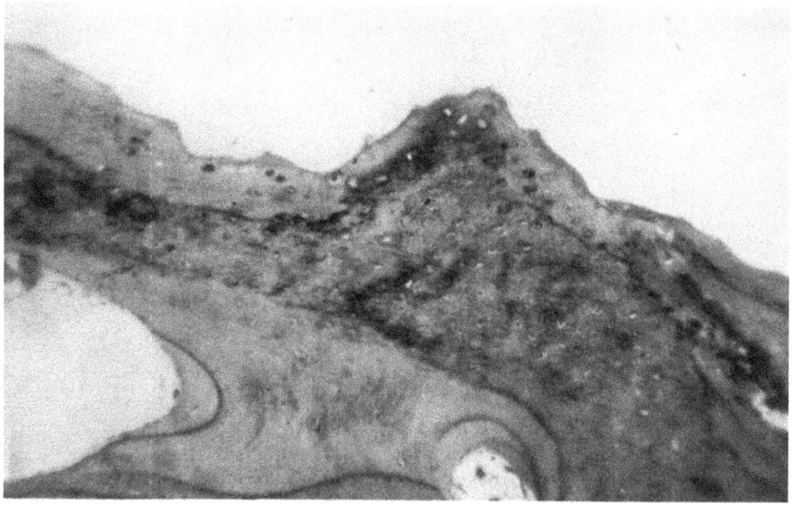

Fig. 4.20. Histology of rectangular field in Fig. 4.19 at higher magnification. Scalloped outline of weight-bearing cement surface. Living cells very much like chondrocytes. Acetabulum

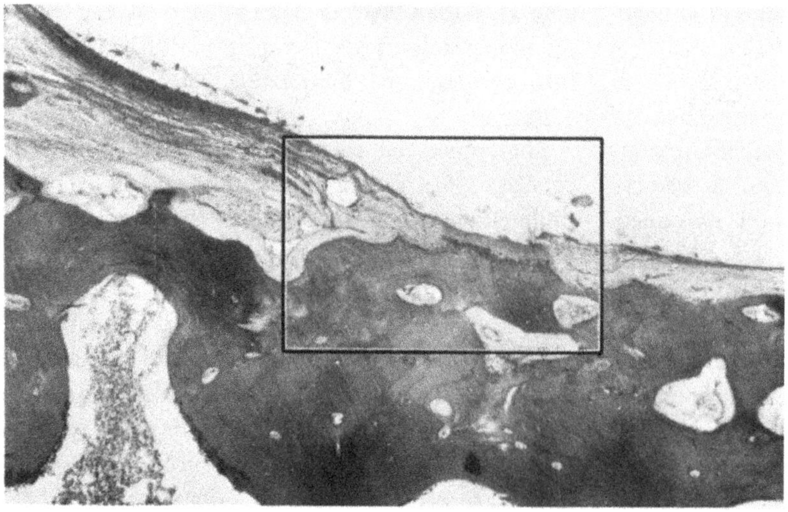

Fig. 4.21. Soft tissue unfit for load bearing on left and right of section passing into central load-bearing zone on lining of acetabulum

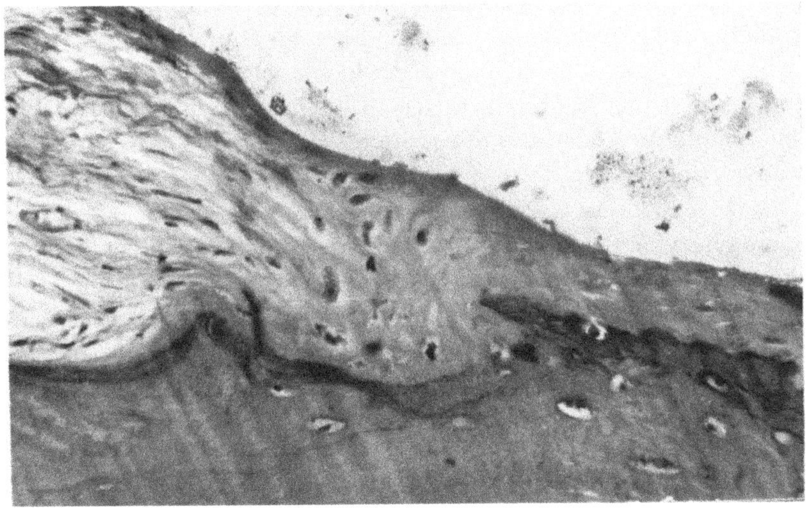

Fig. 4.22. Load-bearing zone in rectangle of Fig. 4.21 seen as fibrocartilage developing out of fibrous tissue

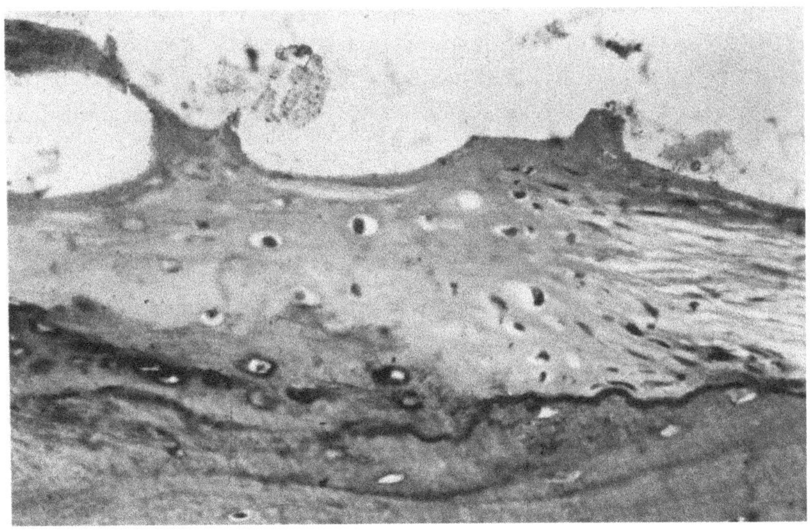

Fig. 4.23. Pink-staining ground substance appearing between fibres of fibrocytes. Nuclei of fibrocyte swell and assume the shape of chondrocytes. H.E.

cytes, and that the cellular bodies of the fibrocytes swell up to assume the shape of chondrocytes. These appearances are seen in Fig. 4.23.

Conclusions

The histological appearances of the cement-bone interface differ whether this is in the medullary cavity of the femur or the acetabulum.

In the medullary cavity of the femur in the author's specimens the appearances are almost universally encouraging. When a fibrous intersection occurs it is usually thin and it never completely lines the whole endosteal circumference. Load transmission occurs between cement and bone through caps of changed bone which appear to be composed of fibro-cartilage, or of demineralised bone matrix, perhaps unique to this situation. No tissue of any kind is interposed between the cement at these load-bearing points and the caps of changed bone. Where a cement surface presents to an intertrabecular space, where load transmission obviously is impossible, the marrow cells are separated from the cement by a membrane of fibrous tissue which is often of extreme delicacy. It is postulated that the delicacy of this membrane, and the fact that the impressions of cement spheres at load-bearing points are clear-cut, indicates perfect fixation of the cement in relation to the skeleton. Evidence of macrophage reactions passing to granulomatous formations was not seen in the shaft of the femur, though it did occur in restricted zones of bone resorption in the region of the medial femoral neck; but this is not discussed in this study.

In the acetabulum appearances were not as encouraging as in the femur but there were grounds for optimism. Collagenous fibrous tissue was present in laminae parallel to the bone surface and occasionally these were separated by monocellular sandwiches of histiocytes. The surface of tissue in contact with the cement frequently was covered with a layer of amorphous, caseous debris. In the most encouraging specimens the layer of fibrous tissue was interrupted by zones where a matrix, or ground substance, characteristic of cartilage had appeared between the strands of collagen and cells closely resembling chondrocytes had formed by the swelling of the cytoplasm of fibrocytes. In these zones direct contact between a cartilage surface and cement was revealed and the cartilage zone obviously transmitted load directly to the underlying bone.

The final conclusion is that histology gives grounds for satisfaction with cement in the femur, but indicates the need to avoid complacency regarding the cement technology used in the acetabulum in the era when these pateints were operated on. The best appearances of cement-bone interfaces in the acetabulum suggested that it ought to be possible to achieve these routinely once a better cement technology has been developed. In all the acetabula of this collection of post-mortem material the technique of using the cement is now regarded as rudimentary. Irrigation, for instance, was never used. These findings therefore are not considered to be discouraging if seen in the light of the improved details of technique and socket design described in this book.

Chapter 5

Long-Term Clinical Results

Six different long-term studies carried out at Wrightington of the **clinical results** of the LFA operation are presented. The chapter is divided into three parts. This is to bring together the studies made on the prospective group of patients and distinguish these from studies on later groups.

Part I comprises four studies on the prospective group of patients. Studies 1 and 3 concern the results of the first year from November 1962 to the end of December 1963; studies 2 and 4, the results of all three years from November 1962 to December 1965.

Part II is a retrospective study of patients operated upon in 1967 and 1968.

Part III is a study of the secondary operations generated by over 10,000 LFA operations performed between January 1966 and December 1976 and it is confined to failures needing revision for aseptic loosening of cement.

Average Quality of Clinical Results by Numerical Notation

The numerical system of grading the quality of a clinical result, on a six-digit scale, and categorising under prefixes A, B and C is described in Chapter 3. Without this system it would have been impossible to conduct this long-term study.

A convenient feature of using the numerical notation to represent clinical quality is that an average figure for each of the three parameters of pain, function and range of motion can represent a group. If a group averaged 2.5 for pain before the operation and 5.9 afterwards this gives some idea of the magnitude of the improvement. If a group is composed of only two numerical grades with contiguous digits, such as grades 6 and 5, it is useful to calculate the average to the second place of decimals because if the result were (say) 5.56 this would mean that 56% of cases would be grade 6 and $100-56=44\%$ would be grade 5. If the group of contiguous numerical grades is large and there are a few grades not contiguous, the same procedure will give an approximate idea of the proportion of the two common grades.

Part I. Prospective Group

The prospective study was initiated in November 1962, when HMWP was first introduced as material for the hip socket, and the group was closed at the end of December 1965. During this period a total of 773 total hip replacements were performed but after exclusions, to confine the study to LFA operations with cemented sockets, the original number of primary interventions was 338. Excluded were 244 cases where the HMWP socket was encased in a metal cup inserted into the acetabulum without cement (these are mentioned briefly on p. 87). Excluded also were 140 revision operations for previous total hips using Teflon (PTFE) sockets.

The patients in the prospective group were recalled to the hospital annually for clinical examination and X-ray for as long as they were able, or agreeable, to attend. Figure 5.1 summarises the three long-term clinical studies[14, 15, 16] which have already been published from this unit.

Resumes of studies 1, 2 and 3 will not be given because study 4 brings the prospective group up to date and so supersedes these previous studies. Nevertheless these previous studies are very important because they are additional checks to ensure that if mechanical failures had occurred but did

	No. 1.	No. 2.	No. 3.
Year of study	1970	1970	1972
Year of publication	1971	1972	1973
Author	Eftekhar	Charnley	Cupic
Follow-up years	7–8	4–5	9–10
Period of operation	Nov. 62– Dec. 63	Nov. 62– Dec. 65	Nov. 62– Dec. 63
Original number of operations	205	338	185
Hips available for study	138	210	106
Comment on selections	–	Only primary LFAs	–
Pain			
Pre-op.	2.2	2.5	–
Post-op.	5.8	5.9	5.9
Function			
Pre-op.	17 Cat. A	46 Cat. A	11 Cat. A
Post-op.	14 Grades 6&5 2 Grade 4 1 Grade 2	5.9	6.0
Range of motion			
Pre-op.	2.2	2.3	–
Post-op.	5.3	5.1	4.9
Loose sockets	2=1.4%	2=1.0%	2=2%
Loose femoral prostheses	0	0	0
Sepsis	3.6%	3.8%	4.3–6.6%

Fig. 5.1. Summary of long-term results already published from Wrightington

not survive the 12–15 years of study 4, they have not been overlooked.

Clinical Study No. 4

12–15-Year Follow-Up

This study of the work of all the 3 prospective years (Nov. 1962 to Dec. 1965) was undertaken by the author in November 1977 specially for this book. Unlike clinical study 2, which also covers this same period, this study includes 58 LFA operations performed for previous surgery (osteotomies, femoral prostheses, Smith-Petersen cups, etc.) raising the original total number of primary LFA operations from 338 to 396. Thus 14.6% of the LFA operations in this study were for previous surgery of the types specified.

Seventy-seven hips were available for clinical examination in 68 patients. There were therefore 9 bilateral LFAs. There were also 7 LFAs which were bilateral by reason of a 'press-fit' socket on the other side also 12–15 years after operation. This explains the apparent incompatibility of a total of 77 LFAs in 68 patients with a total of 16 bilateral operations. In other words 23.5% of the patients in study 4 had bilateral arthroplasties for 12–15 years (Fig. 5.2).

Losses from Clinical Study 4 (CS. 4)[1])

The 77 LFA hips reviewed by attendance at hospital in November 1977 for clinical examination and X-ray represent only 19.4% of the original 396 LFA operations of the prospective study. The reasons for failure to attend are tabulated in Fig. 5.3.

12–15-year follow-up: average 13.2 years	
Nov. 1962–Dec. 1965	338 prim. LFA 58 sec. LFA
	396
77 hips 9 bilateral	68 patients
7 bilateral LFA	press-fit
16 bilateral in	68 patients 23.5%

Fig. 5.2. Summary of clinical material in 1977, 12–15-year clinical review

This chapter is concerned solely with the rate of clinical success or failure. In Chapter 6 it will be shown that long-term X-rays are of more significance for ultimate success than mere clinical examination, because patients can perform remarkably well with X-ray appearances which indicate quite clearly that failure will certainly occur after the lapse of several more years.

Despite the fact that only 19.4% of the original group were available for clinical assessment of suc-

[1]) To show that sub-headings relate to a particular clinical study and not to the chapter in general they are designated CS. 4, etc.

Hips 12–15-year follow-up 1977		
Examined	77	19.4%
Letter and X ray	38	9.6%
Infected	14	3.5%
Revised	9	2.3%
Died	164	41.4%
Follow-up 9–11 years	33	8.3%
Follow-up 4– 8 year	32	8.0%
Follow-up less than 4 years	29	7.3%
	396	99.8%

Fig. 5.3. Summary of attendances and failures to attend 12–15-year clinical review

cess or failure, the **absolute failure rate** of the original series of 396 hips can be fairly judged from the number of cases developing infection and the number of cases which have had to be revised for mechanical failure over the succeeding 12–15 years. It is true that there might have been cases where the patient was physically unfit for a revision operation and therefore to judge failure rate by the number of revision operations actually performed could underestimate the situation. Of the patients who are still alive only one such failure is known to us, as reported on p. 52 of this chapter.

Of the hips from the original prospective series which have been revised, the author is mainly interested in loosening of cement fixation, because this is the central and fundamental problem to which all other reasons for revision are of secondary importance. Of the nine hips requiring revision only five were for loose cement. The remaining four revisions were: two for fractured femoral prostheses; one for recurrent subluxation; one for unexplained pain with no mechanical explanation found and with pain persisting after replacing both components of the implant.

Including the patient described on p. 52, who was physically unfit for revision, the total number of clinical failures by loosening of cement is therefore only six (1.5%) over a period averaging 13.2 years after operation. The failure rate of 3.5% by infection reflects the operating room conditions prevailing from the end of 1962 to the end of 1965 but this rate in no way applies today. As will be shown later in Part III of this chapter, a mechanical failure rate of 1.5% in the prospective series is much higher than the failure rate over the 10,000 LFA operations performed subsequent to the prospective series.

Diagnoses (CS. 4)

There were 22 rheumatoid hips and 2 hips in ankylosing spondylitis, a total of 24 (31%). The overwhelming majority of the remainder were cases of osteoarthrosis (67.5%), there being only two patients with congenital subluxation and one with Perthe's disease.

Age Distribution (CS. 4)

At the time of the operation the distribution of ages, and diagnoses, is shown in Fig. 5.4. The average age for rheumatoid arthritis was 55 years and for osteoarthrosis, 62.

Duration of Follow-Up (CS. 4)

The duration of follow-up ranged from 12 to 15 years and the distribution is indicated in Fig. 5.5. The average follow-up was 13.2 years.

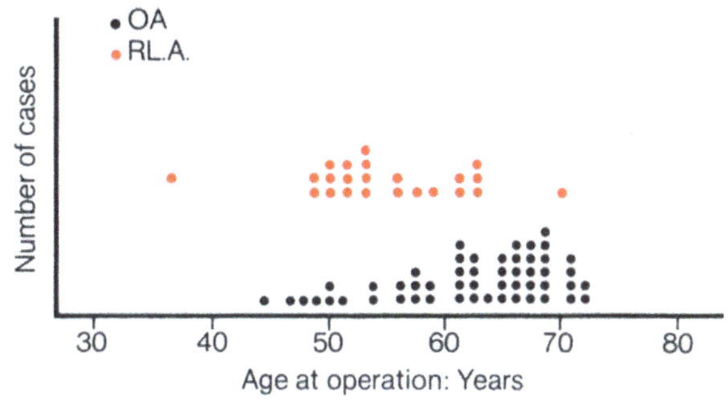

Fig. 5.4. Age distribution and diagnoses in 12–15-year review

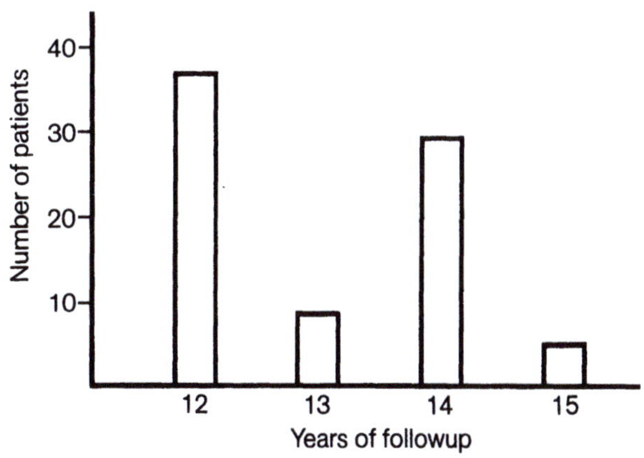

Fig. 5.5. Duration of follow-up in 12–15-year review

Clinical Categories (CS. 4)

The hips were distributed among patients in the following proportion of categories:

Category A	10
Category B	47
Category C	20
	77

Quality of Clinical Results (CS. 4)

Pain

Relief of pain is a well-recognised and reliable characteristic of this operation. Seventy-seven hips were examined clinically, and only 5 of the patients involved were in grade 5 for pain (which corresponds to discomfort or intermittent pain and is a satisfactory result for patients who were all grade 4 or worse for pain before operation). Only one patient remained in grade 4. Success for pain relief over an average period of 13.2 years is therefore 97.4% if grade 5 is accepted as relative success, or 90.9% if only grade 6 cases are included. This corresponds to an average post-operative grade 5.9 for pain.

Function of Walking (CS. 4)

A critical test of the function of walking is the post-operative quality of the category A patients, i.e. unilateral arthroplasties in patients with no factor other than the arthroplasty to complicate the quality of walking. In the present group the ages of the 10 category A patients must be considered because function in any category obviously must be related to the age of the patient: what is normal for a patient of 80 would not be normal for patients of 40 or even 60 (who normally, if required to do so, should be able to walk 10 miles in a day). Because in this series category A forms a small group of patients, the ages, diseases and functional grades are presented in full in Fig. 5.6.

An even greater test of total hip replacement is the function of walking in **bilateral hip arthroplasty** when the patient otherwise is physically fit. Because many bilateral LFA operations involve patients with widespread rheumatoid disease those most significant for assessing the quality of gait are bilateral operations in osteoarthrosis. There were five patients with bilateral LFAs in osteoarthrosis and five bilateral LFAs where one side was a press-fit socket (i.e. without cement). Figures 5.7 and 5.8 show the clinical grades of both these groups. To complete the data on clinical quality

No.	Disease	Years since op.	Age at review	Cat.	Grade
16882	O.A.	14	85	A	6 6 5
18924	O.A.	12	84	A	6 6 5
19334	O.A.	12	84	A	6 6 5
16032	O.A.	14.5	83	A	6 6 5
18494	O.A.	13	80	A	6 6 6
17101	Rh.A.	14	76	A	6 6 6
18104	O.A.	12	75	A	6 6 6
17190	Rh.A.	14	63	A	6 6 6
20565	Rh.A.	12	63	A	6 6 6
20588	O.A.	12	62	A	6 6 6

O.A., osteoarthrosis; Rh.A., rheumatoid arthritis.

Fig. 5.6. Functional grades of all patients in category A in 12–15-year review

No.	Disease	Years since op.	Age at review	Cat.	Grade
15166	O.A.	14	81	B	6 6 5
15781	O.A.	14.5	77.5	B	6 6 5
15787	O.A.	14.5	79.5	B	6 6 4
19170	O.A.	12	79.5	B	6 5 4
17282	O.A.	12.5	84.5	B	6 5 5

Fig. 5.7. Clinical grades of bilateral LFA operations in 12–15-year review. OA

No.	Disease	Years since op.	Age at review	Cat.	Grade
16000	O.A.	12.5	62.5	B	6 6 5
19348	O.A.	12	78	B	6 5 5
16885	O.A.	13.5	67.5	B	6 6 5
19582	O.A.	12	93	B	6 5 5
16415	O.A.	12	60	B	5 5 5

Fig. 5.8. Clinical grades of bilateral operations where one side was press-fit socket in 12–15-year review. OA

No.	Disease	Years since op.	Age at review	Cat.	Grade
18997	Rh.A.	12.5	62.5	C	6 3 4
16695	Rh.A.	14	78	B	6 6 5
15130	Ank.Sp.	14	50	B	6 5 4
16911	Rh.A.	13.5	66.5	B	6 6 5
16752	Rh.A.	14	84	B	6 6 5
15362	Rh.A.	14	67	C	5 2 5

Fig. 5.9. Clinical grades of bilateral operations in rheumatoid arthritis in 12–15-year review

of bilateral LFA operations the results in five bilateral patients with rheumatoid arthritis and one in ankylosing spondylitis are shown in Fig. 5.9.

Range of Motion (CS. 4)

The average value for post-operative range of motion was 4.9.

Revision Operations (CS. 4)

The two revision operations for fractured prostheses are not included because these represent a different problem and concern a type of femoral prosthesis which is now obsolete. There was one revision for recurrent dislocation and one revision for unexplained pain where no loosening was found and the symptoms were not cured by changing both components of the implant.

The revision operations for loosening of cement in the 12–15 years subsequent to the original operation will be presented here in some detail. There were five revisions actually performed and to these must be added the patient with a prolapsed socket who was medically unfit for revision, as reported on p. 52.

396 LFA 12–15 years

Revisions: loose cement

4 Sockets
1 Femoral prosthesis
1 Unfit for revision

6 = 1.5%

Figure 5.10 shows the dates of the original operations and the subsequent number of years before revision was carried out.

The essential clinical data of the five patients who underwent revision are presented because it will be noted that two out of the five revisions were for failures of previous surgery and another was the first LFA performed by the author for congenital dislocation. Therefore only 50% of the revisions (including failure unfit for revision) were originally uncomplicated primary interventions.

M.P., 15131, female, aged 57. Bilateral highly destructive arthritis of obscure origin (Fig. 5.11a); radiologically more like Rh.A. than O.A. but no other joints involved, and no other symptoms of polyarthritis in subsequent 14 years. General health excellent but decidedly overweight (160 lb, 72 kg). Bilateral LFA operations within

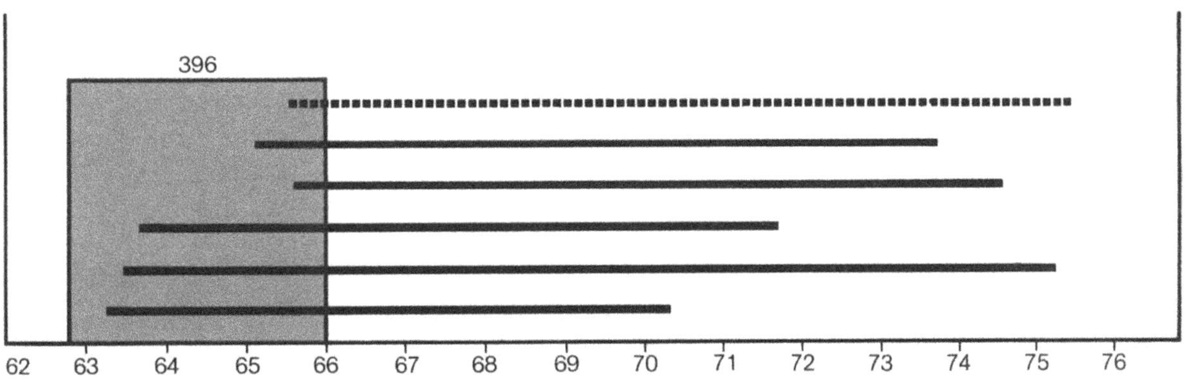

Fig. 5.10. Showing time interval between operations (November 1962 to end December 1965) and revision of the five failures in the prospective series. The *dotted line* represents patient unfit for revision surgery

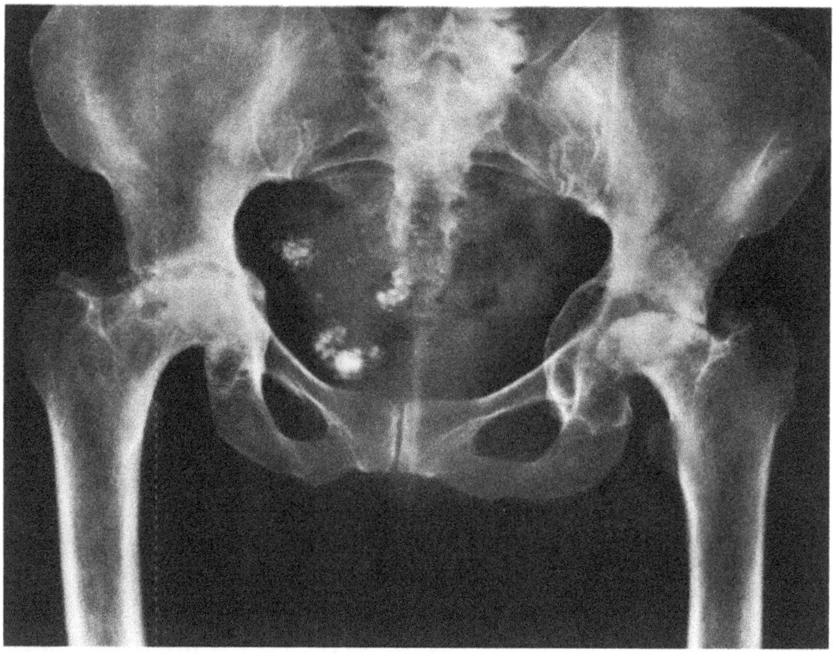

Fig. 5.11. a Pre-op. 1963

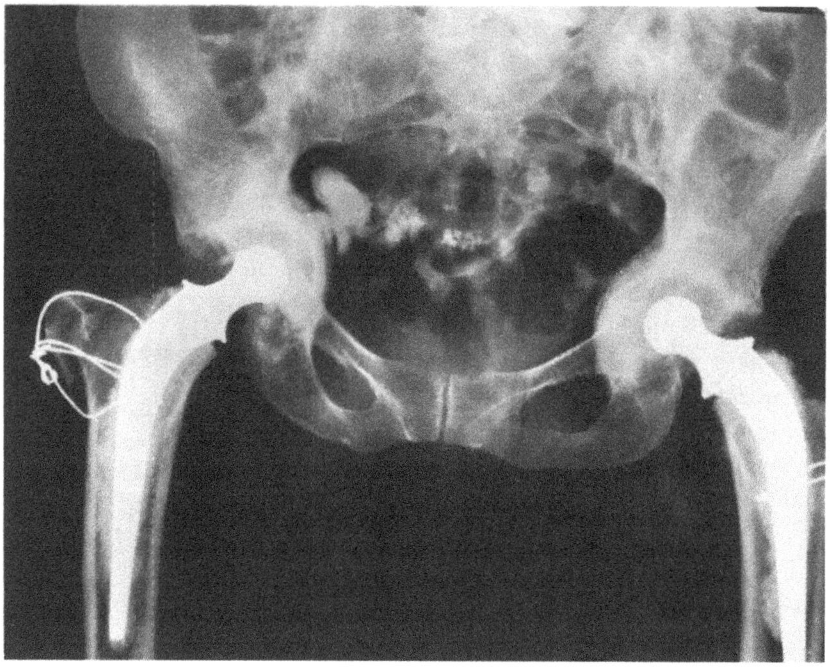

Fig. 5.11. b Post-op. August 1963

3 months of each other in 1963 (Fig. 5.11b). Patient had a very perfect clinical result at 4 years (Fig. 5.11c) but bilateral loosening. Prolapse of both sockets at 7 years (Fig. 5.11d). Right hip later revised with bone graft in floor but further prolapse of this side since. Still gets about quite well. The prolapsed left socket has not been operated on. Present grading October 1977 B. R 4.3.4. L 5.3.4.

F.M., 16751, female, aged 40. Right Judet prosthesis 13 years previously (Fig. 5.12a). Original diagnosis presumed to be secondary osteoarthrosis or osteochondritis on congenital dysplasia. LFA right July 1963, press-fit LFA left August 1963 (Fig. 5.12b). Good result and returned to full duties as school teacher. Had swollen knees and slight discomfort in hips so graded C. R 5.4.4. L 5.4.4. After 11 years symptoms increased in right hip associated with severe wear of socket and cement demarcation (Fig. 5.12c). Was contemplating marriage and revision of hip advised. Revision right May 1975. Cavity present in roof of right acetabulum due to acrylic

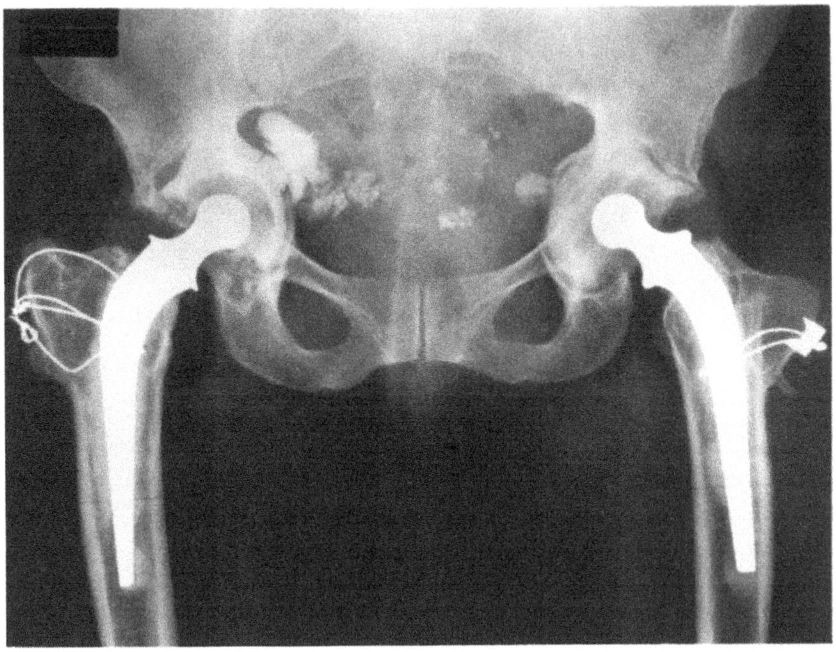

Fig. 5.11. c March 1967

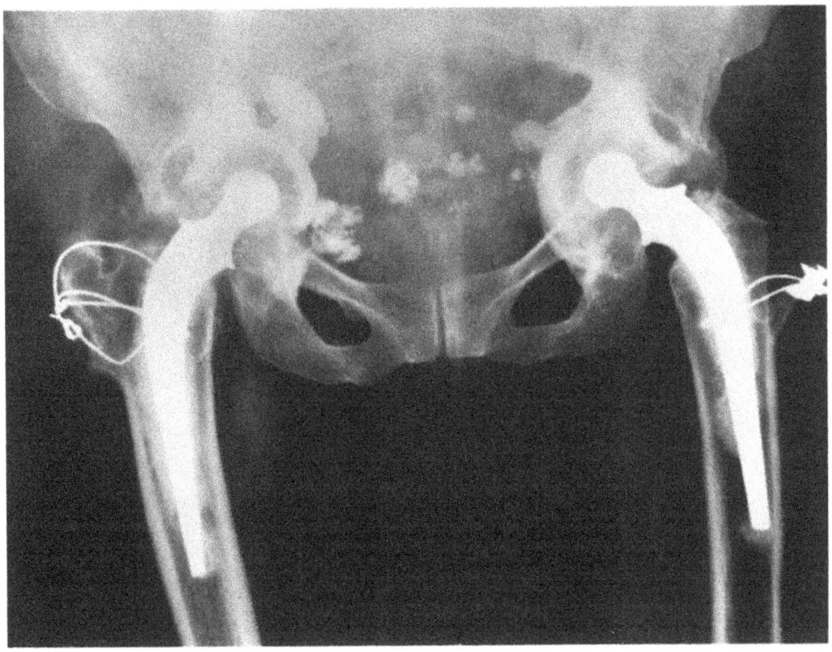

Fig. 5.11. d March 1970. Unusually destructive bilateral osteoarthrosis with unusual bilateral loosening and migration of both sockets. Patient heavy; exceptionally athletic result for first 4 years

granuloma from previous Judet. Asked for left hip to be revised and this performed in June 1975. Present result excellent; now better than before and happily married. Knees still not good. October 1977 C. R 6.5.5. L 6.5.5.

E.G., 18825, female, aged 29. Bilateral CDH. (Fig. 5.13a). Left side LFA August 1965, bone graft of slices of bone from head with bone paste applied to superior lip of left acetabulum. Excellent result. In subsequent years, despite superb function lifting and nursing two small children, left socket obviously migrating and tilting. Condition 5 and 9 years after operation (Figs. 5.13c, d), still minimal symptoms but advised to have revision, performed July 1974. Floor of acetabulum found to be merely membrane separating from abdominal contents. Iliac grafts laid in bottom of acetabulum. New socket cemented in with rim resting on lips of acetabulum. Result adequate but seems likely to fail again. Patient still only 41. November 1977 B. R 5.3.5. L 6.3.5.

Failure here thought due to excessive reaming of acetabulum with a fracture through floor of acetabulum.

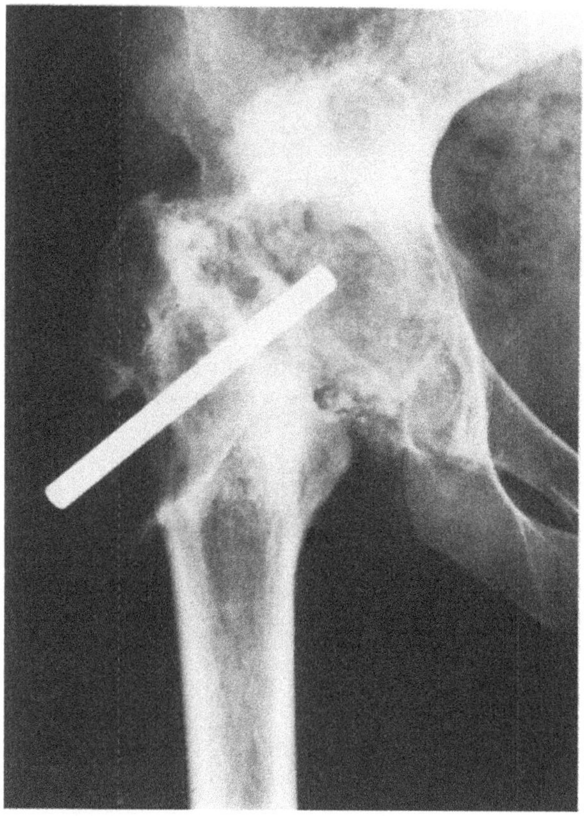

a

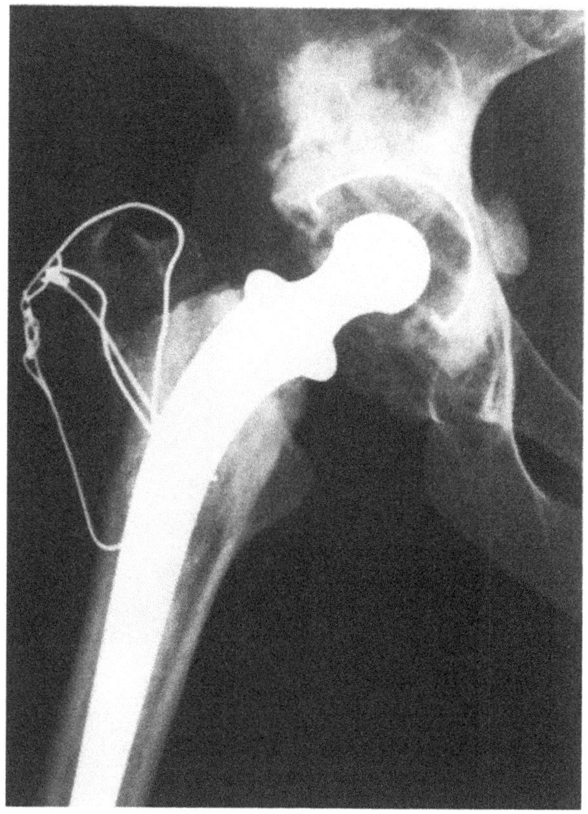

b

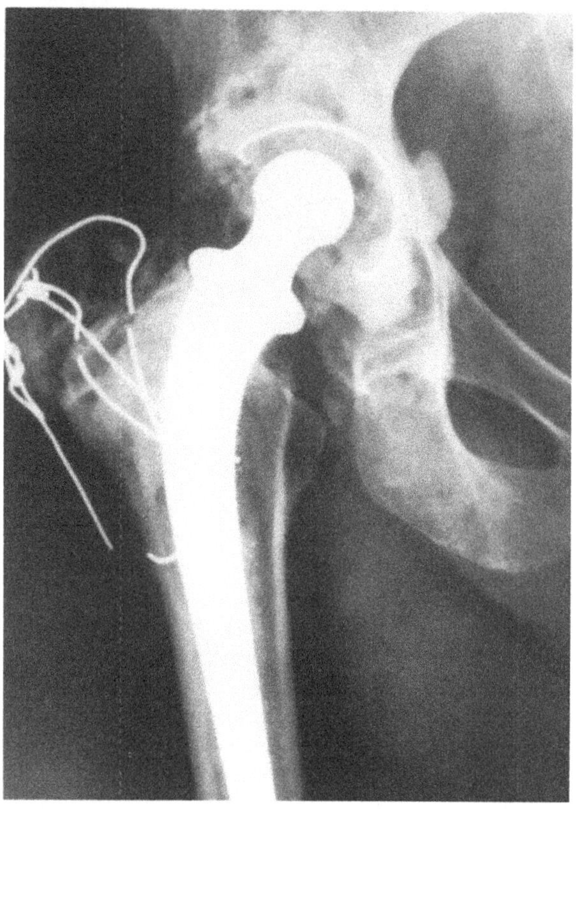

c

Fig. 5.12. a Pre-op. July 1963. **b** Post-op. July 1963. **c** May 1975. Judet prosthesis at original operation

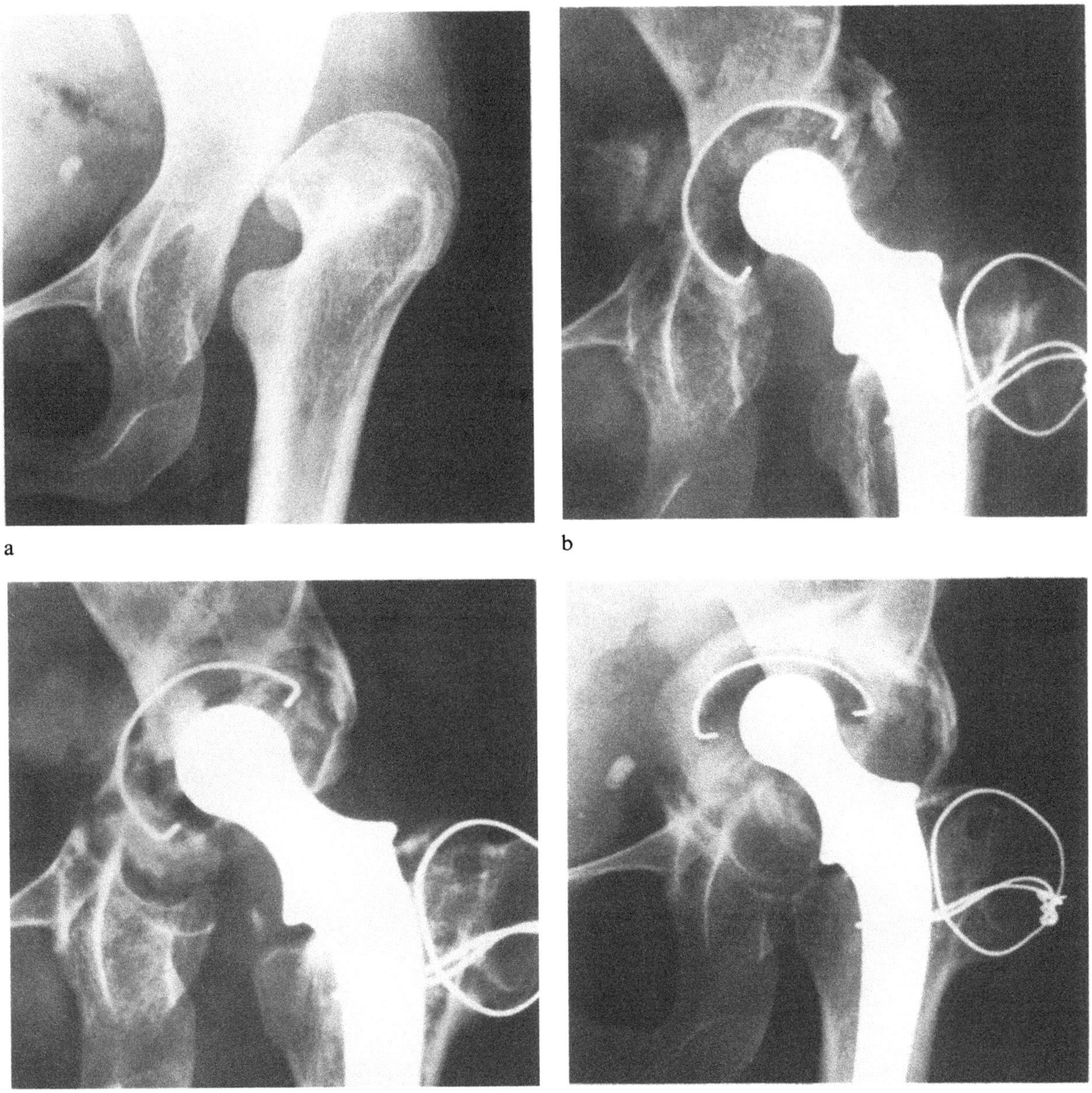

Fig. 5.13. **a** August 1965. **b** Post-op. September 1965. **c** September 1970. **d** July 1974. The first CDH attempted with too large a socket; acetabulum probably fractured

Socket was ordinary small socket and much too large, as subsequent experience has shown.

A.P., 18611, female, aged 35. Left Judet prosthesis at age 21 for osteoarthrosis; changed at age 31 to Thompson prosthesis (Fig. 5.14a). LFA February 1965 acetabulum flat and shelving (Fig. 5.14b). Despite difficulty in completely containing socket in deepened acetabulum a superb clinical result for 9 years, A. 6.6.6. Cavity in bone of acetabulum first noticed 4 years after operation (Fig. 5.14c) had enlarged at 9 years and was now invading the pubic ramus (Fig. 5.14d). Still no symptoms and perfect result. Advised to have exploration for diagnostic reasons (?tumour). Re-operation September 1973. At first examination socket thought to be firm in bone and offered some resistance to extraction but cavity under socket full of dry yellow caseous debris. Part of floor of acetabulum merely membrane against abdominal contents. Curetted and new socket cemented in. Result at first rather disappointing; moderate discomfort. Result in 1977 had improved to be graded A 5.5.6. Histology showed granuloma with minimum of HMWP particles and considered to be result of acrylic cement.

M.H., 16385, female, age 74. Destructive osteoarthrosis. LFA April 1963. Symptoms 1967. Cavitation in

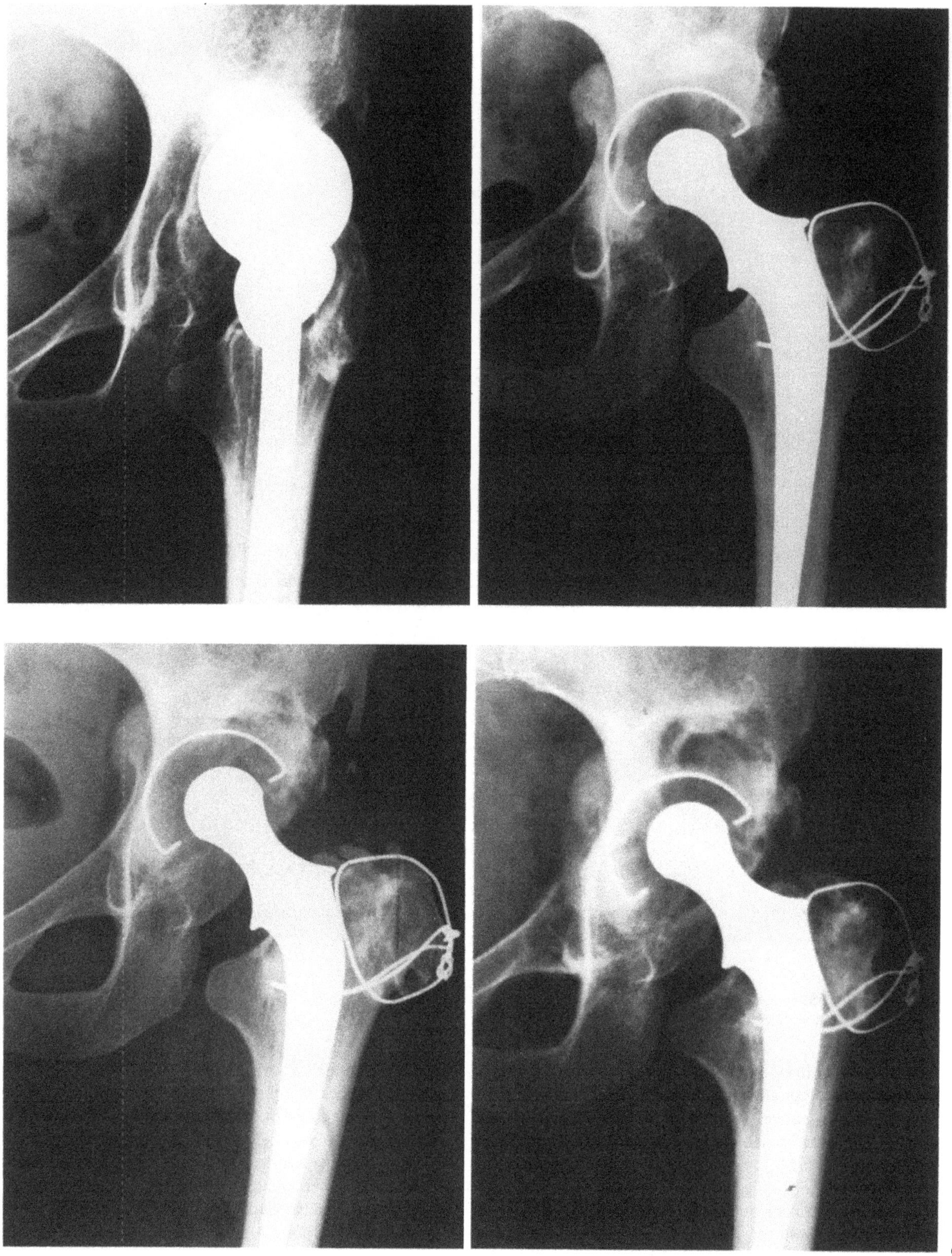

a b c d

Fig. 5.14. a Pre-op. February 1965. **b** Post-op. February 1965. **c** March 1969. **d** September 1973. Judet prosthesis and later Thompson prosthesis. Cavitation of acetabulum spreading into symphysis pubis. Inspissated foreign-body granuloma

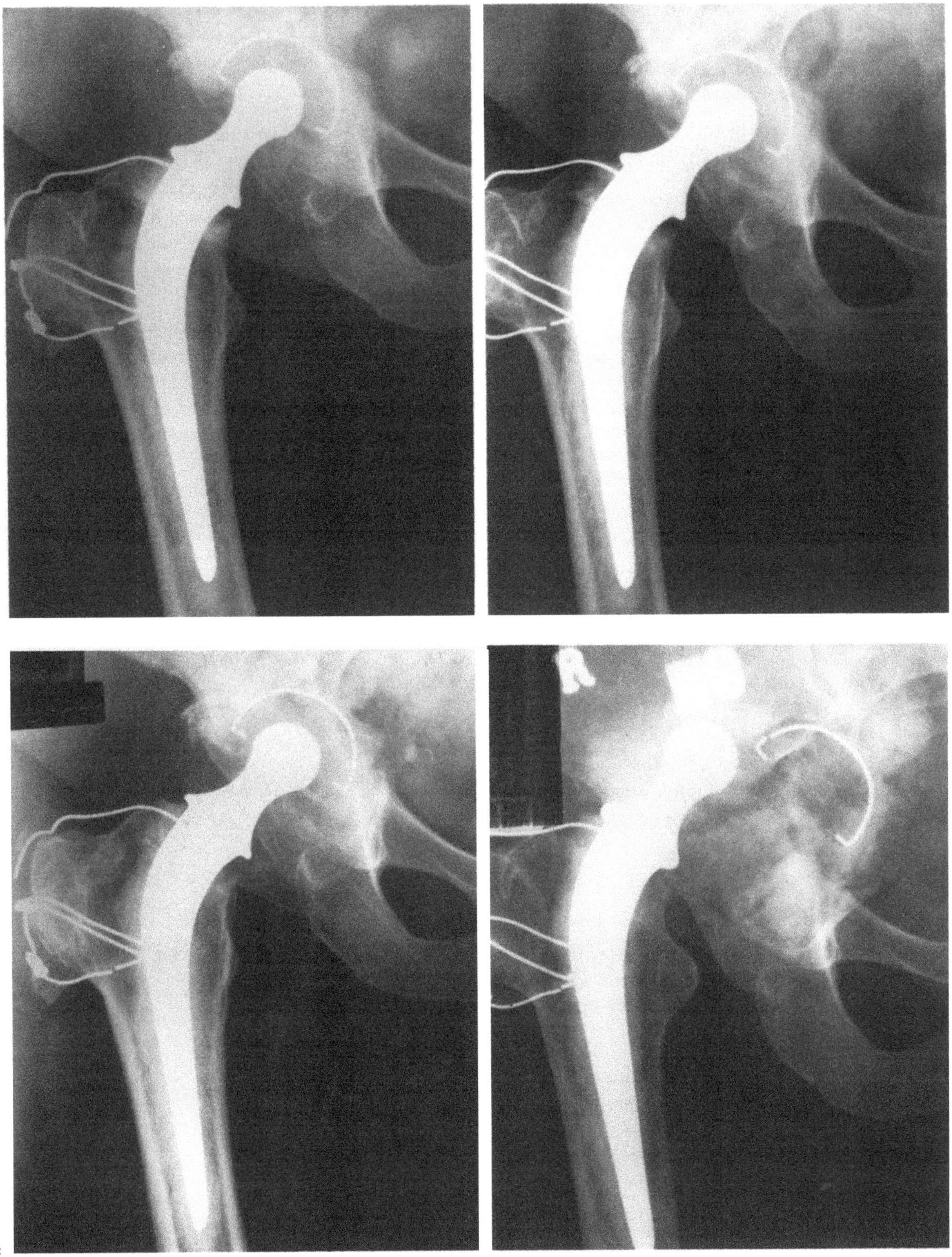

a b c d

Fig. 5.15. a 6.5 years after operation. **b** 7.5 years. **c** 8.5 years. **d** 9.5 years. Unique late migration of socket at 9.5 years. Other side perfect at 10 years femur thought possibly infected. This X-ray was published 1968 (Charnley, Follacci and Hammond) as Fig. 7, p. 827 **Journal of Bone and Joint Surgery.** Explored August 1971 in Johannesburg. Femoral prosthesis quite loose. No infection. Re-cemented with good result.

The following case history relates to the failure not considered medically fit for revision surgery:

A.H., 18995. A female patient with bilateral LFA for osteoarthrosis, 72 years of age at operation, showed slight demarcation of the right socket early and the patient was seen annually and graded as clinically excellent at every review (Fig. 5.15a, b, c). At 9.5 years the right socket suddenly subsided through the floor of the acetabulum without trauma or any other explanation and without prodromal symptoms (Fig. 5.15d). The opposite hip had an identical operation the year previously which still remains excellent and without demarcation. This patient unfortunately could not be explored because she was hypertensive with a blood urea of 80/mg% and was considered unfit for surgery. The ESR was only 2 mm/h so that infection seems unlikely.

Summary of Clinical Study No. 4

Year of study	1977
Year of publication	This volume
Author	Charnley
Follow-up	12–15 years. Average 13.2 years
Period of operations: prospective series	November 1962 to end of December 1965
Original number of operations	396
Hips available for clinical examination	77
Comment on selection	Includes 58 (14.6%) secondary operations
Pain post-op.	5.9
Function post-op.	10 category A all grade 6 10 bilateral in osteoarthrosis 5.5
Range of motion post-op.	4.9
Loose sockets	5 (1.26%)
Loose femoral prostheses	1 (0.25%)
Sepsis	3.5%

Part II. Clinical Study 5
8-Year Results

This is a retrospective study (Griffith, Seidenstein, Williams)[17] of the LFAs performed in 1967 and 1968. The year 1966, immediately following the prospective series, was excluded because of certain changes in the method of manufacture (but not design) of the hip implant. During the years 1967 and 1968, 1359 LFAs were performed and, excluding infections (2.2%), 547 patients were recalled and examined with current X-rays. A special feature of the study was emphasis on looking for radiological abnormalities in cement-bone junctions (reported in Chap. 6) but in this chapter the quality of the clinical results alone will be discussed. The duration of follow-up ranged from 7 to 9 years (mean 8.3 years).

Age Distribution (CS. 5)

Ages ranged from just under 30 years to 80+ (Fig. 5.16).

Years	No.	%
0–29	13	2.4
30–39	11	2.0
40–49	33	6.0
50–59	112	20.5
60–69	266	48.6
70–79	109	20.0
80+	3	0.5

Fig. 5.16. Age groups

Categories of Patients (CS. 5)

Category A patients, 18%; category B, 45%; category C, 37%.

Diagnoses (CS. 5)

Osteoarthrosis represented 62.0%; rheumatoid arthritis, 12.0%; protrusio acetabuli, 11% and failed osteotomy and hemiarthroplasty, 9.0%.

Clinical Results (CS. 5)

The clinical results for pain, function of walking and range of motion are as follows:

Pain (CS. 5)

Pre-operative pain averaged 3.20 and post-operative 5.83. Post-operatively 86% of patients were entirely free from pain (grade 6) and 11% had

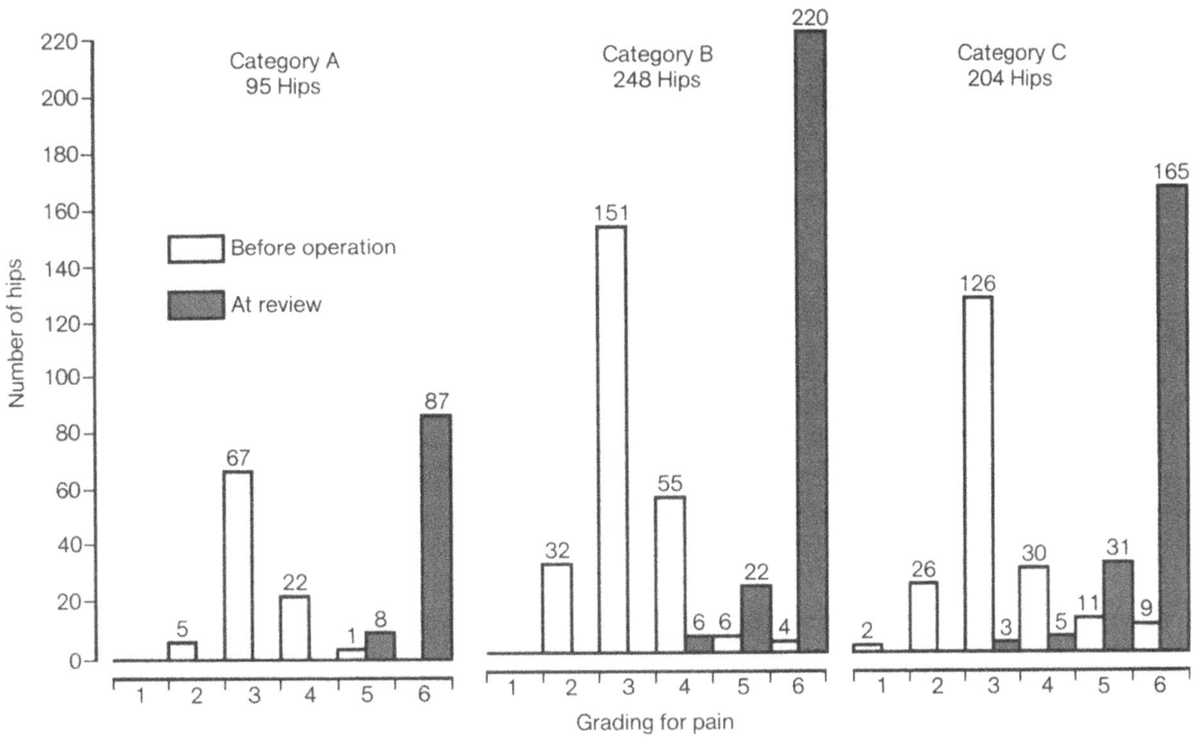

Fig. 5.17. Pain; before and after operation

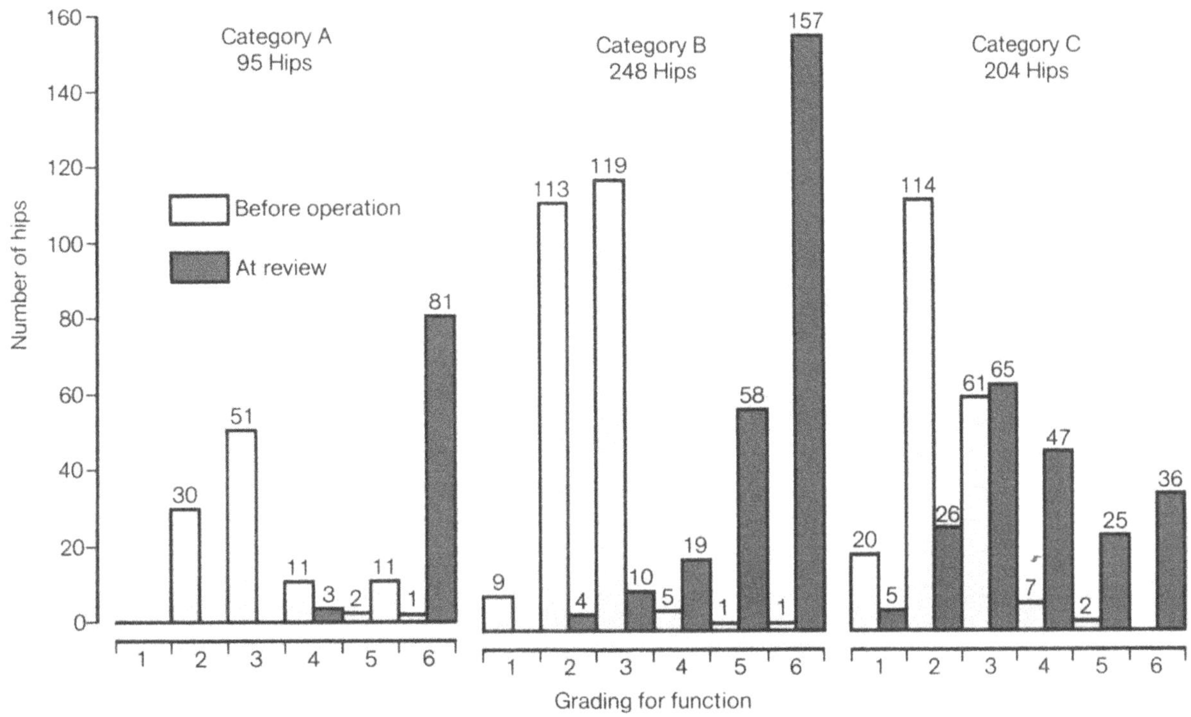

Fig. 5.18. Function; before and after operation

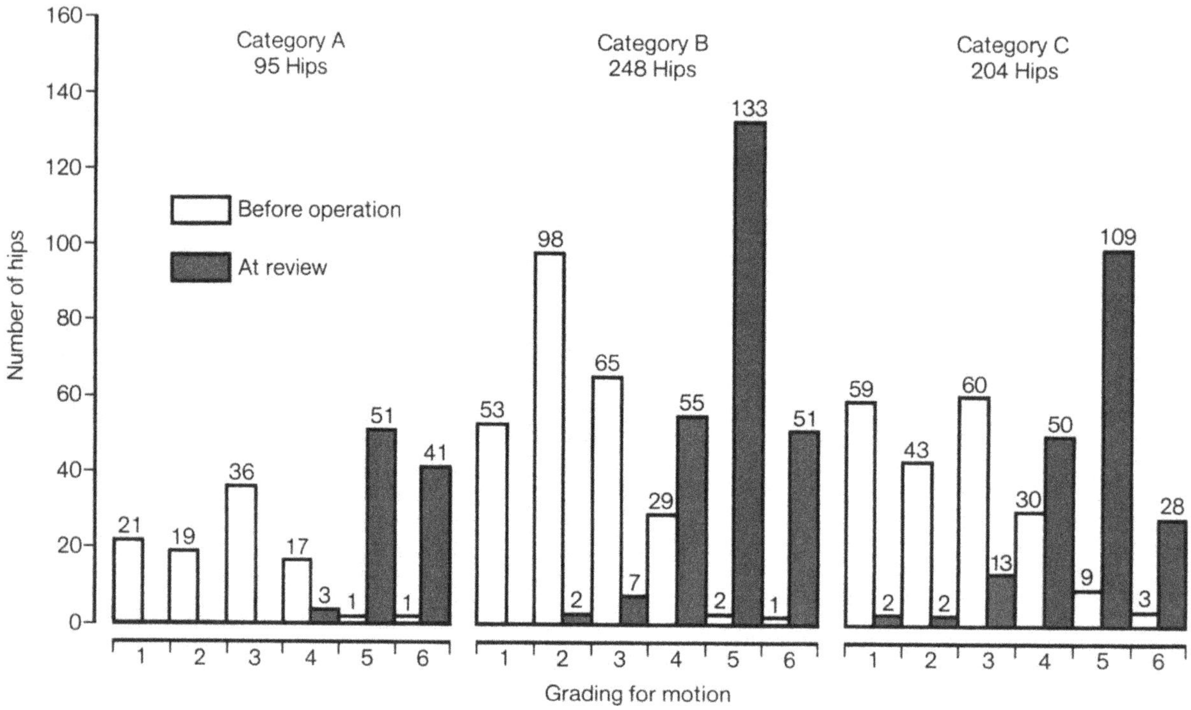

Fig. 5.19. Motion; before and after operation

slight or intermittent pain (grade 5) (Fig. 5.17). This represents 97% success.

Function (CS. 5)

Assessment of the function of walking of a total hip is most easily made in unilateral conditions (category A) though bilateral hip arthroplasties (see below) are an even more rigorous test.

There were 95 hips in category A: the average pre-operative function was 2.87 and post-operative 5.82. Eighty-one patients (82%) had completely normal function.

In Category B there were 248 hips with unilateral arthroplasty. The average pre-operative grading for function was 2.51 and post-operatively, 5.43. The post-operative function in this group was limited by disease in the untreated contralateral hip as shown by the fact that better function, 5.7, was obtained after bilateral arthroplasties (see below).

In Category C there were 204 hips where conditions other than hip disease affected function after operation: the average pre-operative grading for function was 2.30 and post-operatively improved to 3.83 (Fig. 5.18).

Motion (CS. 5)

The average pre-operative value was 2.41 and post-operative, 4.91 (Fig. 5.19).

Bilateral LFA in Osteoarthrosis (CS. 5)

Of the 121 patients with bilateral arthroplasties in osteoarthrosis with the second side operation performed before the end of 1968, function was normal (grade 6) in 94 (78%) and good (grade 5) in 24 (20%). These results are shown in the histogram, Fig. 5.20.[2])

LFA in Rheumatoid Arthritis (CS. 5)

In rheumatoid arthritis the results of this operation have been gratifying despite the bone destruction and osteoporosis in the acetabulum which is not

[2]) There are some inconsistencies in the statistics of this paper by Griffith et al., relating to bilateral operations in category B patients with osteoarthrosis. Of the 121 bilateral patients, 69 had the second side operated on after 1968. This does not change the quality of results for function as shown in Fig. 5.20.

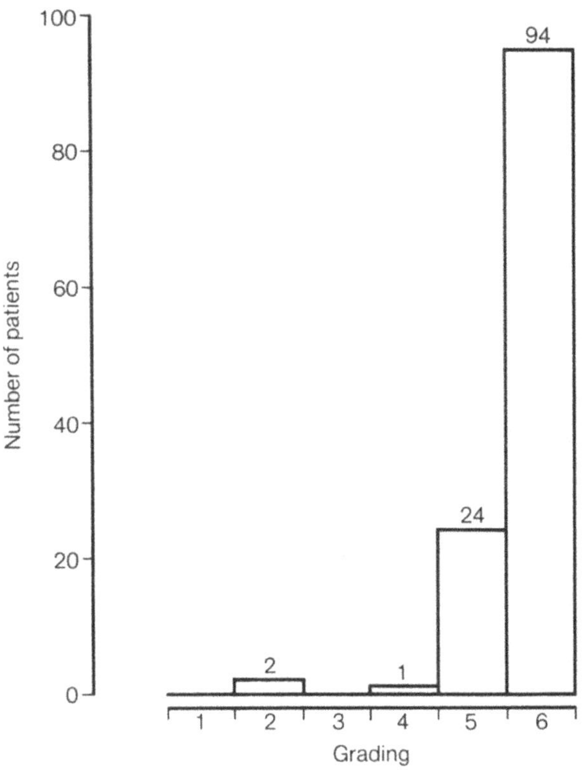

Fig. 5.20. Function after operation in 121 patients with bilateral operations for osteoarthrosis

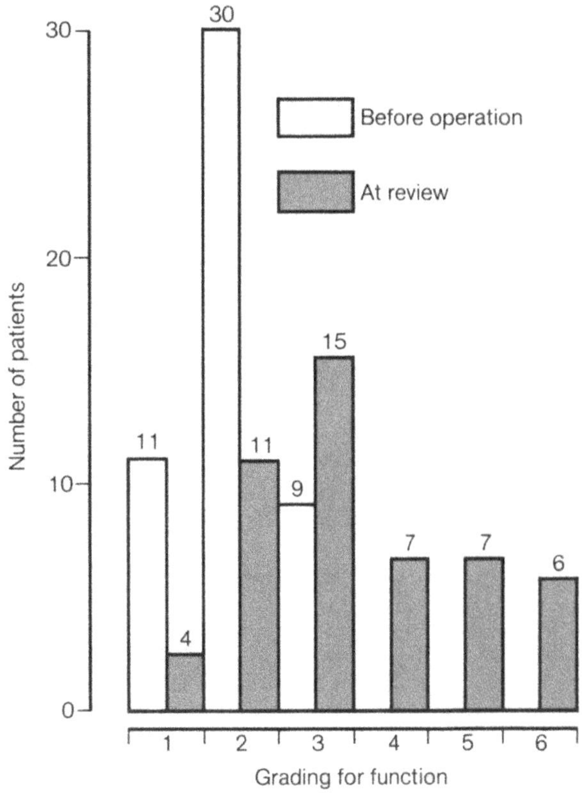

Fig. 5.21. Function before and after operation in 50 patients with bilateral operations for rheumatoid arthritis

uncommonly encountered. The incidence of mechanical failure has been only slightly higher than in osteoarthrosis and sometimes this has been explained by mild infection as proved at a secondary operation. The infection rate in rheumatoid arthritis would seem to be significantly higher than after primary operations for osteoarthrosis (i.e. 1.5% compared with 0.5%) (p. 157).

Bilateral LFA in Rheumatoid Arthritis (CS. 5)

The results of bilateral LFA in rheumatoid arthritis have been gratifying. Thus Fig. 5.21 in 50 bilateral operations for rheumatoid arthritis shows that the average grading for function was raised from 1.96 before operation to 3.4 after operation. Only 13 patients (26%) attained grades 5 and 6 post-operatively, but before operation 41 patients (82%) were in the lowest categories for function, that is to say 22% were grade 1, i.e. bedridden or chairbound, and 60% were grade 2, i.e. could cover limited distances with walking aids. One of our most remarkable long-term successes in bilateral rheumatoid arthritis is shown in Fig. 5.22. This patient M.R. (16695), now aged 78, attended the 1977 review, 14 years after the operation and walked unaided.

Fracture of the Femoral Prosthesis

There were five fractures of the femoral prosthesis in this series. Three occurred prior to the survey. All were in men who had normal function (grade 6) and all weighed over 173 lb (78 kg). Two fractured prostheses were recognized radiologically as a result of recall for this study. Both walked into the clinic with minimal discomfort.

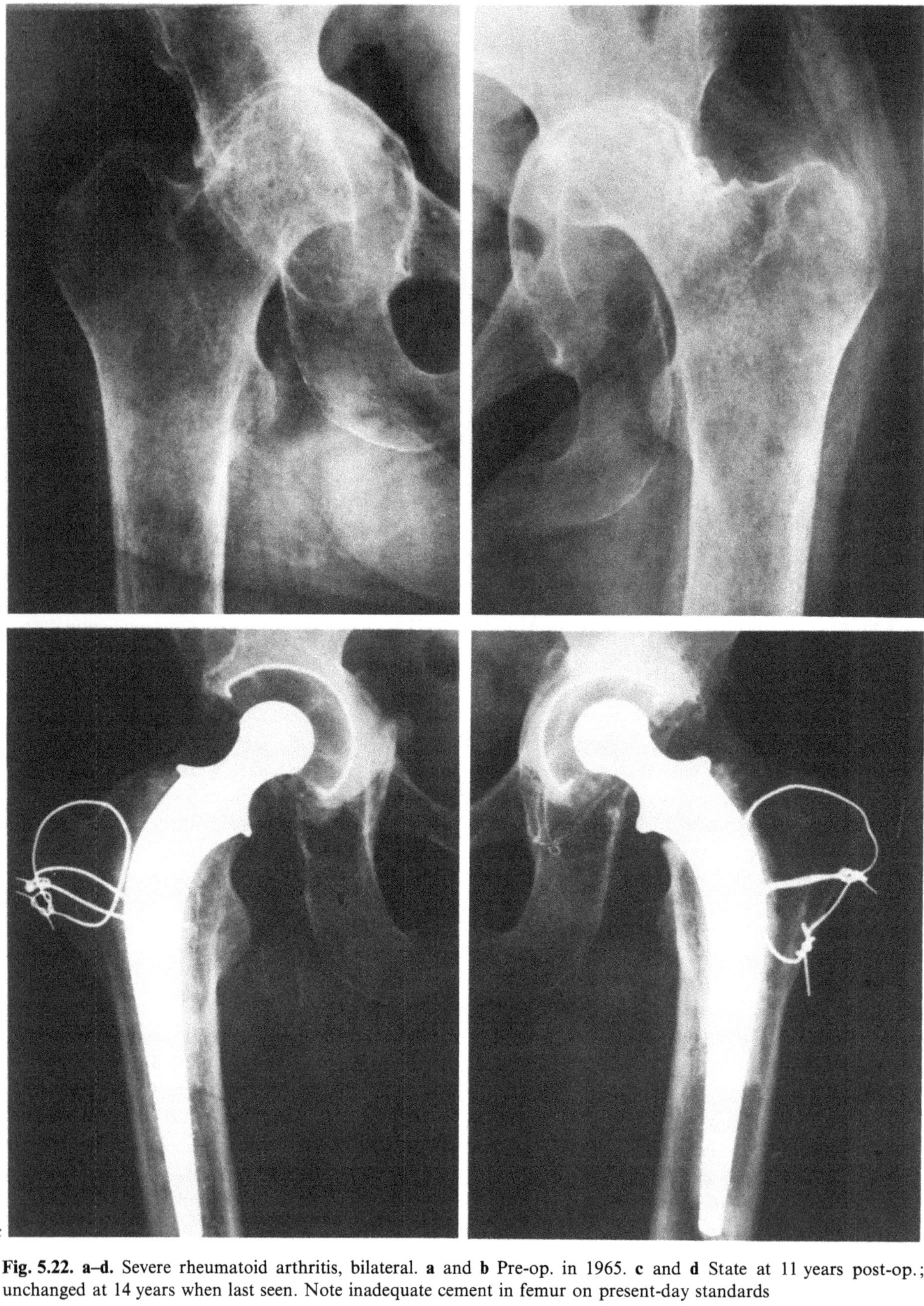

Fig. 5.22. a–d. Severe rheumatoid arthritis, bilateral. **a** and **b** Pre-op. in 1965. **c** and **d** State at 11 years post-op.; unchanged at 14 years when last seen. Note inadequate cement in femur on present-day standards

Summary of Clinical Study 5

Year of study	1976
Year of publication	1978
Authors	Griffith, Seidenstein, Williams and Charnley
Follow-up years	7–9 years. Average 8.3
Period of operations	January 1967 to December 1968
Original number of operations	1359
Hips available for study	547
Comment on selection	Includes 9.0% previous operations
Pain	
Pre-op.	3.20
Post-op.	5.83
Function	95 category A
Pre-op.	2.87
Post-op.	5.82
Range of motion	
Pre-op.	2.41
Post-op.	4.91
Loose sockets already revised	3 (0.22%)
Loose femoral prostheses already revised	5 (0.36%)
Sepsis	2.2%

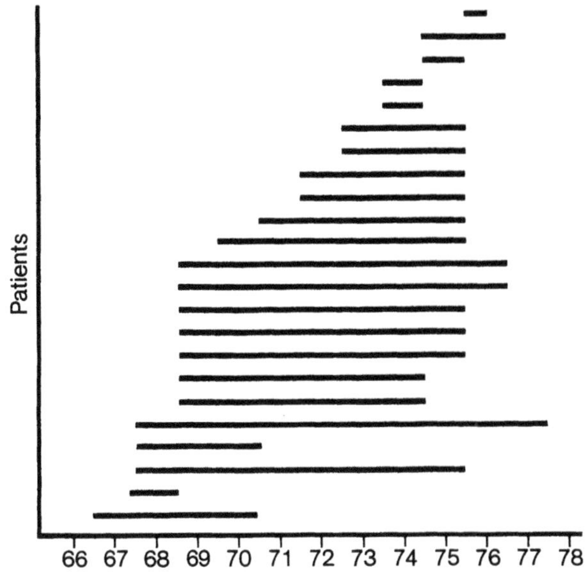

Fig. 5.23. Time interval between original operation and revision in 23 patients requiring revision surgery for loose cement, between January 1966 and December 1976

Part III. Clinical Study 6

The study of mechanical failure by the incidence of revision operations is a fairly accurate parameter because readmission to hospital is another source of information for the records department. This section studies the revision operations for loosening of cement arising out of more than 10,000 LFA operations performed in the 11 years from January 1966 to December 1976 inclusive (including the revisions already reported in study 5 of 1967 and 1968). There were 23 revision operations for loose implants (in two of these both acetabular and femoral prostheses were found to be loose; there were therefore 25 loose implants). This gives a total rate of revision operations for loosening of 0.23% (or 0.25% for the number of loose implants). Sockets and femoral implants loosened in the proportion of 10 sockets to 15 femoral prostheses.

Figure 5.23 displays data on the 23 patients who required revision operations for loose cement, showing the year of the original operation and the period intervening before revision.

Causes of Loosening Demanding Secondary Operations (CS. 6)

It is only rarely possible to identify the cause of loosening in a specific case but many of our loosenings followed when the original operation was not typical of a primary intervention or when there was a clear defect in the original surgical technique which could explain the loosening. Thus out of the 23 re-operations for loosening (excluding the 5 already described from the prospective series before the end of 1965) there are 8 (34.8%) where special circumstances might explain failure. It is of interest to present the essential features of these eight cases.

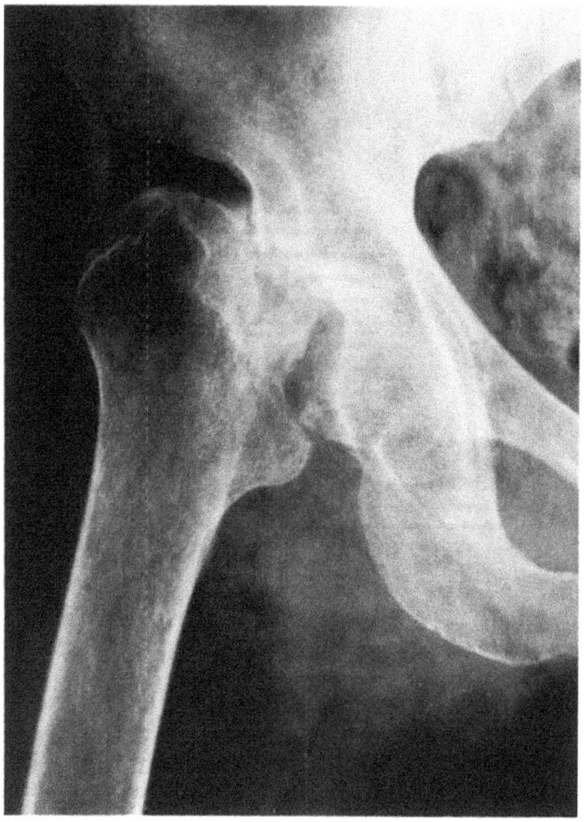

5.24a

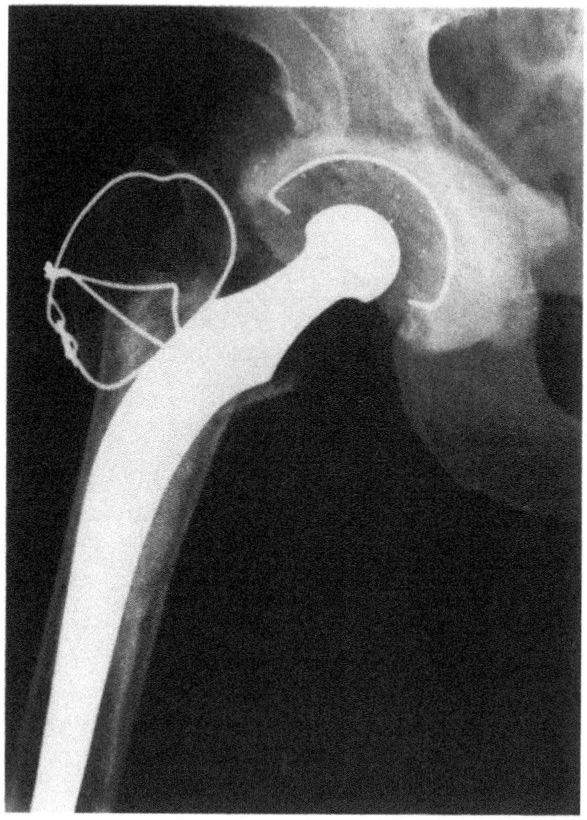

b

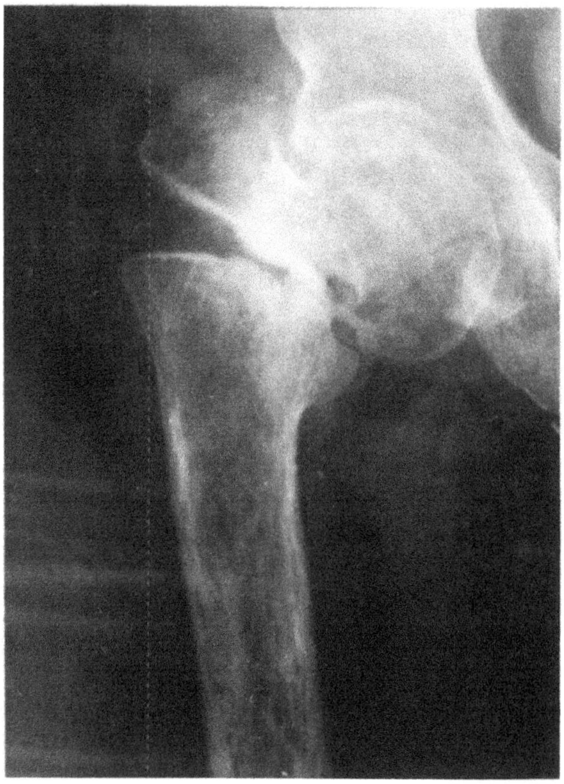

5.25a

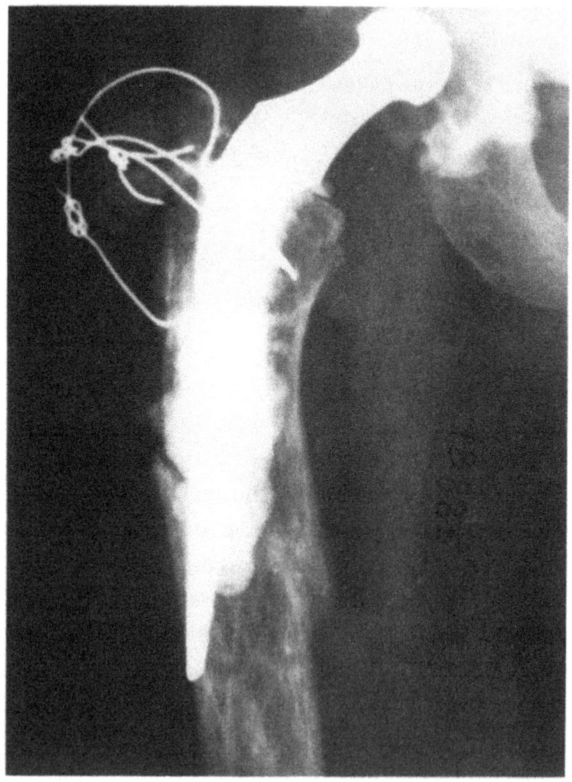

b

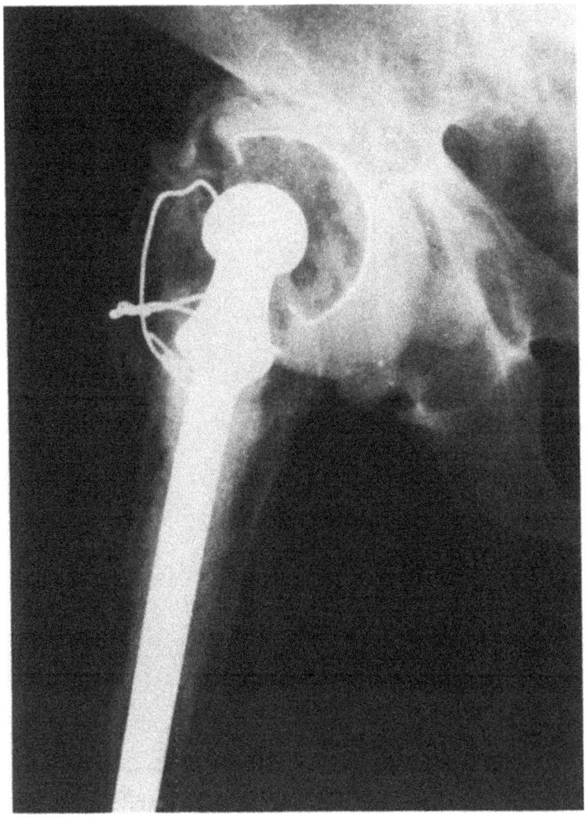

c

N.D., 21915, female, aged 63. Rheumatoid with fracture of neck of right femur (Fig. 5.24a). This was a very difficult operation (September 1966) by reason of a defective exposure resulting from obesity and gross flexion contracture of both hips and knees; the acetabulum was never properly defined and the socket was cemented too superficially (Fig. 5.24b). Complete dislocation of cemented socket out of the acetabulum occurred 3.5 years later (Fig. 5.24c).

Fig. 5.24. a Pre-op. Fracture neck of femur in rheumatoid arthritis. **b** Post-op. September 1966. **c** April 1969. Failure due to poor technique in difficult case

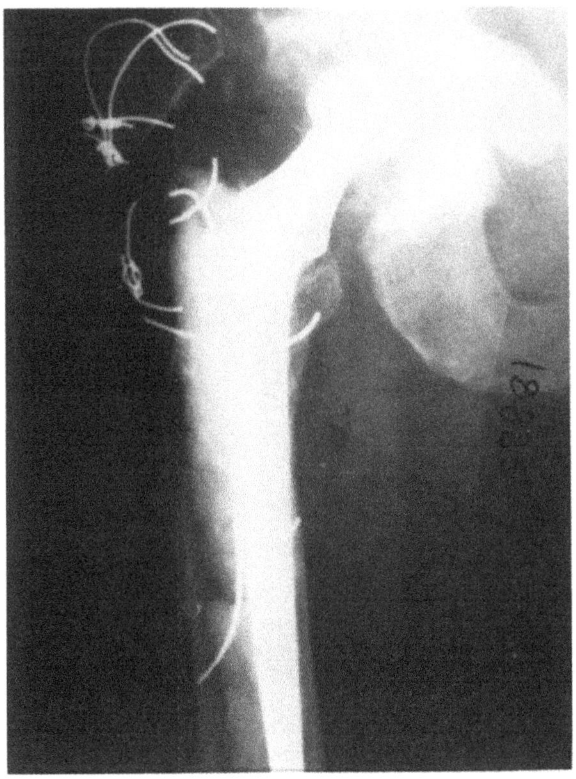

c

L.C., 18885, female, aged 59. Failed osteotomy with internal fixation and later removal of plate (February 1966). Extreme osteoporosis (Fig. 5.25a). Femur fractured during LFA operation May 1967 (Fig. 5.25b). Operation technical failure and prosthesis loosened. Revision August 1968. July 1977 functionally a remarkably good end result (Fig. 5.25c). B. R 6.4.5. L 6.4.4.

Fig. 5.25. a Pre-op. **b** LFA operation May 1967; femur fractured. **c** Revision operation 1968; condition in July 1977—quite good function

J.R., 24048, male, aged 60. Osteoarthrosis. Operation August 1967. Patient's hip never absolutely perfect—yet a first-class personality. Femoral prosthesis subsiding (Fig. 5.26) shows state in 1969 with good function (despite discomfort). Grossly inadequate amount of cement at medial femoral neck; current technique would not tolerate this. Replaced 1975 and found to be quite loose with almost no cement at medial femoral neck. Excellent result 1977 A. 6.6.6.

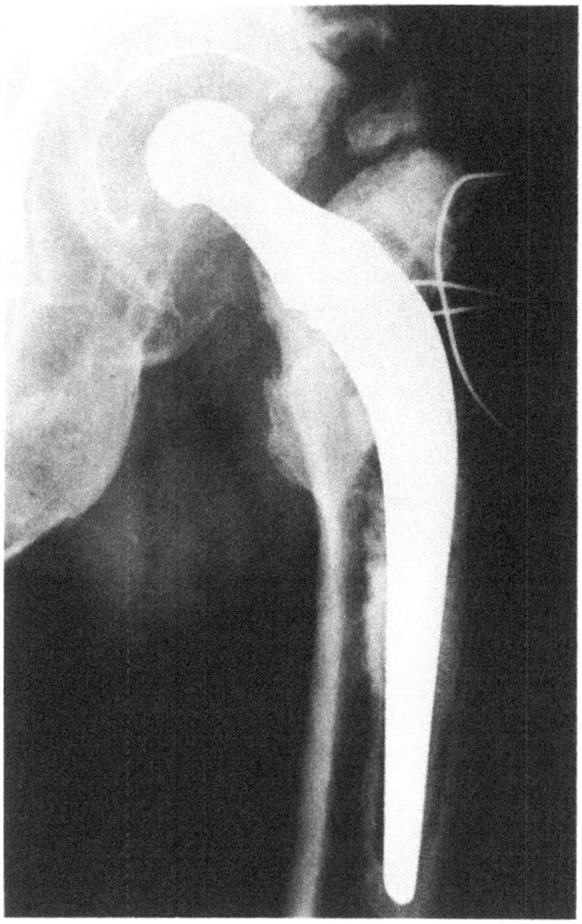

Fig. 5.26. 6 years post-op. Good function but discomfort. Note inadequate cement in femur on present-day standards

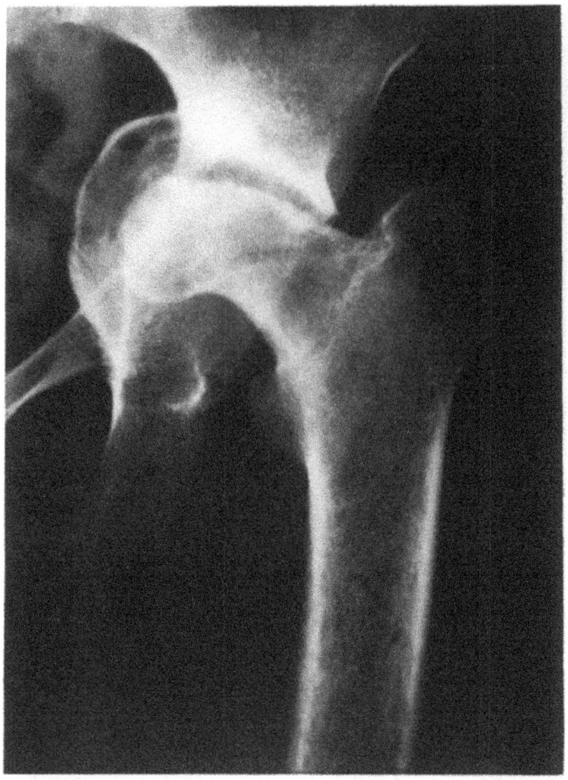

a

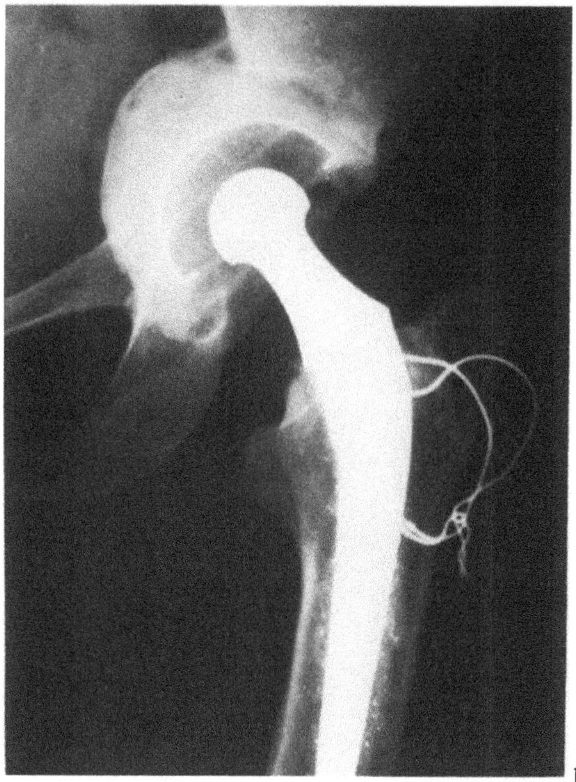

b

Fig. 5.27. a–c. Protrusio acetabuli (bilateral) in rheumatoid arthritis. **a** Pre-op. left side. **b** Operation November 1968; post-op. appearance. **c** Prolapse of cemented socket

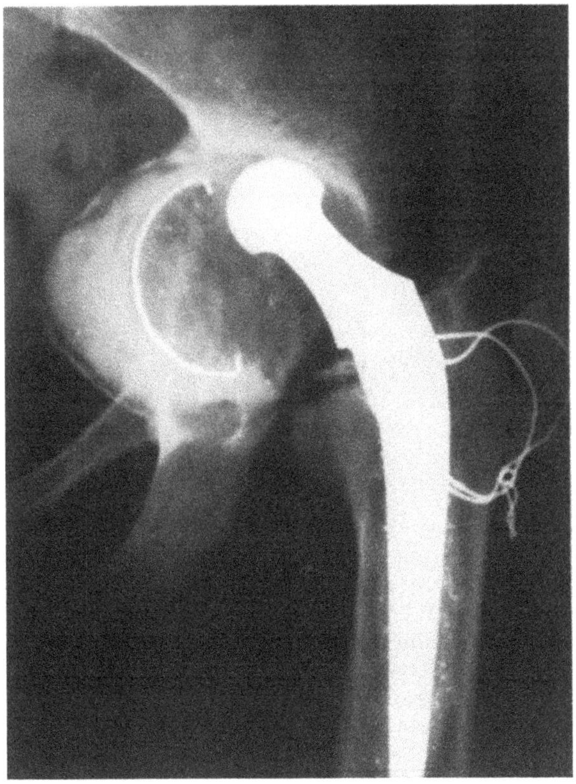

c

M.C., 26827, female, aged 38. Bilateral protrusio acetabuli in rheumatoid arthritis (Fig. 5.27a). Extremely thin floor on left side. Operation left November 1968 (Fig. 5.27b). Prolapse of cemented socket, other side excellent (Fig. 5.27c).

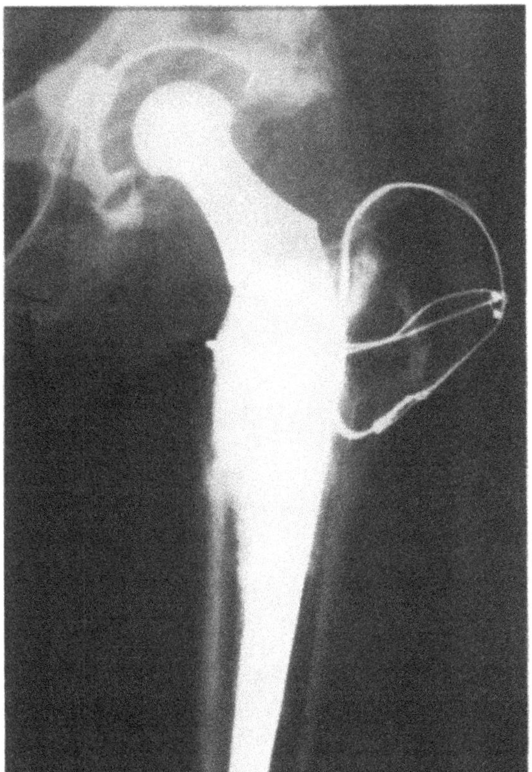

I.P., 31441, female, aged 64. Failed osteotomy for osteoarthrosis. LFA April 1971. At operation very difficult to dislocate and a large fragment of medial femoral neck fractured and discarded; also a defect of the cortex on lateral side of femur under plate (Fig. 5.28). Satisfactory result for 4 years and then pain. Explored March 1975 and prosthesis found only very slightly loose. Still has pain.

Fig. 5.28. Difficult LFA after previous osteotomy; medial femoral neck had been fractured and loose fragment resected

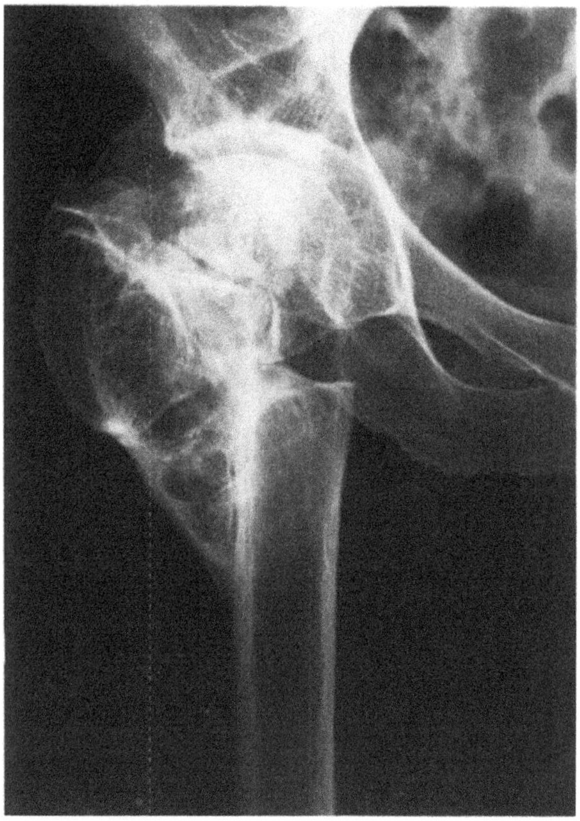

a

M.C., 19159, female, aged 58. Grossly displaced osteotomy for fracture of neck of femur 4 years previously (Fig. 5.29a). Very difficult personality. LFA July 1965—complained of pain always; (Fig. 5.29b) had two explorations for extreme pain; at first femoral prosthesis found retroverted and replaced; at second socket considered to be loose after arthrogram but no relief when changed and looseness not convincing

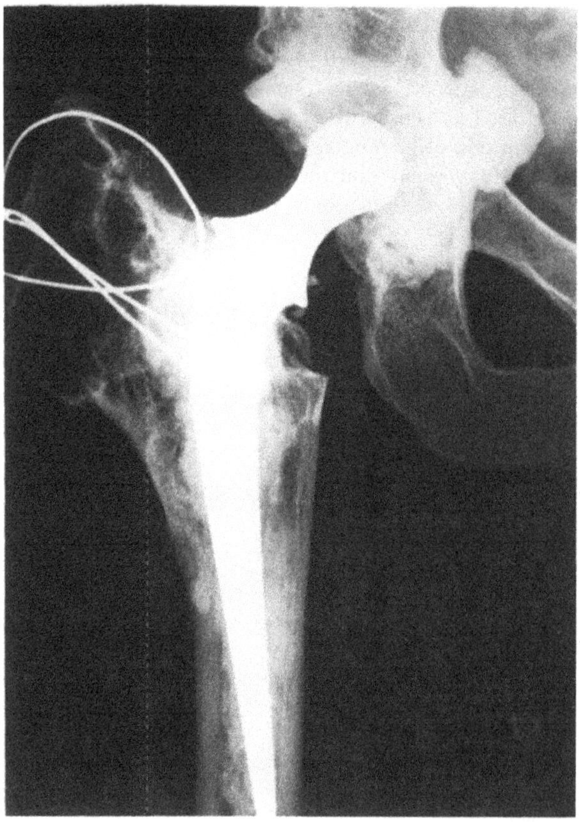

b

Fig. 5.29. a Pre-op. Old osteotomy for fracture of neck of femur. **b** Post-op. result with pain of unknown origin. See text

A.H., 36205, female, aged 62. Uncomplicated osteoarthrosis. LFA June 1973 but socket obviously incorrectly inserted (Fig. 5.30a). Socket and cement migrated laterally 1 year later (Fig. 5.30b).

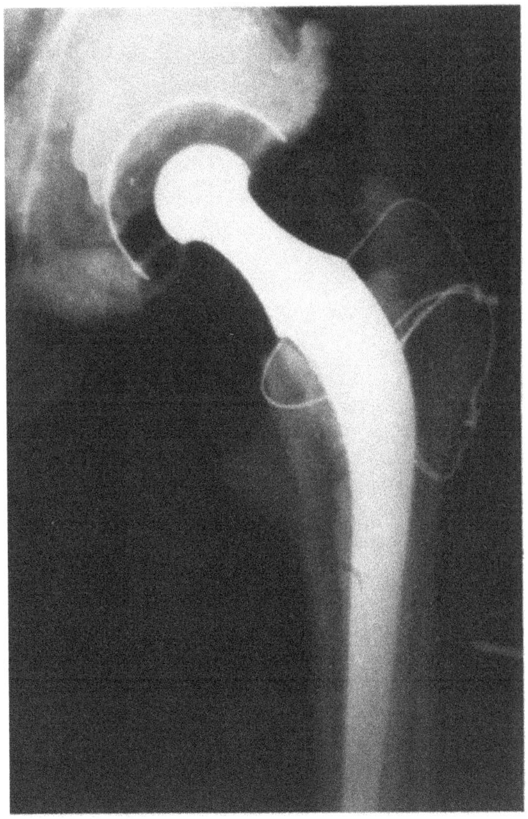

a

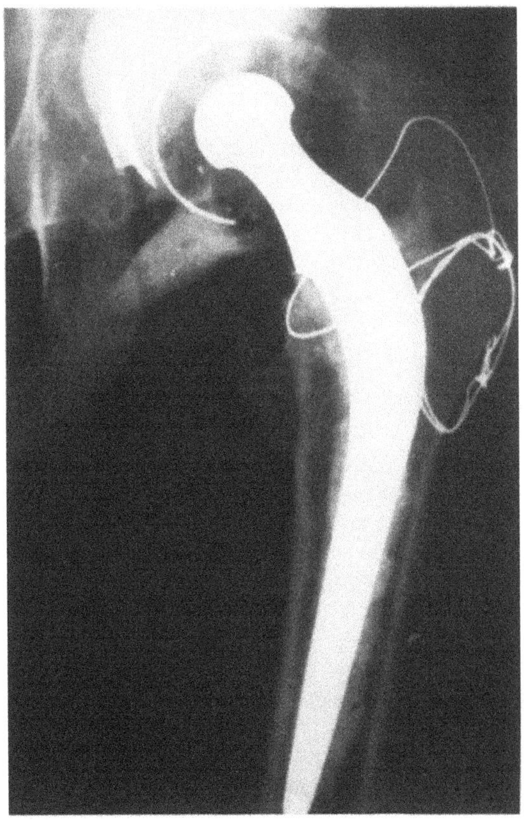

b

Fig. 5.30. a Post-op. June 1973; socket incorrectly sited, too lateral. **b** One year later. Socket dislocated from acetabulum. Poor technique

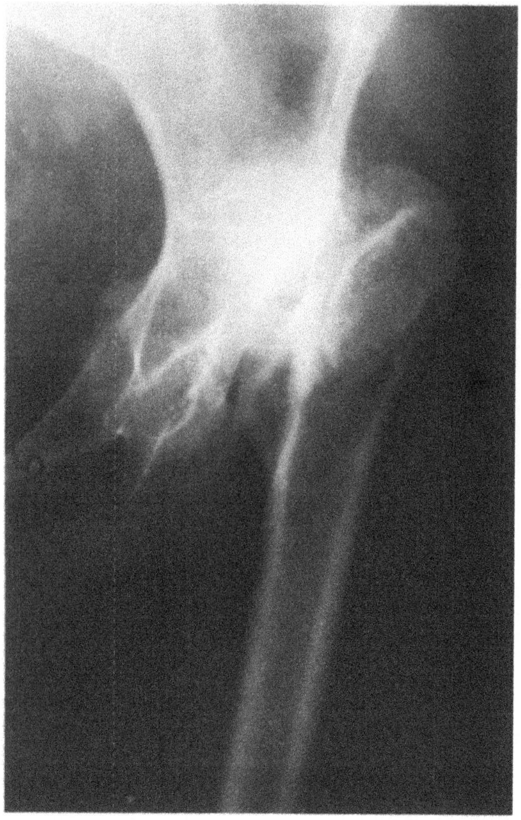

a

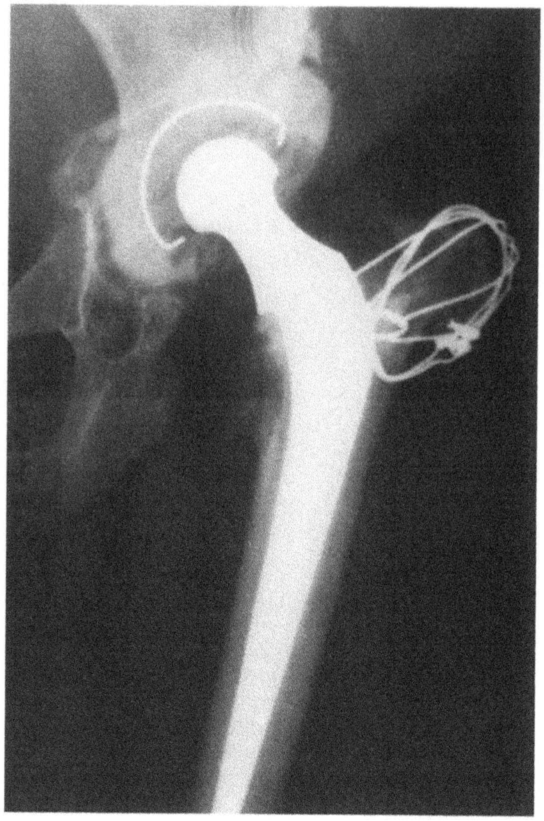

b

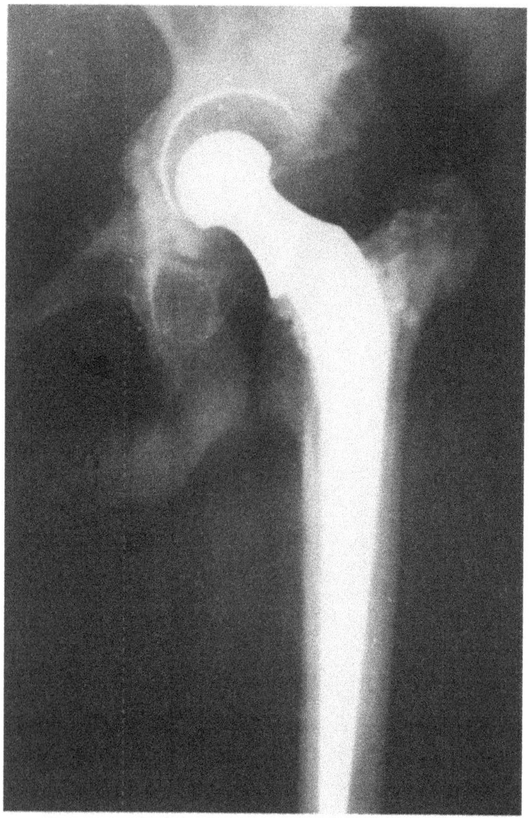

c

M.P., 43285, female, aged 47. Bilateral CDH (Fig. 5.31a). LFA left May 1975 (Fig. 5.31b). Socket too large (43-mm outside diameter). Gross loosening and symptoms, revision with small cup (outside diameter 35 mm, offset bore) December 1975 (Fig. 5.31c).

Fig. 5.31. a Pre-op. Left hip in bilateral CDH. **b** Post-op. May 1975 showing loosening of socket within 6 months of operation. Socket too large for small acetabulum **c** Post-revision December 1975 using extra-small socket with offset bore

Discussion

As yet the literature contains few long-term studies of the results of total hip replacement exceeding 5 years. Dissatisfaction with the many varieties of the basic type of operation which have been used over the last 10 years is suggested by attempts to avoid (1) the use of acrylic cement, e.g. by the use of expanded or porous surfaces, and (2) to avoid using femoral endoprostheses by the 'double cup' technique. The essential source of dissatisfaction is the loosening of cement.

Muller, who after the author has the longest experience of total hip replacement, reported even as recently as 1975[18] a failure rate of 1% per year and was of the opinion that a failure rate of 10% in 10 years was to be expected. He warned against total hip replacement in patients under 60 years of age and advised that it should be done only as a last resort and in younger patients when an intertrochanteric osteotomy was not possible.

Stuhmer[19] reported the loosening of total hip implants in a multi-centric study organised by the Swiss Society of Orthopaedics. The percentage rate of loosening is not stated but if the 48 loose Muller prostheses relate to the quoted total of 2577 operations this corresponds to a loosening rate of 1.9%. This is of the same order as our 1.5% revisions for loosening for the first 396 LFA operations performed at Wrightington before the end of 1965.

If we consider the Wrightington series from the beginning of 1966 to the end of 1968 (Fig. 5.23) the revision rate was 0.66% (12 revisions in 1807 operations). Taking the 10,913 LFA operations performed between the beginning of 1966 and the end of 1976, the 23 revisions resulting from this series correspond to a revision rate of 0.21%. This latter figure certainly will have to be raised with the lapse of more time because at the moment of writing it allows only 2 years since the last of the operations in that decade. As can be seen in Fig. 5.23 the average time elapsing before revision is 6 or 7 years. On the other hand this delay of about 7 years before revision applies mainly to patients operated on before the end of 1969 and as can be seen in Fig. 5.23 the revisions since about 1971 have been performed with a much shorter delay (average about 2.5 years). This does not necessarily mean that failures in recent years have occurred earlier than in previous years; it might indicate that we are nowadays prepared to explore defective results earlier than was the case previously. Therefore for this reason alone the 0.21% of revisions currently recorded for the 1966–1976 period will probably not rise higher than the 0.6% before the end of 1968, but taking into account the improvements in surgical technique which have developed most especially in the 3 or 4 years since 1975 there is hope that in future years it may remain low.

As regards the relative incidence of loosening of the different components of the total hip, in the Swiss report in 46 Muller total hips requiring revision Stuhmer[19] found: 2 loose sockets; 5 loose sockets with loose femoral prostheses; and 39 loose femoral prostheses. Therefore, according to the method of calculation, there was a ratio of 1 loose socket to 18 loose femoral prostheses; or 1 loose socket to 6.3 loose prostheses if the five cases with both components loose are considered as individual loosenings. In the experience of our first 396 operations before the end of 1965 we had 5 loose sockets to 1 loose prosthesis, but in the 23 revisions in 10,000 between 1966 and 1976 the proportions were reversed, the femoral prostheses now being 1.5 times more commonly loose than the sockets.

The relative incidence of loosening of femoral prostheses in the Swiss report suggests that our technique of elevating the trochanter as a routine in primary interventions may be responsible for our better figures. The incidence of relative loosening in our series of femoral prostheses as 1.5 times more common than loosening of sockets, is the result of the **clinical** review of the rate of revisions for failure from this cause. In Chap. 6 radiological signs of cement loosening are the essential criterion, and it will be seen that in the absence of clinical failure socket loosening is much commoner than loosening of the femoral implant by the time the 12–15-year X-rays are analysed.

Chapter 6

Long-Term Radiological Results

This section concentrates on the **radiological** behaviour of the cement-bone interface as found in various long-term studies at Wrightington. The long-term **clinical** results have already been presented in Chapter 5. All cases of known sepsis are excluded. Eight studies of various aspects of the radiological behaviour of cement, all derived from the prospective series of hips operated on between November 1962 and December 1965 are summarized and agreements and disagreements are tabulated at the end of the chapter. A ninth radiological study of cement, this one retrospective for the hips operated on in 1967 and 1968, is also included. Most of these studies have been published in **Clinical Orthopaedics and Related Research**, and references to the original papers are appended.

Radiological Study 1

7–8-Year Results (Eftekhar 1971)[14]

Eftekhar studied 138 hips (in 120 patients) with cemented sockets in the first year of the work between November 1962 and December 1963. The radiographs were inspected for abnormalities at the cement-bone interfaces, as listed by Eftekhar, and the only abnormalities he found were: one femoral prosthesis with unusual cortical thickening of the femur appearing 1 year after the operation but not progressive and with a good clinical result at 8 years (seen again in 1977); one patient with two radiologically loose sockets after bilateral surgery but still with a reasonably good clinical result after 7 years (seen again in 1977). No loose femoral component was found.

Radiological Study 2

9–10-Year Results (Cupic 1973)[15]

This was the same series of patients studied 2 years previously by Eftekhar at 7–8 years. By this time

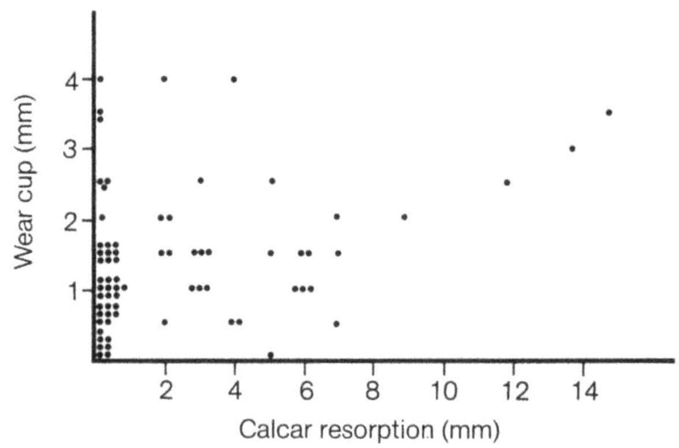

Fig. 6.1. Showing no correlation between wear of HMWP socket and resorption of calcar (Cupic)

only 106 hips with cemented sockets were available for study (85 by personal attendance and 21 by questionnaire and X-ray). The same two loose sockets in one patient were again encountered (one by now having been re-operated) and one loose femoral prosthesis was now found. Resorption of the medial femoral neck in 93 hips was:

3– 4 mm (78.5%)
5–11 mm (18.2%)
12–15 mm (3.2%)

The most extreme neck absorptions (14 mm right and 15 mm left) occurred in a bilateral case of ankylosing spondylitis and was illustrated in the paper, and it did not progress after 5 years. In two bilateral cases there was a marked difference in absorption of the stump of the neck on opposite sides (one patient had 0 mm on one side and 6 mm on the other: another had 2 mm on one side and 6 mm on the other). A search for a relationship between medial femoral neck resorption and the amount of socket wear was made lest resorption were to be the result of wear particles of HMWP, but no correlation was found (Fig. 6.1). No cavities were reported at bone-cement interfaces. The rate of wear of sockets measured in this study is reported in Chapter 20.

Radiological Study 3

Fractures of Acrylic Cement in Relation to the Stem of the Prosthesis (Weber 1975)[20]

Weber made a study of fractures of radio-opaque acrylic cement associated with the stem of the femoral prosthesis. The primary object of the study was the incidence of transverse fractures of the cement near the tip of the prosthesis made possible by the use of radio-opaque cement (Fig. 6.2). These were found in 1.5% of patients and were usually evident at the 6-months post-operative review.[1]) Apart from transient symptoms in the thigh in a minority of patients during the first 6 months there were no symptoms. It was concluded that slight subsidence of the prosthesis resulted in a new and final position of stability. If separation of the fracture exceeded 4 mm the prognosis was doubtful and chronic deep infection might be suspected.

Weber studied the X-rays relating to some 6649 hips operated on between October 1961 and June 1972, no case being followed up less than 1 year. Ninety-nine cases of subsidence of the femoral prosthesis were encountered (1.5%) (Fig. 6.3) but this group is not identical with the 99 cases of fracture of the cement. Twenty-nine patients with fracture of the cement showed no subsidence and 8 patients without fracture of the cement did show subsidence. Weber did not find that fracture of cement near the tip of a femoral prosthesis was related to a patient's weight or sex. Subsequent papers do not put fracture of femoral cement and subsidence of femoral prostheses as low in frequency or as unrelated to the weight of the patient as does this study.

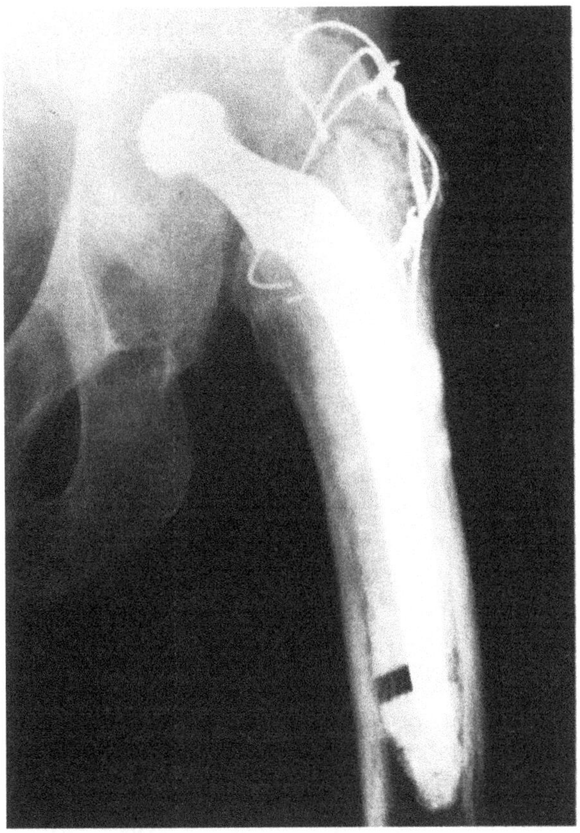

Fig. 6.2. Fracture of tip of cement made evident by radio-opaque cement (Weber)

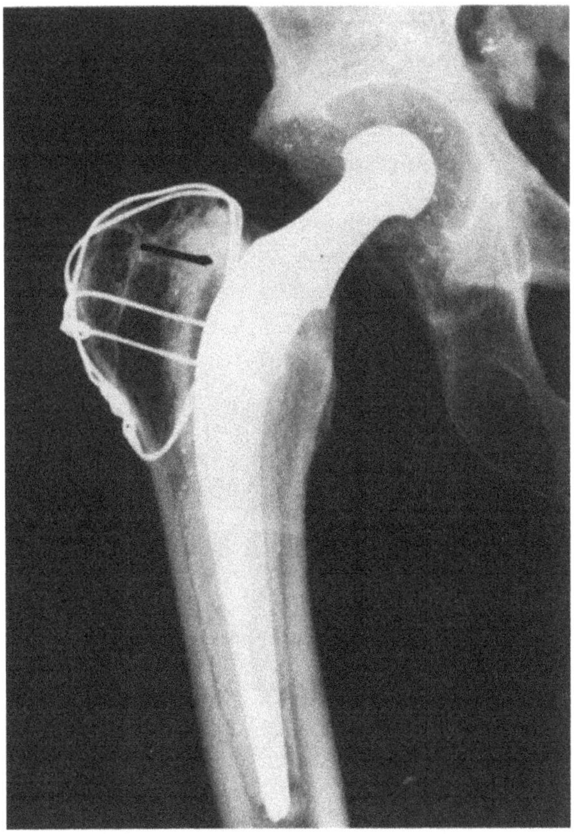

Fig. 6.3. Marked example of subsidence of prosthesis; in this case associated with fracture of tip of cement

[1]) Routine 6 months review was changed in 1972 to 3 months

Radiological Study 4

10-Year Study of Socket Demarcation
(DeLee, 1976)[21]

DeLee studied acetabular cement in 141 cemented sockets available from the prospective study between November 1962 and December 1965. Average follow-up was 10 years. Forty-four hips (31.3%) showed no demarcation of the cement from the bone of the acetabulum; 85 hips (60.3%) showed demarcation but no migration. In 10 the demarcation had increased over the years but seemed to have become stationary for 2 years at the time of the study and it was concluded that progression had stopped.

DeLee introduced an attempt to classify types of demarcation in relation to load-bearing quadrants (Types I and II) and the whole circumference (Type III) (Fig. 6.4). An extended use of the classification has proved its value. In the author's opinion DeLee's Type II is difficult to particularise and he now concentrates on Types I and III, and migration now called Type IV. DeLee reported 9.2% incidence of migration of sockets, the average time to the start of migration being 5.4 years. Seven of the migrating sockets were in rheumatoid arthritis, i.e. approximately 50%. In six cases DeLee found technical details in the operation notes, such as excessive deepening of the acetabulum or a very thin floor, which might explain migration. In only four could he find no such explanation.

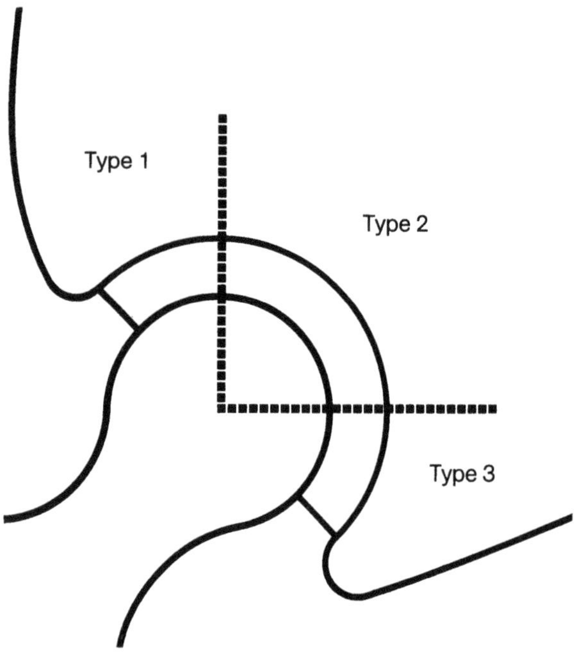

Fig. 6.4. DeLee's figure for types of socket demarcation. Type III involves whole hemisphere as well as especially lower and medial quadrant

A case of sudden collapse of the cement and the socket through the floor of the acetabulum was encountered in this study and is still unique in our total experience. When originally reported[21] we thought that there was no radiological change in the acetabulum for 9.5 years until the moment of sudden collapse, but a second study now indicates that slight subsidence had been occurring progressively without the ordinary signs of marked demarcation of Types I and III preceding the final sudden collapse. This case is in a quite different category from the report of three McKee operations followed by spontaneous fracture of the acetabulum after about 1 year (Evans, Freeman, Miller and Vernon-Roberts, 1974)[22] and is different also from the report of nine cases of fracture of the pelvis occurring 14–18 months after McKee and Ring operations (Miller, 1972).[23]

Radiological Study 5

4-Year Study of Cement in Femur
(Follacci and Hammond, 1966)[24]

This was our first study of cement in the medullary cavities of 190 femurs in 174 patients after the cement had been in situ for 3–8 years (averaging 4 years). In 81% the texture of the bone of the femur remained normal and 4.7% showed some atrophy. In only two cases did the atrophy exceed 10% of the thickness of the cortex. In 2.6% improvement was noted in the thickness of the cortex from previous atrophy. Fusiform enlargement of the shaft with normal texture of bone occurred in 9.4% and was considered to be a physiological response (Wolff's Law). In four cases (X-rays illustrated as Figs. 5, 6, 7 and 8 of their published paper) the appearances suggested sepsis and in three proof was established later. One of these we are now certain was an infection with spontaneous healing, because the socket later became radiologically involved [this patient is still free of

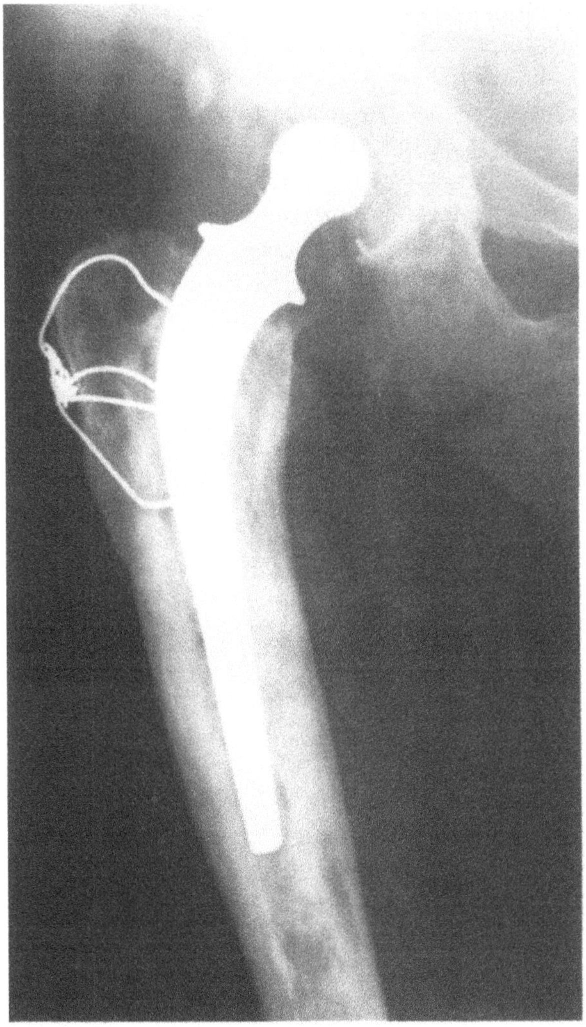

Fig. 6.5. Healed infection. Clinically excellent 14.5 years later. Note 'cloaca' round wire as it emerges through lateral cortex. 'Charnley's sign' of infection

symptoms and the X-rays after 14.5 years (1977) are shown in Fig. 6.5].

Slight condensation of cancellous bone in the medullary cavity on the external surface of the cement near the tip was found in 44.8% of cases. This was mainly restricted to the distal 30–40 mm of the cement. Absorption of the femoral neck averaged 3 mm (maximum 10 mm) in 37.2% of cases in this 4-year study. Twelve cases were studied in which cement had been used twice in the medullary cavity (conversion of cemented femoral head prostheses to a total hip replacement). Eleven of these retained normal cortical bone 4 years after exposure to the second reaction of polymerisation.

Radiological Study 6

10-Year Study of Cement in the Femur

Blacker[25] scrutinized the bone of 169 femora of the prospective group operated on between November 1962 and December 1965, at an average time of 10 years after the original operation. The results were surprisingly similar to the previous study of Follacci et al. at 4 years, especially if one considers hypertrophy as a physiological sign. Hypertrophy is defined in all these studies as a thickening of the cortex with retention of normal cortical texture. Hypertrophy is usually centred on the tip or lower end of the prosthesis. It is considered to be a manifestation of Wolff's Law caused by artificially raised stress at the point of sudden transition from the flexible distal femur to the artificially stiffened proximal femur containing prosthesis and cement.

In the 4-year results of Follacci and Hammond, 81% of the femora were unchanged and 12% showed hypertrophy; in the 10-year results of Blacker, 66.5% were unchanged and 28.8% showed hypertrophy. If we combine unchanged with hypertrophic the combined figures show 93% at 4 years and 95.3% at 10 years. Atrophy in thickness of the cortex occurred in 4.7% at 4 years (Follacci and Hammond) and 4.8% at 10 years (Blacker). This is a remarkable agreement over a period of time from two quite separate studies.

In order to extend the period of observation of cement in contact with the femoral shaft, Blacker examined the radiographs of 31 patients who originally had had Teflon acetabular sockets later revised to HMWP. The duration of cement in the femoral shafts in this group averaged 12.9 years ranging from 10 to 15 years. At the revision operations in 24 (77.4%) a new femoral prosthesis was hammered down the old cement track without adding new cement. In some of these splitting of the cement must have occurred, but the late results show that this caused no harm. In 7 patients (22.6%) a second dose of cement was used after reaming and enlarging the old cement track; in 18 (58.1%) there was no change in the bone of the femoral cortex; 9 (29%) showed hypertrophy and only 4 (12.9%) showed some atrophy.

Blacker found 34% of cases up to 10 years showing slight condensation of bone round the cement

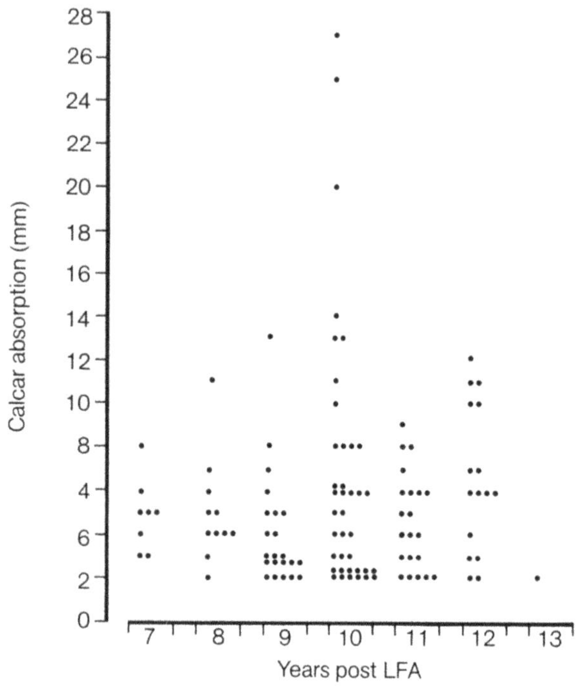

Fig. 6.6. Distribution of medial femoral neck resorption in relation to time after operation in 117 patients (Blacker)

in the region of the tip of the cement in the medullary cavity. In only 2.4% of the cases did this extend above the level of the mid-point of the cement. In no case did this condensation of bone extend round the whole circumference of the cement as seen in the antero-posterior projection as would be expected if loosening were present. Blacker also found that resorption of the medial femoral neck averaged 5.5 mm in 70% of the 167 hips examined over an average period of 10 years. The time of onset averaged 13.1 months from the time of the operation. The resorption ranged from 4 to a maximum of 27 mm. Occasionally cystic areas were noticed without impairment of function. The distribution of medial femoral neck resorption in relation to time in 117 cases is presented graphically in Fig. 6.6.

Radiological Study 7

Changes in the Medial Femoral Neck in Relation to Cement Technology

Bocco and Langan (1977)[26] studied absorption of the medial femoral neck in the light of a new detail of technique introduced in 1969 and developed over 2 or 3 years to become standardised by early 1974. The new technique comprised three factors: (1) a rather exaggerated degree of valgus alignment of the prosthesis; (2) curettage of the medial femoral neck to remove poor-quality cancellous bone, but not completely to denude the endosteal surface to the cortex; and (3) consequent on 1 and 2, an increase in thickness of cement intervening between the prosthesis and the medial femoral neck.

Prior to the introduction of the fully developed valgus technique the femoral prosthesis often had a tendency to lie in slight varus with only a thin shell of cement intervening between the metal and the bone of the medial femoral neck. The radical difference in the preparation of the upper end of the femur in the two techniques is shown diagrammatically in Fig. 6.7.

A problem in this study is the difference in duration of follow-up in the two series. The average follow-up in series II was only 2.1 years (ranging from 1.6 to 2.6 years) whereas the average follow-up in series I averaged 5.6 years (ranging from 4 to 8 years). A special feature of selection was the decision to confine the study to male patients. This was because only in the males was it common to have an exaggerated degree of valgus as a result of the wider medullary cavities in male patients. Cases with less than 1 cm of cement between the calcar and prosthesis were deliberately excluded in series II to make any effects of this feature more evident.

Figures 6.8 and 6.9 are examples of series I and series II appearances. In series I the most valgus position of the prosthesis was modest compared with the valgus of series II. In series II, by definition, all prostheses were valgus and none varus or neutral as in series I. In series I the average thickness of cement at the calcar was 4.5 mm and in series II was 13.2 mm.

There were 119 hips in 87 patients in series I and 97 hips in 83 patients in series II. As seen in Fig. 6.10 there was a reduction in serious destructive changes in the medial femoral neck in series II to one-tenth of that in series I. (Grades III A, III B and III C were serious resorption; grade II, new bone formation; and grades I A and I B, nil and minor degrees of resorption.) There was also a

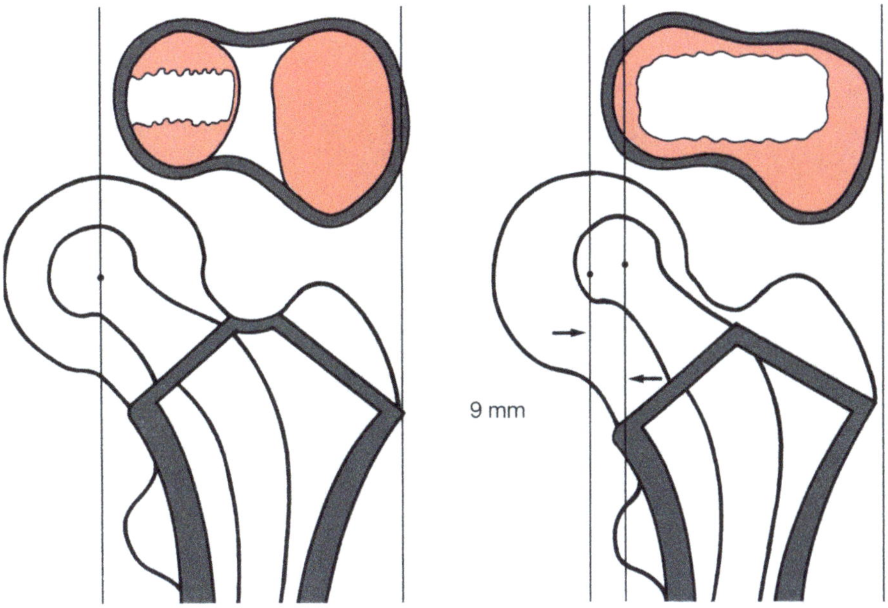

Fig. 6.7. Change in technique of reaming femoral cavity: before 1969 working through cut femoral neck; later invading the area of the detached trochanter and enlarging medullary cavity for 'two-thumb' technique of inserting cement and more valgus position of prosthesis

reduction to one-quarter of moderate changes associated with new bone formation (column II in Fig. 6.10.). Fracture of cement at the tip of the prosthesis was noted in 20.2% of series I compared with only 3.1% in series II. Demarcation of the convex lateral border of the prosthesis (suggesting slight subsidence) occurred in 12.6% of series I and not at all in series II.

This study is encouraging, though it compares only 2.1 years results with 5.6 years results. It proves, at least, that a thick layer of cement between the medial femoral neck and prosthesis is not harmful from the point of view of thermal or chemical reaction. The principle of encouraging the presence of a sound layer of cement between the medial femoral neck and the concavity of the femoral stem is inherent in the technique described in this manual. It must be emphasised, however, that it is no longer considered necessary or desirable to put the prosthesis into such valgus that at least 1 cm of cement must intervene. For mechanical reasons concerned with the 'offset' of the prosthesis (Chaps. 16 and 21), it is now considered best to aim for a neutral position of the axis of the stem of the prosthesis, and this still enables an adequate layer of cement to intervene between metal and the bone of the medial femoral neck.

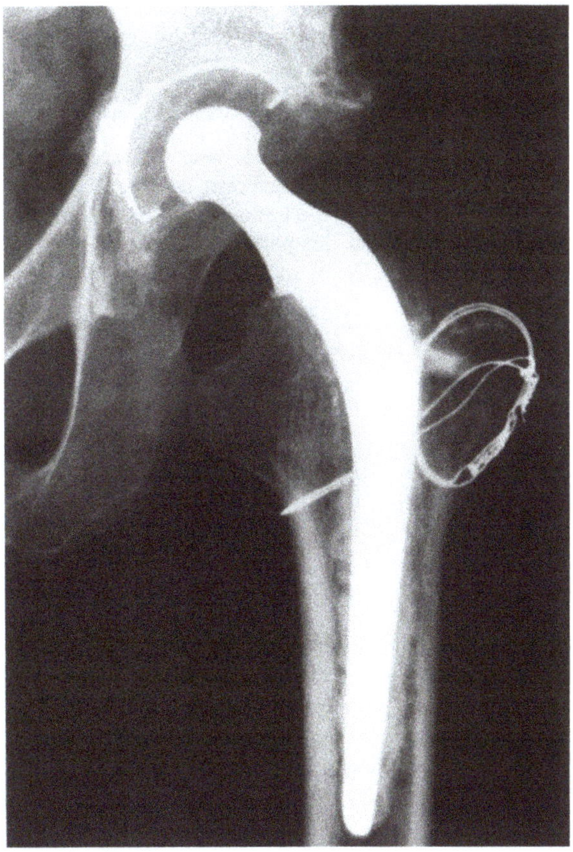

Fig. 6.8. Moderate valgus of series I before 1969. Note small amount of cement in medial femoral neck region

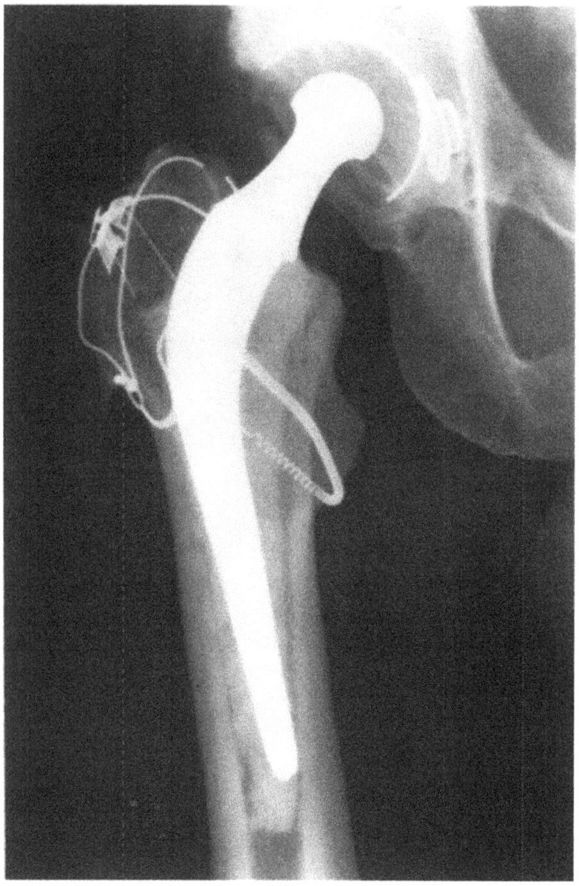

Fig. 6.9. Marked valgus of series II after 1970. Note thick cement in region of medial femoral neck (this amount possible in males and by definition series II had not less than 1 cm of cement at this point)

	IA	IB	II	IIIA	IIIB	IIIC
Series I	21.8	31.1		5.8	7.6	7.6
(%)	52.9		26.1	21.0		
Series II	39.2	52.6		2.1	0	0
(%)	91.8		6.1	2.1		

Fig. 6.10. Severe degrees of calcar resorption and cavitation (IIIA, IIIB and IIIC) reduced 10-fold in series II with thick cement at calcar. Moderate calcar resorption with new bone formation (grade II) reduced four-fold. All figures in percentages (Bocco and Langan)

Radiological Study 8

8-Year Results 1967–1968 (Griffith, Seidenstein and Williams, 1977)[17]

This was primarily a search for radiological evidence of pathological changes in cement-bone interfaces, especially in patients who were clinically successful. The idea of this study was to counteract over-optimism as regards long-term extrapolation and so give priority to adverse radiological appearances over good function and patient satisfaction. By this means it was hoped to get some idea of the worst that might be expected 20 years or more after one of these operations. The study was to be a check in particular on the figure of 9.2% for migration of the socket reported in the paper by DeLee.

A new group of patients was required and therefore a retrospective study was made of patients operated on in 1967 and 1968. Out of 1359 operations in this period it was possible to study 547 hips in 461 patients, with an average follow-up of 8.3 years.. (The **clinical** results of this study are reported in Chap. 5 and the rate of wear of the sockets in Chap. 20). In this study radiological abnormalities considered not important were:

1) Fusiform enlargement of the shaft of the femur of a physiological nature (Wolff's Law) occurring in 19%
2) Condensation of medullary new bone round the cement at the tip of the prosthesis (a very faint shell) in 7.9%
3) Transverse fracture of cement near the tip of the prosthesis in 47 hips (8.6%)

Definite Radiological Failure of Cement-Bone Interface (RS.8)[2]

Pathological changes in cement-bone interfaces so advanced as to constitute true radiological failure are shown in Fig. 6.11. This table includes hips for which revision surgery for loose cement had already been performed prior to the study, as well

[2]) In radiological studies 1–7 there are no sub-headings to confuse the reader, but studies 8 and 9 have multiple sub-headings. These will all be designated RS.8 or RS.9 to make quite clear that they belong purely to that section and not to the chapter in general.

	Revised prior to review		Discovered in review: probably will need revision		Totals
	No.	% of 1359	No.	% of 547	%
Socket loosening	3	0.22	2	0.36	0.58
Femoral subsidence	5	0.36	2	0.36	0.72

Fig. 6.11. Total failure rate (i.e. revision for loose cement only) 1967 and 1968 operations

as pathological cement-bone interfaces found in the study such that revision surgery at some time in the near future would seem certain.

Incipient Radiological Failures at Cement-Bone Interfaces (RS.8)

Radiological appearances interpreted as being possibly signs of incipient failure, the special terms of reference of this study, were:

1) Subsidence of the femoral prosthesis
2) Demarcation of the socket plus suspicion of tilting, or migration of the socket in the acetabulum
3) Cavitation of bone in the acetabulum
4) Cavitation of the medial femoral neck
5) Cavitation of the endosteal surface of the femur

Because the special objective of this study was to search for any evidence suggesting that future trouble might develop at cement-bone junctions, the problem was how to separate truly 'minor' radiological abnormalities from those abnormalities which could very well signify trouble during the next 10 years (i.e. perhaps 18–19 years after the operation).

Subsidence of Femoral Prosthesis (RS.8)

The measurement, and even the detection, of subsidence of a femoral prosthesis, when only 1–2 mm is concerned, can be difficult. The appearance of a gap between the convex, lateral surface of the upper end of the prosthesis and the adjacent radio-opaque bed of cement probably underestimates the true incidence of this feature. The only way to study this accurately would be to centre the X-ray beam over the hip with special precaution to ensure that the upper end of the femur is in neutral rotation, but this was not possible in this study. McLeish and his colleagues[27] have shown that the straight, distal portion of the stem can transmit loads of 675–2025 lb (3000–9000 N), a load capacity greater than most estimates of the hip joint load; '... this maximum load requires prior slip of the prosthesis up to 0.6 mm to provide self-locking of the taper necessary for load transmission to the cement ... The system will come into equilibrium with the load partly transmitted by the straight position of the stem and partly by the calcar.' It was therefore decided to ignore subsidence of less than 2 mm because small amounts of subsidence permit the tapered stem of the pros-

Degree of Subsidence	Present at 2 years but did not later increase	Present at 2 years and later increased	First appeared after 2 years	Total incidence at 8.3 years
2 mm	27	0	1	28 (5.1%)
2–5 mm	8	8	1	17 (3.1%)
5 mm	2	2	0	4 (0.7%)
Total	37 (6.7%)	10 (1.8%)	2 (0.4%)	49 (8.9%)

Fig. 6.12. Incidence of femoral subsidence in 547 X-rays, giving the benefit of any doubt to subsidence

	Patients with subsidence (49 hips)	Total series (547 hips)
Sex	Males 39%	Males 28% 157
Average age	64 years	62 years
Average weight	167 lb (76 kg) (108–203 lb) (49–92 kg)	147 lb (66 kg) (84–244 lb) (38–110 kg)

Fig. 6.13. Relation between weight of patient and subsidence of femoral prosthesis

thesis to take up a better load-transmitting position at the lower level.

The total incidence of subsidence, giving the benefit of any doubt to subsidence, is shown in Fig. 6.12. The relationship of subsidence to weight of the patient is shown in Fig. 6.13.

Socket Demarcation (RS.8)

Another difficult decision concerns the amount of socket demarcation which could be ignored. All cases with demarcation involving the whole of the frontal profile (grade III) were recorded as incipient failure. If grade III demarcation had reached 2 mm or more in thickness this would have been considered a definite stage in socket loosening and had any of these occurred in this study (which they did not) they would have been reported as failures in the Table in Fig. 6.11 even without gross migration or tilting of the socket. The total incidence of socket demarcation is shown in Fig. 6.14. It was decided to ignore socket demarcation of 1 mm or less because of its common occurrence in the absence of symptoms (50.6%) in this study. Our previous 9–10-year studies had suggested that demarcation of this small amount did not often increase.

Types	I	II	III	%
<1 mm	141	53	83	50.6%
1–2 mm	2	7	8	3.1%
>2 mm	0	0	0	0
				53.7%

Fig. 6.14. Incidence of socket demarcation at 8.3 years (average) in 547 X-rays, giving the benefit of any doubt to demarcation

Cavitation of Cement-Bone Interface (RS.8)

All cases of erosion and cavitation of bone were included because these must be regarded as caused by granulomata produced by histiocyte reactions and therefore harmful on a very long-term basis.

There were two very small (2-mm) cavities on the endosteal surface of the femur and there was one cystic cavity involving the superior lip of the acetabulum (Fig. 6.15) in an energetic female with osteoarthrosis, completely devoid of symptoms and with a perfect result. Compare with the other instance in Fig. 5.14c, d.

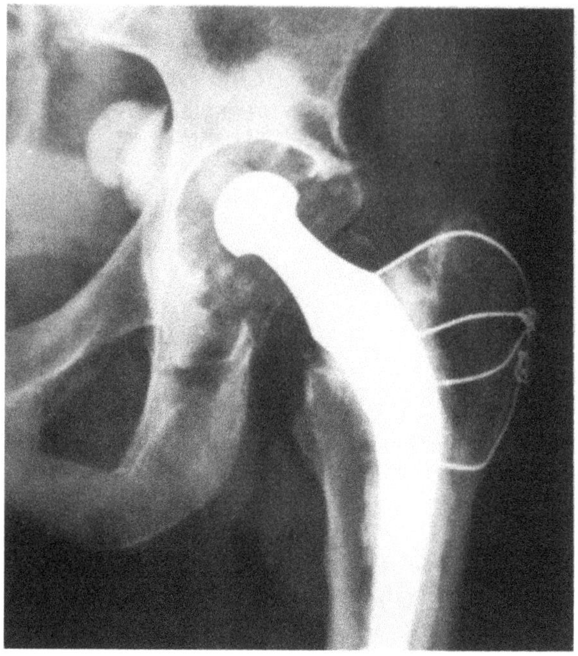

Fig. 6.15. Cyst in bone-cement junction in region of superior lip of acetabulum. No symptoms at 8 years

Incipient Pathology at the Cement-Bone Interface (RS.8)

The total incidence of these selected types of incipient failure is presented in Fig. 6.16. It must be emphasized that these criteria for recording incipient defects of the cement-bone interface in clinically successful patients after an average period of 8.3 years, are more 'hair-splitting' than any we know to have been published so far. **These figures are intended as criteria against which the results of future research into improved techniques of using cement can be tested.** These figures need not be viewed pessimistically; indeed, the author interprets them optimistically because during the period of this study (1967 and 1968) the technique of using cement was still quite unsophisticated in the light of our present knowledge and in the light of technical advances which are described in the practical part of this book.

This 1967–1968 study did not confirm the incidence of 9.2% of socket migration reported by

	No.	%
Femoral subsidence over 2 mm	21	3.8
Socket demarcation over 1 mm but not more than 2 mm	17	3.1
Cavitation of calcar femoris, all grades	25	4.5
Cavitation of bone of acetabulum, all grades	1	0.18
Cavitation of endosteal surface of femur, all grades	2	0.36
	66	12.0

Fig. 6.16. Incidence of signs of incipient failure at cement-bone interfaces after an average period of 8.3 years

DeLee[21] in the prospective study prior to 1966 (though DeLee's findings are confirmed on the same patients in the 12–15-year study of the prospective group). It is to be noted that DeLee in his reading of operation notes and inspection of X-rays in the prospective group suspected excessive deepening of the acetabulum and it is possible that a more conservative attitude to deepening had become general by 1967 and 1968. In the early years, deepening of the acetabulum was a central dogma of the author's teaching and residents frequently overdid the teaching in efforts not to defect in this direction. The amount of deepening was judged by palpation with the tip of the index finger through the 'pilot hole' in the floor of the acetabulum and this test was frequently unreliable. The present method of 'deepening by eye' (stages 49–62, pp. 218–226), so keeping the floor of the acetabular fossa intact, is now an essential technical detail. Moreover, removal of eburnated bone in the roof of the acetabulum also was a dogma in the prospective group because it was held that cement must always be applied to cancellous bone, but in later years the eburnated bone in the roof was retained and this becomes inevitable in the technique of 'low-siting' of the socket.

It is to be emphasized that though cavitation of bone is a specific complication of acrylic cement it is almost certainly a sequel to movement between cement and bone. If cavitation were to be a purely 'biological' reaction to cement one would expect it to be more common than it is. Improved cement injection technology, to avoid slight mechanical loosening being present from the start, ought to prevent cavitation.

Radiological Study 9

12–15-Year Results

Specially for the purpose of this book the author in November 1977 made another clinical and radiological study of those patients of the original prospective study who were still available in their twelfth to fifteenth post-operative years. In order to increase the number of long-term observations of cement in the femur, patients with uncemented sockets were included in the study (press-fit sockets, see below).

For the 12–15-year study of cement-bone junctions in the acetabulum up-to-date X-rays were available for the 77 hips described in clinical study 4 (Chap. 5) plus 38 X-rays received in reply to a questionnaire. This made a total of 115 current X-rays of cemented sockets and cemented femoral prostheses, to which is added 58 patients with press-fit sockets and therefore the same number of cemented femoral prostheses (i.e. current X-rays of 115 cemented sockets and 173 cemented femoral prostheses). The general clinical data of diagnoses, ages and average follow-up are as for the clinical study of the same group in Chap. 5.

The Femora

Apart from resorption of the medial femoral neck, which in various degrees was almost (but not entirely) universal, the condition of the bone of the shaft of the femur in all 173 femora was remarkably good. Typical examples are illustrated in Fig. 6.17a, b, c, d. Resorption of the medial femoral neck up to 0.5 cm was very common but it was notable that the edge of the resorption was more clearly demarcated than we have been accustomed to seeing in post-operative reviews at shorter periods of follow-up. The remaining bone of the medial femoral neck had a density in keeping with the rest of the femur.

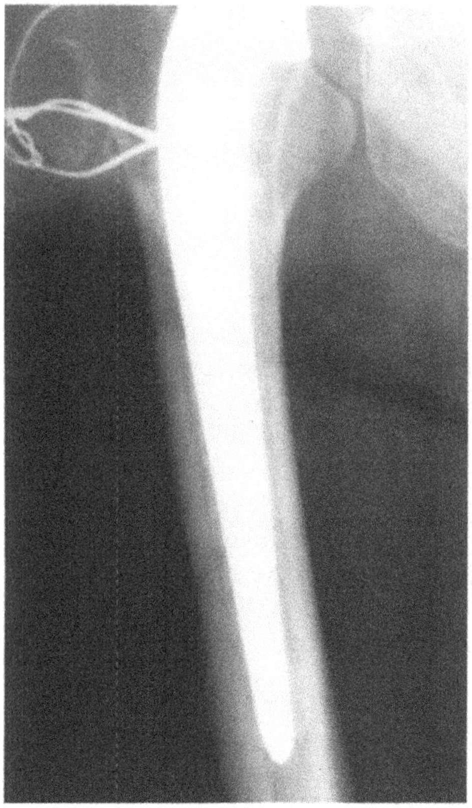

a

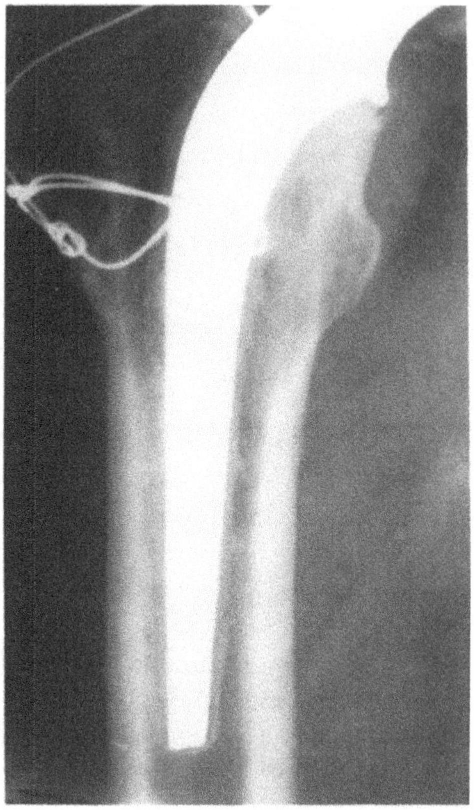

b

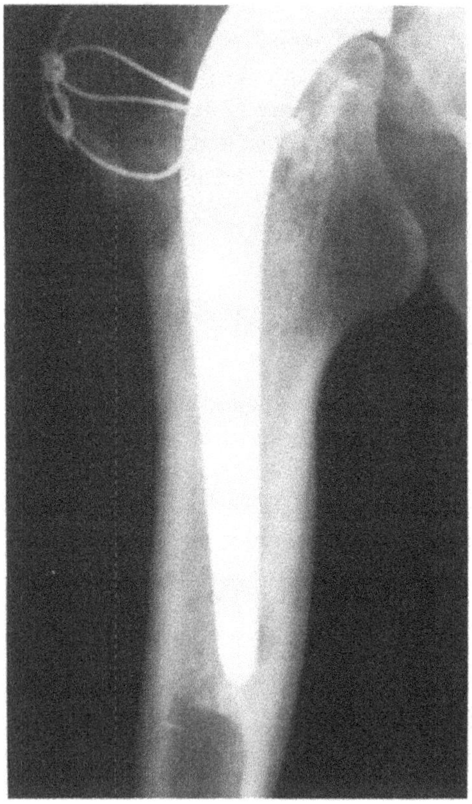

c

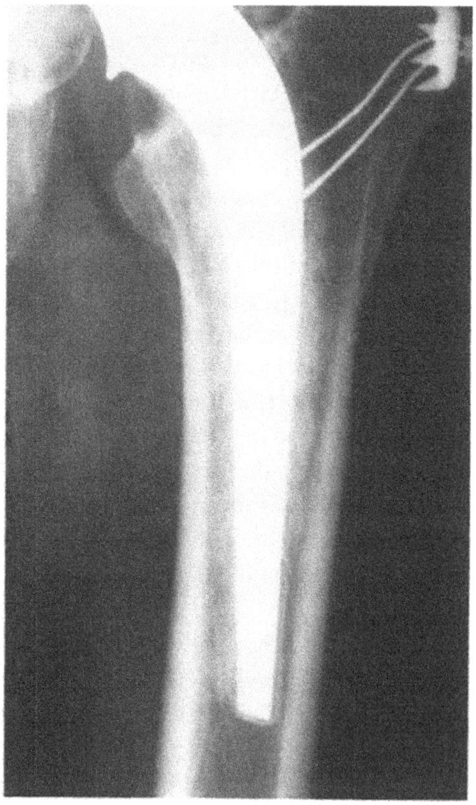

d

The amount of resorption of the medial femoral neck was estimated as:

0 – 5%
0.5 cm – 55%
1.0 cm – 35%
1.5 cm – 5%.

There were no examples in this group of resorption of over 20 mm as had occasionally been encountered in previous studies. The general appearances as indicated in the examples shown in Fig. 6.17 suggested that the process of resorption had probably become stationary. The examples of femora in Fig. 6.17 obviously have to be selected to demonstrate typical appearances but those with good femoral cortices greatly outnumber those with osteoporotic cortices. There was no evidence of resorption of the femoral neck being part of an extensive process of osteoporosis, such as some have predicted would be the result of the rigidity imposed by the implant and the by-passing of the physiological stimulus of load-bearing. The facts supported the idea that load is transmitted to the endosteal surface of the medial femur in a physiological direction, being received by the cut ends of trajectories of cancellous bone in the medial femoral neck as illustrated in Fig. 21.10a, p. 336. There was nothing to suggest that permanent load transmission could possibly occur from the prosthesis to the cut surface of the femoral neck through the medium of a metal collar on the prosthesis.

Endosteal Bone Cavities (RS. 9)

There were two endosteal bone cavities measuring about 4 mm in diameter, one situated lateral to the tip of the femoral prosthesis and the other medial (Fig. 6.17c) and with slight erosion into the endosteal surface of the cortex. There were no symptoms and after 12 years progress must have been very slow.

Healed Infection (RS.9)

One patient showed extensive thickening of the femoral cortex with an abnormal texture compatible with the appearance of a healed osteomyelitis already mentioned in Fig. 6.5. This patient had been illustrated in a previous publication (Follacci and Hammond[24], p. 827 of that paper); at that time the cause of the abnormal cortical bone at 4 years after the operation was obscure, in the absence of any clinical suspicion of infection in the post-operative period. Now 14.5 years after the operation she is clinically 100% at the age of 75.5. The socket shows migration and it seems almost certain that this was originally a mild infection which healed without antibiotics.

Another patient exhibited a thickened femoral cortex with a slightly different texture: for this appearance the term 'onion skin' seems not inapt, indicating that the thickening seemed to be caused by a layer of periosteal bone separated from the underlying femur by a more porous layer (Fig. 6.18a). The difference from the appearance of physiological hypertrophy in accordance with Wolff's Law is seen in Fig. 6.18b.

Summary of Appearances in the Femur (RS.9)

The 12–15-year radiological appearances of the cortical bone in these 173 femora were indistinguishable from femora in normal patients of the same age with the same pathological background. That is to say in cases where osteoporosis was present it had been present from the start and was consistent with the patient's function. It is to be emphasized, from the up-to-date clinical examination of the 135 of these patients who attended hospital in person, that their function was consistent with their age. The function of the whole group, with 22 patients over 80 years of age (19%) was so good that it seemed almost to represent an elite who enjoyed keeping in contact with the hospital and demonstrating their function.

◄

Fig. 6.17a–d. Examples selected as typical of the average appearance of 173 femora after 12–15 years. **a** Perfect radiological appearance plus no calcar resorption. **b** Slight condensation of bone on medial aspect of distal part of prosthesis stem. **c** Shows slight cavity formation medial to tip of femoral prosthesis, but hypertrophy of medial cortex is considered to be typical of Wolff's Law and not a reaction indicating osteitis; cavitation of medial femoral neck. **d** Typical resorption of calcar with sound fixation of stem

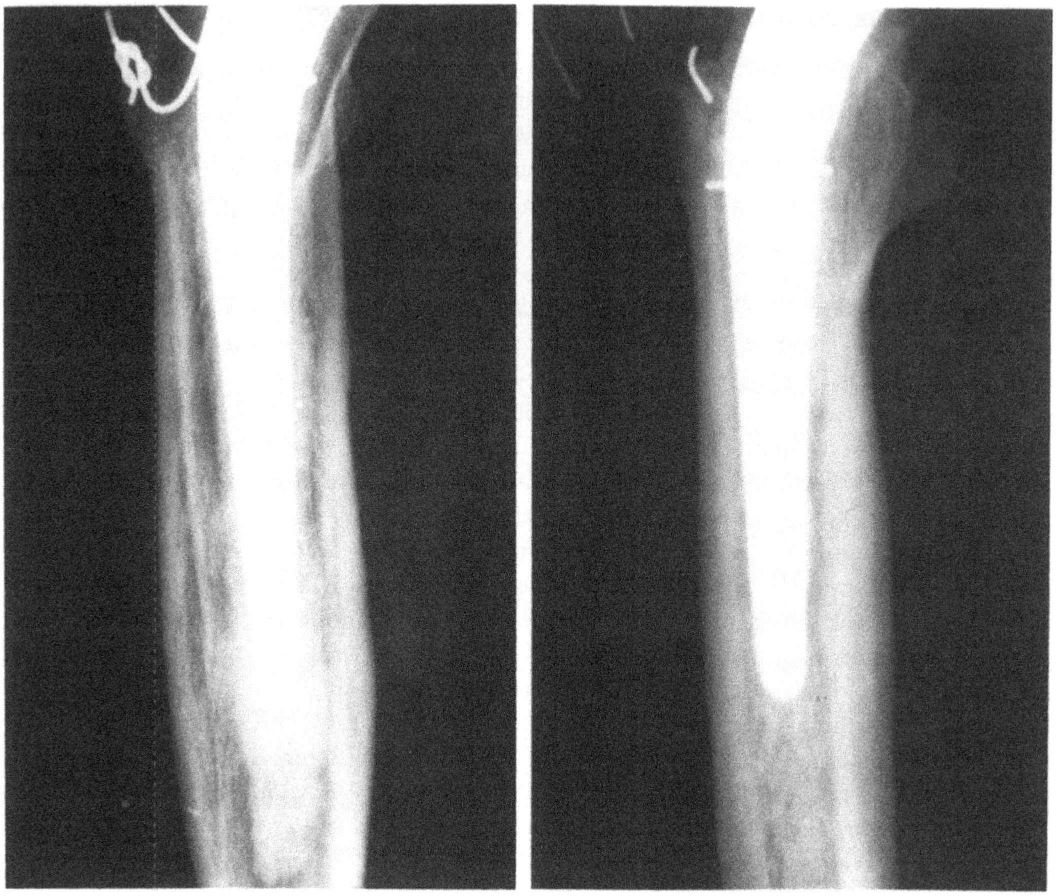

a b

Fig. 6.18. a Unusual appearance of hypertrophied cortex compatible with excellent function and with no history of infection. 'Onion skin' appearance. **b** Compare with physiological hypertrophy

Cemented Sockets

The radiological appearances of cement-bone interfaces in the acetabulum were extremely informative because they were not all as impressive as those in the femur. Many showed amounts of demarcation, and even migration, which were surprising in view of the universally excellent clinical results.

Clinical Material (RS.9)

For the study, 115 cemented sockets with up-to-date X-rays were available, 77 in patients who attended personally for clinical examination and 38 in patients who returned our questionnaire and sent in a new X-ray.

Perfect Acceptance of Cement (Grade I)

There were 47 acetabula (41%) with no demarcation of the radio-opaque cement from the bone of the acetabulum. Four examples are shown in Fig. 6.19a, b, c, d.

Slight or Moderate Demarcation (Grade II)

The amount of demarcation accepted for this category of 'slight or moderate' is shown typically in the four selected cases illustrated in Fig. 6.20a, b, c, d. There were 39 examples of slight or moderate demarcation (34%). Demarcation in this group affected the upper quadrant (grade I) only.

By definition no case in this group showed an appearance under the lowest part suggesting slight upward migration of the socket. It is important always to look for this because slight upward migration can be overlooked if the upper pole alone is scrutinized. (This factor could have been responsible for the conflicting interpretation of the X-rays in the case reported in detail on p. 57.) Upward migration probably obliterates demarcation at the upper pole by compressing these tissues (indeed demarcation at the upper pole might almost be proof that upward migration is not taking place).

Severe Demarcation (Grade III)

In this group demarcation involves the whole circumference of the socket and the gap need not be wider than 1 mm to be in this category if it

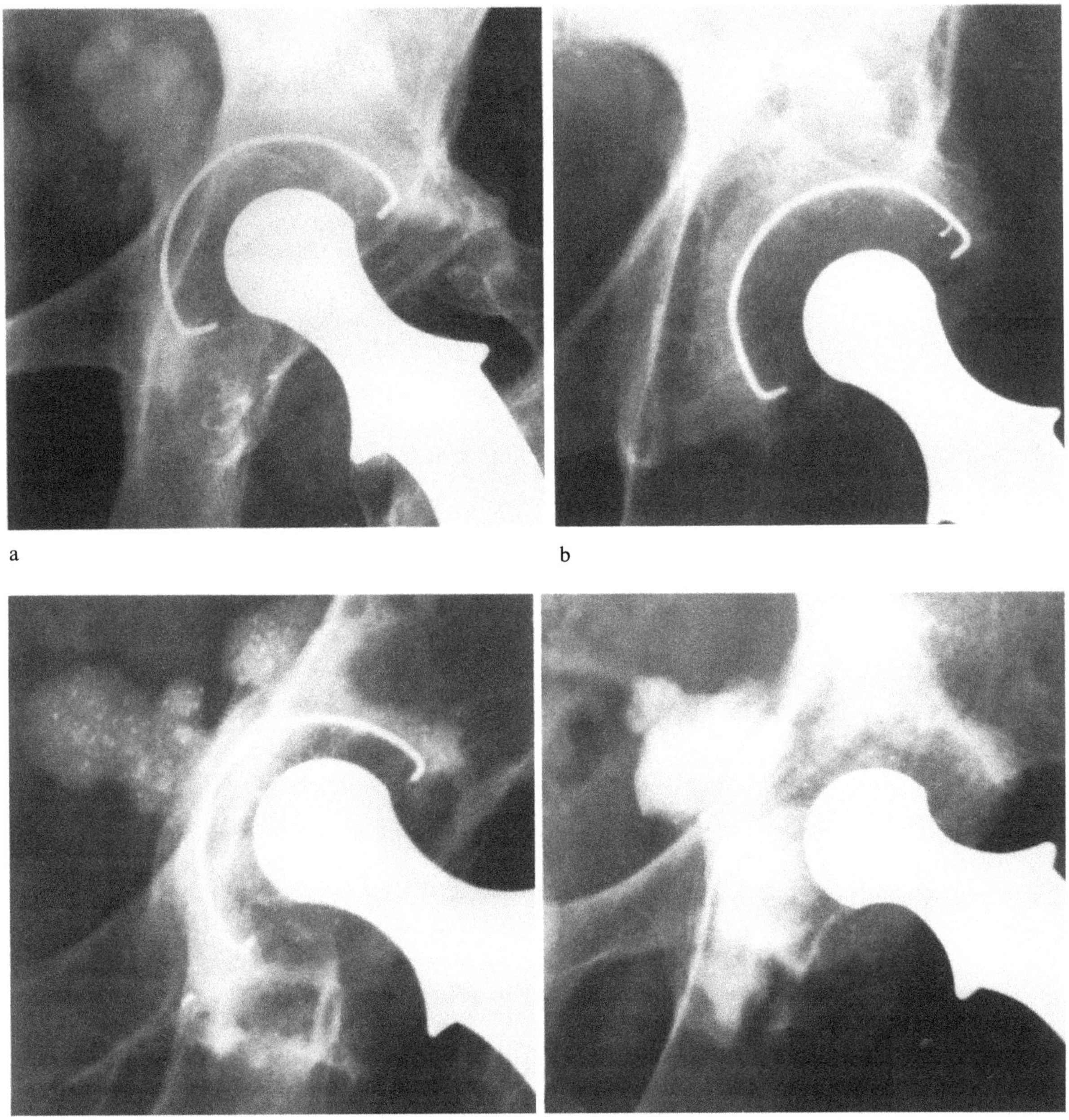

a b c d

Fig. 6.19. a–d Four typical examples **a**, **b**, **c** and **d**, of 'perfect' acceptance of cement by the bone of the acetabulum (41%)

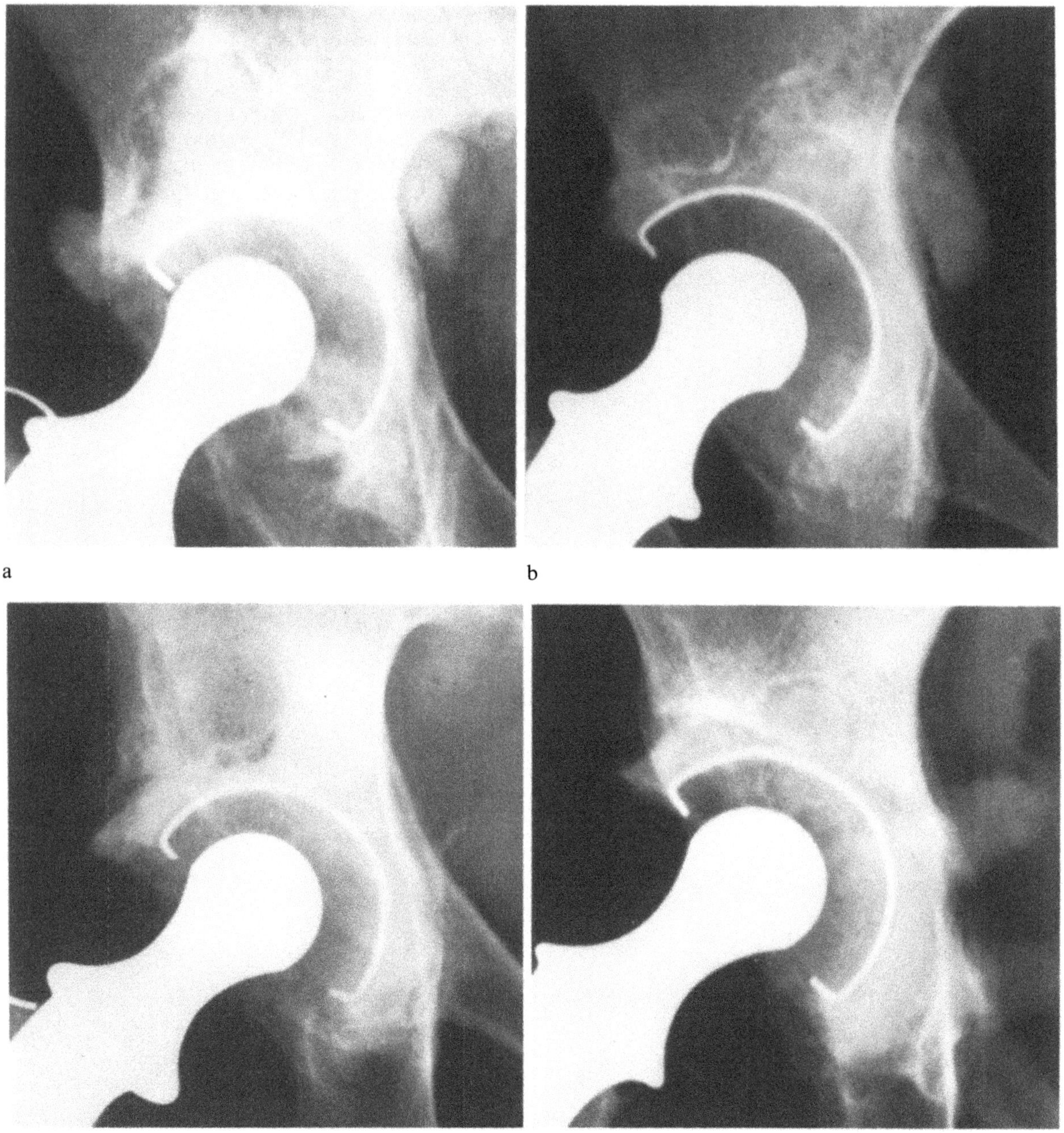

a b c d

Fig. 6.20 a–d. Four examples **a**, **b**, **c** and **d**, of 'slight' or 'moderate' demarcation of cement from the bone of the acetabulum (34%)

involves the whole circumference. Examples are shown in Fig. 6.21 a, b, c, d. There were 16 examples of category III demarcation (14%). In some cases of severe demarcation, incipient upward migration may be suspected by the suggestion of a slight gap below the lower part of the cement.

Migration (Grade IV)

The feature which decides grade IV is a very definite gap between the lower part of the cement and the lower part of the acetabulum. This is possible even without a gap superiorly in the grade I and grade II position as already mentioned. Examples of this are shown in Fig. 6.22 a, b, c, d.

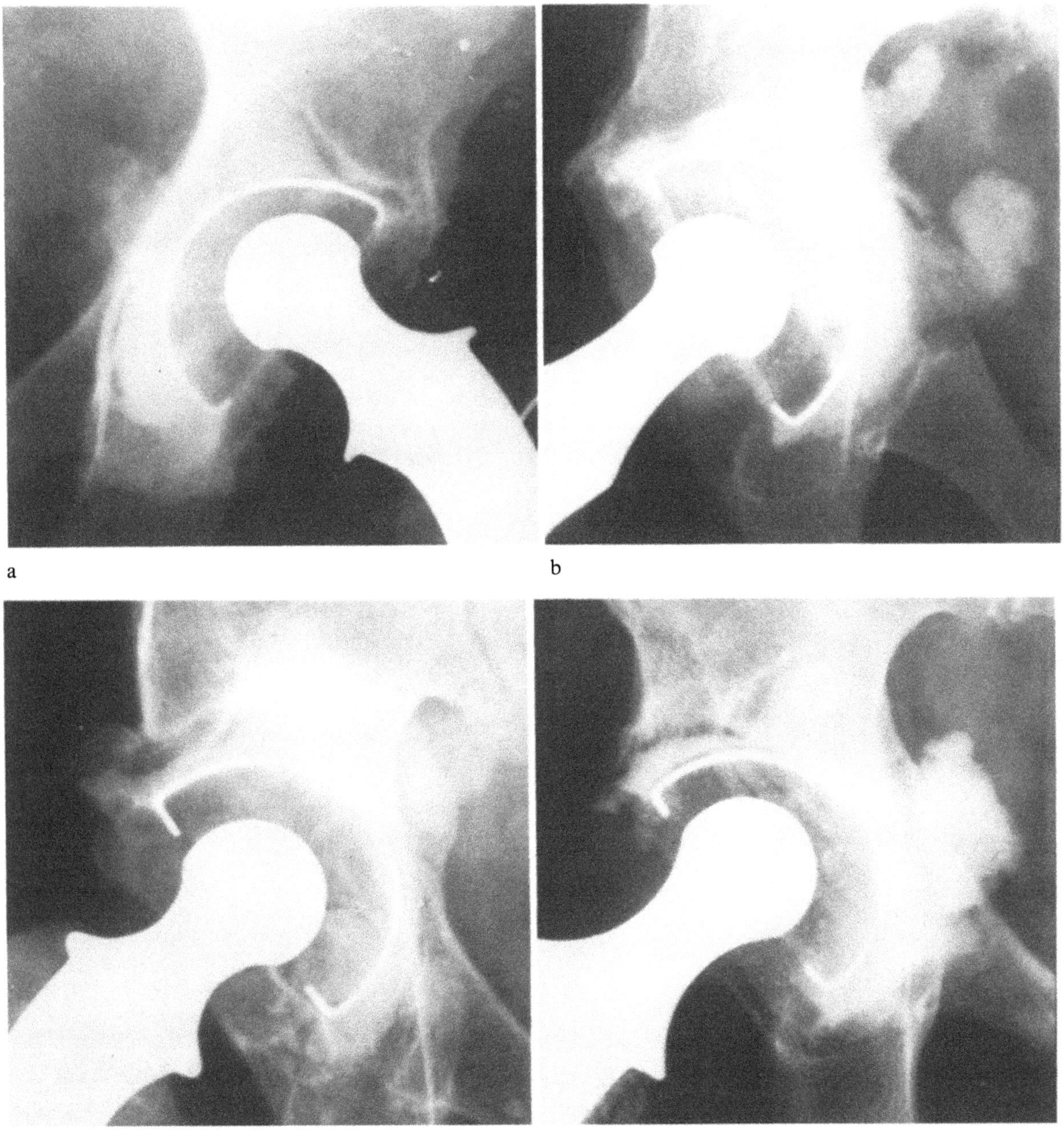

a b c d

Fig. 6.21 a–d. Four examples **a**, **b**, **c** and **d**, of 'severe' demarcation of cement from the bone of the acetabulum without migration (14.0%). Perhaps **b** suspicious of upward migration

Migration can be assessed by the level of the lower end of the semicircular wear marker in relation to the 'tear-drop' or to the pelvic part of Shenton's line. There were 13 examples of grade IV demarcation (11%). In all cases of migration in this series the movement of the socket was mainly in an upward direction. There were no instances in this study of medial prolapse of the socket. One case of migration was sufficiently gross to suggest that future re-operation might have to be recommended despite excellent function. This patient, M.C. 20588, was a female, 50 years of age at operation for osteoarthrosis (OA); she is now only 62 and is graded A. 6.6.6 (Fig. 6.22d).

The table below summarizes the incidence of the four grades of cement demarcation in the aceta-

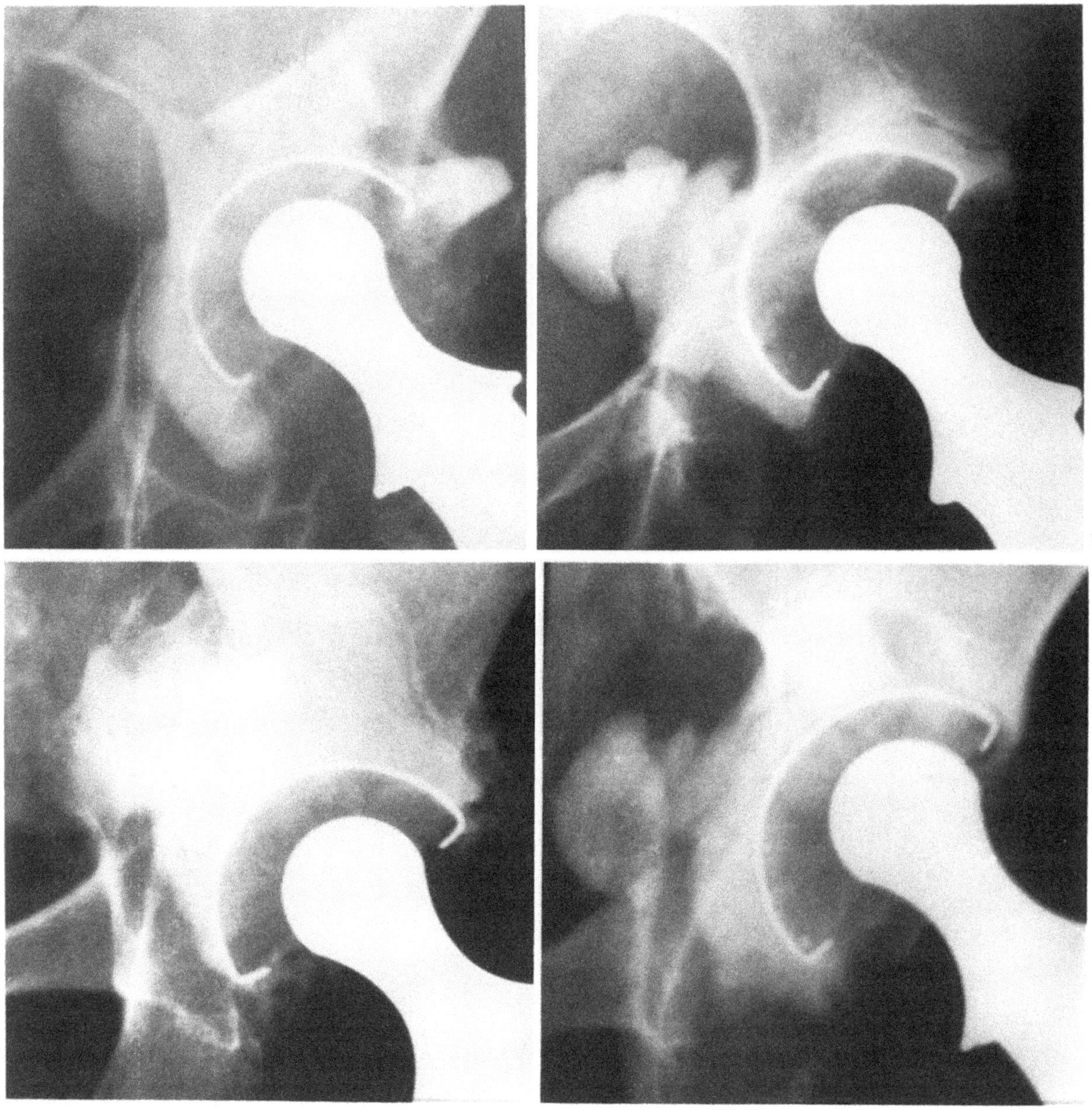

a b c d

Fig. 6.22 a–d. Four examples **a**, **b**, **c** and **d**, of migration of cemented socket in the acetabulum (11.0%). Note how migration is upwards and indicated by gap below cement and only small gap at the superior pole

bulum encountered in the 12–15-year study, all with excellent clinical function.

Grade	Number of Sockets	% of 112	
I	47	41%	75%
II	39	34%	
III	16	14%	25%
IV	13	11%	

Pseudo-Migration (RS.9)

This appearance has been seen two or three times and occurred once in this series and it is worth special comment. The appearances are shown in Fig. 6.23a, b, comparing the early post-operative state with 14 years later. The main feature is the appearance of what looks like a cavity below the cement, suggesting upward migration, but comparison of the level of the lower part of the semicircu-

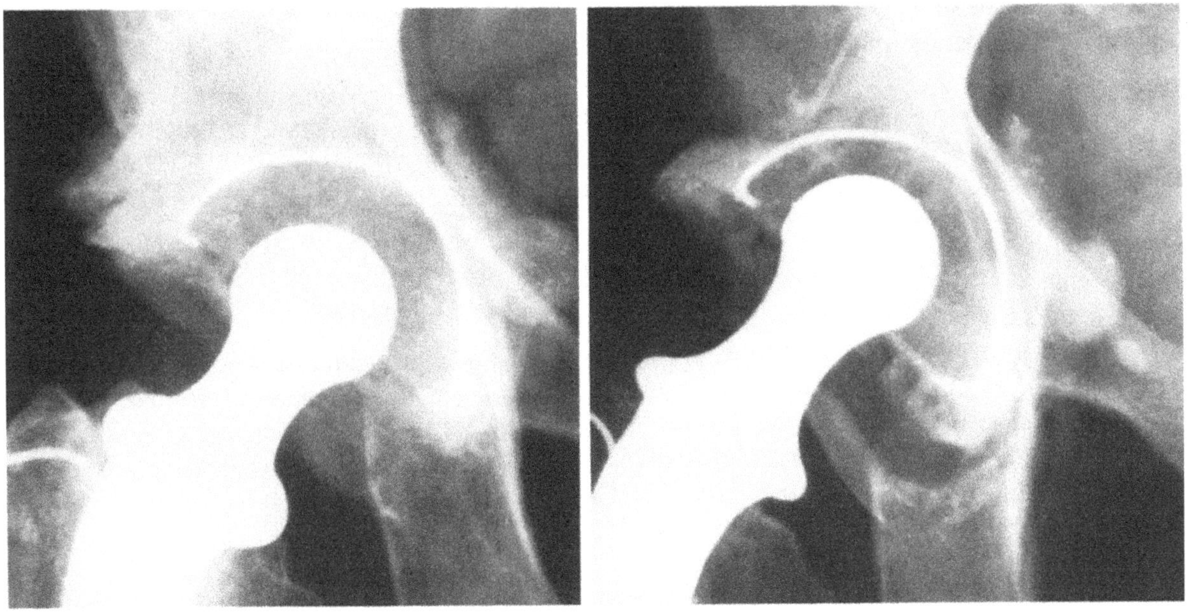

Fig. 6.23. a, b 'Pseudo-migration'. **a** Post-op. state. **b** Appearances 14 years later. Rheumatoid arthritis. Excellent function

lar wire marker with the level of the 'tear-drop' does not confirm upward drift. Post-mortem specimens suggest that this appearance can be produced by new bone growing from the lower part of the rim of the acetabulum and creating the appearance of a cavity below the acetabulum without upward migration of the socket. In this patient (17099) the grading was C 6.2.4., the disability being a severe rheumatoid arthritis but the quality of the hip was excellent.

It must be emphasized again that in all the radiologically loose sockets in this 12–15-year study there was neither pain nor defect of function. In other words, the radiological appearances of looseness or migration would never have been suspected on grounds of clinical behaviour.

Cavitation of Cement-Acetabular Interface (RS.9)

There were two examples of small cavities involving the cement-acetabular interface typified in Fig. 6.24 but these seemed to be merely cystic examples of ordinary demarcation with the bone of the acetabulum condensed and resisting invasion. This appearance of a cavity differs from invasion without condensation of the cancellous bone to resist it, as has been observed on two occasions in the acetabulum (see Figs. 5.14 and 6.15). Note that the appearance of severe wear of HMWP is probably an artefact caused by tilting of the socket.

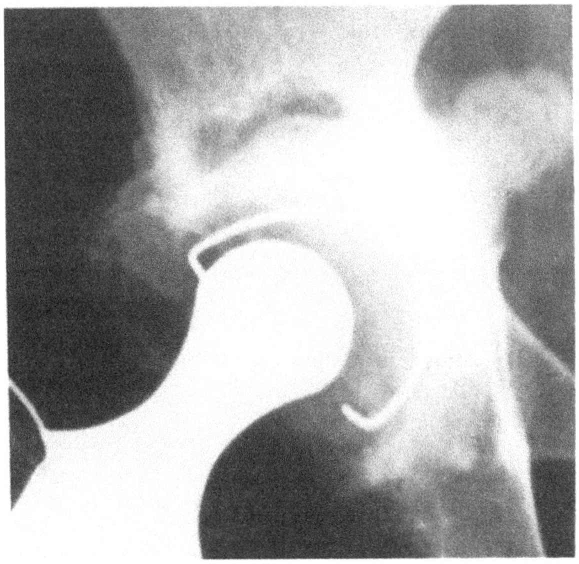

Fig. 6.24. Cystic state of superior pole of cement-bone interface. Absence of migration by appearances of lower pole. Note that appearance of severe wear in this case is almost certainly artefact by plane of wire marker not being in coronal plane – shown by radiolucent ellipses of HMWP visible outside wire above and below

Extended Series of Long-Term Radiological Observations—Sockets

In order to scrutinize as many long-term X-rays as possible in the search for evidence of cavitation at cement-bone interfaces and for more information regarding severe socket demarcation and migration, the Wrightington follow-up system was used to find the X-rays and clinical records, at their last attendance, of patients in the prospective series who were not available for the 12–15-year study. Figure 6.25 shows the source of these additional 149 long-term patients of the prospective series with records and X-rays for 5–11 post-operative years. It is to be noted that these additional cases do not necessarily reduplicate clinical studies 1 and 3, both of which relate only to the first year's work (November 1962 to end of December 1963) nor do they reduplicate clinical study 2, which was only a 5-year study.

Extended Radiological Study—Socket Migration

In order to examine the effect of time, and the nature of the disease (rheumatoid arthritis or osteoarthrosis) on severe socket demarcation (grade III) or migration (grade IV) the number of X-rays was increased to a total of 264 by adding the 115 of the 12–15-year study to the extended group as in Fig. 6.25.

Annual follow-up	9–11 years	33
Annual follow-up	5–8 years	43
Died but follow-up	5–11 years	64
Discharged but follow-up	5–11 years	9
1977 follow-up	12–15 years	115
		264

Fig. 6.25. Origins of follow-ups of 5 years and over: clinical gradings and X-rays available at last attendances

264 hips 5–15 years	Hips	III+IV	
Rheumatoid arthritis	80	17	21.25%
Osteoarthrosis	184	21	11.4%
	264	38	

Fig. 6.26. Demarcation of sockets to grade III and migration IV according to disease

Disease and Demarcation

As regards the effect of rheumatoid and osteoarthritic conditions, Fig. 6.26 shows that the percentage of patients with rheumatoid arthritis which demarcated to grade III and IV over the whole 5–15-year period was 21.25%, whereas only 11.4% demarcated to this degree in the osteoarthrosic cases.

Time and Demarcation

As is shown in Fig. 6.27 for both rheumatoid and arthrosic conditions combined, from a percentage of 4.5% of sockets demarcating to grade III and IV in the first 5 years, the proportion rose to 24% in the second 5 years.

Acceleration of Migration with Time

An important observation, derived from 12 of the migrating sockets in the 12–15-year study, was that migration appeared to accelerate after about 10 years. It is very difficult to establish whether or not slight migration is taking place **until about 7–8 years have elapsed.** From the moment that migration is first definitely established the process often seems to accelerate. This undoubtedly explains the increased number of demarcations in the 12–15-year study compared with the study of DeLee, which averaged 10 years. The acceleration of demarcation with time is obviously something which is to be expected because increasing movement at the cement-bone interface will increase the abrasive action of the rough surface of the loose cement. There are cases where perfect radiological fixation appears to be present over the first 2–3 years, yet the case can end 14 years later with severe migration; but the numbers of observations of this kind are too small to permit statistical analysis.

264 hips 5–15 years	Hips	III+IV	
5–10 years	131	6	4.5%
11–15 years	133	32	24%
	264	38	

Fig. 6.27. Demarcation of sockets to grade III and migration IV according to time after operation

Retrospective study of the X-rays of those cases eventually showing severe migration suggests that the process has been continuous throughout the whole period: it can be very slow and even unrecognisable during the first 5 years; becoming manifest in the second 5; and accelerating during the third 5 years.

It is put forward as a suggestion (which obviously will take years to verify or disprove) that slight demarcation (up to 1 mm) in the region of the upper pole (grade I) is not as sinister as no demarcation in the upper pole region when combined with slight gap under the lowest part of the cement. This combination suggests that early upward migration is compressing and obliterating a gap which otherwise would be revealed as a granulomatous process at the upper pole.

Extended X-Ray Series – Femoral Cement

In the 5–11-year X-rays of the 149 additional cases derived as in Fig. 6.25 there was only one notable pathological condition in the femur (Fig. 6.28). This was a cyst in the cancellous bone medial to the upper end of the femoral prosthesis. The patient was a male with severe bilateral osteoarthrosis, who was aged 62 at the time of the operation. The illustration represents the state at the 9-year follow-up. There were no symptoms. There is in this case a notable lack of radio-opaque cement in the important load-bearing region of the medial femoral neck (cf. Fig. 6.9). This appearance is identical with that illustrated in Fig. 9.7, in this case a press-fit socket without cement, which was explored to prove the presence of inspissated caseous material of a foreign-body granuloma.

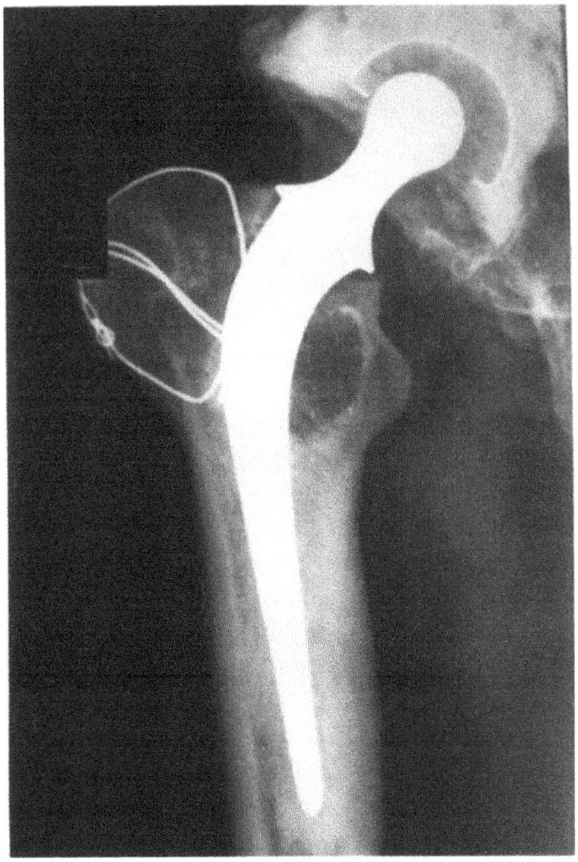

Fig. 6.28. Cavitation in region of medial femoral neck when last seen 9 years after operation. No symptoms

Massive Lysis in the Femur

Extensive cyst-like erosion of the endosteal surface of the femur related to the cement of a femoral prosthesis has been illustrated and called 'massive lysis' by Harris et al.[28] in four cases where infection or tumour had been excluded as possible causes. At revision it was noted that '... the femoral components were not rigidly fixed but were only slightly loose'. Though we are familiar with these radiological appearances we cannot recall a case developing in our own clinical practice and certainly there were none in the long-term studies reported here.

Discrepancies in Different Studies

In the nine different studies reported here of different aspects of the long-term radiological behaviour of cement (presented in tabular form at the end of this chapter) there are some discrepancies. Some discrepancies relate to different groups of patients: studies 1 and 3 relate to the work of the first year only of the prospective group and study 8 is a retrospective study of patients operated on in 1967 and 1968. This latter study was specially concentrated on searching for minute radiological evidence of trouble at the cement-bone interface after an average interval of 8.3 years. This study did not confirm the high incidence of serious socket migration found in the prospective study recorded as 9.2% by DeLee after 10 years and raised to 12.5% by the author after 14 years. An explanation has been offered in the possibility of less radical deepening of the acetabulum after the initial 4 years of experience.

There are conflicts on the incidence and magnitude of radiological subsidence of femoral prostheses. In study 8 there was an incidence of 3.8% of subsidence of more than 2 mm and patients with subsidence weighed 9 kg more than the average. In study 7 an incidence of 12.6% of subsidence was reported in 119 hips operated on by the pre-1970 techniques, and a zero incidence in 97 hips operated on after 1974 when an extreme valgus technique was started with a thick (1-cm) layer of cement between calcar and the concave surface of the prosthesis. Patients with subsidence in this study also were 8 kg heavier than average. The high incidence of 12.6% of subsidence in series I of study 7 might be explained by this study being restricted to male patients. The figures in this study also were not large (216 hips) and statistical errors could be present. The high rate of radiological subsidence of femoral prostheses is not supported by a high rate of revision surgery because only 0.15% of revisions were actually performed for loose femoral prostheses in 10,000 cases.

Final Remarks

The long-term radiological study of the behaviour of bone in contact with cement is a more important criterion of long-term success than is the satisfaction of the patient. The long-term radiological behaviour of cement in the femur has been gratifying apart from resorption of the cut end of the femoral neck, which seems to be self-limiting, and this is consistent with the low rate of revision surgery for loose femoral prostheses. We attribute this success to elevation of the trochanter, which removes all obstacles to packing in cement and to inserting the prosthesis in a rehearsed, straight line without having to 'push it round the corner'. Also the greater enlargement of the entrance to the medullary cavity (Fig. 9.14, p. 123) made possible by elevating the trochanter and the use of rotary reaming, with the facility thereby for using the 'two-thumb' method of injecting cement, also must contribute. In the original prospective series the average amount of cement in the femur was quite small compared with that currently being used, so that it seems reasonable to expect even better long-term radiological results in the femur in the future.

Improvements in cement technology in the acetabulum we hope will reduce the demarcation and migration of cement encountered in 25% of the 12–15-year results of the prospective series and less frequently in the 8-year results of the 1967–1968 series. The improvement in the latter series could be the result of avoidance of excessive deepening and the result of retaining eburnated bone in the roof of the acetabulum.

The progression of severe demarcation and migration (grade III and IV) of sockets with passage of time, and with some but not invariable dependence on the rheumatoid process, are disturbing facts. That **clinical failure** by socket loosening might be delayed and prevented from making itself manifest for at least 14 or 15 years as a result of the low frictional torque of the small head, does not solve the fundamental problem. The long-term behaviour of the socket, as described in this book in cases operated on before 1966, certainly does not establish as proved the author's belief that it is reasonable to expect successful results after 25 years in vigorous patients operated on at 45 years of age. Nevertheless the following facts give cause for optimism:

1) That 75% of the sockets were either perfectly accepted or showed only slight or moderate demarcation, after an average period of 13.2 years using what is now recognized as an unsophisticated technique
2) That the technique of using cement in the acetabulum has been significantly improved by the new methods advocated in this book
3) That acceptance of cement in the femur in the overwhelming majority of cases was gratifying and even here better technical methods of cementing the femoral prosthesis are now available

Table of Discrepancies

Loose prosthesis failure	0.72% (8)				
Loose socket failure	0.58% (8)	1.4% (1)	1.4% (2)		
Subsidence of prosthesis: no symptoms	1.5% (3)	12.6% Series I 0% Series II (7)	<2 mm 5.1% 2–5 mm 3.1% >5 mm 0.7% (8)	8% (8)	
Migration of socket: no symptoms	1.4% (1)	1.4% (2)	9.2% (4)	11% (9)	
No demarcation of socket	31.3% (4)	41% (9)			
Moderate demarcation: no symptoms	60.3% (4)	>1 mm 50.6% 1–2 mm 3.1% <2 mm 0% (8)	34% (9)		
Resorption of calcar	3–4 mm 78.5% 5–11 mm 18.2% 12–15 mm 3.2% 99.9% (2)	3–10 mm Av. 3 mm 37.2% (5)	4–27 mm Av. 5.5 mm 70% (6)	21% Series I 2.1% Series II (7)	0 mm 5% 5 mm 55% 10 mm 35% 15 mm 5% (9)
Fracture tip of cement	1.5% (3)	20.2% Series I 3.1% Series II (7)	8.6% (8)		
New bone at tip of cement	44.8% (5)	34% (6)	7.9% (8)		
Hypertrophy of cortex femur	0.7% (1)	9.4% (5)	28.8% (6)	19% (8)	
Atrophy of cortex femur	4.7% (5)	4.8% (6)			
Cysts of cortex femur	0.3% (8)	1.2% (9)			

Press-Fit Socket Without Cement

In attempting to decide whether the demarcation and migration of a cemented socket is inherent in a histiocyte reaction specifically evoked by acrylic cement, it is interesting to compare results when a socket is implanted without cement.

The press-fit socket (Fig. 6.29) was made of HMWP encased in a stainless steel shell, almost identical with a Smith-Petersen cup and differing only in the addition of a projecting spigot of plastic to engage with the pilot hole used for reaming the acetabulum. The idea of the spigot was to prevent tilting. The socket was hammered into position and because of the precise size of the acetabulum produced by reaming with the expanding reamer an 'interference' fit was usually obtained in primary interventions. The external diameter

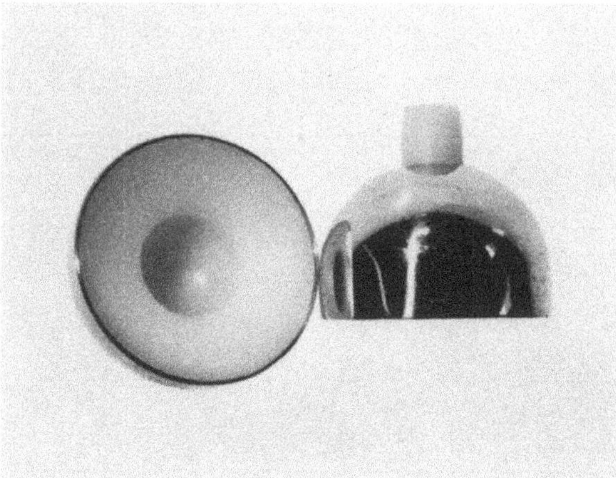

Fig. 6.29. Press-fit socket used without cement

of the metal shell encasing the socket was 50 mm. The theory was that the difference in diameter between the exterior of the 50-mm-diameter socket and the 22.25-mm-diameter metal head would encourage the socket to remain stationary while the femoral head rotated under load. Experience showed that eventually almost all these sockets rotated freely on their axis of symmetry and the mechanical situation became rather like the trunnion design of hip arthroplasty which shares its movement at two sliding surfaces.

The reason for introducing the press-fit socket was the recognition, by mid-1963 (i.e. rather more than 6 months after the HMWP LFA operation had been introduced on a regular basis), that demarcation between radio-opaque cement and the bone of the acetabulum was becoming a common radiological occurrence. In the femur radiological demarcation of radio-opaque cement was considered to be practically non-existent in the 5 years of experience in the femur which had already been acquired. It was felt that early demarcation of cement in the acetabulum spelt ultimate failure.

Demarcation of cement in the acetabulum was postulated as the result of a too-abrupt transition from the elastic modulus of the cement mass (considered stiff in this situation) to the more elastic cancellous bone lining the reamed acetabulum. During this epoch we always excised eburnated bone from the roof of the acetabulum believing that cancellous bone offered a better bed for fixation of cement than a smooth eburnated surface in the roof of the original acetabulum. It was feared, if demarcation ended in loosening, that the rough external surface of the cement might act like a rasp and progressively abrade away the acetabulum. The solution at that time seemed to be to abandon any attempt to make a fixed interface between two substances with different elastic moduli. To effect a compromise the principle of Smith-Petersen seemed ideal: a polished metal surface, under load and slight movement, would cause fibrous tissue to metaplase into hyaline cartilage and so create a physiological interface; the absence of roughness would avoid mechanical attrition.

We performed 35 of these operations in 1963; 158 in 1964; 99 in 1965. No more were performed after this because (1) demarcation of the cemented sockets did not seem to be progressing beyond the amount visible at the end of the first year; (2) though the press-fit sockets were excellent when they were mechanically sound, they were often not quite as good as the cemented sockets when compared in the other hip of the same patient (i.e. the patient usually preferred the cemented side though still pleased with both); (3) when not mechanically firm at the operation this was the result of factors outside the surgeon's control and the results were unreliable; finally (4) a high rate of tilting and migration of the press-fit sockets occurred and in subsequent years became a serious problem. Over the first 7–8 years about 15% of the press-fit sockets had to be changed to cemented sockets because of tilting and the start of recurrent dislocation.

In the 12–15-year study, 58 press-fit sockets (in 55 patients) were seen at the clinic and 20 (35.5%) had tilted or migrated (Fig. 6.30a, b). This rate was nearly three times the migration rate after 12–15 years (11%) of the cemented sockets! A constant feature of migration of the press-fit sockets was the direction of tilt; this invariably was in the direction to 'open' the mouth of the socket (i.e. changing it from 45° downwards and laterally, to vertical). It seemed likely that this was due to the direction of the joint force not being directed axially into the socket but loading the superior lip of the socket. When press-fit sockets had to be explored because of tilting and migration, it was found that the lining of the acetabulum had never generated a continuous surface of hyaline cartilage. The surface of the acetabulum

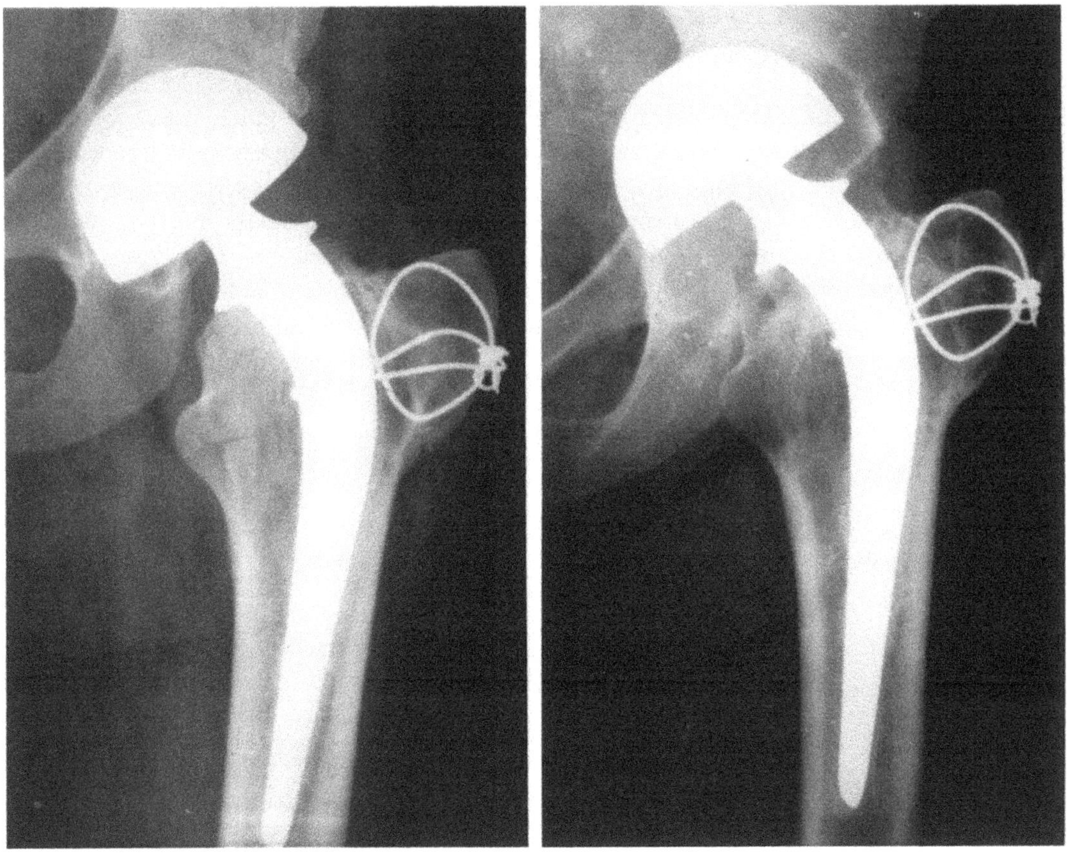

a b

Fig. 6.30. a Press-fit socket after operation in 1964. **b** Press-fit socket at review in 1977. Good clinical result but serious migration is present. Femur excellent. Typical resorption of medial femoral neck after 13 years

always presented a mottled appearance with cartilaginous patches interspersed with red areas of fibrous tissue. Histologically (after 7–8 years, which was the commonest time for re-operation) the lining was always impregnated with particles of HMWP. Apart from the giant-cell reaction to be expected in this case there was no evidence of an active destructive process to explain the migration and there were no local accumulations of caseous debris invading the acetabular surface.

Abraded Plastics Particles and Expanded Surfaces

The high incidence of migration of the press-fit sockets makes one wonder whether the free ingress of abraded particles of HMWP to the moving interface between socket and acetabulum, continuous with the synovial cavity, might have played a part in promoting migration compared with the less free ingress of abraded particles in the cemented cases. The possibility of ready access of abraded plastics particles to spaces between implants and bone may have significance in relation to the use of expanded surfaces to effect a direct bond with bone without cement. If a perfect bond is established between a porous surface and living tissue then all will be well because there will be no pumping action to suck particles into the interfaces between implant and living tissue. But if the porous bond at the interface is imperfect, especially at the ends presenting to the synovial cavity such as at the base of the femoral neck or at the rim of the socket, invasion of the interface with abraded particles from the surface of the socket might perhaps be worse than with cement.

Total and Long-Term Failure Rates

It is not out of place to re-emphasize the difference in significance of the 'total' failure rate and the 'long-term' failure rate after hip replacement.

The **total failure rate** can be assessed before 5 years have elapsed, because it comprises factors such as death and sepsis, and mechanical failures (dislocation, recurrent subluxation, trochanteric problems, etc.). The latter are in part attributable to the skill and experience of the operator. The total failure rate for operations performed at Wrightington before the end of 1968 has been estimated at between 8% and 10% but the accuracy of this figure is no longer of very great interest in view of the much lower total failure rate currently being experienced, and which alone will be the figure by which to assess this operation. It is possible that the current total failure rate is not more that 2%.

The long-term failure rate is fundamental to total hip replacement because it concerns the acceptance of acrylic cement by the living tissues. It is this aspect of the subject which dominates Chaps. 5 and 6.

Chapter 7

Hip Sockets – Theory

In this chapter the limitations of conventional designs of hip socket are discussed and a new socket which has been designed specifically for use with acrylic cement is described.

Acrylic Cement in the Acetabulum

In clinical studies of the cement-bone interface (Chap. 4 and 5) radiological demarcation of cement in the acetabulum was observed in roughly 60% of cases. The corollary that about 40% of hips show no demarcation, even after an average period of 14 years, is important because if demarcation were caused by a basic problem such as too great a discrepancy between the elastic moduli of cement and bone, then 100% of sockets ought to demarcate. The fact that 40% of sockets bond perfectly could be explained by some factor of better technique in the perfect cases. Even though minor degrees of radiological demarcation in the acetabulum do not necessarily presage clinical failure, we cannot consider ourselves in control of the situation until we can find a method of significantly reducing the incidence to make it as rare as in the femur.

Unsophisticated Cement Technology in the Acetabulum

It is necessary to examine what we now consider were defects in cement technique as used in the acetabulum 10 years ago (and also in some respects until quite recently).

Anchor Holes

Before about 1969 the theory of low frictional torque so dominated our ideas of anchoring cement in the acetabulum at Wrightington that it seemed unnecessary to make multiple recesses for keying the cement into the bone as was being done by McKee and Müller. On the theory of low frictional torque the roughness of the cancellous bone itself was sufficient to resist rotatory movement. There is no reason to doubt the truth of this because demarcation in the acetabulum could start as the result of loading in a purely vertical direction, without any rotatory element; frictional torque transmitted to the socket to accelerate loosening is obviously most important when cement bonding is imperfect. The absence of high torque could explain **clinical** success persisting after 14 years despite radiological evidence of migration of the socket (Chap. 6).

Before 1969 we removed eburnated bone from the roof of the acetabulum in order to expose the cancellous bone, which was considered to be the ideal bed for cement. When later we started to deepen the acetabulum transversely, eburnated bone was left intact in the roof of the acetabulum and it seemed a good policy to conserve eburnated bone looking ahead to the time when replacement of the socket might be necessary. The cement was anchored by three anchor holes 0.5 in. (12.5 mm) in diameter in the superior, posterior and ischial directions in addition to the central pilot hole of the same diameter.

Now, in addition to the three 12.5-mm holes (superior, pubic and ischial) and the central pilot hole, we advocate that a multiplicity of 6-mm holes (0.25 in.) should also be made. The 6-mm holes are distributed randomly over the acetabulum but in particular in areas of dense eburnated bone.

Six to 12 of these 6-mm holes can be distributed over the lining of the acetabulum. It is essential that the drill should have a collar to prevent penetration deeper than about 6 mm.

Irrigation

In the past it was never our custom at Wrightington to irrigate the acetabulum with water or saline. We concentrated on repeated packing with a sequence of dry gauze swabs and the cement was inserted with as short an interval as possible, during which blood could start to accumulate, between removing the last dry pack and inserting the cement. The 'cement restrictor' has also been re-designed to prevent its being pulled out of the acetabulum when the last gauze pack is being removed and so interrupting the smooth sequence of steps immediately before the cement is inserted. In the present technique assiduous irrigation with a syringe and sucker is strongly advocated. Irrigation removes blood and replaces it with a less viscous fluid, which is theoretically more easily displaced into cancellous spaces by the pressure of the cement dough. Irrigation also renders remnants of fibrous tissue visible. These show up as white, slimy strands which cannot be distinguished from cancellous bone when wetted with blood. Swabs soaked in hydrogen-peroxide (10 vols) frequently have a useful styptic action on bleeding.

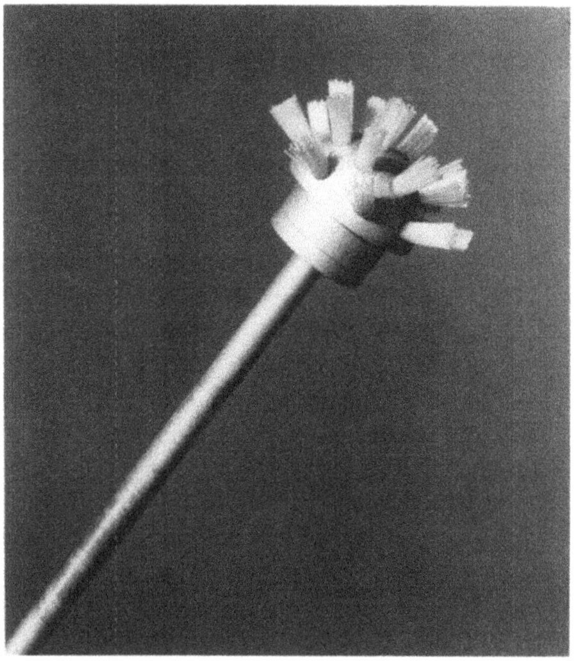

Fig. 7.1. Nylon rotary brush for use in power tool for cleaning cancellous bone of acetabulum

Rotary Brush

Experiments with a power-driven rotary nylon brush appear to be encouraging in helping to remove fibrous tissue (Fig. 7.1). It also cleans out soft marrow tissue from cancellous spaces to leave the cancellous bone with a coarser texture to accept the cement.

Socket Design

Defects of Simple Hemispherical Designs

The basic shape of most hip sockets is a hemisphere. This has two disadvantages: (1) a simple hemisphere is unable to exert injection pressure on acrylic cement unless the rim of the socket fits the mouth of the acetabulum rather closely, and (2) being of necessity loose in the acetabulum before the cement is inserted a hemispherical socket can continue to wobble while the cement is soft.

If a simple hemispherical socket is to exert uniform pressure on cement it must be pressed into the acetabulum in a direction perpendicular to the face of the socket so that the excess cement extrudes evenly round the close-fitting rim (Fig. 7.2). Most hip sockets in their final position are inclined at about 45° to the long axis of the body and therefore they must be pressed into the cement-filled acetabulum in a 45° headward direction if the cement is to extrude evenly round the rim. This is perfectly acceptable if there is no need to deepen the acetabulum, but if we need to deepen an acetabulum this will have to be done also at 45° in a headward direction, if the rim of the socket is to remain concentric with the rim of the acetabulum to preserve injection pressure. This may cause the site of the centre of rotation of the socket to be higher than the anatomical level (Fig. 7.3a, b, c).

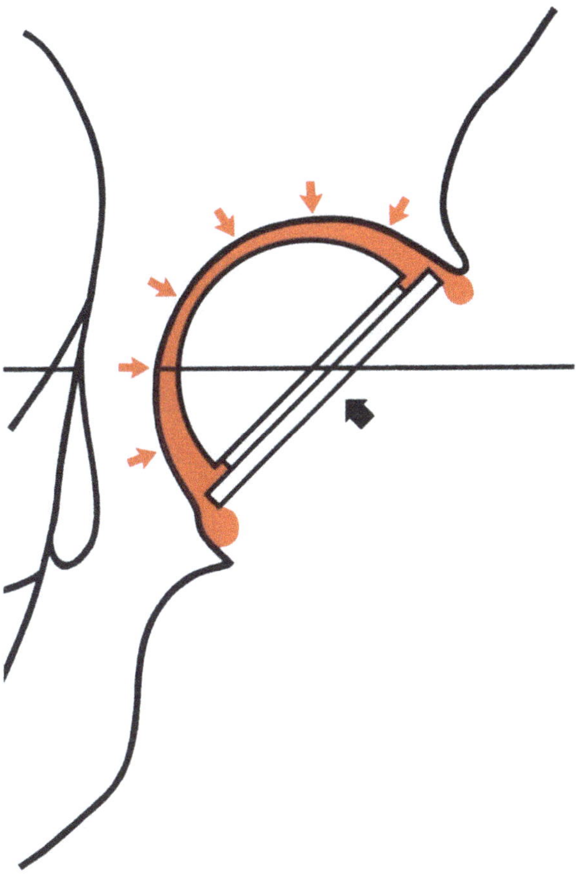

Fig. 7.2. Even pressurisation of cement with force acting perpendicular to face of socket (45° to long axis of body)

There are disadvantages in failing to keep the centre of a socket down to the anatomical level. Our experience prior to 1970 suggested that siting of the socket too high contributed to failure to restore full limb length and this predisposed to post-operative dislocation because normal tension may not be restored in the fascial structures of the thigh (Chap. 19).

Transverse Deepening of the Acetabulum

We now advocate that deepening the acetabulum should be performed in a direction transverse to the long axis of the body to keep the centre of rotation of the socket at the anatomical level. This also counteracts upward migration of the head of the femur in a destructive arthritis produced by erosion of the superior lip of the acetabulum. The same applies in congenital subluxation.

When an acetabulum is deepened transversely the rim of an ordinary socket no longer fits the rim of the acetabulum like a piston; a crescentic gap always presents between the roof of the acetabulum and the superior lip of the socket (Fig. 7.3 c). When the socket is pushed transversely into the cement the excess cement no longer extrudes uniformly round the circumference of the rim but

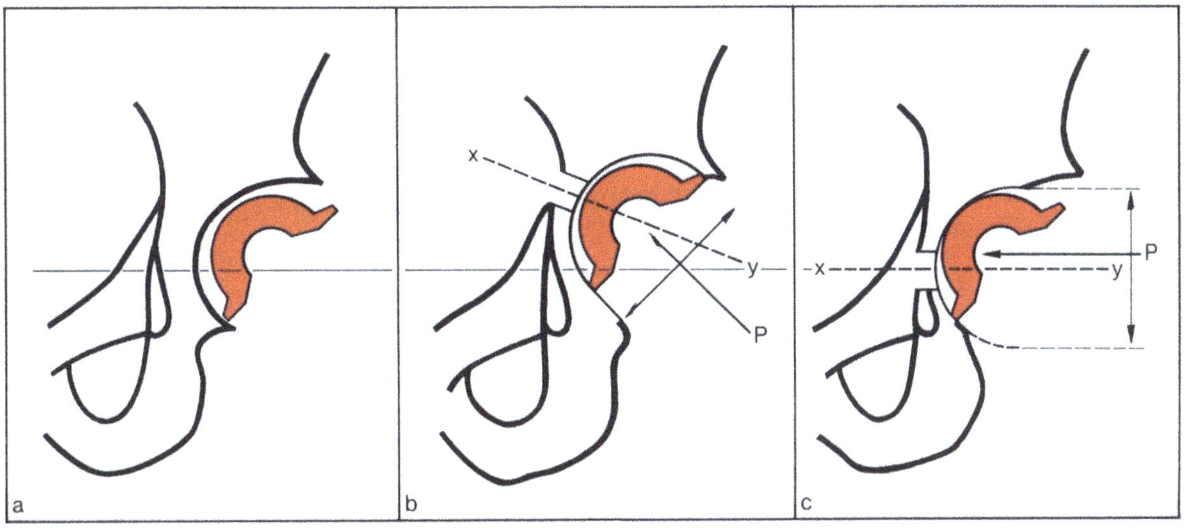

Fig. 7.3. a Socket in acetabulum which will fit socket better when deepened. **b** Deepening at 45° keeps rim of socket concentric with rim of acetabulum; good for pressurisation of cement; but centre of rotation raised above anatomical level. **c** Socket deepened transversely to keep centre of socket at anatomical level; but renders rim of socket eccentric to rim of acetabulum; bad for pressurisation of cement in roof of acetabulum

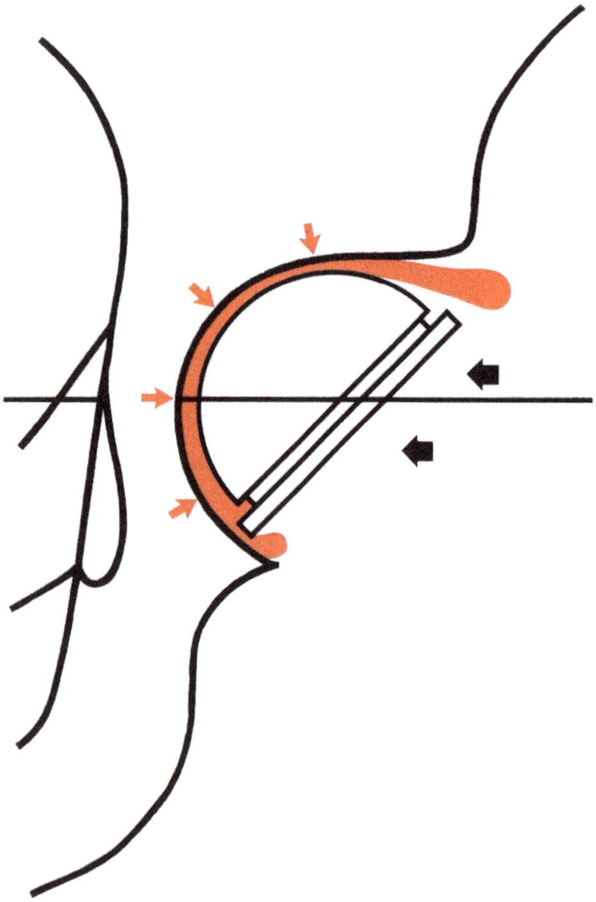

Fig. 7.4. When acetabulum is deepened transversely, cement escapes over summit of socket without uniform, hydraulic pressure being developed in the cement

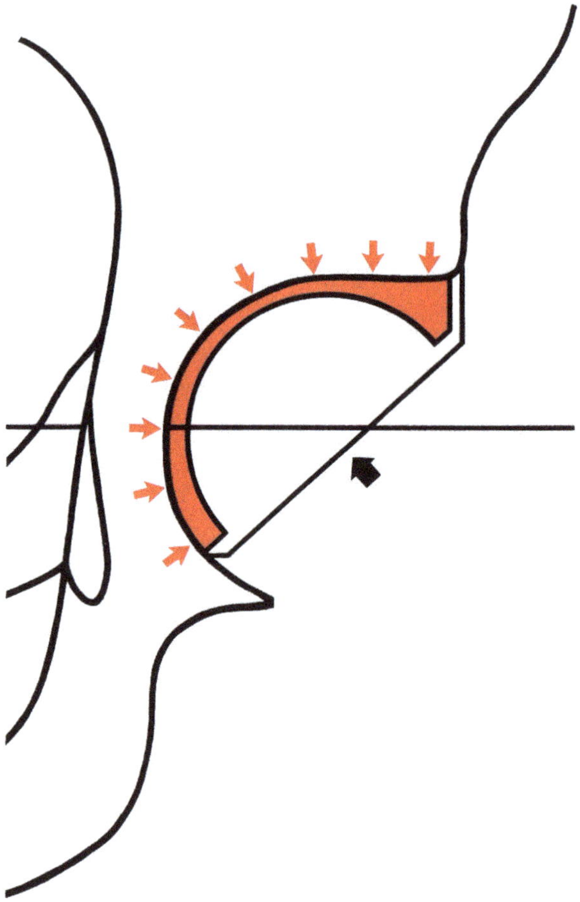

Fig. 7.5. Pressure injection (PIJ) rim socket prevents escape of cement over summit of socket, after transverse deepening of acetabulum, with generation of uniform hydraulic pressure in the soft cement

escapes over to the summit of the body of the socket into the low-pressure region of the crescentic gap (Fig. 7.4). Attempts to press the extruded cement back into the crescentic gap cannot achieve the same uniform hydraulic pressure produced when the rim of a socket fits the acetabulum like a piston.

In attempting to resolve this problem the first idea that comes to mind is to make the face of the socket oval (a 45° section through a 50-mm-diameter cylinder). In practice this does not work because if the face of the oval socket is flat, the upper margin of the oval face projects outside the superior lip of the acetabulum (unless very gross deepening is possible); and the cement therefore will not be pressurized. The solution is to design the socket with an oval rim inclined at 45° away from the face. This makes the superior part of the rim vertical when the face of the socket is inclined at 45°. The oval rim will then be entirely contained inside the acetabulum (Fig. 7.5).

Cutting the Rim of the PIJ Socket

The rim of the pressure injection (PIJ) socket is about 1 mm thick and can be trimmed with strong serrated scissors to fit a large range of different sizes and shapes of acetabulum. When an acetabulum of **average diameter** has been deepened transversely, the superior rim of the injection socket is cut to reach to about the same height as the body of the socket when the face of the socket is inclined at 45° (Fig. 7.6a).

When an acetabulum is **grossly enlarged** by erosion of the superior lip and the acetabulum has been deepened transversely at the anatomical level,

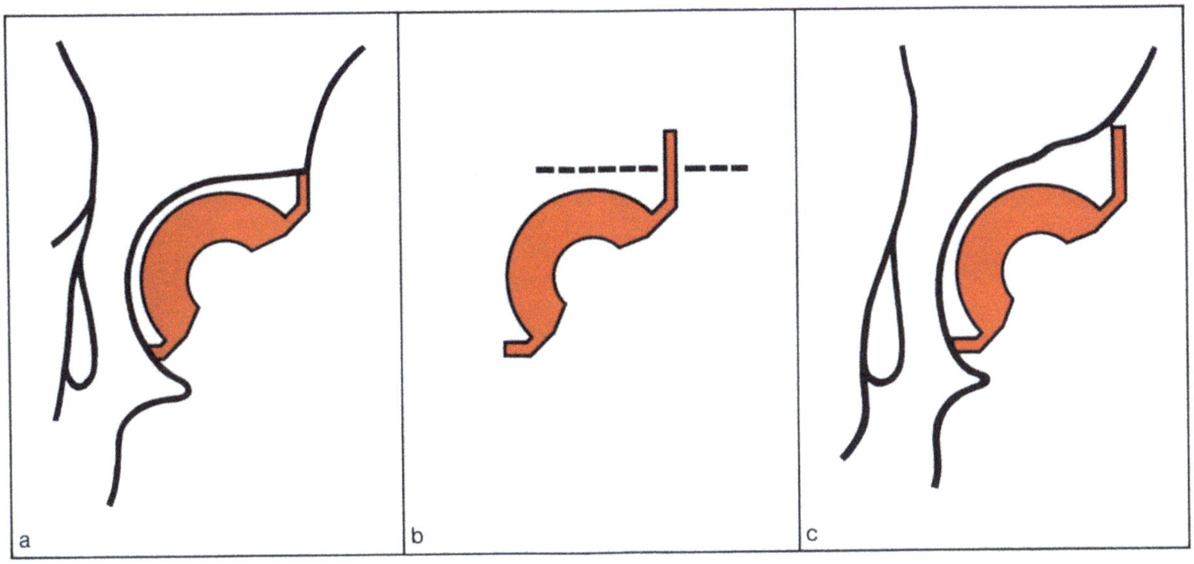

Fig. 7.6a–c. Length of the superior lobe of the rim of the socket is cut to different heights, in relation to the level of the summit of the body of the socket: **a** in an acetabulum of normal size, after deepening; **c** in a large acetabulum with erosion of the roof

an inclined surface of eburnated bone extends above and lateral to the deepened zone. In this case the superior lobe of the rim of the PIJ socket must be kept longer than in the previous case so that it will reach to a higher level than the body when the face of the socket is inclined at 45° (Fig. 7.6c). The extended superior rim will then pressurize the wedge of cement applied to the roof of the acetabulum. The same situation exists in congenital subluxation.

Socket Stability

Because space must be available in the acetabulum to contain the cement, a simple hemispherical socket is mechanically unstable in an empty acetabulum and can wobble in the acetabulum while the cement is soft. The surgeon is therefore faced with the strenuous task of attempting to hold a socket without its wobbling for 5–10 min while waiting for the cement to harden. It is possible that this may be a frequent source of imperfect cement fixation in the acetabulum because the patient's pelvis may be moving with respiration and it is humanly impossible to hold the socket completely immobile.

When the rim of the PIJ design of socket is correctly trimmed to fit the acetabulum, at least three points of contact will be established between rim and acetabulum to make it stable against wobble (Fig. 7.7a, b). Stability can be demonstrated when the socket is being tested in the empty acetabulum in the following way: with the 'pusher' exerting pressure on the face of the socket-holder, the friction generated between the rim of the socket and the rim of the acetabulum will offer sufficient resistance for the horizontally projecting handle of the socket-holder not to fall under its own weight if the surgeon releases his hold on it. If this test does not demonstrate complete stability, due to a slight error in trimming the rim, stability ought still to be possible by applying a gentle force to the handle of the socket-holder in rehearsed direction.

When a socket is inserted into soft cement, adhesion of soft cement to the exterior of the socket is always greater than adhesion to the wet bone of the acetabulum. If the socket is able to wobble there is therefore a tendency for the cement to be pulled away from the wet acetabulum. In the dough state cement is too viscous to flow round the sides of a socket from high-pressure to low-pressure sides. On the high-pressure side (i.e. the side towards which a socket is moving) dough is

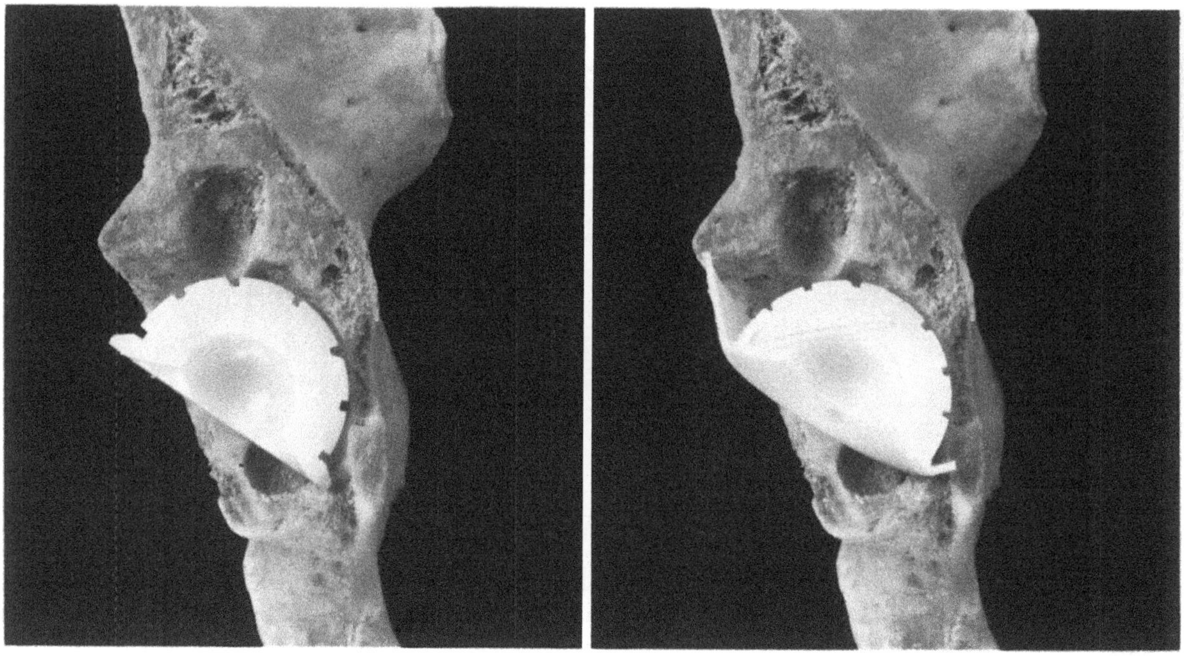

a b

Fig. 7.7. **a** Standard socket in acetabulum before cement inserted. Unstable. **b** Contact of periphery of rim of the trimmed PIJ socket renders socket stable before cement is inserted and during time the cement is still soft

extruded externally because it cannot be sucked back to the low-pressure side between the sides of the socket and the acetabulum. Stated in another way, when soft cement loses volume by being transiently compressed by a wobbling socket it never recovers the lost volume when the socket moves back to the original position. When back to the original position the lost volume produces a gap between cement and wet bone though this gap may be only a matter of micrometres.

Pressure Injection

In addition to stabilising a socket in the acetabulum while the cement is soft, the PIJ rim exerts an element of hydraulic pressure on the cement during insertion. It is particularly in a large osteoarthrosic acetabulum, and in congenital subluxation, that effective pressurisation of cement in the superior quadrant of the acetabulum is difficult to achieve with ordinary designs of socket.

The original idea of the pressure injection socket was for the rim to make contact with the periphery of the acetabulum before the body of the socket touched the floor of the acetabulum. The cement would thus be trapped by the rim and would then be pressurized by deflection of the semi-rigid rim when the body of the socket was pushed to full depth. In practice this ideal situation arises only rarely and the rim and the deepest part of the body of the socket usually make contact with the acetabulum simultaneously. But even so, injection pressure rises significantly in the last few moments of insertion as the gap between rim and acetabulum is progressively narrowing and progressively increasing the resistance to escape of viscous cement.

It is undesirable to achieve such a perfect seal between the rim of the socket and the acetabulum that a very high injection pressure can be maintained for a period of minutes rather than seconds. Early experiments using a flexible, self-sealing rim showed that seals can be made too efficient with the result that the socket cannot be made to sink through the viscous cement. It is essential that excess cement should be able to escape to permit the body of the socket to reach its rehearsed depth. The essence of the exercise therefore is to slow down the rate of escape rather than to stop it too effectively.

Experience has show the most practical design to be a semi-rigid rim which restricts escape of excess cement during the 5–10 s needed to settle the socket into its rehearsed position in the acetabulum. In this short period the injection pressure is much higher and much more uniformly distributed than anything a conventional hemispherical socket can achieve. Very important is the fact that as the injection pressure falls with the escape of excess cement, it is supplanted by the stabilizing action of the semi-rigid rim making contact with the lips of the acetabulum. The cement then polymerises with the socket stable in the rehearsed position.

PIJ Socket

In its simplest form (i.e. with the plain face and without the long posterior wall feature) the PIJ socket (Fig. 7.8) has a rim with an oval lobe designed to contact the superior lip of the acetabulum. This design is reversible for left or right hips. The PIJ socket can be trimmed to fit all sizes of acetabulum from the average size (50-mm diameter) to one with an ovality of 56 mm in the antero-posterior diameter and 64 mm in a longitudinal diameter. A PIJ socket is available also in the extremely small size (35-mm diameter with offset bore). The PIJ design is not available at the moment for acetabula between 35 mm and 50 mm because acetabula requiring the ordinary small socket rarely need much deepening and the small undeepened acetabulum is adequately treated with a conventional socket fitting concentrically and pressed into the cement in a 45° direction.

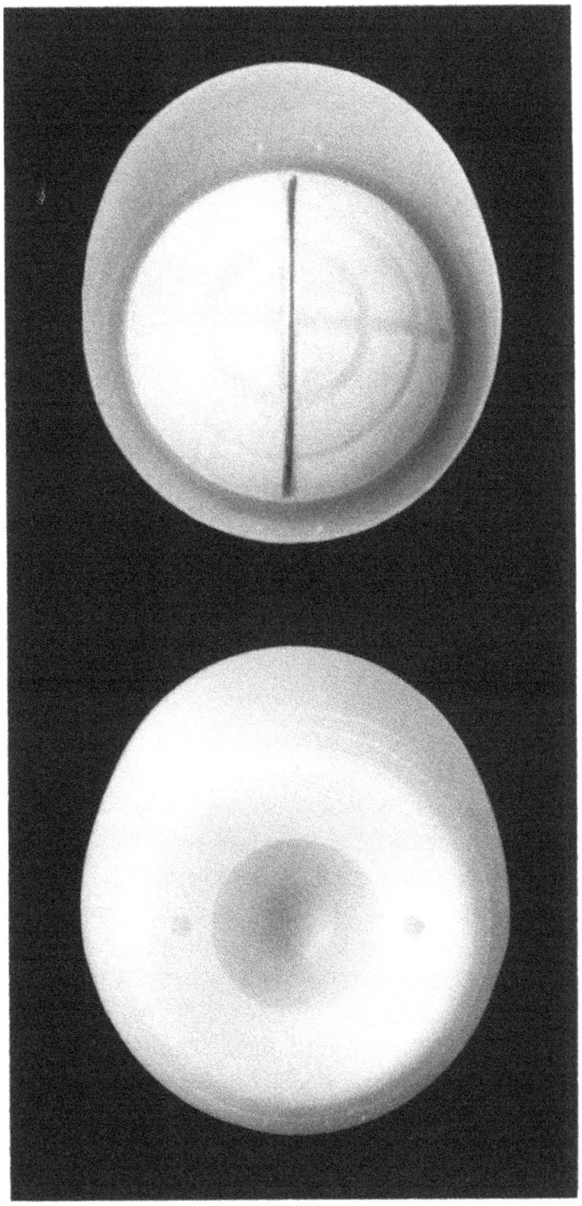

Fig. 7.8. Standard PIJ, or flanged, socket (i.e. without long posterior wall)

Trimming Technique

The first step in trimming a PIJ socket is to concentrate on the antero-posterior diameter. This is estimated by testing socket size-gauges in the acetabulum. For a large acetabulum it is useful to have a 52-mm diameter socket size-gauge in addition to large 50 mm and small 47 mm.

On the face of the PIJ socket two circular rings are engraved to act as guides for cutting the rim for the estimated *antero-posterior* diameter of acetabulum. The inner ring is 50 mm in diameter; the outer ring is 54 mm in diameter. The maximum *antero-posterior* diameter without cutting is 56 mm. When reducing the *antero-posterior diameter* of the rim it is convenient to start by making two straight, parallel cuts removing excess of rim from the front and back of the socket (Fig. 7.9a). These straight cuts will be tangents to the desired diameter of circle estimated from the rings engraved on the face of the socket.

The distal, or inferior, part of the rim is cut by following the appropriate engraved ring (Fig. 7.9b). It is advisable not to shorten the distal

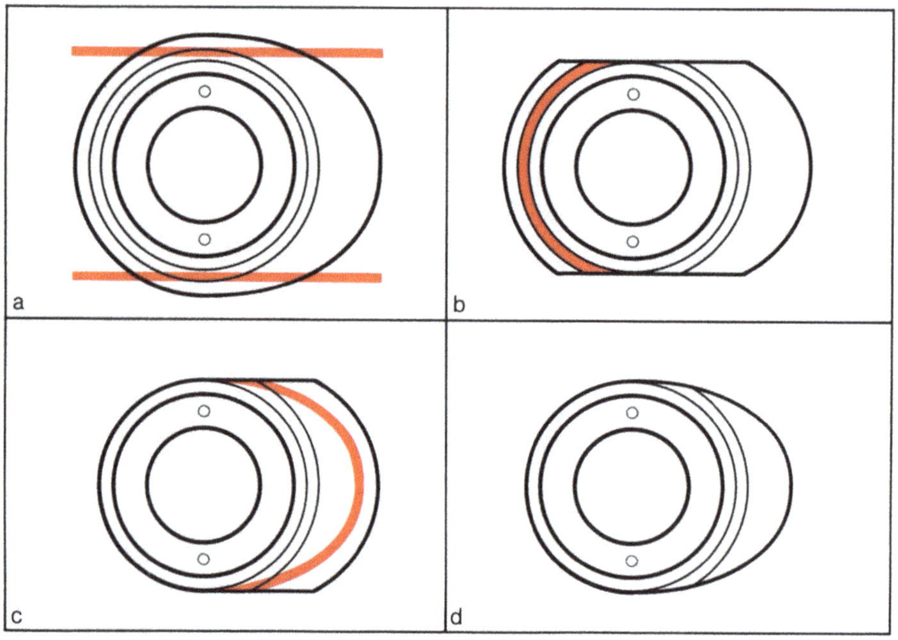

Fig. 7.9. **a** Cutting antero-posterior diameter to antero-posterior dimension of acetabulum. **b** Cutting distal curvature according to appropriate inscribed circle. **c** Trimming superior, oval lobe for roof of acetabulum. **d** End result

rim too much; practical experience shows that if the radial length of the rim is a little longer inferiorly than the antero-posterior radial lengths a more stable fit is obtained. The final step is to trim the oval superior lobe to fit under the roof of the acetabulum (Fig. 7.9c). This is done bit by bit, with trials in the acetabulum with the socket mounted on the socket-holder. The radial length of the superior lobe is correct when it fits under the superior lip of the acetabulum with the face of the socket at 45° to the long axis of the body (judged by the position of the handle of the socket-holder).

Before the length of the superior lobe is finalised the antero-posterior diameter must be able to enter the acetabulum. To be sure of this the bony rim of the acetabulum must be rendered clearly visible by good retraction. When adjusting the radial length of the superior lobe, it should start by being a little too long. This is indicated by the socket-holder tending to take up a position 10° or 15° below the horizontal (i.e. the face of the socket being directed too much towards the patient's feet, in what is sometimes called the 'closed' position). In this situation the handle of the socket-holder can be pushed towards the transverse position provided that strong pressure is maintained with the pusher on the face of the socket-holder to prevent the socket-holder disconnecting from the face of the socket. The superior lobe will deflect with a lateral concavity, this being in the situation for maximum pressure on the superior cement. It is not imperative that this type of fit should always be achieved.

Inserting the Cement

Once the PIJ rim is correctly trimmed and insertion into the empty acetabulum has been rehearsed, the procedure with cement differs not at all from the standard method.

The socket is pushed into the cement-filled acetabulum at first with the face directed slightly towards the patient's feet. When the inferior part of the rim has achieved full depth the socket-holder is moved to the transverse position (pressing firmly with the pusher on the face of the socket-holder during this change of direction so that the socket-holder does not disengage at a critical moment). Blood and air will be extruded through the small vent holes in the superior lobe as the socket is pressed into the cement.

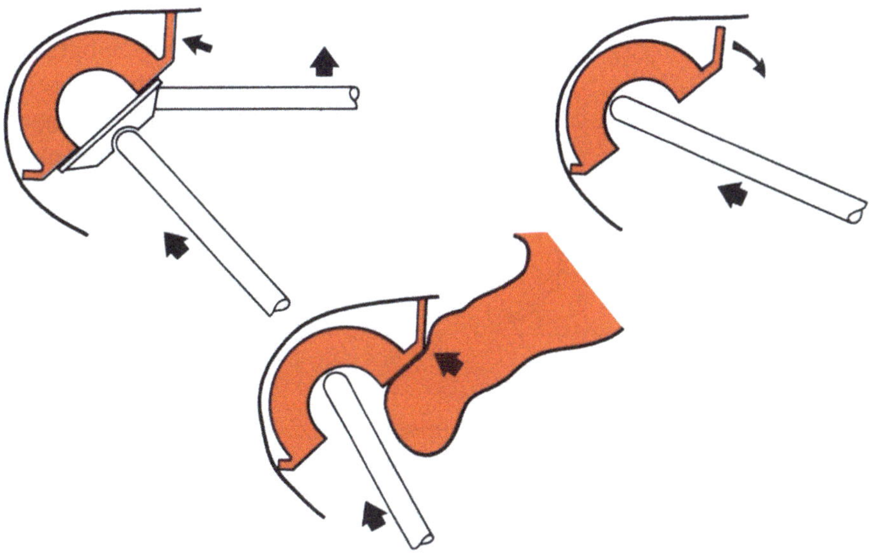

Fig. 7.10. Method of detaching socket-holder (only the 'self-ejecting' design will fit this socket). *Top left:* about to detach holder. *Top right:* holder has just been detached; pressure of cement and elastic recoil of the superior lobe of the rim is tending to tilt the socket into 'closed' position. *Bottom:* surgeon's thumb applies pressure to superior lobe of socket *immediately* after etaching socket holder and held until cement is hard

Having achieved transverse alignment of the socket-holder, the handle of the socket-holder is given to the assistant to hold for 3–4 s while the surgeon gives two or three quick, but quite light, blows with a mallet on the pusher before immediately resuming his hold on the handle of the socket-holder. These short, sharp blows 'coin' the cement into irregularities on the surface of the acetabulum and, **very important,** also ensure that the socket reaches the rehearsed depth and has not hitched against some trivial obstruction obscured by the cement and not detected during the rehearsal. The surgeon continues to apply strong force to the pusher and, because of the stabilizing action of the PIJ rim, this force can be exerted perpendicular to the face of the socket without pushing the socket too high in the acetabulum. The stability of the socket-holder at this stage under pressure from the pusher is noticeably greater than when a conventional socket is used. Nevertheless it is always possible to make a small change in alignment of the socket if the rehearsed position has not been immediately achieved.

It is unnecessary to remove excess of soft cement at an early stage; it is better to wait till the socket-holder is to be removed because then the excess cement will come away in one piece as the result of the excess cement having been severed from the deep cement by the 'knife-edge' contact between the narrow rim of the socket and the acetabulum. The socket-holder should be detached while the cement is soft and truly plastic and before the 'rubbery' stage of setting is reached.

A most important detail after the socket-holder is detached is immediately to apply thumb pressure to the upper part of the socket (Fig. 7.10) and hold thumb pressure till cement has set. This prevents the face of the socket tilting into the 'closed' position, under the influence of cement pressure and elastic recovery of a deflected superior lobe. Under pressure of the thumb the rigidity of the socket in the acetabulum is impressive.

Long Posterior Wall Design of Socket Face

The long posterior wall (LPW) design of socket (see Chap. 8) has contributed to the almost total disappearance of post-operative dislocation (Chap. 19). An ordinary socket is shown diagrammatically in Fig. 7.11a, with the head of a pros-

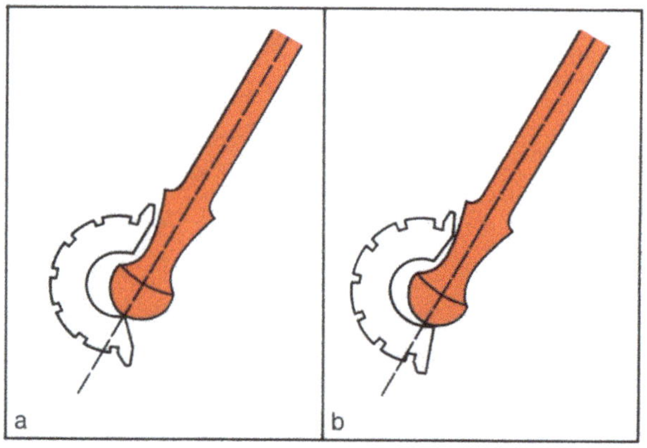

Fig. 7.11. a, b. Showing how LPW socket (**b**) offers some millimetres of platform to prevent head slipping posteriorly when the femoral prosthesis is at an angle which is critical for the standard design (**a**)

thesis poised at the 'water-shed' for dislocation; this is compared with an LPW socket with a prosthesis at the same angle to show how some millimetres of platform are still present to support the femoral head posteriorly before the summit of the sphere reaches the critical point of instability.

When using an LPW socket it must always be implanted with the long wall **posterior** (or **inferior** if the patient is visualized as being horizontal on the operating table). If a surgeon has not previously used the LPW socket he may be apprehensive about what appears to be an added complexity. He can be reassured, because should it happen that when finally cemented in situ the orientation is recognized as being incorrect it is an easy matter to cut away the excessively projecting wall with a sharp chisel, knife or gouge. When the LPW feature is cut away the socket reverts to the plain face of the original design and the dislocation rate for this was very low if the other technical details were correct. It is even possible by this means to correct a socket which has been put in back-to-front!

Anteversion of Sockets

The LFA socket should not be anteverted. This has been standard teaching since the very earliest days. Absence of anteversion combined with retention of the anterior capsule is an important element in preventing anterior dislocation in external rotation (Fig. 19.6, p. 318).

When using the LPW socket it is specially important to avoid anteversion because this would increase the projection of the posterior wall and could cause impingement against the back of the neck in the fully extended position of the hip.

LPW Socket Combined with PIJ Rim

If the single-lobed PIJ rim were to be combined with the LPW feature it would be necessary to

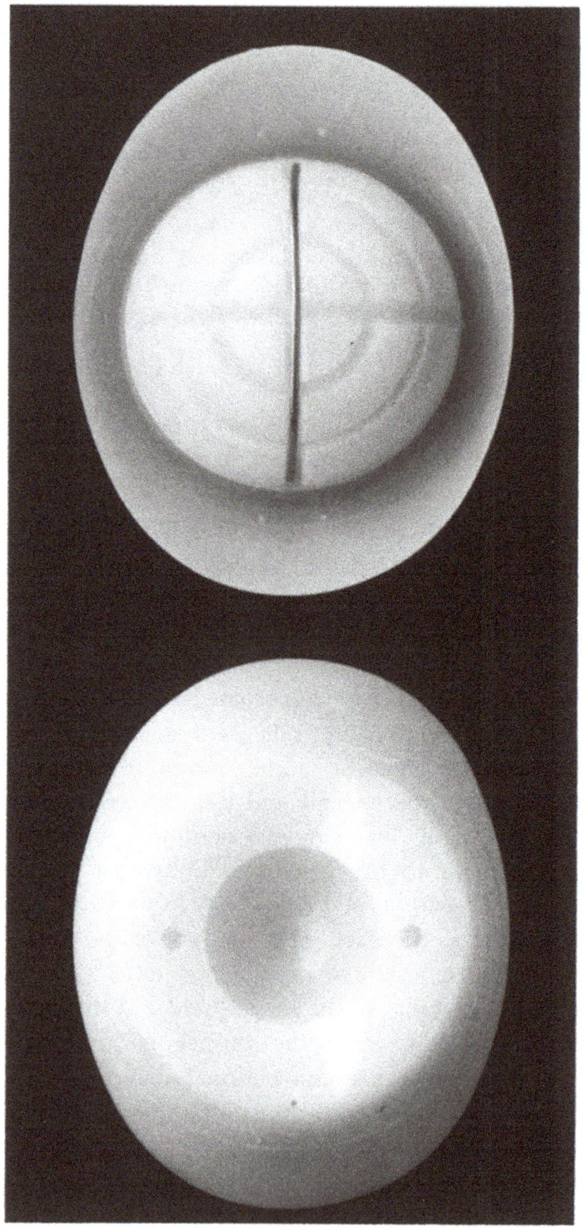

Fig. 7.12. LPW design combined with PIJ rim (three-dimensional view)

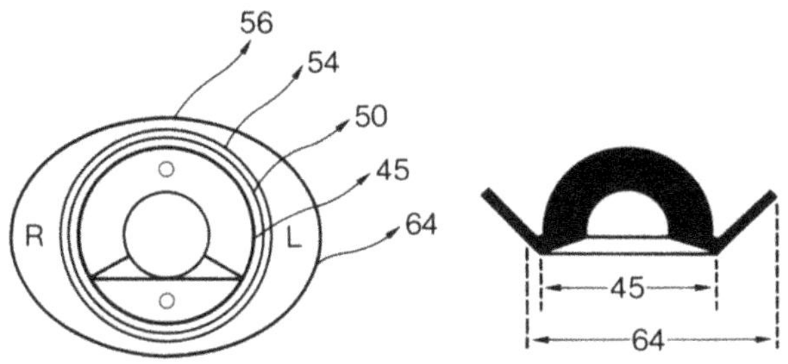

Fig. 7.13. Dimensions of PIJ design

provide sockets for right and left hips. To avoid this the PIJ socket with LPW is double-ended, with one lobe marked L and the other R (Fig. 7.12). If required for a right hip the lobe marked R is retained and the lobe marked L is cut away as a preliminary to cutting the rest of the rim to size. Preservation of the lobe marked for the operated side helps to guarantee that the LPW will be correctly orientated posteriorly; it is hardly conceivable that the long superior lobe

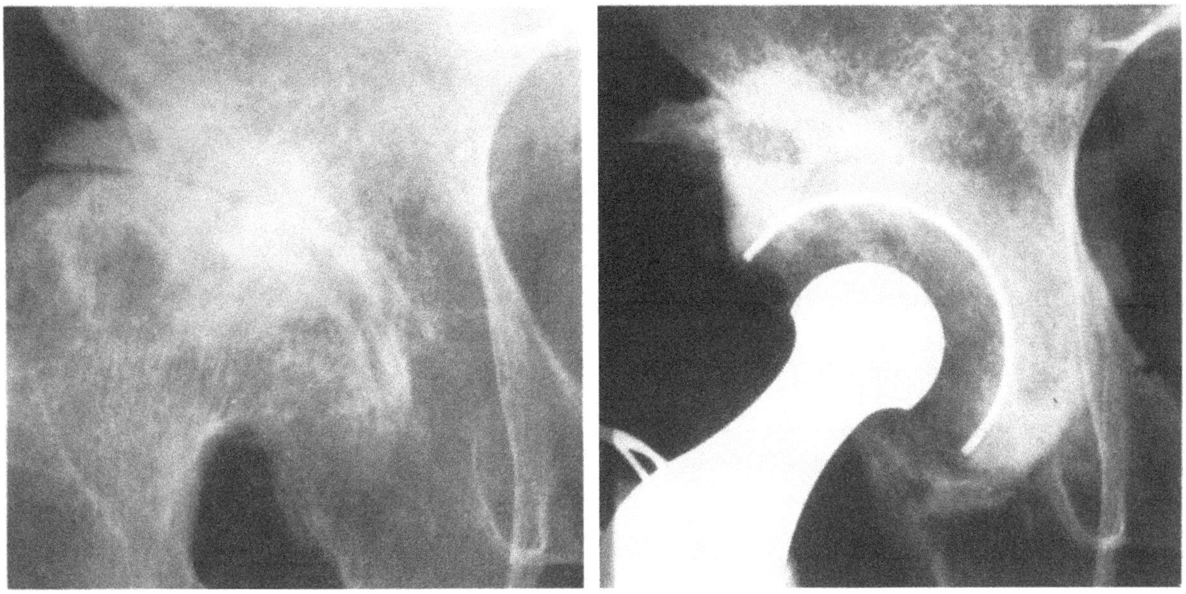

a b

Fig. 7.14. a Pre-op.; large femoral head and acetabulum. **b** One year post-op.; no demarcation of cement

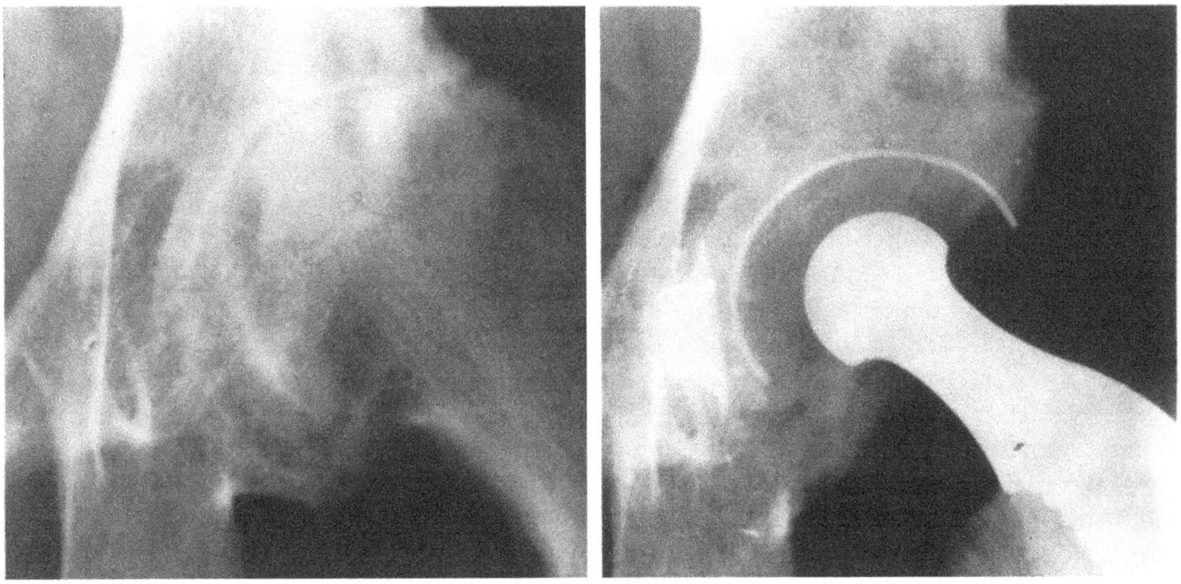

a b

Fig. 7.15. a Pre-op.; large femoral head and acetabulum. **b** One year post-op.; no demarcation of cement could be accommodated in an acetabulum elsewhere than superiorly!

Figure 7.13 shows the various diameters which are available when this socket is trimmed to fit. It will cover antero-posterior diameters from 45 mm to 56 mm, and a longitudinal ovality of 64 mm. Once the unwanted lobe (R or L) is cut away the method of trimming is identical with the technique described for the PIJ socket with plain face as described previously.

PIJ Socket in Position

Figure 7.14a, b and 7.15a, b show the PIJ socket in position 1 year after the operation in hips which both had large femoral heads.

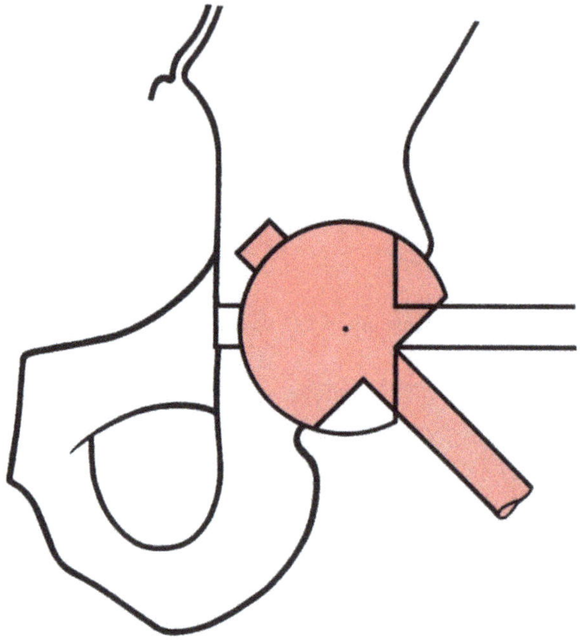

Fig. 7.16. When the object of reaming an acetabulum is merely to size it, **without deepening,** it is not important whether the reamer is directed transversely or at 45° headwards

Conventional, Hemispherical Socket Technique

The correct technique for implanting the original design of Charnley socket is described here for situations when the PIJ socket may not be available.

A simple hemispherical socket can effectively pressurize cement if it is concentric with the rim of the acetabulum and if it can be pressed into the cement with a force acting perpendicular to the plane of its face. These conditions commonly exist when the acetabulum is small. A hemispherical socket therefore can be used when a socket does not require deepening or when only slight deepening is required.

All sockets benefit from use of the expanding reamer because this ensures that the acetabulum is sized to accept the socket concentrically. When using the expanding reamer purely for sizing, without deepening, the rule to make the pilot hole with the pilot drill transverse to the body is no longer essential, because the object is merely to produce a hemispherical socket in the same position as the original socket (Fig. 7.16).

In these conditions the socket is introduced into the cement-filled acetabulum in the same attitude as will be the final orientation of the socket. The excess cement extrudes evenly round the rim.

Hemispherical Socket in a Large, Deepened Acetabulum

This is the situation where the PIJ socket is ideal but there may be occasions when a PIJ socket is not available. The following was the original routine before the introduction of the PIJ design. When the acetabulum is very large the socket must be kept low and must not be pushed in a headward direction. Transverse deepening helps to keep a socket low in a large acetabulum because the body of the socket lodges in the deepened part even when the upper part is unsupported.

Technique of Inserting Ordinary Sockets into Cement

1) The socket on its socket-holder is introduced 'edgeways' into the cement in the acetabulum with the face of the socket directed more towards the patient's feet (the 'closed' position) than will be the case in the final position (Fig. 7.17a).

2) When the deep part of the rim has reached the floor of the acetabulum the cement which has been extruded between the roof of the acetabulum

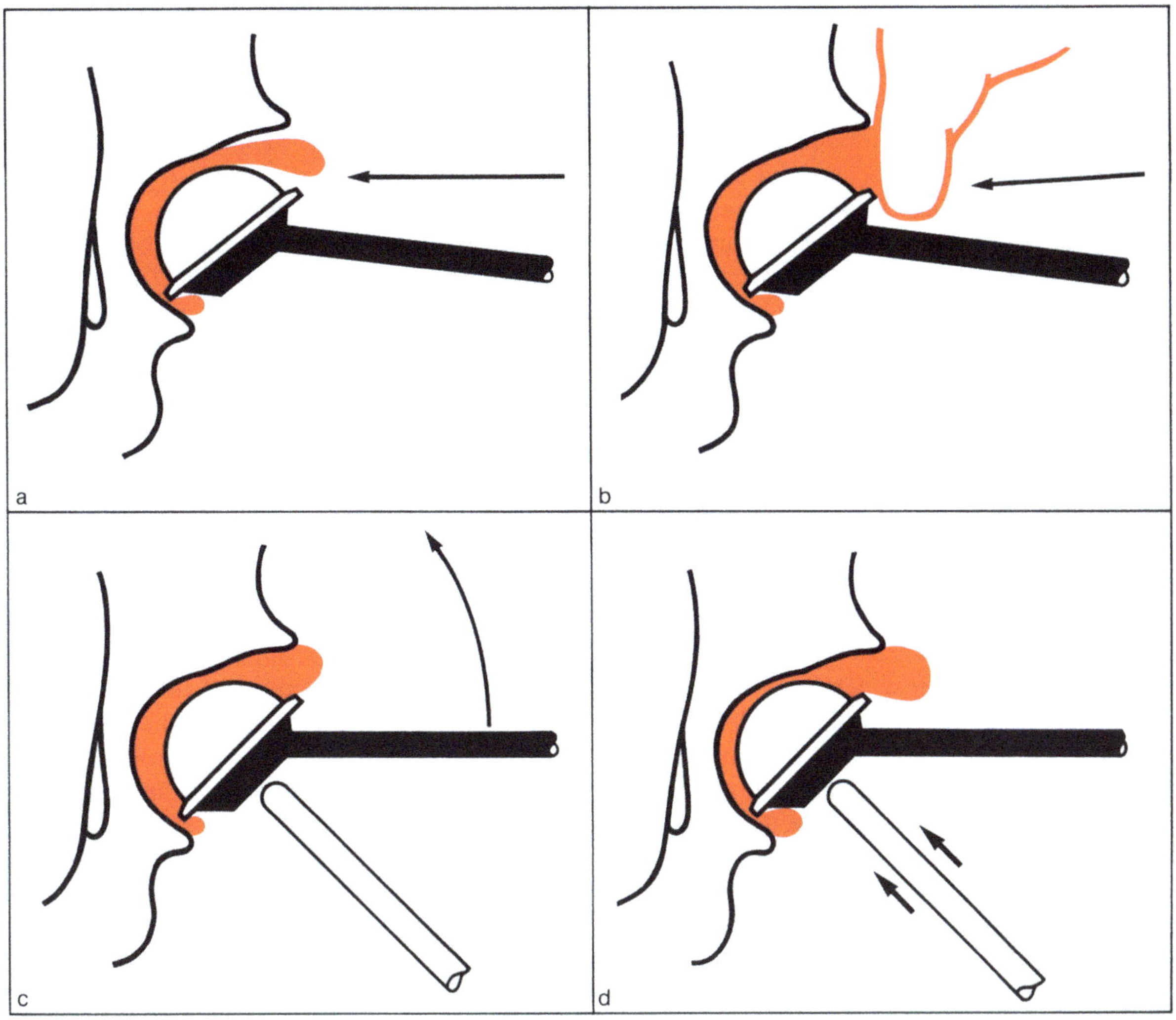

Fig. 7.17. **a** Standard socket inserted into cement with face of socket directed slightly to patient's feet. **b** Cement which has extruded from above socket is pressed back with surgeon's thumb. **c** Pusher is applied to face of socket-holder and handle is brought to transverse position. When doing this pressure on the pusher is relaxed a little to allow the socket to 'float' and draw cement into the space between it and depths of acetabulum. **d** Coining the socket in position. To be done **only when a layer of cement intervenes** between socket and floor of acetabulum

and the superior lip of the socket is pressed back into position with a finger or thumb (Fig. 7.17b).

3) The pusher is then applied to the face of the socket-holder and the handle of the socket-holder is brought to the transverse position (face of the socket at 45° with neutral anteversion). When doing this it is advantageous for the pressure on the pusher to be relaxed in order to permit the socket to 'float' a few millimetres away from the depth of the acetabulum and permit the rotating socket to carry some of the superior wedge of cement deep to the acetabulum (Fig. 7.17c).

4) The handle of the socket-holder is given to the assistant for a matter of seconds while the surgeon applies two or three short sharp taps with a hammer on the pusher, to coin the cement into minute irregularities on the surface of the acetabulum. These blows are important to ensure that the socket was not accidentally hitched against an obstruction and failed to reach the rehearsed depth in the acetabulum (Fig. 7.17d).

It is a mistake to hammer too powerfully, or too repeatedly, when performing this coining action because, if the deepest part of the body of the socket has reached the bottom of the acetabulum, hammering can do only harm by knocking the socket sideways in the cement and leaving a gap between cement and the wet lining of the acetabulum. Coining is effective only while a cushion of cement exists between socket and acetabulum; therefore a light quick tap with the mallet **early in the procedure** is recommended. Coining should not be left to the last act as the author originally used to teach. (With the PIJ socket coining cannot knock the socket sideways because the rim of this design of socket is making circumferential contact with the acetabulum.)

5) The surgeon waits for the cement to start to show signs of becoming stiffer than when received. **A 10-min clock and an operating room with a constant air temperature are important requirements.** This phase of waiting for setting is the difficult period. It is difficult to hold the conventional socket stationary in the acetabulum against respiratory movements of the patient's pelvis and without involuntary movements of the surgeon's hands. **A useful trick to enhance stability is for the surgeon to extend the index finger of the hand holding the socket-holder to touch the drapes on the wound edge to provide a fixed point as a steady.**

6) The socket-holder must be detached before the cement is reaching the rubbery stage. **Cement must never be allowed to harden with the socket-holder in position.**

The reason for detaching the socket-holder while the cement is still plastic is that it is quite impossible with conventional designs of socket to avoid small movements while the socket-holder is still attached. When the cement becomes rubbery the cement is no longer a viscous fluid; it has become an elastic solid; and tensile forces can now be transmitted from the socket to the cement to pull the rubbery cement away from the wet surface of the acetabulum. This cannot happen while the cement is still truly plastic and behaving as a viscous liquid. If the socket-holder is kept attached to the socket till polymerisation has started the cement already may be microscopically loose in the acetabulum even before the operation is ended. When cement in the 'key' holes of the acetabulum has hardened **it may seem to be completely rigid** on crude manual tests, but there may still be microscopic movement between cement and bone when the amplitude of movement is viewed in terms of histological dimensions. It is therefore important to detach the socket-holder while the cement is still plastic and thereafter steady the socket with the 'pusher' applied to the cavity of the socket. The tip of the Charnley pusher is much smaller in diameter than the concavity of the socket so that point-contact exists between pusher and socket. Small movements of the patient's pelvis or of the surgeon's hand therefore cannot be conveyed as angulatory movement to the socket.

Fear that the point-contact of the small end of the pusher will damage the socket is quite without foundation. All sockets must be slightly larger than the diameter of the femoral head in order to avoid the catastrophe of them ever being too tight on the prosthetic head; this discrepancy is further increased as the socket expands when attaining body temperature (the coefficient of thermal expansion of HMWP being much greater than that of metal). Therefore all sockets of HMWP have to adapt to the exact diameter of the femoral head by a combination of wear and plastic deformation, and a small depression caused by the small-radius end of the pusher (if any) will soon be eliminated.

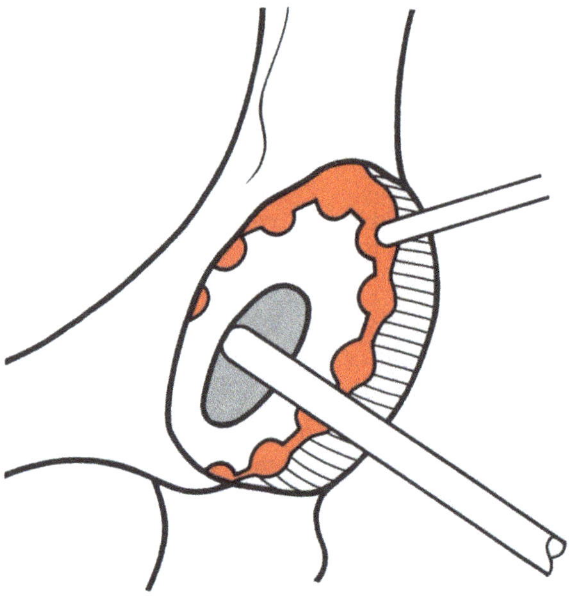

Fig. 7.18. The final step of packing the cement where it bulges out of the scallops round the rim of the socket while holding the socket in position by pressure with the pusher

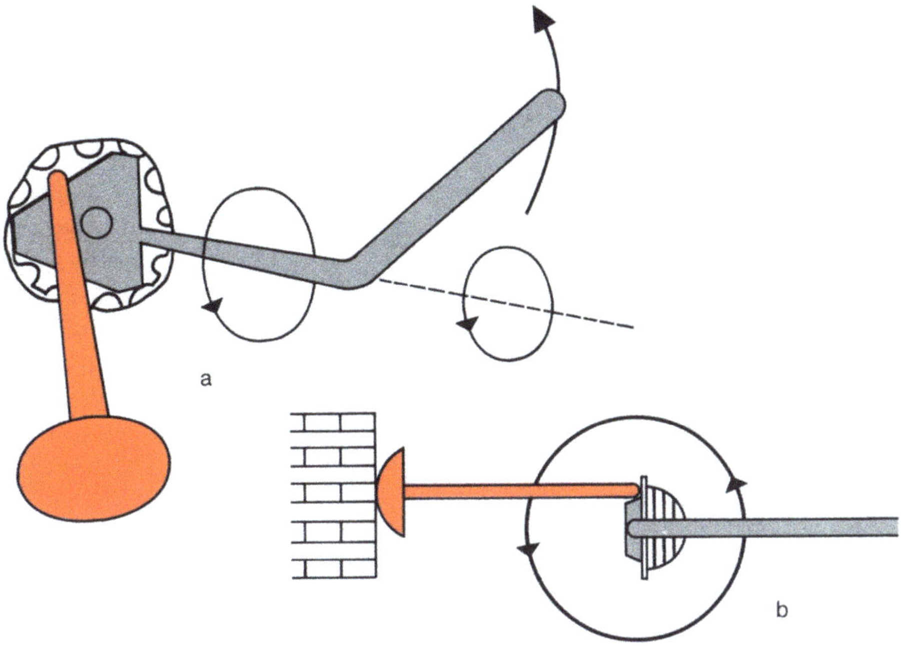

Fig. 7.19. a The pusher transferred from the face of the socket-holder to the face of the socket. **b** The pusher acts as a fixed stop while the socket-holder is peeled off the face of the socket by pronation of the hand holding the socket-holder

7) While waiting for final polymerisation the surgeon enhances the packing of the cement round the lips of the acetabulum with a small flat-ended instrument (a closed Kocher's forceps is useful). The packing is done by pushing the cement back into the scallops in the rim of the Charnley design of simple hemispherical socket (Fig. 7.18). **This is a very important stage** in the technique of using a conventional socket.

Detachment of Socket-Holder

Errors in the technique of detaching the original pattern of socket-holder from the original design of socket can pull the cement away from the wet bone of the acetabulum and so precipitate loosening even before the operation is complete. In this respect the self-ejecting socket-holder is a great advance, because it permits the pressure of the pusher to be maintained even in the moments when the socket-holder is being freed from the face of the socket. All sockets are now available with the faces drilled to accept the self-ejecting socket-holder but the original socket-holder cannot be used with the PIJ socket.

The **correct method of detaching the original socket-holder** (which grips between three studs on the holder and the scallops on the rim of the socket) follows the following sequence of movements:

1) The tip of the pusher is transferred to the exposed surface of the plastic socket anterior to the triangular plate of the socket-holder (Fig. 7.19a).

2) The surgeon 'locks' his arm and the hand which is holding the pusher in three-dimensional space by holding his shoulder muscles rigid. The tip of the pusher is thereby merely applied to the face of the plastics socket without exerting pressure against it. The pusher thus acts as a **fixed stop** to prevent the socket moving towards the pusher during the next step.

3) The surgeon's other hand (the one holding the socket-holder) is now pronated. This peels the holder away from the surface of the socket because the pusher, acting as a fixed stop, prevents the socket following the socket-holder in the direction of pronation (retroversion) (Fig. 7.19b).

The two common errors are: For the surgeon (1) to rotate both hands in the same direction, or (2) to push too hard with the fixed stop and so rotate the socket in the opposite direction (anteversion) after the holder is detached. Because the right hand holds the socket-holder for a left hip, and the left hand for a right hip, detachment of the socket-holder for both right and left hips always involves pronation of the hand holding the socket-holder. The self-ejecting socket-holder avoids all these problems.

Final Cautionary Note

When handing the socket-holder to the assistant, for the surgeon to be free to coin the socket into the cement, always warn the assistant not to angulate the holder in the direction of the patient's head (towards the 'open' position). This is a very common assistant's error. It is very bad to have to bring the handle of the socket-holder back to the transverse position if the assistant has pulled it towards the patient's head, because this will pull the cement away from the wet bone in the roof of the acetabulum. It is better for the assistant to err in the direction of angulating the socket-holder towards the 'closed' position, because then to assume the final position the cement would be compressed against the roof of the acetabulum.

Chapter 8

Types of LFA Hip Socket

This section describes the different types of Charnley hip socket. It is hoped that the whole range of sockets in time will be replaced by one single type and size of PIJ design which can be cut down to suit all sizes of adult acetabulum. The very small (35-mm-diameter) socket with offset bore will be the only exception. Until this policy comes into action it is necessary to describe the range as it exists at the moment (1978).

There are two series of sockets, one has the LPW configuration of face and the other the plain face. In the author's practice the LPW series is used exclusively, but the plain face is available for surgeons who have been satisfied with this design and see no reason to change. The smallest of the sockets (the 35-mm-diameter 'offset bore') at the moment does not have an LPW version (Fig. 8.1).

All the sockets have a semicircular wire wear marker. The shape of the semicircular wear marker shows in the X-ray whether the socket is of the plain face series or whether it is an LPW series: in the plain sockets the semicircular wire terminates in short right-angled bends turned inwards towards the femoral head: in the LPW sockets the ends of the semicircular wire are straight (Fig. 8.2). All sockets are drilled on the face to enable them to be used with the two pins projecting from the face of the self-ejecting socket-holder. The original design of socket-holder can be used only with the original large and small sockets with the scalloped rims.

With one exception it is possible to attach a socket to the socket-holder in an erroneous orientation and therefore precautions must be observed. All sockets should have the semicircular wire marker in the same plane as that of the two right-angled limbs of the handle of the holder. The LPW socket when on the holder must have the letter L or R visible, corresponding to the side of the hip being operated on (the opposite letter will be obscured by the holder). With the self-ejecting socket-holder errors of attachment of the socket cannot be less than 180°; therefore the semicircular wire marker can never be out of the coronal plane. When a plain-faced socket is used on the self-ejecting holder this is the special case where it is impossible to make any error of orientation.

With the LPW socket on the self-ejecting holder it is possible to place the socket with 180° of error even though the semicircular wire marker is correctly orientated (the LPW then being anterior rather than posterior) **but this cannot occur if the letter L or R,** corresponding to the side of the hip being operated on, is visible while on the socket-holder.

PIJ sockets cannot be inserted without the self-ejecting holder.

The very small socket with offset bore (35-mm diameter) also needs the self-ejecting holder. A third pin projecting from the face of the holder makes it impossible to attach this very small offset bore socket upside down, i.e. with the thick wall of the socket not in its correct position to accept wear in the roof of the acetabulum. The face of the standard self-ejecting socket-holder unfortunately is too wide for the 35-mm offset bore socket and this means that when trying to use the standard self-ejecting socket-holder with the 35-mm offset bore socket it may be displaced headwards in the soft cement (by about 2.5 mm) at the moment of ejection unless the surgeon has been able to remove bone at the inferior aspect of the acetabulum to prevent this. It is therefore most essential to rehearse ejection in this special case before cement is inserted. A special small-diameter self-ejecting socket-holder is available for the 35-mm socket if required.

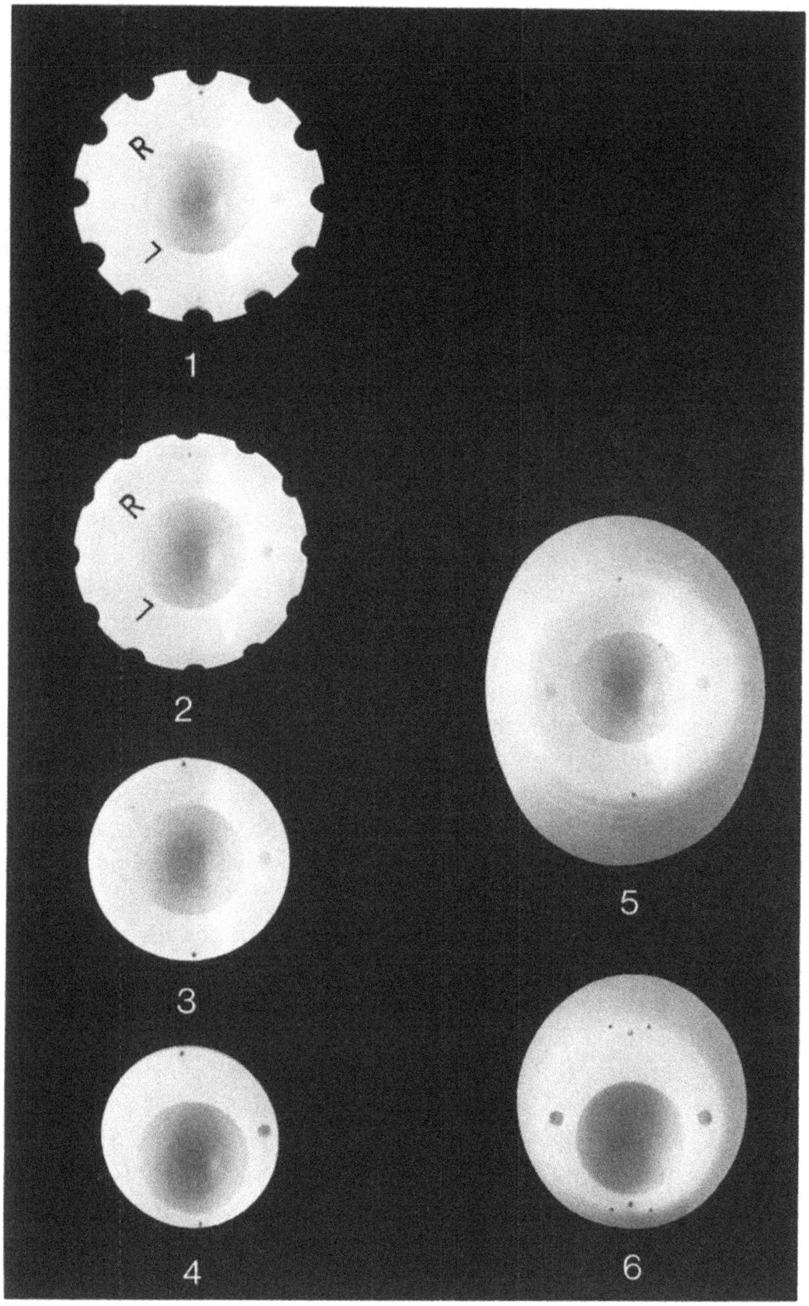

Fig. 8.1a. Lateral surfaces of the sockets currently in use. All except 4 and 6 are of the long posterior wall (LPW) design and though this feature is not clearly visible in these illustrations it lies on the right side

The PIJ version of the 35-mm diameter offset bore socket avoids this problem because when this socket has been trimmed to size and thereby made stable in the socket in a rehearsed position it can be inserted without a socket-holder (i.e. just with the fingers).

All LFA sockets are designed to be inserted without anteversion. Anteversion weakens resistance to anterior dislocation in external rotation of the femur. Absence of anteversion does not block flexion range, in such movements as cutting toenails, etc., because this movement is a combination of abduction and external rotation. Anteversion must be avoided with LPW sockets because this will cause the long posterior wall to project excessively. Anteversion makes the semicircular wire marker invalid for making measurements of the wear of the socket.

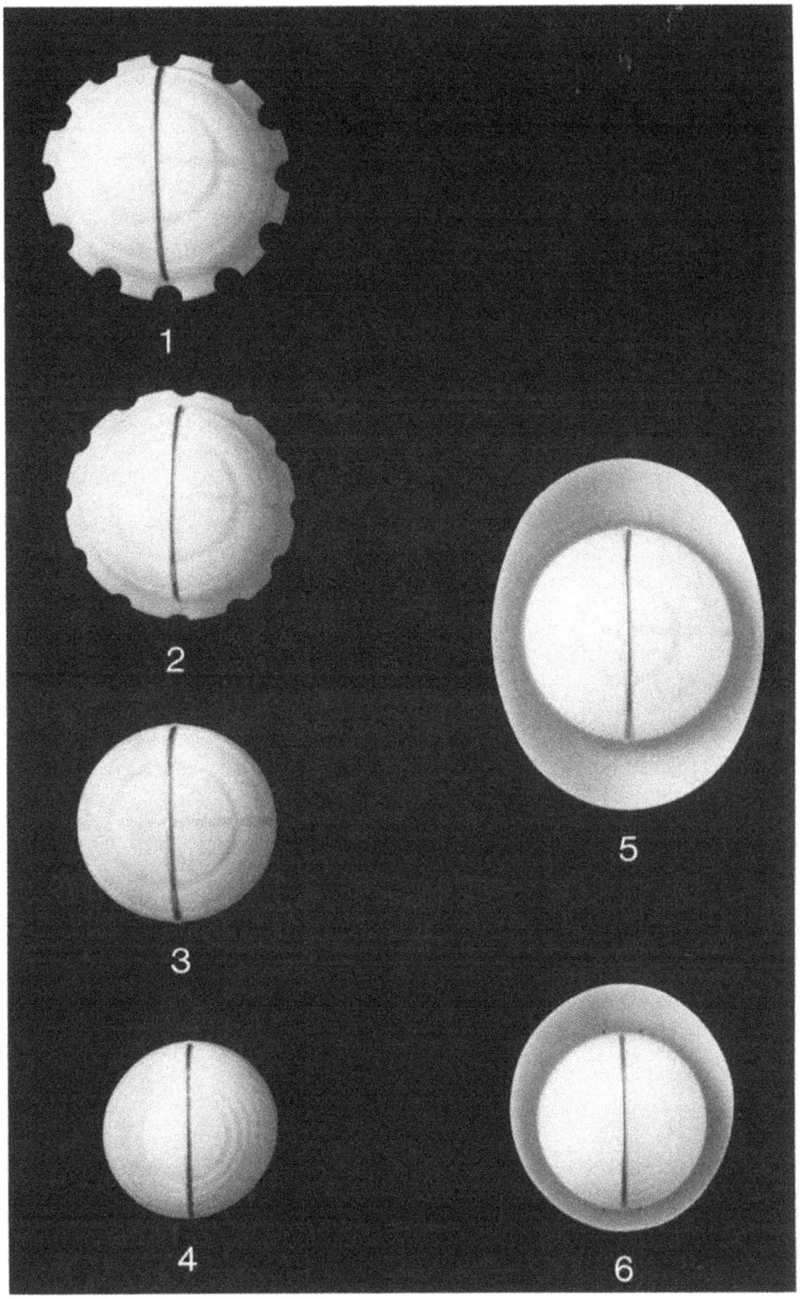

Fig. 8.1 b. Deep surfaces of same.
1 Large-diameter, 50-mm, LPW
2 Small-diameter, 47-mm, LPW
3 Extra-small, 40-mm, LPW
4 Offset bore, 35-mm, plain face.
5 Flanged socket (PIJ) LPW, 45–56 mm a-p diameter, up to 64-mm ovality.
6 Flanged (PIJ) offset bore, plain face, 35–47-mm a-p diameter, maximum ovality 50 mm

Dimensions of LFA Sockets

There are only two important dimensions in sockets: the diameter of the face of the socket, and the diameter of the body (Fig. 8.3).

Original Series (i.e. not PIJ Design)

1) **Large socket (plain face and LPW):** 50-mm-diameter face; 43-mm-diameter body.

2) **Small socket (plain face and LPW):** 47-mm-diameter face; 40-mm-diameter body.

3) **Extra small socket (plain face and LPW):** This latter is the small socket without the rim; therefore the diameter of the face is the same as the diameter of the body, i.e. 40 mm.

4) **Offset bore socket (plain face):** This has no rim and the diameter of the face is the diameter of the body, i.e. 35 mm. In this very small socket

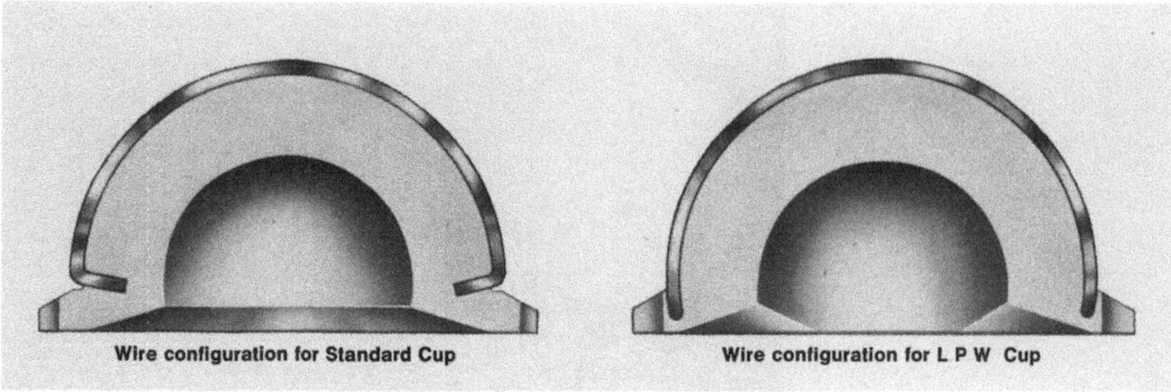

Fig. 8.2. Configuration of wire markers. On left plain face socket; on right LPW configuration

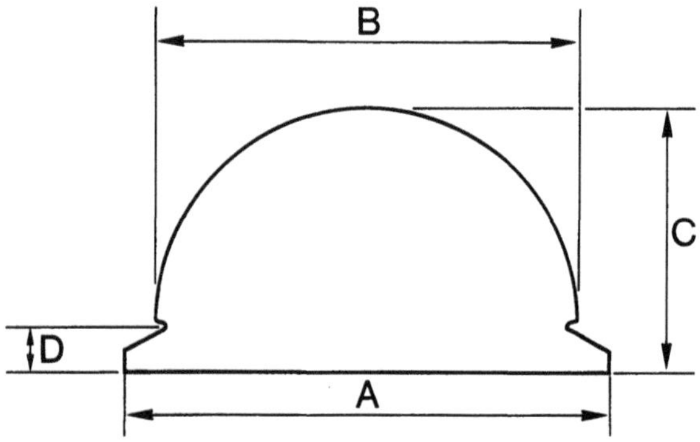

	A	B	C	D
Large **(LPW** and **Standard)**	50	43	28	4
Small **(LPW** and **Standard)**	47	40	26	4
Extra Small **(LPW** and **Standard)**	–	40	26	–
Offset Bore	–	35	21	–

All dimensions in millimetres.

Fig. 8.3. Basic dimensions of non-flanged (non-PIJ) sockets

the thickness of HMWP available for wear in the upper part equals that in the large socket, i.e. about 10 mm, excluding cement grooves.

Pressure Injection (Flanged) Sockets

5) **PIJ socket (plain face):** Single lobe: reversible for right and left hips.

6) **PIJ socket (LPW):** Double lobes marked L and R.

Both these PIJ sockets, single lobe plain face (5, above); and double lobe LPW (6, above); have inscribed circles on the face to guide cutting:

Smallest circle	diameter 50 mm
Largest circle	diameter 54 mm
Without cutting	diameter 56 mm
With all rim removed	diameter 43 mm

Maximum ovality 64 mm

7) **35-mm offset bore with PIJ rim:** Body diameter 35 mm (with all rim removed). Maximum diameter of rim 47 mm. Maximum ovality 50 mm

Serrated Cutting Scissors

Trimming the PIJ rims is greatly facilitated using heavy scissors with serrated cutting edges. These can be improvised from small plaster scissors.

Chapter 9

Femoral Prostheses – Theory

Femoral components in total hip replacement are subject to loosening of cement and fatigue fracture of the stem. The latter is a problem which we hope will become more a matter of historical interest than a continuing problem, because there are still many details (surgical, mechanical and metallurgical) not yet fully explored which hold out hope of a solution.

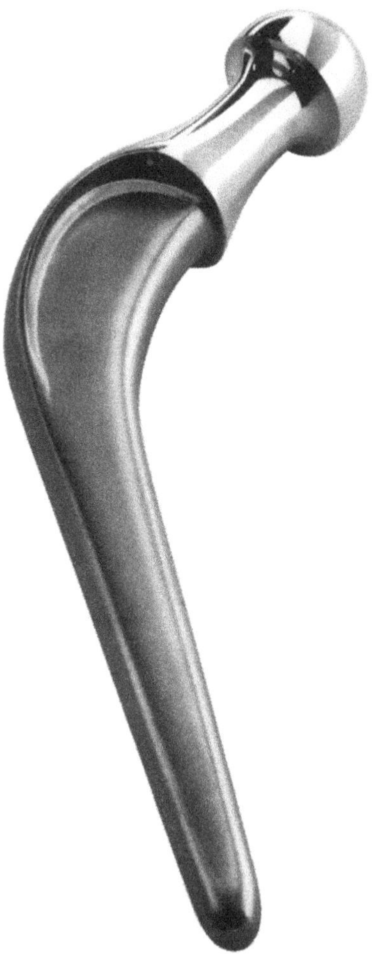

Fig. 9.1. General three-dimensional view of flanged prosthesis

In this chapter a new design of stem is described (the flanged or 'Cobra' stem) whose purpose is to secure optimum use of cement in the upper levels of the medullary cavity. The general appearance of this stem is shown in Fig. 9.1.

Loosening of Femoral Cement

Loosening of cement in the femur can take three forms:

1) Loosening of the whole of the cement-bone interface
2) Loosening of the prosthesis inside the cement with most of the cement-bone interface remaining sound
3) Loosening of the prosthesis and fragmentation of the cement in the upper part of the femur, with the distal prosthesis and cement-bone interface remaining sound

1) Loosening of the whole cement mass is characterised by radiological demarcation of the whole of the cement interface (if the cement is radio-opaque). This picture is sometimes difficult to distinguish from the effects of deep infection (Fig. 9.2) but two features which partially clarify the diagnosis are the sedimentation rate and whether or not the cement-bone bond in the acetabulum also is affected.

A minute degree of loosening sometimes can produce cavities, with clear-cut walls and without periosteal reaction, caused by foreign-body granuloma invading the endosteal surface of the femur. The appearance in Fig. 9.3 preceded a fatigue fracture of the prosthesis; the granulomatous material presumably was produced in the region of the medial femoral neck and migrated distally.

2) Loosening of a prosthesis inside the cement is probably more common than is generally sup-

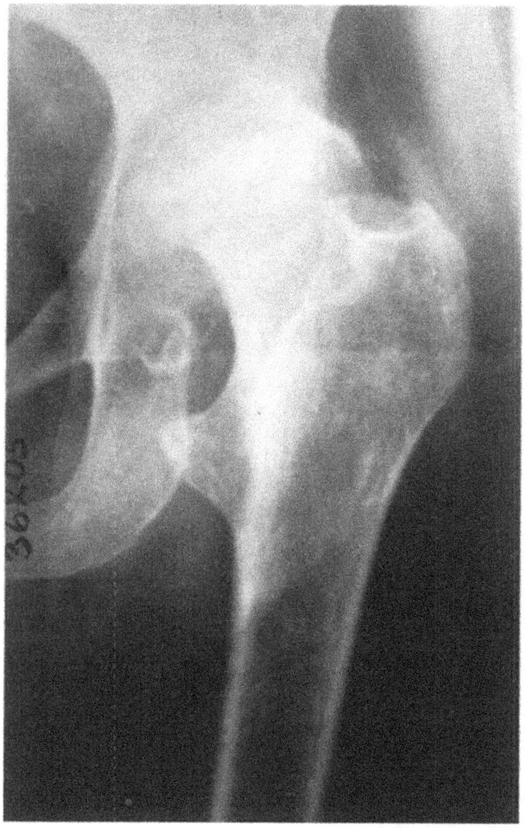

a

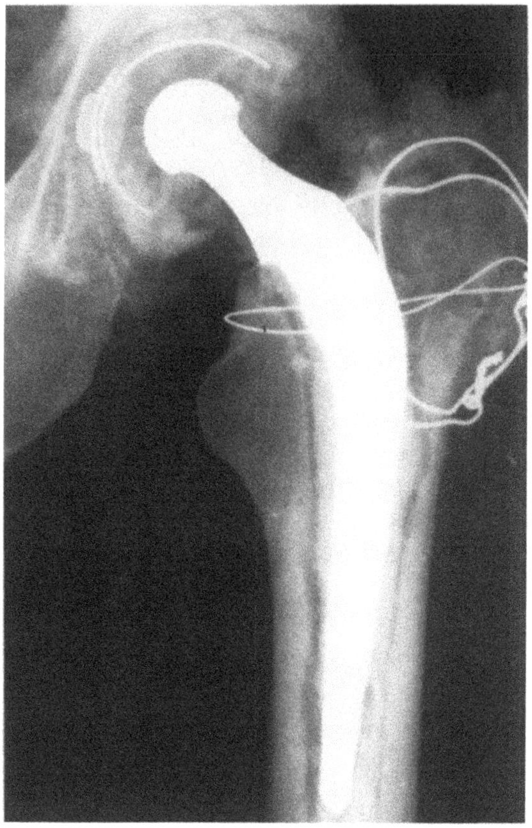

c

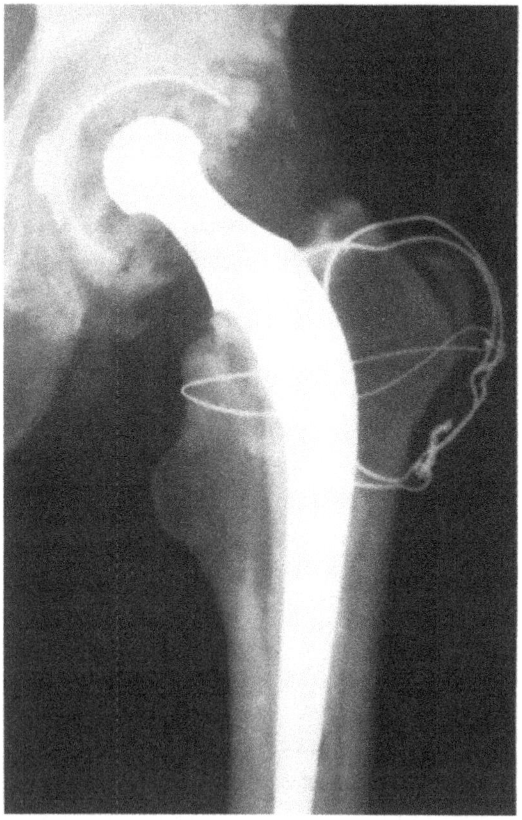

b

Fig. 9.2. a Pre-op.: osteoarthrosis; male patient. **b** One month post-op. Slight symptoms. Socket loose. Bad technique. **c** One year post-op. Symptoms now warrant re-operation. Socket, and now femoral cement, both loose. Very suspicious of infection, but ESR only 5 mm in 1 h; no growth on cultures at re-operation; result of re-operation still good after 2 years. Therefore considered to be simple loosening and not infected (but still could be an infection!)

posed because this state is characterised by the absence of any radiological abnormality of the cement-bone interface. When explored the prosthesis is found to be loose in the cement track but the cement track is firm in the femur. This situation could be the result of defective surgical technique, such as wobbling the prosthesis in the cement, or moving the prosthesis to a last-moment corrected position just when the cement is setting.

One presumes that when pain accompanies this type of loosening it must be caused by an exposed part of the metal stem moving against an exposed area of bone on the endosteal surface of the femur.

3) **Loosening of the upper part of the cement-bone bond**. This is the most serious and probably the most common cement defect. In this case load transmission occurs almost entirely through the distal part of the stem of the prosthesis. At every loading cycle the upper end of the prosthesis will flex elastically in relation to the fixed, distal portion of the stem. These cyclic stressings will be concentrated in the metal stem at the junction of the fixed and moving parts.

If there is an adequate thickness of cement and a good cement-bone bond in the upper levels of the femur the elastic deflection of the upper end of the prosthesis will be reduced in amplitude by the cement but some deflection of the prosthesis must always occur ('stress cannot exist without strain'). The amplitude of deflection of the metal of the prosthesis will be checked by compression of the cement between the prosthesis and the bone of the medial femoral neck and if the cyclic stresses in the metal are below the endurance limit fatigue will not occur. In this situation the prosthesis may survive indefinitely without fatigue fracture even though it may be flexing more than would be the case with a better cement technology.

If the elastic deflection of the prosthesis is so great that it transmits cyclic movement to the cement-bone interface in the medial femoral neck, then the living tissues will respond with a histiocyte (macrophage) reaction. The bone of the medial femoral neck will then start to become eroded by a biological process as opposed to a mere mechanical process of attrition. A vicious circle is then set up: the bone is eroded by the biological process; the cement loses mechanical support from the bone; the cement then fails to reduce the amplitude of elastic deflection of the prosthesis; the upper levels of the cement then become fragmented. The vicious circle continues until cyclic stressing in the metal exceeds the endurance limit for fatigue and it is then merely a question of time before fatigue fracture occurs.

Figure 9.4 shows the upper end of a post-mortem femur from which the cement has been removed by a solvent 8 years after operation. The changed appearance of the cancellous bone over the upper 3 cm indicates an early granulomatous reaction produced by cyclical movement of the cement against the bone. This reaction is not present lower in the femur where the cement fixation was perfect. There was no obviously detectable looseness on macroscopic examination of the specimen.

The crux of the problem lies in the behaviour of the cement-bone **interface** at the medial femoral

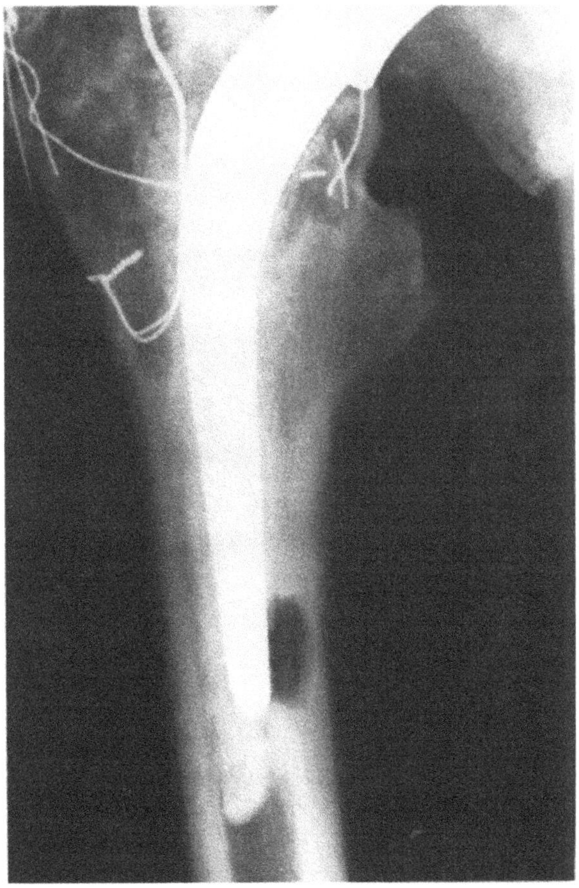

Fig. 9.3. Clear-cut endosteal cavity typical of foreign-body granuloma. This can precede fatigue fracture of a femoral prosthesis, indicating minute movement of cement on bone. Granuloma tracking down from calcar femoris

neck during load transmission. If the cement (1) interlocks perfectly into the endosteal cancellous surface and (2) if the amplitude of cyclical displacement of the cement does not exceed a certain amount, then the displacement can be accommodated within the elasticity of the cancellous bone. In this happy situation relative movement between the cement and the bone of the interface does not occur; the superficial layer of the more elastic substance (the cancellous bone) moves as one with the surface of the less elastic substance (the cement).

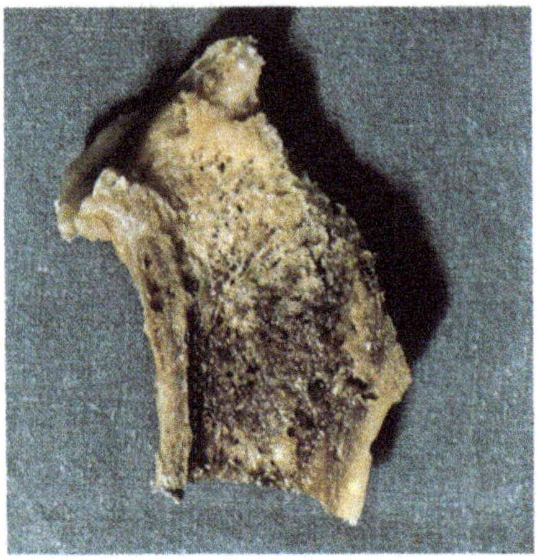

Fig. 9.4. Cement dissolved out of femur after 8 years of excellent function (post-mortem specimen). Note change in appearance of cancellous bone over upper 3 cm. Suggests that cyclical cement movement was inducing granulomatous reaction not present at lower level

This state is easily visualized in compression, but it is in shear that a perfect interlock of the surfaces is essential. In attempting to visualize the situation in shear one must not regard the medial femoral neck as composed of solid cortical bone. The dense bone of the external layers of the cortex grades into cancellous bone on the endosteal surface and this is still the case even when soft, superficial cancellous bone has been curetted away.

It is generally said that there is approximately a 10 times difference in elastic modulus between bone and cement, but it seems unlikely that such a difference exists between **cancellous** bone and cement. Therefore if good cement technology has achieved a satisfactory interlock into an endosteal cancellous surface one can visualize cement and cancellous bone behaving as a composite elastic layer. According to this idea the zone of maximum elastic movement will be sited away from the interface and will lie **inside** the cancellous layer (Fig. 9.5).

If this interpretation of the situation in the cement-bone interface at the medial femoral neck is correct, a histiocyte reaction produced by relative movement between cement and living bone

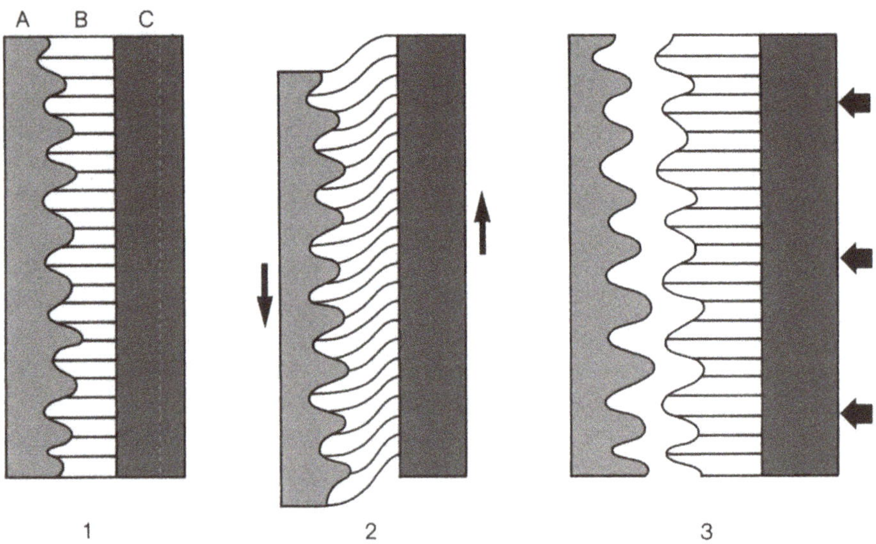

Fig. 9.5. *1 A.* cement; *B*, cancellous endosteal lining of femur; *C*, cortical bone of femur. *2* In shear we visualize elastic deformity taking place within the thickness of the layer of cancellous bone without relative motion occurring at the cement-bone interface. *3* (Surfaces distracted to illustrate absence of adhesion.) When under compressive loads there will be no relative motion between the surfaces

will occur only (1) if the cement-bone interlock was imperfect from the start, and (2) if the amplitude of elastic displacement of the cement is too great to be accommodated within the elastic range of the cancellous layer between cement and cortex in the medial femoral neck.

Plugging the Medullary Cavity of the Femoral Shaft

Methods are currently being employed to improve injection of cement in the distal femoral cavity. The use of cement-guns and the plugging of the medullary cavity distal to the prosthesis stem certainly will improve distal cement injection. Nevertheless because fatigue fractures of femoral prostheses have occurred following unsophisticated cement technology, this suggests that even this was more effective in the distal than in the proximal levels.

Because it is obviously important to achieve a reasonable proportion of the total load transmission from the upper levels of the prosthesis to the upper levels of the femur, one wonders whether to improve distal cement injection might not be counter-productive; it could be argued that we need 'controlled subsidence' of the distal half of the prosthesis stem to enable the cement in the upper end of the femur to maintain load-bearing contact with the cancellous bone. This might break the vicious circle, starting as elastic deformation of the upper end of a prosthesis too effectively supported below, and ending as granulomatous resorption of the medial femoral neck.

If it were to be decided that plugging the distal medullary cavity of the femur is a worthwhile objective, a plug porous to blood, fat and air but impermeable to viscous cement would be a convenient method. Figure 9.6 show such a cement restrictor but a radiolucent device would be more attractive. Certainly the extension of cement for some distance beyond the tip of the prosthesis, when the cavity is not occluded, is cosmetically distasteful.

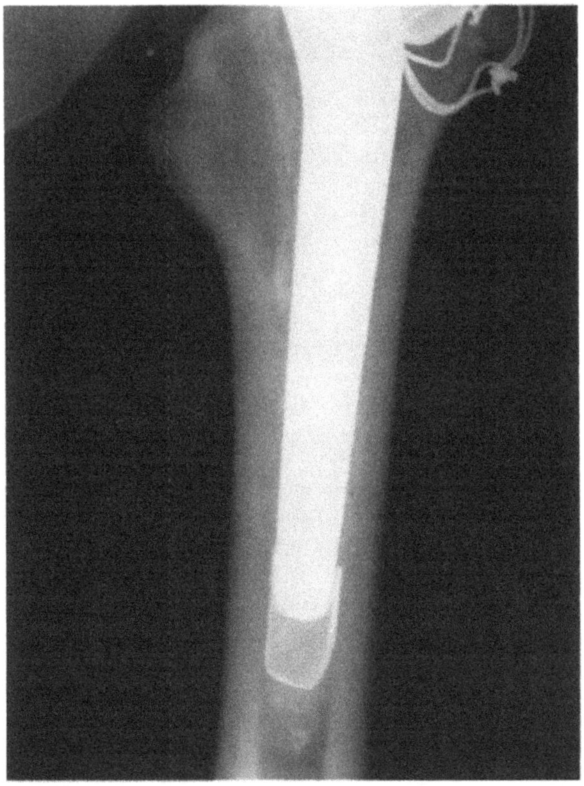

Fig. 9.6. Cement restrictor in situ. Some cement has penetrated the very small gap between the exterior of the restrictor and the endosteal surface of the bone. A radiotranslucent plastics device would be more pleasing

Limits to a Metallurgical Solution of Fatigue Fractures

To avoid fatigue fractures of femoral prostheses many surgeons imagine that all that is needed is for prostheses to be made out of some alloy possessing exceptionally high resistance to fatigue. But, even if this were possible, there would then almost certainly be an increased rate of re-operation for late loosening **if there were no parallel improvement in the surgeon's cement technology**. The patient's problem is to avoid the need for a second operation of any kind, and most especially to avoid a second operation which will be more difficult than the first.

A purely metallurgical solution could lead in the extreme case (i.e. infinite fatigue resistance) to a result such as that illustrated in Fig. 9.7. This patient now aged 74 is still functioning perfectly on this prosthesis 13 years after the original operation but nobody would like to see our 'vigorous male of 45 years of age' develop something like this even if fatigue fracture were never to ensue.

This patient with osteoarthrosis was operated on in February 1964 at the age of 61 years and achieved a near

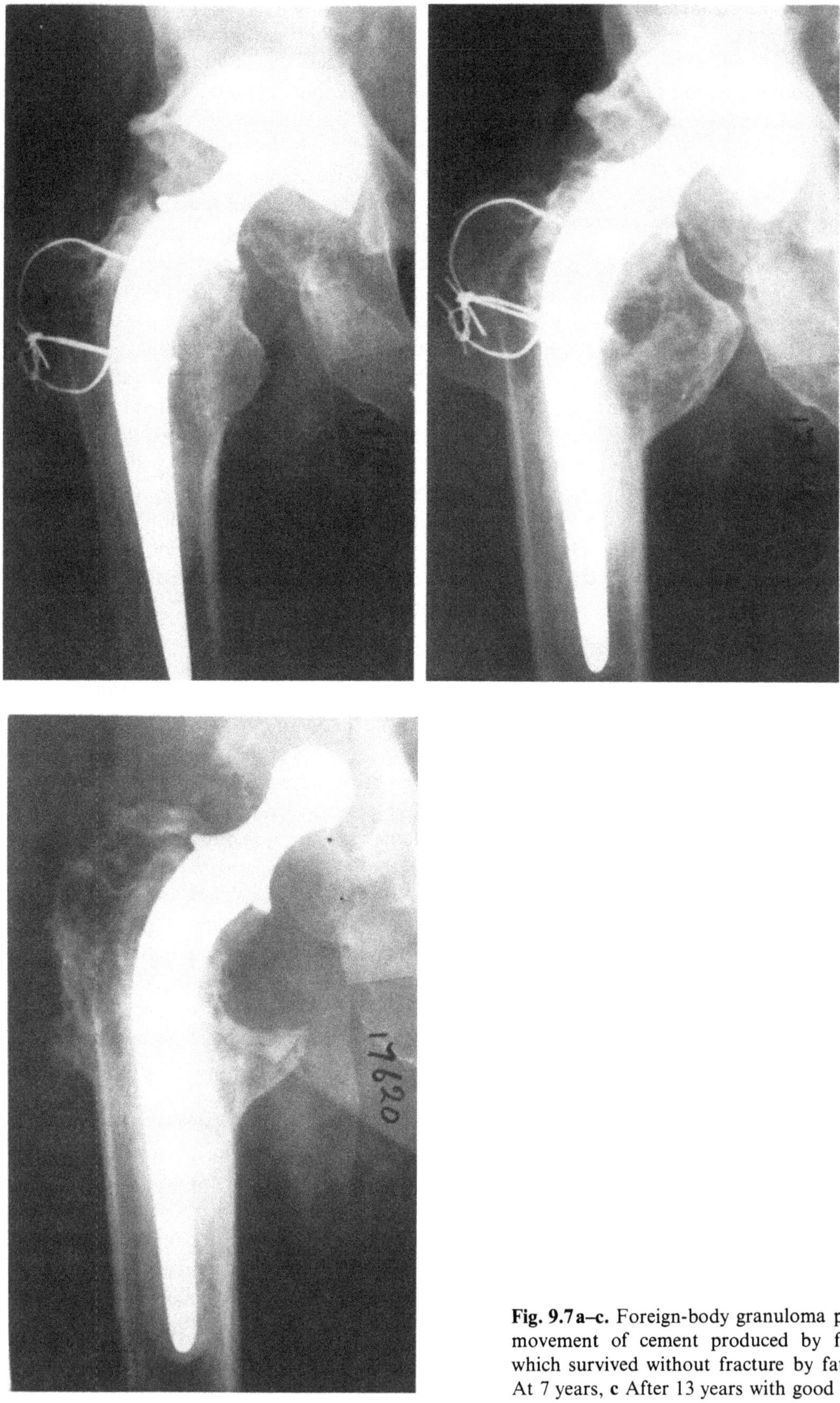

a b c

Fig. 9.7 a–c. Foreign-body granuloma produced by cyclic movement of cement produced by femoral prosthesis which survived without fracture by fatigue. **a** Post-op, **b** At 7 years, **c** After 13 years with good function perfect result. A cavity filled with inspissated caseous material developed in the medial femoral neck as discovered at exploration 9 years later. Because function was good and the patient by now was 70 years of age and frail it was decided to take a chance, leaving it as an excision biopsy.

This case illustrates in an unusual way the destructive effect of a foreign-body granuloma in the medial femoral neck. In this granuloma only a small number of abraded particles of HMWP were found and these were thought probably to be secondary invaders from the synovial cavity, sucked into the cement-bone interface.

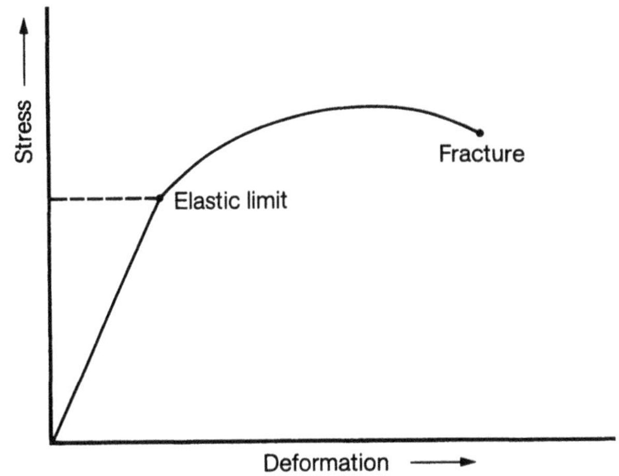

Fig. 9.8. Classic stress-strain curve for metals. Showing perfect elasticity up to stress level corresponding to the elastic limit for that specimen

Stiffness of a Prosthesis

To protect the medial femoral neck from movement at the cement-bone interface it can be argued that a stiff prosthesis would be advantageous. A stiff prosthesis might be defined as one which deflects less, at the junction of its proximal and distal parts, than has been customary with prostheses in the past, when the distal part is soundly implanted in the stiff cortical bone of the shaft of the femur.

To appreciate why it is not possible to stiffen a prosthesis **of a given size and shape** merely by using a stiffer alloy it is necessary to outline some elementary features of metallurgy.

The 'stress-strain curve', basic to all strength-of-materials tests (Fig. 9.8), can be explained in very simple terms in the following way. When a specimen of metal is subjected to increasing tension it will elongate; at first the elongation will be strictly proportional to the tension so that over the early range the graph of elongation plotted against tension will be a straight line. Over this first part of the range of elongation the specimen will return to its original length when the tension is removed, which constitutes perfect elasticity. The slope of the curve in this first part of the graph reveals the elastic modulus of the metal. The term 'elastic modulus' denotes a concept which makes it possible to **measure** that quality which in lay terms underlies the ideas of 'stiffness', 'elasticity', or 'flexibility' when a metal object is bent, short of producing a permanent deformity.

As the elongation under increasing tension continues, a point will be reached beyond which the plot of tension against elongation will no longer continue as a straight line (the elastic limit). Beyond this point the specimen will not return to its original length on removing the load. Beyond the elastic limit, too, the behaviour will differ for different metals and different alloys, but the essential fact in relation to a femoral prosthesis is that the initial slopes of the stress-strain curves for almost all the 'surgical' metals are more or less the same (i.e. their elastic moduli are more or less the same). The main difference is that those alloys with high tensile strength will retain their elasticity over a greater range of elongation than will metals of low tensile strength. The same applies to metals with different abilities to resist fatigue failure; up to their elastic limits the slopes of the stress-strain curves will be almost identical.

The message for the orthopaedic surgeon therefore is that **for a given size and shape** of prosthesis the **stiffness cannot be increased merely by changing the alloy**. The only way to increase the stiffness of an implant is to increase the cross-sectional dimensions. This will have the same effect as reducing the total load on the prosthesis as regards stress in the metal.

To take the argument a little further let us imagine that Fig. 9.9 shows the deflections under load of two **prostheses**, identical in shape and size, but one made of a low tensile metal (L) and the other of a high tensile metal (H). If the maximum load the prosthesis is likely to experience corresponds

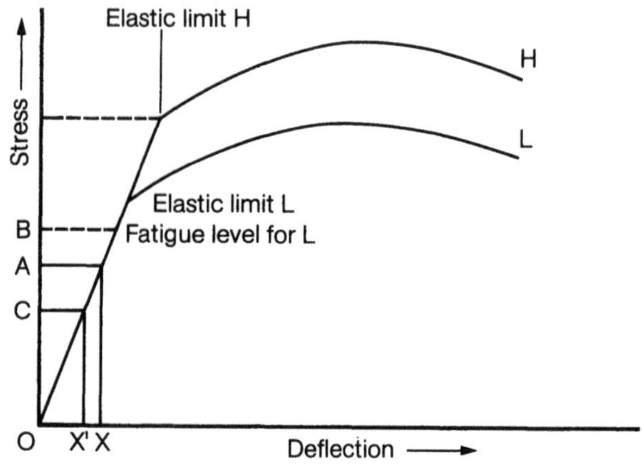

Fig. 9.9. Theoretical schema: to explain how maximum deflection, OX[1], tolerated by cement-bone interface takes precedence over the intrinsic tensile, or fatigue, strengths of the metals. Cross-section dimensions to reduce stress to C are of predominant importance. Note that the 'fatigue level' on this graph is a theoretical concept introduced here for teaching purposes; without specifying the number of reversals of stress it has no place on such a graph

to stress level B then high tensile metal is not needed; but when used **with cement**, in the **living body**, the matter now becomes more subtle. If the elastic deflection 0–X caused by stress A is so great that it will produce movement at the cement-bone interface the higher tensile strength, and even the higher fatigue resistance, of metal H is of no value because the bone of the medial femoral neck will resorb. On the other hand if the maximum elastic deflection of a prosthesis which the cement-bone interface can tolerate is 0–X[1], the only solution is to **increase the cross-sectional areas** of the stems of **both** prostheses. The cross-sectional areas must be increased until under any load neither the L nor the H prosthesis will deflect more than 0–X[1].

With the exception of titanium, the elastic moduli of all the surgical metals are in the range of 200–230 GN/m^2 even though their ultimate tensile strengths are in the range about 520–1700 GN/m^2 and their fatigue strengths about 245–600 GN/m^2 (Swanson and Freeman[13]). The case of titanium needs special consideration in the light of the above argument. Like most metals titanium retains its modulus of elasticity almost unchanged whether pure or alloyed and this is only half (100 GN/m^2) the stiffness of the other surgical metals. Theoretically therefore the cross-sectional dimensions of prostheses made from titanium and its alloys should be greater than with other metals even though the tensile strength and fatigue strength of titanium alloys can be very high.

'Physiological' Flexibility of Femoral Prostheses

The view is held by some that a stiff femoral prosthesis is unphysiological and that a more flexible implant comparable with the modulus of bone would be preferable. The fear is that rigidity of the implant might cause osteoporosis, especially in the region of the medial femoral neck, as a result of the load-bearing function being by-passed to lower levels of the femoral shaft. But osteoporosis within about 1 cm from the cut end of the cortical bone is inevitable because it no longer receives the physiological stimulus of 'end-bearing' loads. On the other hand the cut ends of the vertical trajectories of cancellous bone on the inner surface of the medial femoral neck are specialized for transmitting compressive load to the cortical bone of the femoral shaft, and ought to be able to accept this type of load from the cement in a physiological manner. One can therefore imagine load transmission by this route reaching the cortex rather more than 1 cm distal to the cut end of the femur (Fig. 21.10a, p. 336). In our long-term radiological studies we have not seen progressive osteoporosis in this region.

Resorption of the cut surface of the femoral neck up to 15 years after total hip replacement has been a constant object of scrutiny in this unit because during the Teflon era this was the site where granulomata first caused erosions and fear that particles of HMWP might be doing the same thing has been a constant urge to vigilance (p. 66). This type of resorption was studied by Bocco and Langan[26] and though it can be quite severe it appears to become stationary before 10 years have elapsed after the operation. It ranges from 0 to 1.5 cm (and very rarely to more than 2.0 cm) but the quality of the residual bone in the 10–15-year study appears normal for the particular patient.

Elasticity of Cement

Our concept of the elastic behaviour of acrylic cement affects our ideas on the relative stiffness or flexibility of a femoral prosthesis and also our ideas on whether a thick or thin layer of cement should be interposed between a prosthesis and the medial femoral neck.

Because cement is about 100 times less stiff than metal the view is often expressed that it is not reasonable to hope to support a prosthesis with cement at the medial femoral neck, and in attempting this a thin layer of cement would offer better support than a thick layer. Nevertheless, and regardless of the logic of the foregoing argument, the author believes from surgical experience that a thick layer of cement at the medial femoral neck does in fact protect the bone in this region better than a thin layer. Bocco and Langan (1977)[26] compared 119 hips with an average of 4.5 mm cement intervening between calcar and prosthesis, and 97 hips with an average thickness of 13.2 mm (Figs. 6.8, 6.9, p. 71, 72). The thick layer of cement protected the calcar 10 times better than did the thin one. The comparison is complicated by the fact that a thick layer of cement means a greater valgus alignment of the prosthesis.

The relative merits of a thick or thin layer of cement is another aspect of the question whether it is better to fill the enlarged medullary cavity of the upper end of the femur with metal, leaving only a thin shell of acrylic cement, or to have a prosthesis of rather smaller calibre (though of adequate cross-section to behave with sufficient stiffness) and fill the enlarged medullary cavity with cement to whatever thickness is necessary. A thick layer of the low-modulus material (cement) might be able to absorb elastic deformation of the prosthesis and diffuse it over the cement-bone interface in a way not possible with a thin layer. On the other hand a thin layer of low-modulus material (cement) would be exposed to less elastic deformation if the stem of the prosthesis had a maximum cross-section of metal.

Surface Area of Metal

The surface area of metal through which load is transmitted to cement in the highly stressed region of the medial femoral neck should be as great as possible to prevent splitting of the cement (Fig. 9.10). All designers have now learned to avoid stems with sharp or wedge-shaped cross-sections in this zone. But splitting of cement in the highly loaded area of the medial femoral neck can also be precipitated by failure to centralize the stem in the cement (Fig. 9.11). This can be the result of striving too zealously to avoid anteversion of the neck of a prosthesis (an early dogma of the author, now modified to accept 5° of anteversion, and sometimes even 10°). If the stem of the prosthesis is not centralized the U-shaped layer of cement may be pierced and the prosthesis may come into direct contact with bone so that progressive splitting of the cement may result. The dorsal flange of the author's design of prosthesis centrali-

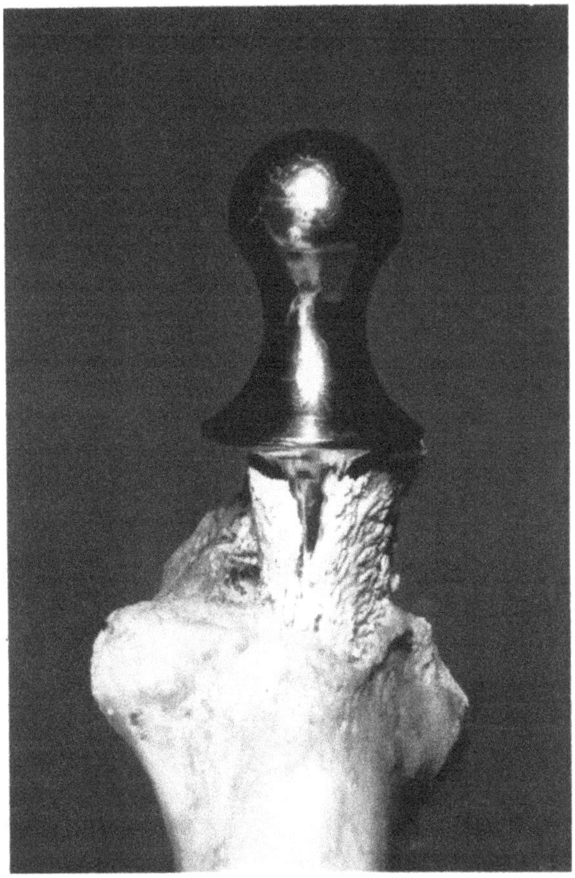

Fig. 9.10. Splitting of cement between medial femoral neck and concave surface of stem of prosthesis even though surface of metal is rounded in cross-section. Splitting here is considered to be result of layer of cement being too thin, with the prosthesis in varus

zes the stem of the prosthesis in the enlarged medullary cavity and fosters a U-shaped bed of cement of even thickness between bone and metal (Fig. 9.12).

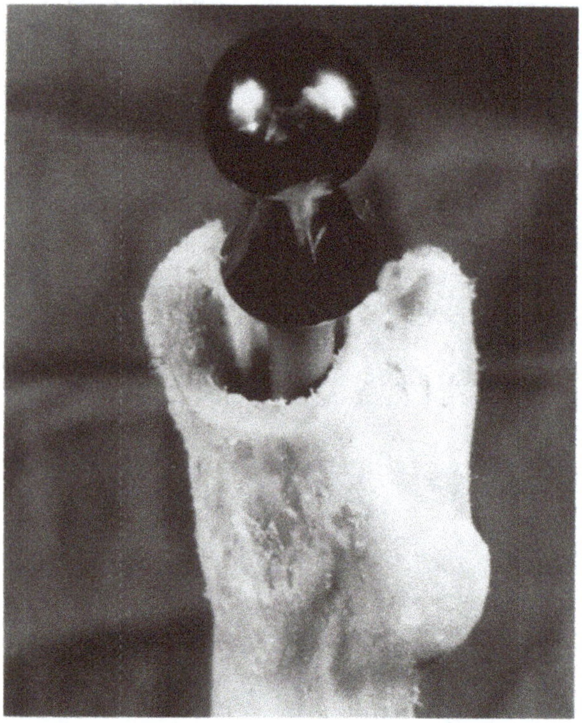

Fig. 9.11. Splitting of cement at medial femoral neck can result from failure to centralize prosthetic stem. In this case this is the result of struggling to avoid anteversion of the femoral neck

When considering the 100 times difference in elastic modulus between metal and cement, a large surface of contact through which load is transferred from metal to cement invites the idea of walking on snow with skis or snow-shoes. The author believes that by distributing load over a large area of low-modulus cement something of this mechanism comes into play with the flanged prosthesis.

Load Transmission to Cement by Dorsal Flange of Prosthesis

The dorsal flange of the femoral prosthesis increases the area of metal transmitting load to the polymerised cement. The dorsal flange transmits load to the cement in front and behind the stem and the cement transmits the load, in shear, to the rough internal surfaces of the bone of the femur in front of and behind the stem. The flange of the prosthesis also stiffens the upper half of the prosthesis against elastic deformation in a rotary direction. This should help to preserve the cement-bone interface in the upper levels of the femur when the hip is loaded in flexion.

Offset of a Femoral Prosthesis

In the Charnley profile, the 'offset' of a femoral prosthesis is a concept rendered clearly visible because of the straightness of the distal three-quarters

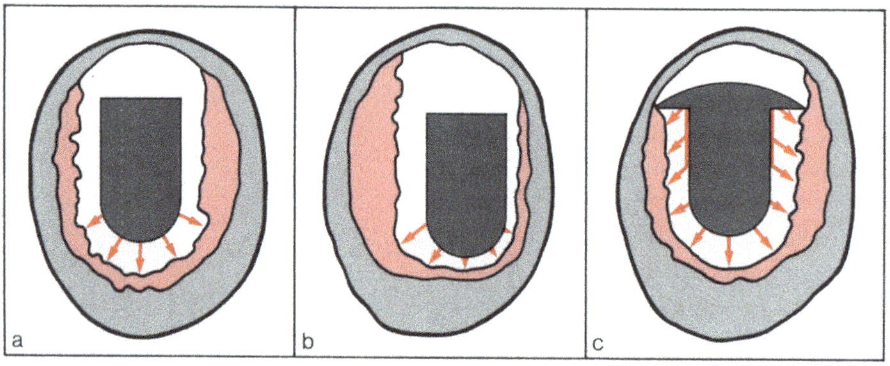

Fig. 9.12 a–c. Load distribution through medium of cement to cancellous bone of medial femoral neck. **a** Ideal arrangement of conventional system. Polished sides of prosthesis, in shear, fail to transmit load to cement. Total load is therefore received by cement in floor of medial femoral neck. **b** Eccentric placement of prosthesis worsens situation by exposing thin layer of cement to initiate fracture. **c** Flanged (Cobra) prosthesis stem puts all the cement under compressive stress even though polished sides of body of prosthesis not capable of transmitting load in shear. Part of load on prosthesis transferred in shear to rough surfaces of cancellous bone in front and behind the stem

of the stem. This renders it easy to locate an axis in the distal part of the stem and deviations from alignment with the axis of the shaft of the femur, in valgus or varus directions, are very noticeable.

The amount of offset is measured as the perpendicular distance between the centre of the head and the axis of the stem (Fig. 21.16, p. 339). In prostheses with curved stems, such as those derived from the original Thompson profile, it is not easy to define varus or valgus alignment. The smaller the offset of a prosthesis, the stiffer and stronger will the prosthesis be, because this will reduce the bending moment of the joint force. The smaller the offset, the smaller also will be the stresses on the cement between the concavity of the prosthesis and the medial femoral neck. Prosthesis offset is discussed in more detail in Chap. 21.

Stem-Neck Angle

Different offsets of the Charnley design of prostheses maintain a constant 50° stem-neck angle (Chap. 21). Different offsets also can be obtained by changing the stem-neck angle; the offset becomes less as the stem-neck angle becomes more valgus.

Weight of Patient—Strength of Prosthesis

In a study of fatigue fractures of femoral prostheses (Charnley)[(29)] a correlation was found between the patient's weight and fatigue fracture, especially in male patients. Ideally a scale should be constructed relating a patient's weight to the calibre of prosthesis stem, but on the other hand this theoretical ideal is rendered unnecessary by the practical policy of always using the heaviest prosthesis reasonably possible. The insertion of heavy-calibre femoral prostheses becomes a simple matter if the trochanter is elevated and if rotary femoral reamers are used.

Rotatory Forces on a Femoral Prosthesis

In the course of fatigue tests on Charnley femoral prostheses the manufacturers (Messrs. Chas. F. Thackray Ltd.) were unable to produce fatigue failures after 10^7 loading cycles in a corrosive environment in what was considered to be a physiological direction. They also failed to produce fatigue failure even when the prosthesis was loaded in a disadvantageous direction, this direction of loading being with the stem of the prosthesis vertical and the load also acting vertically, so exposing the stem to the full effect of the offset.

When however a prosthesis of the first-generation 'flat-back' type was positioned so that the frontal plane of the prosthesis was inclined 15° from the vertical, the force still acting vertically, (as though standing on a hip flexed to 15°), a fatigue fracture could now be produced in a corrosive environment. One explanation was that stress in the stem was increased because the front-to-back dimension of the section, now exposed to cyclical bending, was narrower than the side-to-side dimension in the vertical position. But in the fatigue tests of the flat-back prostheses of the first generation the point of interest in the initiation of the fracture was the effect of the corner joining the flat lateral surface of the stem with the anterior surface. This corner was not sharp; it had a perceptible radius after finishing and polishing[1]). So striking is this feature that it is usually possible to tell (Wroblewski[(30)]) from the inclination of the plane of the fracture whether a fractured first-generation prosthesis with flat back has been in a right or a left hip.

Recognition that rotatory forces can produce fatigue fractures of the stem of a femoral prosthesis might explain how fractures occasionally can occur so low in the stem that bending moments in the frontal plane at this level would seem to be impossibly small (as low as 2.5 cm above the tip) (Fig. 9.13). To prevent rotatory forces being transmitted to low levels in the prosthetic stem these forces must be transferred to the bone at the highest levels of the femur. At these levels the medullary cavity has the maximum internal diameter and hence maximum area of cement-bone interface. At these levels also the radius from the central axis of the femur is maximum, thus offering maximum torque to resist rotary stresses. It should be our

---

[1]) This feature was borrowed from the Austin-Moore design of prosthesis which was never subject to fatigue fracture.

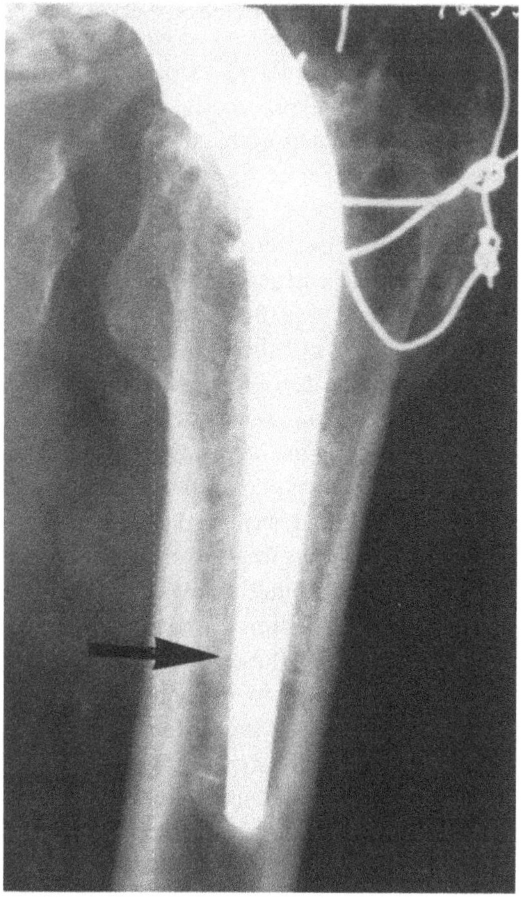

Fig. 9.13. Fracture of stem of prosthesis, with almost no displacement, 2.5 cm above distal end. The fracture is just visible on the *lateral surface only*, at level of *arrow*

aim therefore to make the upper levels of the femoral cement-bone interface work to maximum efficiency.

Nature of the Rotatory Forces

The nature and magnitude of the rotatory forces acting on the head of a femoral prosthesis as yet are still rather ill-defined. Rotatory forces of this kind are physiological and must occur in the intact hip joint. This is indicated by the location of the centre of the area of eburnation of articular cartilage on the head of an arthrosic femur. The centre of the eburnated area will always be found lying anterior to the summit of the femoral head. When a femoral prosthesis is loaded with the hip flexed (as in mounting stairs or sitting down and rising from the sitting position) the direction of the force will tend to cause internal rotation of the femoral prosthesis inside the femoral cavity. Reducing the offset of a prosthesis will reduce the moment arm responsible for generating the torsional stress producing the fatigue fracture. This is therefore another argument for using prostheses with minimum acceptable offset.

Flanged (Cobra) Femoral Prosthesis

This femoral prosthesis is designed to optimise load transmission from the upper levels of the cement to the endosteal surface of the upper part of the medullary cavity. To do this it has certain principles in common with the PIJ socket also designed to optimise the use of cement:

1) The edges of the dorsal flange produce some degree of mechanical stability in an enlarged medullary cavity by establishing points of contact with the bone without obscuring significant areas of bone needed for cement contact. Accidental movements of the prosthesis in the soft cement while waiting for the cement to polymerise are thus minimised.

2) Contact between the edges of the dorsal flange and the endosteal surface of the femur locates the stem of the prosthesis centrally in the medullary cavity of the femur and so ensures that the cement on the load-bearing medial surface has a U-shaped section of even thickness.

3) Contact of the edges of the dorsal flange with the endosteal surface of the femur restricts the escape of cement posteriorly. A more positive injection pressure is therefore developed than was the case with previous designs.

The great increase in surface area of endosteal bone in the upper levels of the medullary cavity employed in recent years and essential when using the Cobra design of prosthesis, compared with the limited area of endosteal surface in the old technique of working entirely through the cut end of the femoral neck, is demonstrated in Fig. 9.14.

Experience has proved that the new technique of reattachment of the trochanter avoids non-union even though the cancellous surface on the femur from which the trochanter has been detached can be quite extensively invaded by prosthesis and cement.

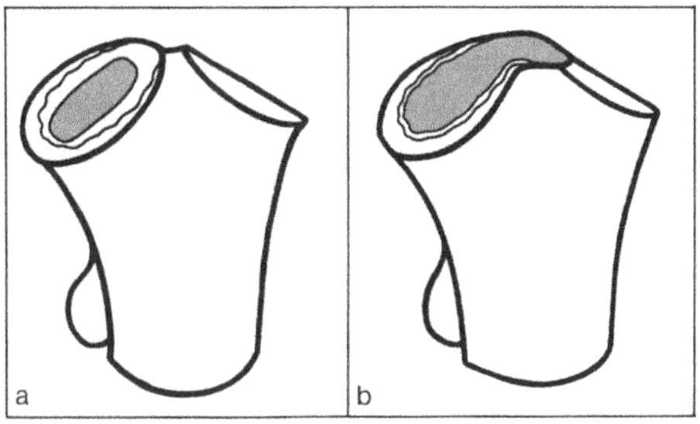

Fig. 9.14 a, b. Showing (**a**) result of old method of 'broaching' the medullary cavity through the open end of the femoral neck compared with (**b**) the current technique of invading the cut surface from which the trochanter was detached with much more extensive enlargement of the medullary cavity

Serrated Medial Border

When the flanged (Cobra) prosthesis was first introduced the author recommended the incorporation of serrations on the upper part of the convex medial border to enhance load transmission to cement in this important region. Serrations were not added to the 40-mm-offset design because there was not sufficient room in which to place them. The theory which prompted the incorporation of these serrations was based on the observation of 'fretting corrosion' on this concave, medial region in first-generation prostheses removed years later at post-mortem. It was thought that the rather exaggerated bend caused by the 45-mm offset could be responsible for cyclical elastic deformation which would tend to separate the metal and cement surfaces at this point when under load, and that the use of serrations would deter this fretting action.

The possibility that the re-entrant angle of the serrations might render the prosthesis fatigue-prone was thought to be unlikely because (1) the serrations were on the compression aspect of the stem, (2) the stem was of heavier calibre than the previous flat-back design, (3) the flat-back element had been removed and (4) fatigue tests in the laboratory were satisfactory.

The recognition of significant rotatory forces acting on a prosthesis and contributing to fatigue fracture now makes it seem possible that serrations could weaken a prosthesis subjected to cyclic rotatory forces and for this reason this feature has now been abandoned. In any case the teaching of this book (see Chap. 21) is to favour the 40-mm-offset prosthesis as a routine and there is no room to incorporate serrations in the reduced length of the concave medial surface in this design.

Fatigue Fracture of Femoral Prostheses

In 1975 the author[29] reported the clinical data associated with the first 17 fatigue fractures of femoral prostheses which had been implanted at Wrightington. The fractures which have presented since that original study still come from the same group operated on before about 1973 and, as before, the type of patient at risk is a heavy male who has had an extremely good result. A change from the clinical pattern originally described is that there is now a lengthening of the interval between operation and fracture, which is not unexpected since the original group at risk is receding into the past.

Countermeasures Against Fatigue Fracture

The factors to be considered in avoiding future fatigue fractures concern:

1) Achieving a stem with maximum cross-sectional area
2) Avoiding stress-raising features on the surface of the stem
3) Reducing the offset but maintaining the moment of the abductor force
4) Improving proximal cement support
5) Metallurgical considerations

1) To reduce stress in the stem by increasing cross-sectional area is of paramount importance taking precedence even over some aspects of metallurgy. Because strength versus weight is not important in this field there is no virtue in subtle shapes of cross-section (e.g. the I-beam). Detachment of the trochanter to permit rotary reaming of the medullary cavity is essential if large-calibre prosthetic stems are to be employed.

2) **Shape of Stem**. The avoidance of stress-raising features on the stem (such as the antero-lateral angle of the flat-back first-generation prosthesis)

has now become of even greater importance since the role of rotary stresses in producing fatigue failure has been recognized. The role of the nature of the surface of the stem in preventing the initiation of fatigue cracks is important.

The importance of the **quality of the surface in preventing the initiation of fatigue cracks** may impose a permanent restriction on the use of expanded surfaces in the femur by which to achieve a direct bond with living bone. If a sound bond were achieved and if the stem of the prosthesis did fracture it would be a formidable matter to extract the distal portion. Fortunately in the author's experience the need to consider expanded metallic surfaces in young patients is less important for the femur than the acetabulum.

3) **The offset**. Originally the author believed that a significant offset was an advantageous feature of design. The rather long concave section of the stem adjacent to the base of the neck was visualized as lying in a gutter produced by the stump of the neck of the femur making the stem of the prosthesis stable against rotatory forces. By contrast, prostheses based on the Thompson and Moore designs, with almost total resection of the neck of the femur down to the lesser trochanter, were considered potentially unstable to rotation.

It is now evident that if the distal half of the stem of a prosthesis is held more rigidly against rotation than is the proximal half, rotatory stresses at the common level for fatigue fracture will be increased by a long offset. Therefore a short-offset prosthesis becomes desirable on all counts and, to get the ultimate in protection against fatigue fracture, may need to be combined with lateral displacement of the trochanter.

4) **Cement support**. The idea of shedding as much load as possible from the prosthesis to the upper levels of the femur, so that less reaches the mid-level of the stem, is as important for rotary forces as for forces in the coronal plane. By achieving a large surface area at the cement-bone interface the stress, both in shear and compression, will be lowered. Because of more extensive curettage of the upper end of the medullary cavity to accept a large volume of cement, more sophisticated methods of re-attaching the trochanter are necessary.

5) **Metallurgical matters**. The development of alloys with outstanding characteristics of resisting fatigue failure is important, but this must not encourage a surgeon to think that in vigorous and heavy male patients he can continue to operate with his original technique depending merely on having his favourite implants made of an improved metal. A prosthesis which is functioning within its fatigue limits but is deflecting elastically under load so much that it is damaging the cement-bone bond is in no way a technical advance.

At the present moment stainless steel for femoral prostheses is tending to be derogated, perhaps unfairly, in favour of expensive alloys containing high proportions of relatively rare metals (i.e. 35% nickel). It would be a pity if this trend should go unchallenged before stainless steel has been fully explored under less highly stressed conditions than has been the case in the past; especially in view of the possibility of future world shortages of rare metallic elements. It is now realized that in heavy patients, in whom the overwhelming majority of fatigue fractures have occurred, the prostheses in the past were much too small in calibre. They could easily have been doubled, or even tripled, in cross-section area had the need for this been realized. The recognition of an important contribution of torsional stress is new knowledge with far-reaching significance in this field.

Chapter 10

Types of LFA Femoral Prostheses

Historical

The first generation of Charnley femoral prostheses is easily distinguished by the flat lateral surface of the stem. This design is now called the flat-back (Fig. 10.1). The flat lateral surface was derived from the Austin-Moore and Thompson prostheses.

There were only three designs in the range of first-generation prostheses:
1) Standard (45-mm offset)
2) Straight thick stem (38-mm offset)
3) Straight narrow stem (38-mm offset)

The straight **narrow** stem (SNS) prosthesis differed from the straight **thick** stem (STS) only in its front-to-back thickness which was 5/16 in. (7.9 mm). The front-to-back thickness of the other two prostheses was $^{3}/_{8}$ in. (9.5 mm).

The straight narrow stem was originally introduced for the revision of failed Teflon operations at a time when the technique of reaming out a cement track in the femur was undeveloped. With more recent methods of reaming cement in the medullary cavity the author prefers always to use thick stems and he deprecates requests from surgeons that the manufacturers should continue to make the SNS pattern available. There is no femur into which the STS prosthesis cannot be inserted by rotary reaming after detaching the trochanter.

To describe the development of the Charnley prostheses historically the current range can be divided into second and third generations.

The second generation is characterized by the addition of more metal to the flat lateral surface of the stem of the first generation to give the design now known as the 'round-back' (Fig. 10.2).

The third generation is characterized by the addition of the 'dorsal flange' added to the round-back of the second generation (Fig. 10.3). The design with dorsal flange is also called the Cobra design.

The range of prostheses with 40-mm offset, introduced in 1975, is now the author's first choice and on grounds of increased strength in his practice has totally replaced the 45-mm offset.

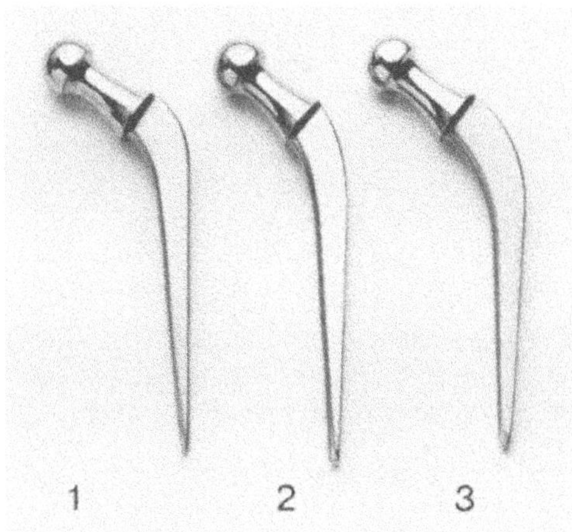

Fig. 10.1. First-generation flat-back designs of prosthesis. (*1*) SNS 38-mm offset. (*2*) STS 38-mm offset. (*3*) Standard 45-mm offset

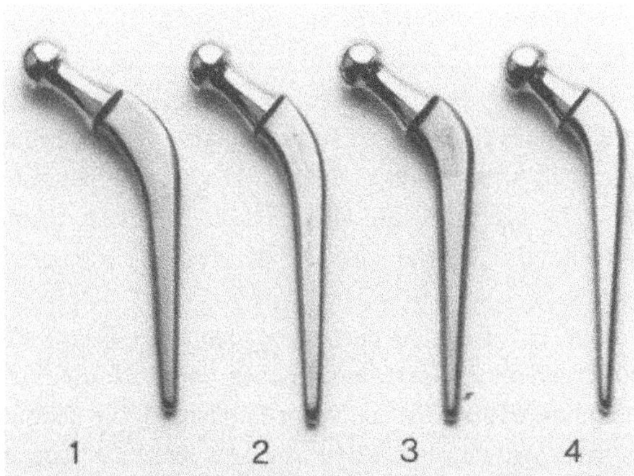

Fig. 10.2. Second-generation round-back designs of prosthesis. (*1*) Standard 45-mm offset. (*2*) 40-mm offset. (*3*) 35-mm offset. (*4*) 35-mm offset $^{3}/_{4}$ neck

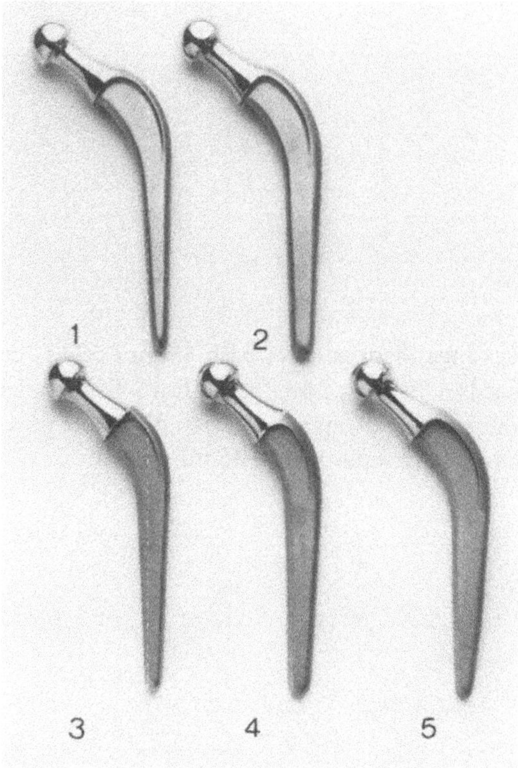

Fig. 10.3. Third-generation flanged designs of prosthesis (Cobra). (*1*) 45-mm heavy. (*2*) 45-mm extra-heavy. (*3*) 40-mm heavy. (*4*) 40-mm extra-heavy. (*5*) 40-mm extra-heavy with taper tip

Heavy Prosthesis – Heavy Patient

The adjective 'heavy' in the nomenclature of these prostheses has proved to be unfortunate but it is now difficult to supplant with any other. During development from the standard flat-back prosthesis of the first generation the obvious adjective was 'heavy', but seen now in comparison with the 'extra-heavy' range introduced later, the stem of the 'heavy' is heavier than in the first generation only by the addition of sufficient metal to round off the flat lateral surface of the original prosthesis.

The point which can be misleading is that the so-called heavy **prosthesis** never was intended for heavy **patients.** The heavy prosthesis of the second generation was intended for the average patient as the flat-back of the first generation. It was the extra-heavy prosthesis which was designed for patients over average weight and most certainly for patients of 168 lb (75 kg) and over.

Factors Contributing to the Strength of the Flanged Design of Stem

Despite the only modest increase in amount of metal in the stem of the so-called heavy prosthesis when comapred with the first-generation flat-back with 45-mm offset, there are a number of factors which now combine to enhance very considerably the strength of this average prosthesis in comparison with its predecessor. These factors are:

1) The 3 mm of metal added to the lateral border of the stem enhances strength by about 10%.

2) A reduction of offset from 45 mm to 40 mm enhances strength by more than 10%.

3) The absence of 'corners' where the lateral surface of the flat-back joined the anterior and posterior surfaces of the stem removes a source of fatigue fracture. The magnitude of this enhancement is difficult to quantitate but it is certainly very significant and could contribute in excess of another 10% in strength.

4) The dorsal flange is intended to make the upper levels of cement function more effectively in load transmission, thereby reducing the amount of stress reaching down to the mid-level of the stem where fatigue fractures are prone to develop. This feature makes what at the moment is an imponderable contribution to strength in the in vivo situation.

5) A system of cold-coining to form the shape of the stems individually is expected to raise significantly the tensile strength over the annealed metal and bring with it an improvement in fatigue resistance.

6) As part of the technique of the surgical operation, slight lateral displacement of the trochanter, to compensate for slight medial displacement of the femur produced by a short-offset prosthesis, can significantly reduce bending moments on the implant (Chap. 21).

Therefore it is possible that taken all together these factors could enhance the strength of the **'Heavy, flanged (Cobra), 40-mm offset'** by well over 100% compared with the first generation **'standard, flat-back, 45-mm offset'** and also do this without any great increase in difficulty of inserting into the femur.

The extra-heavy 40-mm-offset prosthesis incorporates all the preceding features in addition to the very considerable matter of another 3-mm increase in width of the stem as seen in the frontal plane. This extra 3 mm is a lamina the full front-to-back thickness of the stem, whereas the 3 mm added to the flat-back to make the heavy prosthesis was reduced in thickness at front and back in the making of the round-back.

Special Remarks About the 40-mm Offset

Prospective users of 40-mm-offset prostheses, who previously have used only 45-mm offsets, should be aware of two technical details which are not specific to the author's design but which concern any prosthesis with a short offset.

A prosthesis with a reduced offset displaces the shaft of the femur nearer to the midline of the body by the amount of the reduced offset (given that the stem is axial in the femur). Medial displacement of the femur can compress soft tissue between it and osteophytes projecting from the lower margin of the acetabulum, and this may enhance the fulcrum action tending to lever a femoral head out of the socket when the adduction range is being examined during the test reduction.

This situation is encountered only in big patients with big bones, but these are the very patients in whom the extra strength of a short offset is desirable. In a man with big bones it is therefore advisable to be conservative in deepening the acetabulum because excessive deepening in a large acetabulum can cause the inferior rim, already made prominent by osteophytes, to project unnecessarily from the level of the face of the socket. This projection can be cut away (steps 82, 83) but if the socket can be fully contained under the roof of the acetabulum, without deepening the 1 cm (or even the 1.5 cm), which is often possible in such cases, there is no need to do so. The biomechanics of this change of policy towards radical deepening of the acetabulum is discussed in Chap. 21.

If at the test reduction a tendency exists in a patient with big bones for the prosthetic head to be levered out of the acetabulum, there is no need to be alarmed provided that: (1) the test reduction is stable against external rotation and (2) the head of the femur cannot be distracted from the socket under long-axis traction. [Both these features receive enhanced control by the precision inherent in the neck-length jig (Chap. 16)]. With these provisos the hip will be rendered completely stable once the trochanter is reattached. There will be no need to change the post-operative management. The patient can be allowed out of bed at the normal second or third day and thereafter rehabilitate without restraint (certainly if the trochanter is reattached as advised in this text).

Common LFA Prostheses

The author's own day-to-day practice is covered by the following four types of prostheses arranged in order of frequency of use:

1) Extra-heavy, flanged (cobra), 40-mm offset
2) Heavy, flanged (Cobra), 40-mm offset
3) Straight-thick-stem, round-back, 35-mm offset
4) Straight-thick-stem, round-back, three-quarter-length neck, 35-mm offset

1) Extra-Heavy, Flanged (Cobra), 40-mm Offset

Following the general world trend of using the heaviest stem which can conveniently be inserted, this extra-heavy prosthesis is now the one most commonly used by the author, except in obviously small and light-weight female patients.

For patients weighing 160 lb (75 kg) or over, it should be obligatory to ream out the medullary cavity, by whatever means, to take the extra-heavy stem if this cannot be introduced at the first pass. This statement applies especially to vigorous male patients in the younger age group (45 years) who require this operation. Many of these strong patients at 45 years of age have thick femoral cortices and the medullary cavity is not wider than about one-third of the total width of the femur (the normal proportion in an athletic person) and it is important to be forewarned in this matter.

A modification of the frontal profile of the tip of the extra-heavy range has currently been adopted as standard. The blunt end of the original extra-heavy has been tapered a few more degrees over the terminal 2 cm of the stem (Fig. 10.3). This greatly facilitates introduction in a narrow medullary cavity without weakening the prosthesis over the critical zone of the stem.

2) Heavy, Flanged (Cobra), 40-mm Offset

This is the standard prosthesis for all patients up to 140 lb (63 kg). Choice of this prosthesis can overlap with the extra-heavy in the range 140–168 lb (63–75 kg).

3) Straight Thick Stem, Round-Back, 35-mm Offset

This profile (STS, RB, 35-mm offset) was originally designed for conditions of the upper end of the femur where the neck is short or even absent, such as failed intertrochanteric osteotomy, congenital dislocation, pseudarthrosis, etc.

The straight thick stem profile is very important in adults with secondary arthritis from congenital subluxation. When anteversion of the femoral neck is extreme (60°–90°) no attempt should be made to enter the prosthesis through the cut surface of the open end of the femoral neck. The medullary cavity must be approached by piercing the medial cortex of the femoral neck, leaving the open end of the cut surface of the neck of the femur facing forwards in the direction of the patella. The need for a short offset in this situation is therefore obvious.

Extended experience now shows that the STS 35-mm-offset prosthesis must no longer be regarded as intended only for patients with abnormal anatomy at the upper end of the femur, or only for small and therefore light-weight patients. The short offset and the thick stem (round-back) make it a very strong and stiff prosthesis and it has a wide range of usefulness if the surgeon is prepared to displace the trochanter laterally to make up for medial displacement of the shaft of the femur so to maintain the length of the gluteal lever (Chap. 21).

4) Straight Thick Stem, Round-Back, Three-Quarter-Length Neck, 35-mm Offset

The neck here measures 22 mm from base of head to base of neck (compared with 29 mm of the standard neck). Like the previous STS prosthesis this should not be reserved only for patients where the anatomy of the upper end of the femur is grossly destroyed. This prosthesis is useful in small adult patients with normal anatomy of the upper end of the femur. It is chosen from an assessment of the radiograph with X-ray templates.

Because of its short offset it is even stronger than the previous design but could not be used with relatively normal anatomy unless the great trochanter is transferred laterally to balance medial displacement of the shaft of the femur. This combination might be very valuable for reducing stresses to obtain long life in very young patients such as those of 20 years of age with CDH or with traumatic acetabulae (Chap. 22). On grounds of strength this prosthesis would be preferable to the CDH and the extra-small prostheses (described below) if the stem can be introduced after appropriate reaming. It must be emphasized that the CDH and extra-small prostheses (described later) are intended essentially for patients whose bones are not larger than those of early adolescence even though the patient may be of adult age (i.e. Still's disease, etc.).

45-mm-Offset Series

45-mm Offset 'Heavy' and 'Extra-Heavy' Flanged (Cobra)

The distal stems of both these prostheses are identical in calibre with those of the 40-mm offset described above and the profile differs only in the longer curved segment where the base of the neck joins the straight part of the stem.

Some of the prostheses with 45-mm offset in the past were provided with serrations on the concave medial surface. The serrations were intended to give additional grip between cement and metal to support the extra 0.5 cm of offset. This feature has now been abandoned and the 40-mm offset is preferred.

Figure 10.4 shows the excessive valgus alignment of the stem which can result from a 45-mm offset in a patient of slightly smaller than average size. Following our first fatigue fracture in 1969, which was in varus alignment, this ostentatious valgus position was considered eminently desirable.

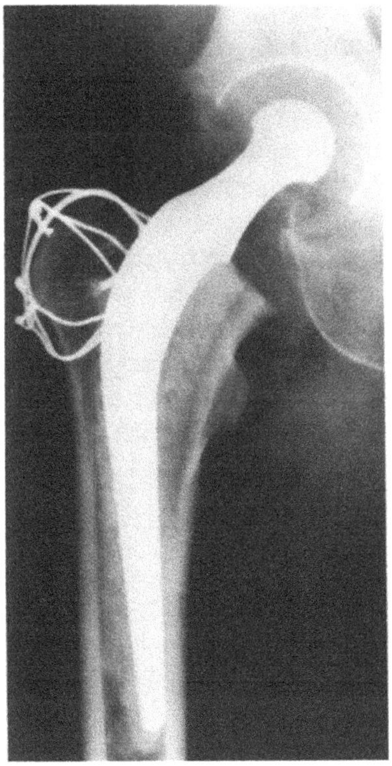

Fig. 10.4. Unnecessary valgus alignment resulting from 45-mm-offset prosthesis in patient slightly smaller than average

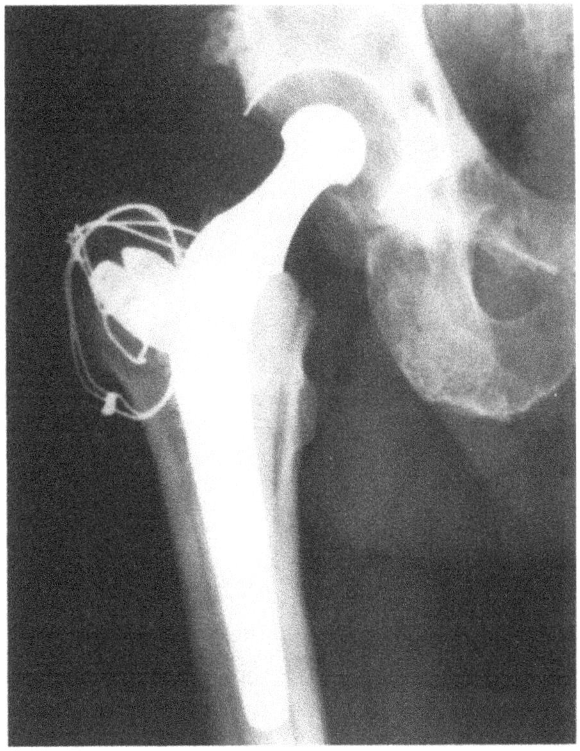

Fig. 10.5. Neutral alignment when 40-mm-offset prosthesis is used in a patient of same size as in Fig. 10.4

Compared with Fig. 10.5, where a 40-mm offset is used, it will be seen that the 45-mm offset presents the stem with an unnecessarily large bending moment (see Chap. 21).

The 45-mm offset is available for surgeons who are accustomed to using the 45-mm offset, which has been normal practice for 15 years and over 10,000 patients at Wrightington. The change to the 40-mm offset is based on theory, to avoid fatigue fractures, but unless the surgeon takes special care in large femora it is rather easy to put a 40-mm offset in varus and impair the value of the reduced offset. The neck-length-jig avoids this problem.

Second-Generation Round-Back Prostheses

The second-generation round-back prostheses now replace the first-generation flat-backs and are available for surgeons who do not wish to use the flanged (cobra) design. In frontal profile they are identical with the first-generation prostheses except for the slight increase in frontal width as a result of the 3 mm of metal (tapering away front and back) added to the lateral surface of the stem. As already stated the process of cold-coining and the addition of metal to give the round-back cross-section add very considerably to the strength of this prosthesis. The round-back series is not made in the extra-heavy calibre.

When the second-generation round-back was first introduced the author did not anticipate that the relatively small amount of metal added to the lateral surface could sometimes make it difficult to insert without elevating the trochanter. A test prosthesis for the small amount of added metal unfortunately was not considered necessary. This experience emphasizes a fundamental rule: **the definitive prosthesis must always be tried in the femoral cavity before cement is introduced.** It is conveniently done to push the wires out of place prior to inserting cement. The true purpose of a test prosthesis is not to test the size of the medullary cavity; it is to check neck length and the stability of the reduction. All prostheses should be loose in the medullary cavity of the femur if an adequate volume of cement is to intervene between the stem and the bone.

Round-Back, 45-mm Offset

This replaces the first-generation flat-back 45-mm offset.

Round-Back, 40-mm Offset

This is suitable in small patients for surgeons who do not elevate the trochanter. The author occasionally uses this prosthesis with detachment of the trochanter in patients (usually female) whose femora are too narrow to accept the flanged (Cobra) design.

Prostheses for Special Purposes

CDH Prosthesis (Fig. 10.6.1.)

This very small prosthesis is designed specifically for congenital dislocation in patients with bones not much larger than adolescents'. It is for problems where the normal neck of the femur is absent and little more than the open end of a tube of cortical bone exists. Attachment of the trochanter in a lateral position can produce a remarkable restoration of anatomy in these cases. It is unlikely that this prosthesis will ever be made with a dorsal flange to improve centring in the medullary cavity because of the unpredictability of the size of the medullary cavity in the conditions where it will be needed.

The length of the femoral neck here is 22 mm measured from the base of the head to the base of the neck (i.e. the same as the three-quarter-length neck prosthesis). This prosthesis often requires the extra-small socket (40-mm diameter) and often the 35-mm offset bore socket (p. 108). The diameter of the head is the standard 22.25 mm.

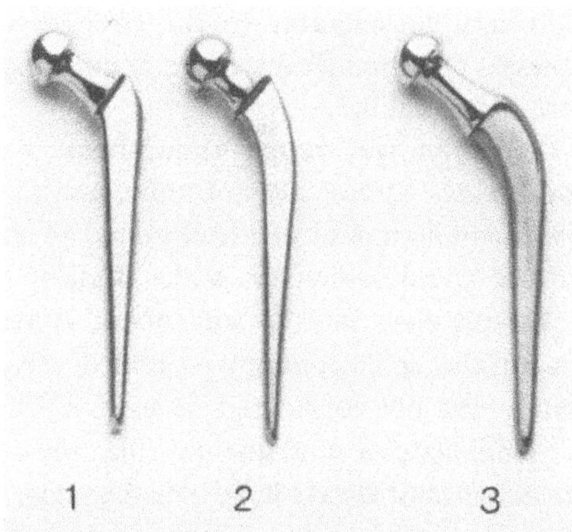

Fig. 10.6. (*1*) CDH prosthesis. (*2*) Extra-small prosthesis. (*3*) Heavy 40-mm offset, for comparison of size

Extra-Small Prosthesis (Fig. 10.6.2.)

This is another pattern of very small prosthesis: the neck here measures 16.5 mm from base of head to base of neck. The curvature of the stem is designed for patients with bones of adolescent size which have retained the anatomy of the femoral neck, as for instance in Still's disease. The stem of this prosthesis is more slender than the CDH design and on grounds of strength the CDH design is preferable if it can be inserted. This prosthesis will usually be used with the smallest sizes of hip socket. The femoral head is the standard 22.25-mm diameter.

Note: On grounds of strength it is to be emphasized that the two very small prostheses (CDH and the extra-small) are advised only if the straight thick stem with three-quarter neck, combined with rotary reaming of the femur, is out of the question.

Femoral Prosthesis with Extra-Long Stem

In the early manufacturer's catalogues this prosthesis acquired the misnomer of 'Intramedullary' prosthesis (Fig. 10.7.6). This is essentially a round-back prosthesis with an extra-long stem – 15 in. (38 cm) compared with 5 in. (12.5 cm) of the standard. The offset is 40 mm because this prosthesis is most commonly needed in difficult secondary operations where the neck of the femur usually is shorter than normal. In the future a 35-mm offset configuration may be available because of its usefulness in difficult problems and because of the increased stiffness of the 35-mm offset.

This long-stemmed prosthesis was introduced about 1965 to cope with spiral fractures of the shaft of the femur incurred during the operation when dislocating a hip with a femoral shaft weakened by the removal of an osteotomy plate. Spiral fractures used to be sustained before the importance of dislocating by pure adduction was recognized and before the danger of using external rotation force before the femoral head was out of the acetabulum was recognized.

This design of prosthesis is in effect a standard prosthesis with an intramedullary nail added. The idea was to permit a total hip operation to be completed if a femoral shaft fracture had been sustained and facilitate holding alignment during 8–10 weeks of traction while waiting for the fracture to heal under conservative methods. Cement was restricted to the upper end of the femur without any attempt to inject cement to the level of the fracture line. No attempt was made to encourage weight-bearing before the shaft fracture was clinically united (10–12 weeks).

Since recognizing the factors responsible for producing fractures of the femur during the operation the original purpose now only rarely applies but it is always a useful device to have in stock. It has a special application in secondary operations where the stem of an ordinary prosthesis is too short and where a stem of 7 in. (or 18 cm) or more would be advantageous. Without the need to hold a large stock of prostheses with stems of different lengths any desired length can be obtained by cutting down the 15-in. stem. This can be done prior to surgery in the hospital workshop or, if required without warning during an operation, a sterile bolt-cropper can be used. This tool can be obtained from hardware stores and it should be capable of cutting $^3/_8$-in.-diameter mild steel bar; it is kept for emergencies in a sterile pack and when needed a circulating male assistant operates the handles.

The extra-long prosthesis unfortunately has been abused by surgeons allowing patients to walk with full load on the leg before a fracture is soundly consolidated, with predictable bending of the prosthesis. Several instances have been reported where surgeons have used this slender prosthesis in error for the much stronger resection prosthesis when the upper 5–6 in. of the femur have been excised for tumours, etc.

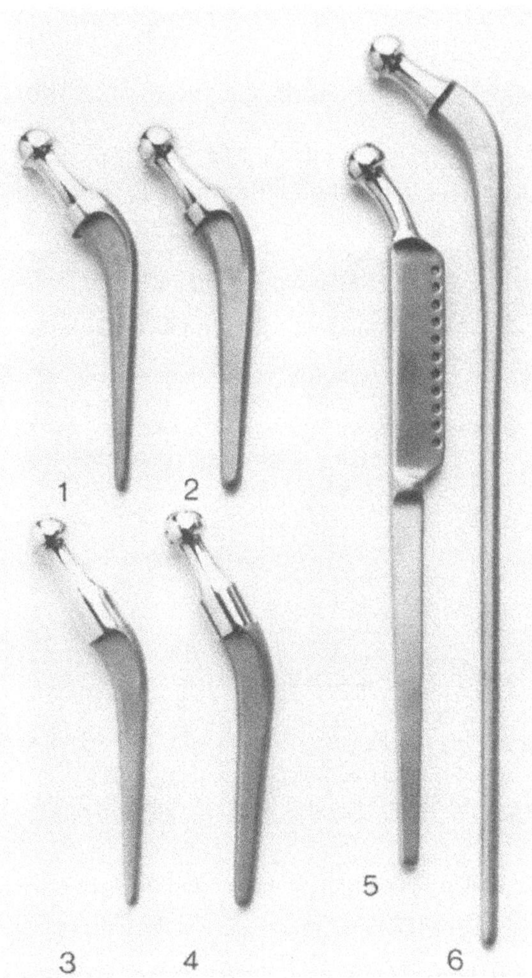

Fig. 10.7. Extra-long prostheses: (*1*) 1-cm extra-long neck – ordinary stem. (*2*) 1-cm extra-long neck – extra-heavy stem. (*3*) 2-cm extra-long neck – ordinary stem. (*4*) 2-cm extra-long neck – extra-heavy stem. (*5*) Resection prosthesis with muscle plate. (*6*) Extra-long stem 15 in. (38 cm)

Resection Prosthesis with Muscle Plate

This heavy-calibre prosthesis is designed for patients with bone pathology necessitating resection of the upper 5–6 in. (75–150 mm) of femur and where long-term survival is not expected (Fig. 10.7.5).

It is important that the intermuscular septa in the thigh should be anchored to the perforations of the 'muscle plate' by non-absorbable sutures in order to restrict excessive rotation of the pros-

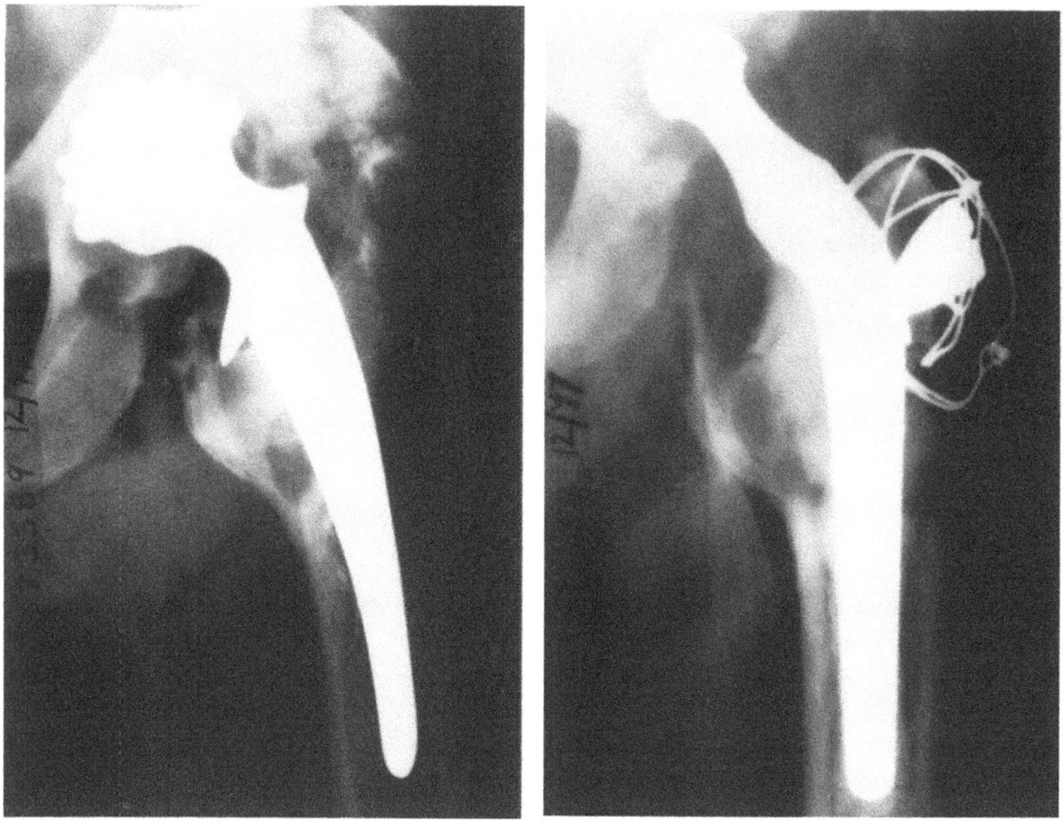

a b

Fig. 10.8. a Failed McKee–Farrar and (**b**) 1-cm extra-long neck prosthesis

thesis and thereby avoid dislocation. Ideally the muscle plate ought to be sited posteriorly, because the fibrous intermuscular septa of the thigh converge on the linea aspera which lies posterior on the femur; but this would require right and left prostheses. The results have been good even with the laterally sited muscle plate and it is convenient to hold a single prosthesis of this design to cope with these rare cases because, when they do require the operation, they need it with minimum delay.

When using this prosthesis no attempt is made to attach the abductor muscles to the metal of the prosthesis because the tendinous insertions of the abductor muscles, which alone are capable of holding heavy sutures, are usually lost in the resection (if for tumour). The abductor muscles are therefore best allowed to reattach themselves to the fascia lata with the hip held in abduction for some weeks. Insertion of the abductor muscles into the fascia lata produces a longer and more effective abductor moment arm than any attempt to suture to points of reattachment on a prosthesis. Three months in full abduction is advisable, ending in a short hip spica plaster cast.

If a resection prosthesis is required for a non-metastasizing tumour a heavier design would be preferable; the rather abrupt change of cross-section in this design exposes the stem to the danger of fatigue fracture unless the patient's activity or survival is limited.

Extra-Long Neck, 1-cm and 2-cm, Flanged (Cobra)

These prostheses offer extra lengths of neck by the introduction of a cylindrical section of metal 1 or 2 cm in length between the base of the standard neck and start of the stem (Fig. 10.7.1–4).

These two prostheses are useful in a number of special applications:

1) When the bone of the femoral neck has been lost, as in revision operations for a Moore prosthesis or a pseudarthrosis (Fig. 10.8).

2) In replacing a fractured femoral prosthesis when the medial femoral neck has been eroded. One can thus avoid the temptation of trying to build up the eroded region with cement.

3) The 1-cm extra-long prosthesis can save an embarrasing situation during a primary intervention if the ordinary prosthesis does not achieve a satisfactory 'tight' reduction (perhaps as the result of cutting the stump of the femoral neck too short and/or placing the socket too high in the acetabulum). In such a case the prosthesis with 1 cm extra length of neck will probably be too long but the too-much shortened femoral neck can be shortened a little further and stability achieved.

In order to avoid extra-long necks creating excessive offsets and so weakening the prosthetic stems by increased bending moments, the neck-stem angles are made more valgus than the standard 50° of the rest of the range. The 2-cm extra-long neck is even more valgus than the 1-cm extra-long neck. If these prostheses are held in the standard prosthesis neck-holder (with protective plastics head caps) because the neck-axis angle is not the standard 50°, the handle of the holder will not align with the stem of the prosthesis and allowance must be made for this.

Chapter 11

Pre-operative Measurement of X-Rays

Much study at Wrightington has gone into attempts to enhance the precision of total hip replacement by making pre-operative measurements of the X-rays with radiographic templates. Provided that certain limitations are recognized (particularly errors in transverse dimensions caused by external rotation of the femur) these radiographic techniques have their uses and hip surgeons should be familiar with the information they can reveal.

Radiographic Magnification

In making measurements with radiographic templates X-rays must have a standard magnification. With the film casette in its standard position, which is about 2 in. (5 cm) below the top of the X-ray table, and a 40-in. (1-m) tube-to-film distance the magnification will be about 1.2 times. This can be checked by measuring the total length of the image of a Charnley prosthesis in a clinical X-ray: this should measure about 19 cm on the film compared with the real length of about 16 cm, when measured as a chord from the tip of the stem to the top of the head. The scale on Thackray radiographic templates is in divisions of 1.2 cm so that direct measurements on the film can be made using these divisions as centimetres on the patient. The templates available for this purpose are shown in Fig. 11.1.

Simple Radiographic Measurements

The simple but useful pre-operative radiographic measurements made with a template are:

1) **Size of hip socket.** Most particularly this relates to deciding when a small socket (40-mm outside diameter of the body) will be preferable to the large socket (43-mm outside diameter of the body). It is to be noted that the semicircles on the radiographic templates represent the outlines of the semicircular socket wear-markers and therefore the external surfaces of the bodies of the sockets. The diameters of the rims, or faces, of these sockets are larger than the diameters of the bodies, i.e. 47 mm for the small, and 50 mm for the large sockets.

2) **Thickness of bone in floor of acetabulum.** This is a useful guide for the possibility of deepening or of not deepening the acetabulum. The measurement is made by taking the lateral, or superficial, cortex of the 'tear drop' as denoting the deepest level of the floor (Fig. 11.2 a).

3) **Level of roof of acetabulum.** From this one can estimate whether a 'crescent' of cement will have to be present between the top of the socket and the outer part of the roof of the acetabulum. This estimate is made by superimposing the socket template over the acetabulum with the lower end of the semicircle representing the wire marker about 0.5 cm above the lowest part of the tear drop. In this position a crescentic gap between the upper part of the socket and the roof of the acetabulum will indicate the thickness of the crescentic layer of cement which will be required above the socket (Fig. 11.2 b).

4) **Protrusio acetabuli.** If the socket template is placed at the bottom of a protrusio acetabuli, it will become evident whether the ordinary prosthetic femoral neck will displace the femur away from the side of the pelvis more than in the pre-operative state. In the ordinary grade of protrusio acetabuli this test usually shows that even when the socket is at the bottom of the protruded acetabulum the standard length of neck of the femoral prosthesis will still displace the femur laterally 0.5–1 cm from its pre-operative position (Fig. 11.3).

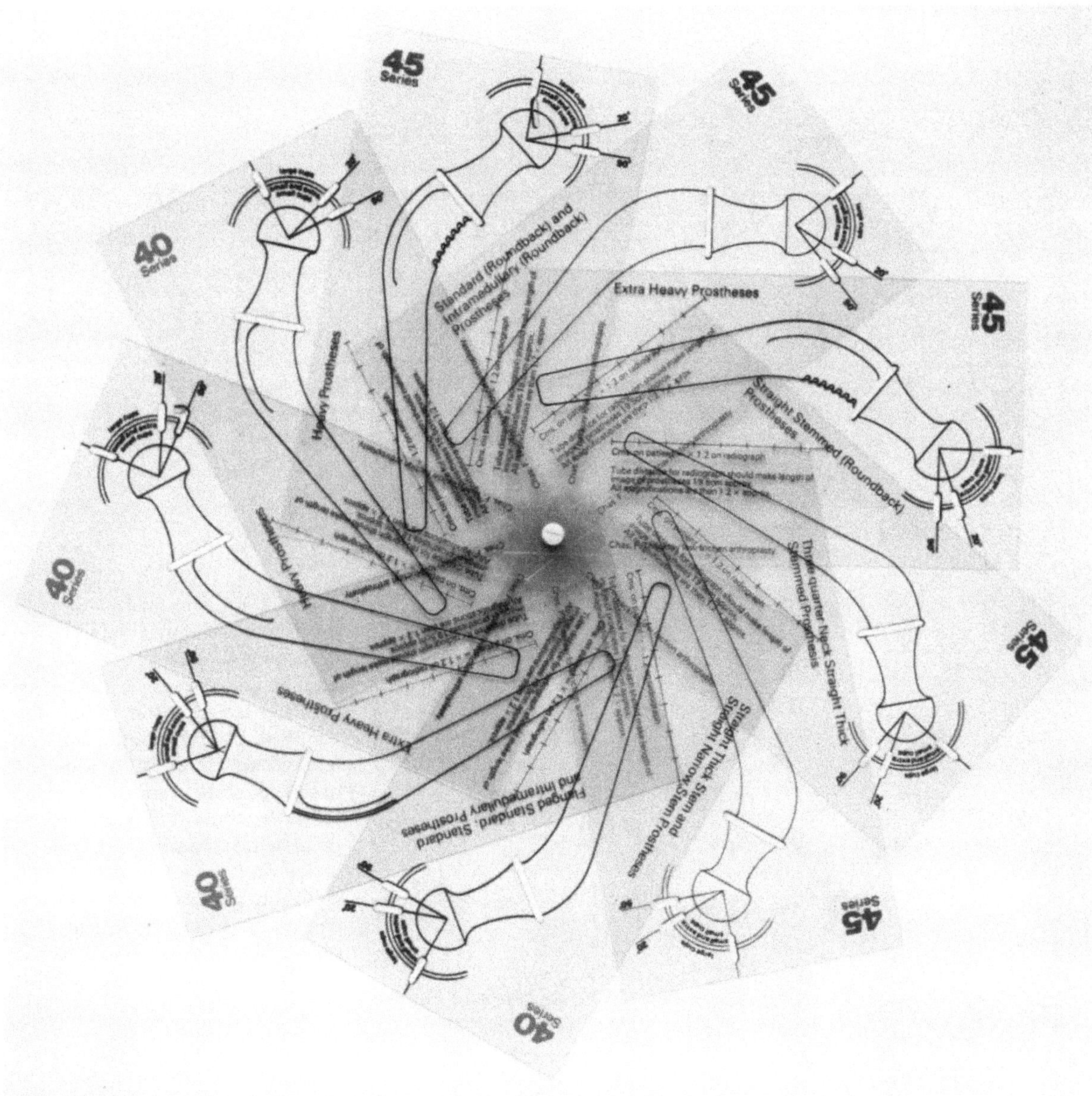

Fig. 11.1. Templates for different prostheses for use at magnification of 1.2 ×. These templates have been arranged in spiral fashion in this picture; each template is a separate item

In estimating how much lateral displacement of the femur from the side wall of the pelvis can be obtained if the socket is placed at the bottom of the protruded acetabulum, the optimum level for cutting the neck of the femur must be taken into account. Sometimes rather more length of stump of femoral neck can be retained with advantage than in the ordinary case. Only rarely will the template show a need for a special layer of cement, or for a bone graft, or other device to lift the socket towards the mouth of the acetabulum. In many patients with protrusio acetabuli an acceptable range of flexion is still present even before operation, though there may be no rotation and very little abduction. In such cases only a small increment in lateral displacement of the femur is needed.

5) **Diameter of medullary cavity of femur.** a) Very narrow femoral medullary cavities are common in congenital hip dysplasia. The radiological tem-

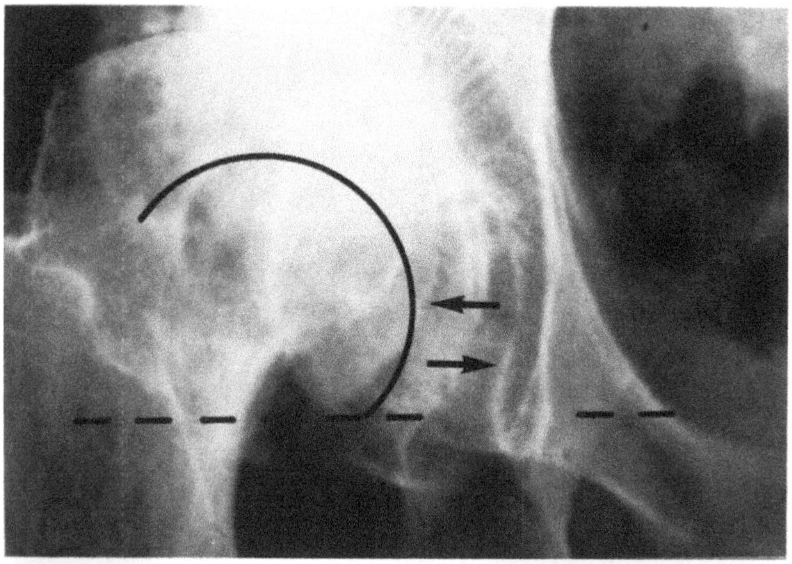

a

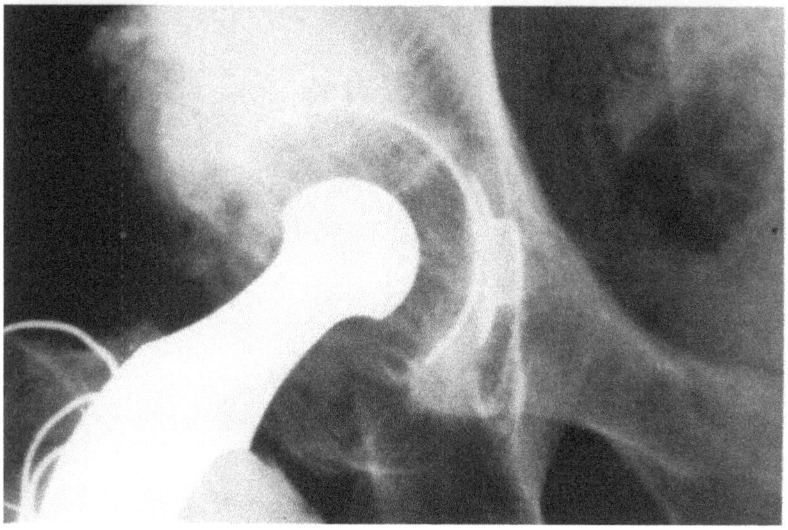

b

Fig. 11.2. a Lateral cortex of 'tear drop' marks the maximum deepening possible in an acetabulum. Pre-op.: *bottom arrow* indicates lateral cortex of tear drop; *top arrow* indicates outline of femoral head. Lowest limit of outline of socket template is placed correctly, about 0.5 cm above lower point of tear drop. Upper limit of socket outline then reveals a crescentic gap between it and roof of the acetabulum. **b** Cement restrictor is flush on lateral cortex of tear drop. Gap above socket filled with cement

plates can give warning that power reaming may be needed and this can turn an arduous operation into a straight-forward procedure. b) In heavy men in whom it is proposed to use the extra-heavy prosthesis the width of the medullary cavity at the level of the tip of the prosthesis can be tested against the template of this prosthesis. (Note the new profile of extra-heavy, 'taper-tip', Fig. 10.3.5.)

6) **Length of femoral neck.** In small adults the standard neck length may be too long and the three-quarter neck may be preferable.

7) **The 40-mm offset series** can be tested on the X-ray to assess how much medial displacement of the femur must be achieved. This is merely of general interest if one has decided to use this profile as a routine (as is now recommended). Conservative deepening of the acetabulum (see Chap. 21) in conjunction with the 40-mm offset can also be studied in relation to a particular case.

8) **Straight-stem prosthesis.** Radiographic templates will indicate whether the standard profile of stem should be replaced by the straight profile. This is particularly the case when the neck of the femur is very short, or is absent as a result of previous surgery. Occasionally a straight-stem profile (now called 35-mm offset) may be chosen in an anatomically normal hip for special strength and trial with the template is useful here.

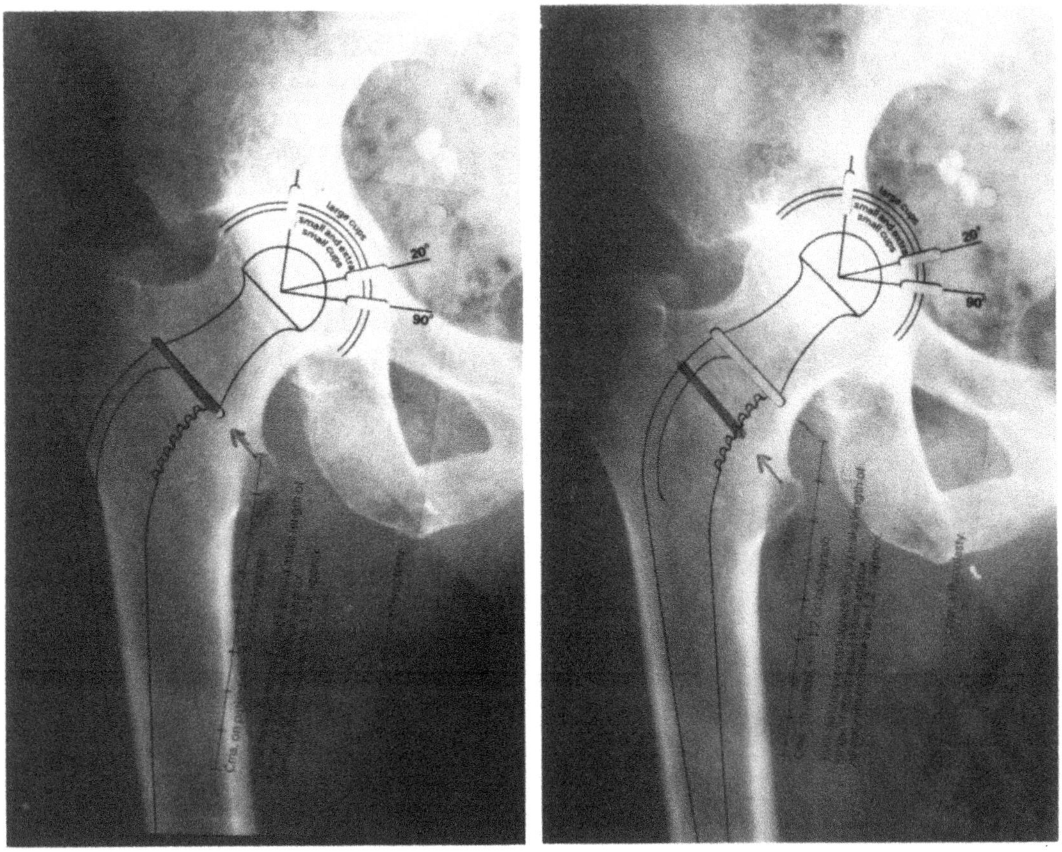

a b

Fig. 11.3 a, b. Protrusio acetabuli of moderate degree. **a** Socket outline placed at bottom of protruded acetabulum. Shaft of femur seen to lie medial to stem of prosthesis (45-mm offset). *Arrow* indicates level of base of neck of prosthesis; this level would mean resection of too much bone of femoral neck. **b** Template centred on femur with level of base of neck of prosthesis in correct position; this indicates that when the socket is at bottom of acetabulum the femur will be displaced laterally from side of pelvis

Stable Reduction and Limb Length

An important objective of radiographic templates when first introduced was to avoid unstable reductions resulting from failure to restore full limb length. In this context an unstable reduction is defined as one where the prosthetic head can be distracted from the acetabulum at the test reduction when long-axis traction is applied to the femur. The stable reduction which comes from inability to distract the prosthetic head from its socket is analogous with stability in 'unconstrained' knee arthroplasty when the capsular structures are restored to normal tension by inserting implants of appropriate thickness to replace eroded cartilage and bone.

We discovered in 1970 that dislocation after LFA was often associated with shortening of the lower extremity which had not been fully restored by the operation (Chap. 16) and it was noticed that this shortening was often caused by the socket being placed higher than the anatomical level in the acetabulum (Fig. 11.4). This is clearly revealed by the level of the lower part of the semicircular wire marker in relation to the tear drop.

Measuring Longitudinally

The possibility of predicting final limb length from the pre-operative X-rays depends on the fact that longitudinal measurements made from X-rays can be reasonably reliable; on the other hand attempts

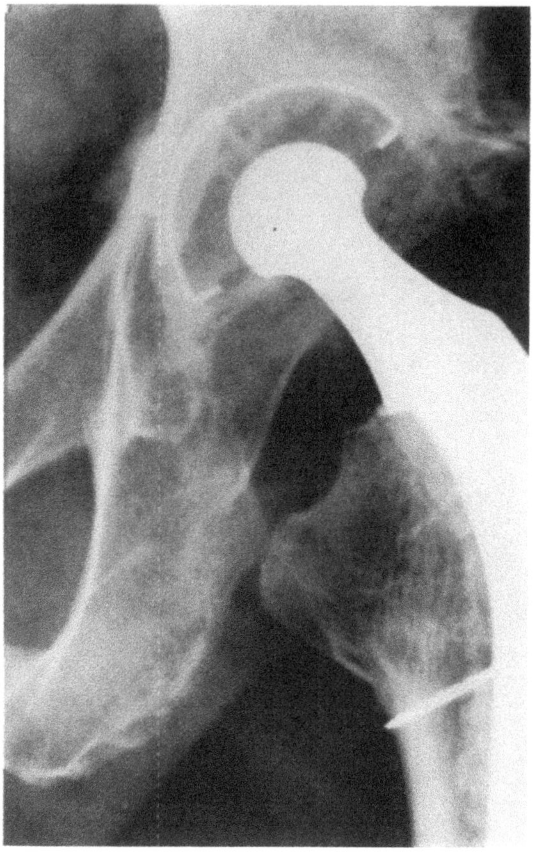

Fig. 11.4. Socket too high in acetabulum. Lower end of semicircular wire marker should be only about 0.5 cm above lower limit of tear drop. Shortening of lower extremity is not corrected and there will be risk of post-operative dislocation

to make transverse measurements can be frustrated by fixed external rotation of the femur.

The basic idea in making longitudinal measurements is to imagine a femoral prosthesis with its socket as one intact unit, and not as two separate items (Fig. 11.5). It will reproduce the outline of the head and neck of an average femur. Taking a femur of average size it is evident from Fig. 11.5 that the centre of the prosthetic femoral head of a 45-mm offset prosthesis will coincide with the centre of a pre-operative femoral head when the infero-medial angle at the base of the prosthetic neck lies on a line passing transversely through the vastus lateralis ridge (there are exceptions to this however and the 40-mm-offset prosthesis is a better average dimension than the original 45-mm 'standard' profile).

Because we are dealing only with **levels**, all measured in a **longitudinal direction**, these are not altered by external rotation of the femur. Therefore the level of the base of the prosthetic neck can be located on a transverse datum line through the vastus lateralis ridge even when the femur is in gross external rotation (Fig. 11.6)

We therefore superimpose the radiographic template so that the infero-medial angle at the base of the neck lies on this datum line and then compare the level of the top of the semicircle represent-

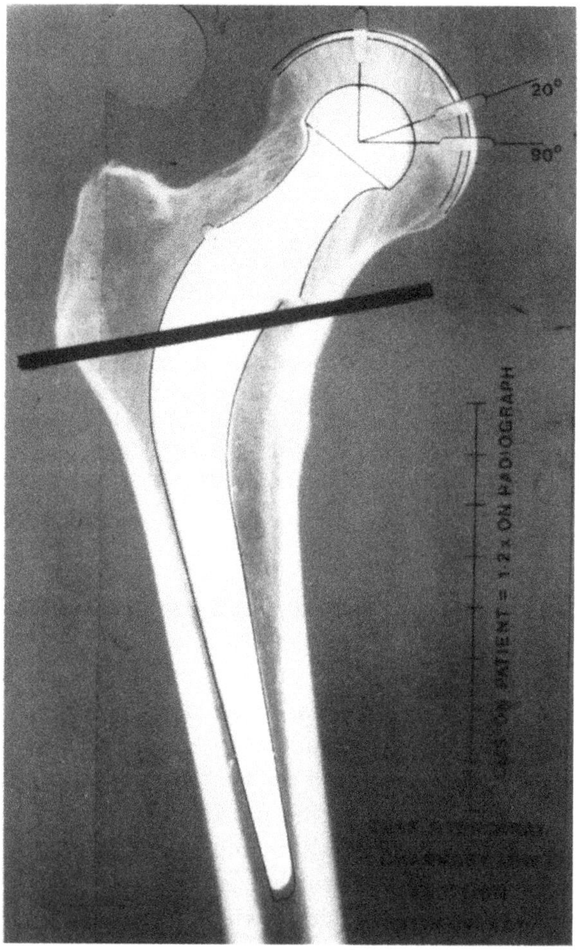

Fig. 11.5. Femoral prosthesis and socket visualised as one unit; not as two separate components. In this case the 45-mm-offset prosthesis is a little too much for this 'average' femur: the stem is in slight valgus; a 40-mm-offset prosthesis would have been in neutral position and a stiffer and stronger implant

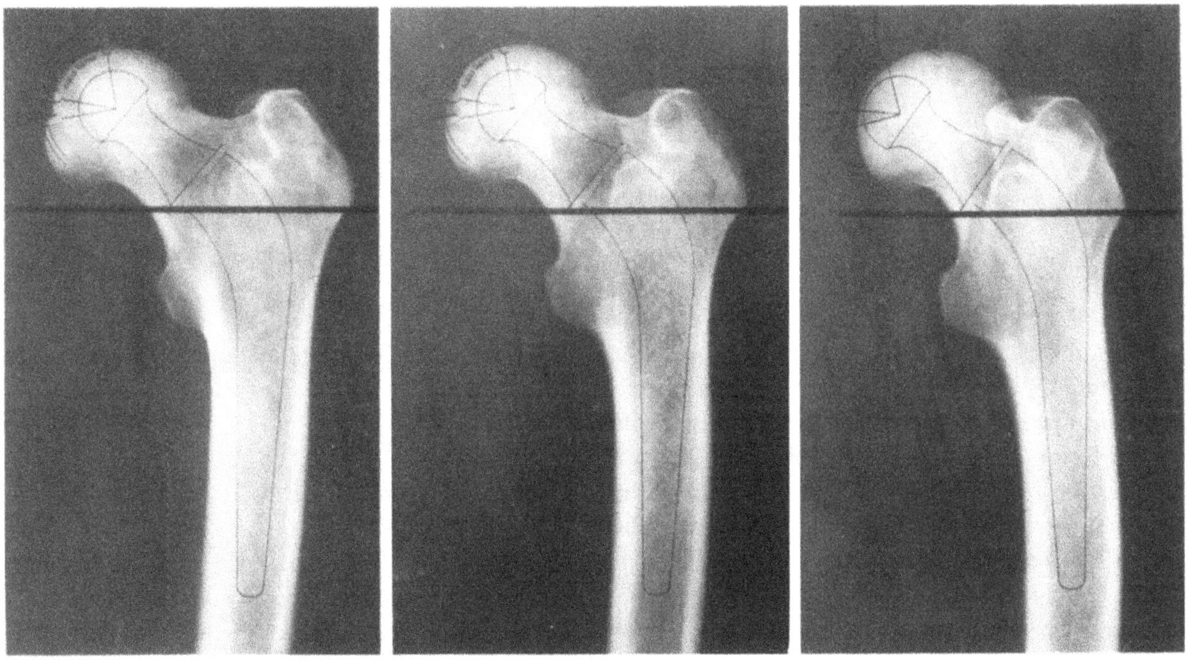

a b c

Fig. 11.6a–c. Template applied to femur in different degrees of external rotation. Datum line passes through vastus lateralis ridge and is transverse to long axis of femur. **a** Neutral. **b** 20°. **c** 40°

ing the exterior of the socket with the level of the roof of the acetabulum. We can always compare **levels** even though the template of the socket may be **dislocated laterally in relation to the acetabulum**.

Broadly speaking two situations will present themselves: 1) the highest level of the semicircle representing the socket will lie at the level of the roof of the acetabulum. This represents the normal hip and if the neck of the femur is sectioned according to routine (Fig. 15.37, p. 210) a stable hip with normal length of extremity should result. 2) The highest level of the semicircle representing the socket will lie above the roof of the acetabulum. If the difference in these levels equals the amount of shortening then full length will be obtained when the socket is placed under the roof of the acetabulum.

When the roof of the acetabulum is destroyed by erosion, or deformed by congenital subluxation, the correct level of the socket can be located by placing the lower end of the wire marker about 0.5 cm above the lowest point of the tear drop (Fig. 11.2). Shortening can be estimated on the X-ray as the difference in levels of the medial and lateral arcades of Shenton's Line. Alternatively, and as a check, shortening can be measured by the difference in levels of the lesser trochanters.

Neck-Length Jig

It must be admitted that attempts to predict from the X-ray the correct level of section of the neck of the femur in order to achieve a stable reduction are occasionally inaccurate; therefore one tends to leave a little extra length on the stump of the neck of the femur when resecting the head to allow for shortening at the time of the test reduction. The use of the 'neck-length jig' (Chap. 16) now makes this stage of the operation a matter of some precision making pre-operative radiographic measurements unnecessary as well as supplanting the need for a full range of the test prostheses during the operation.

Chapter 12

Detachment and Reattachment of the Great Trochanter

If it could be guaranteed that a great trochanter would unite within 3 weeks when reattached, and without imposing restrictions which would impede rehabilitation, few surgeons would fail to avail themselves of the easy and beautiful access to the hip joint provided by the lateral approach. The author has never minimized the disadvantages of failing to achieve osseous union of a detached trochanter. The fact that non-union of a trochanter only rarely interferes seriously with function, and X-rays can reveal detached trochanters which were never suspected, does not advance the science of hip surgery. A disadvantage of non-union of the trochanter with complete separation, is that it can precipitate early and late dislocation. If associated with discomfort and broken wires non-union can be damaging to a surgeon's reputation.

Reattachment of a trochanter certainly tests a surgeon's natural mechanical instincts, but it is a general principle in any orthopaedic procedure that inability to teach consistent success always indicates that there must be something basically wrong in the method. In a study of trochanter union at Wrightington (Boardman and Bocco, 1977[31]) a total of 5% of radiological failure of union of the trochanter was revealed and postgraduates in training had a failure rate 2.3 times higher than the consultants even though the latter in secondary interventions had more difficult cases.

The main reason for the author's withholding publication over the last 10 years of the detailed LFA technique has been the testing of many different methods of reattaching the trochanter. Only since 1974, with the development of the method to be recommended here, is it believed that the problem of the trochanter has been truly solved; or at least solved for those surgeons who are prepared to follow with understanding the technique described.

Theory of Union of the Trochanter

The trochanter is composed of cancellous bone and has an excellent blood supply; therefore it is well suited for rapid union under ideal conditions of mechanical fixation.

In the very early days of total hip replacement at Wrightington (Teflon, 1958–1962) the author used to produce complete lateral displacement of the trochanter applying it to the lateral, cortical surface of the femur (Fig. 12.1). The area of bone contact was only small and fixation was by a single horizontal loop of wire. For the first 3 weeks these patients were nursed in hip spica plasters, without weight-bearing, and despite the very primitive fixation there were no cases of non-union. Non-union only started to manifest itself when early rehabilitation was introduced.

Failure to achieve 100% osseous union of the trochanter indicates: failure to achieve perfect fixation; and failure to maintain perfect fixation during a critical period. This critical period could be as short as the 3 weeks immediately following the operation.

It is curious that we seem to refuse to acknowledge that the abductor muscles must exert an extremely powerful force on the trochanter when walking activity is encouraged. If the abduction force in the post-operative phase were to be only half that in normal activity this would still be about equal to the weight of the body, because in normal activity the abductor muscles contract with a force about twice body weight. These forces are truly enormous when compared with the forces the internal fixation of a fractured long bone is likely

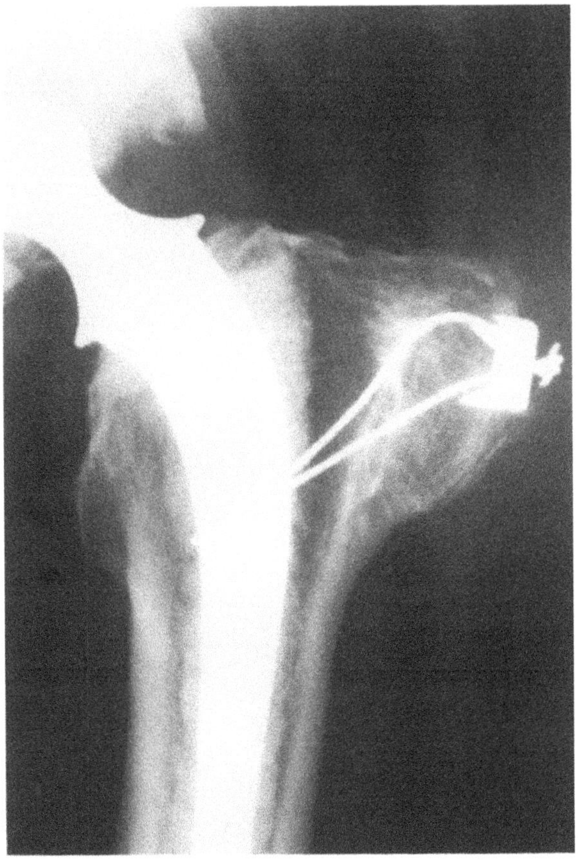

Fig. 12.1. Extreme lateral displacement of trochanter used 1958–1962

to experience during the first 3–4 post-operative weeks.

That the trochanter must possess strong natural powers of union, despite the powerful forces acting on it, is shown by the fact that a multitude of different wiring techniques, none of which can possibly maintain truly rigid fixation, at the worst do not produce more than about 10% of failures. Surely this must suggest that it requires only a little more understanding of the factors causing defective fixation in this particular site for consistent success to be possible.

Psychology and Reattachment

Surgeons disillusioned by failure to secure consistent union of the trochanter cannot be blamed for disliking this anticlimactic stage of total hip replacement. If a surgeon believes that union of the trochanter is out of his control he will not be interested in new techniques. On the other hand when a surgeon feels that he is in control of union then other factors combine to stimulate his interest; such as to improve the biomechanics of the hip by slight lateral displacement of the trochanter (Chap. 21); to guarantee, almost, that patients will not dislocate post-operatively (Chap. 19); and to encourage rehabilitation as vigorously as if the trochanter had not been elevated (or even more vigorously).

With these objectives in mind reattachment of the trochanter then becomes almost the most interesting part of the operation, especially when the wide exposure removes all problems in cementing the implants in perfect alignment and with a good bonding technique.

Biomechanics of Failure to Unite

In the past it was considered that the only force to be counteracted when reattaching the trochanter was the pull of the abductor muscles (gluteus medius and minimus). These muscles were never envisaged as acting otherwise than with the hip in the anatomical position: i.e. extended as in standing or walking.

If the abductor muscles pulled only in the extended position of the hip, a simple calculation will show that most wiring techniques ought to be able to resist the available force. If the traction force of the abductors in the period of rehabilitation were no greater than body weight (as previously suggested) there still would be a safety factor of at least four to six times if four to six strands of wire cross from trochanter to femur [each strand of 18 s.w.g. wire is capable of taking 100–150 lb (45–68 kg)] and muscle tension can be estimated at the strength of one strand.

Resistance to Shearing Motion

An important feature contributing to fixation of the trochanter is the interlocking of the rough cancellous surfaces of the osteotomy under the compression produced by tightening the wires. The frictional resistance so produced can resist very powerful shearing movements in the plane of the osteotomy.

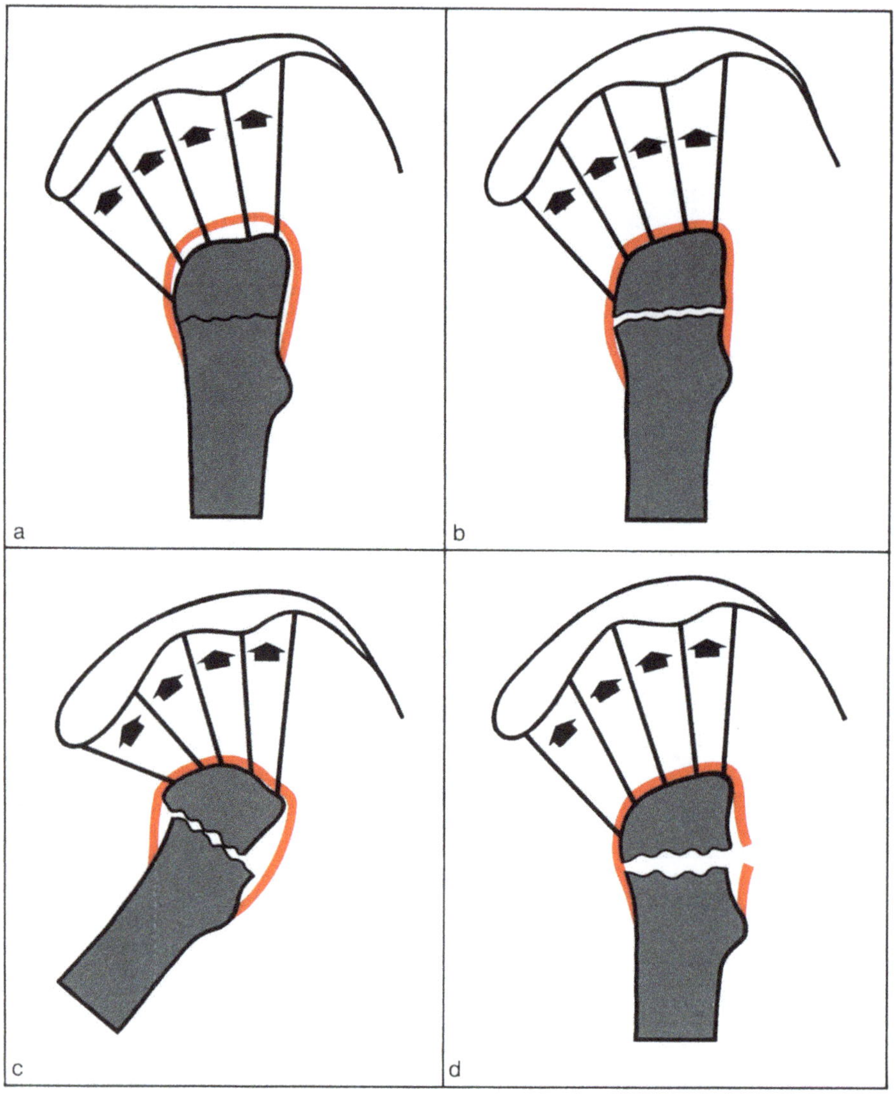

Fig. 12.2 a–d. Mechanism of loosening of wires: **a** Soft tissue trapped between wire and cortex of trochanter. **b** Soft tissues necrosing; osteotomy separates. **c** Frictional resistance against shearing lost; trochanter slides forwards. **d** Trochanter pulled back in extended position; wires fatigue and fracture

In the sequence of events which leads to failure of union it is suggested that there are two phases. **In the first phase** the tension of the abductor muscles acts in the long axis of the femur (as when standing or walking) and tends to separate the surfaces of the osteotomy, to disengage the interlocking of the asperities and so to reduce resistance to shear. Soft tissues clothing the external surface of the trochanter (fibrous tissue, periosteum, and some tendon fibres) are trapped between the loops of wire and the underlying cortex of the trochanter (Fig. 12.2a) and these start to necrose. The pull of the abductor muscles is then able to separate the osteotomy by the thickness of the necrosed tissue (Fig. 12.2b) and so the rough surfaces of the osteotomy become truly disengaged.

The second phase concerns changes in direction of pull of the abductor muscles in relation to the position of the hip joint. In actions such as mounting a staircase, sitting down, or rising from sitting, the pelvis remains more or less horizontal so that the abductor muscles continue to act in a vertical direction even though the hip may be in flexion.

Fig. 12.3 a–c. Test apparatus. **a** General view. Load pulling vertically; hip in flexed position. **b** Hip extended; load still pulling vertically; clock micrometer at zero position. **c** Hip flexed; load pulling vertically; trochanter has moved forward; micrometer indicates distance moved

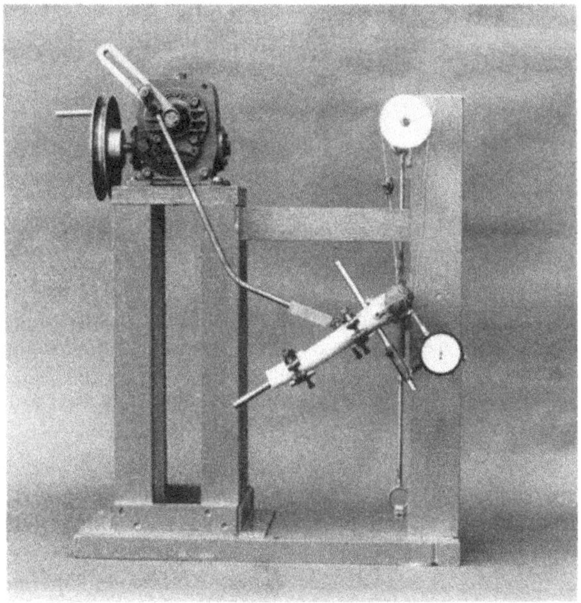

a

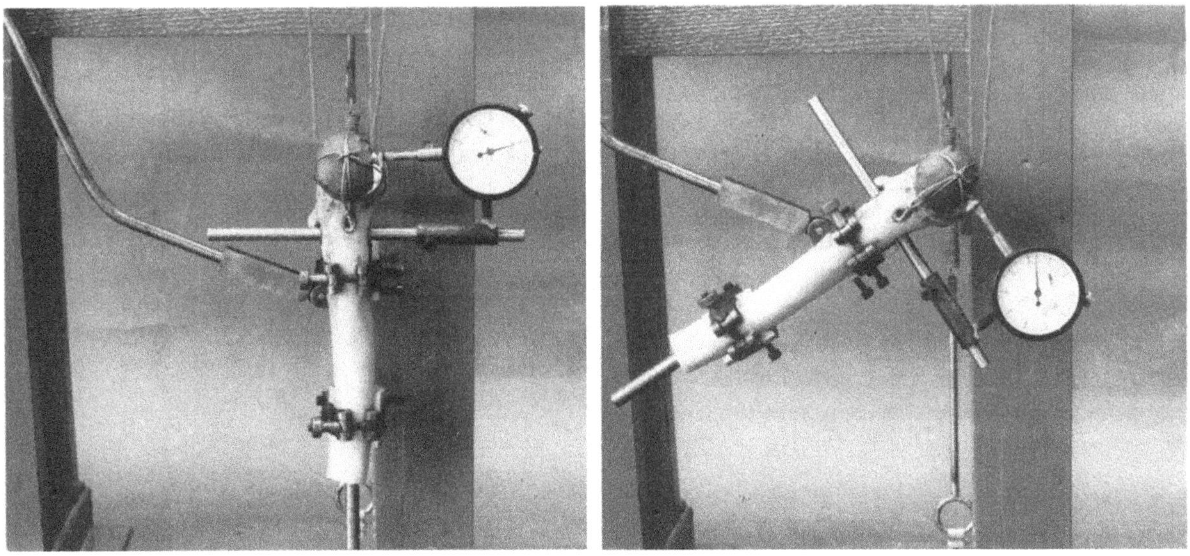

b c

The line of abductor muscle pull will therefore change from being in line with the axis of the femur in extension. In flexion of the hip the abductor muscles will tend to pull the trochanter forwards in relation to the axis of the femur and produce a shearing force on the osteotomy (Fig. 12.2c). If frictional resistance at the osteotomy is lost (as a result of the slight separation following necrosis of soft tissues as described above) the trochanter will move forwards in relation to the femur. As the flexed hip returns to the extended position the trochanter will be pulled back again, into alignment with the femur. Repeated backward and forward movement of the trochanter abrades the surfaces of the osteotomy and the gap of the osteotomy further increases. A vicious circle starts: the increasing width of the osteotomy gap permits longer lengths of wire to cross between trochanter and femur permitting a greater range of backward and forward movement. Fatigue fracture of the wires then ensues. After the first fatigue fracture the amplitude of movement increases still further to be followed by fatigue fractures of the remaining wires (Fig. 12.2d).

This process has been simulated in a test rig and it has been demonstrated that all the elementary wiring systems can be fatigued and broken in a matter of 3–4 h (at 120 cycles/min) depending on the amount of abductor tension imposed (Fig. 12.3a, b, c).

This test apparatus incorporates certain subtleties not immediately obvious. It is designed specially to test fixation when the osteotomy line has lost frictional resistance against shear, even though the wiring may still be tight. This is achieved by using a trochanter made of hard wood (or plastic) with the cut trochanteric surface on the femur protected by a smooth metal plate cemented in position (partially visible in Fig. 12b). The drill holes in the femur through which the wires are passed are lined with metal tubes cemented in position; without this the wire loosens very quickly by cutting into the edges of the holes and repeated tests become impossible. The artificial trochanter is covered with a 2-mm-thick layer of rubber to simulate periosteum, etc. The abductor muscle tension is applied (Fig. 12a) by a loop of Bowden cable passing over a plastic pulley on one end of a lever; the other end of the lever is pulled downwards with a spring of adjustable strength. The pulley enables the specimen to flex and extend without altering the tension in the front and back wires of the loop. The backward and forward shearing of the trochanter is measured by the clock micrometer; in this case a movement of 0.018 in. has occurred during the range of flexion and returns to zero when the specimen returns to vertical. An electric motor can be connected by V-belt to the reduction gear to perform fatigue tests at 120 cycles/min.

This experimental rig has demonstrated the importance of developing **a mechanism which will resist backward and forward movement of the trochanter**.

Criticism of Bolts and Screws

A number of techniques have employed bolts or screws with the object of applying a compression force perpendicular to the plane of the osteotomy. This has the following mechanical weaknesses:

1) It is difficult to estimate an end-point for the tightening of a compression bolt, because of the cancellous nature of a trochanter. To overtighten will crush the egg-shell-thin cortex of the trochanter and seriously weaken the whole assembly.

2) A spring washer under the head of a bolt or screw will mitigate the danger of crushing the egg-shell cortex of a trochanter, but it will produce a projection in the centre of the surface of the trochanter which takes part in the sliding mechanism of the trochanteric bursa. Large projections of metal from the lateral side of the femur are not uncommon in different types of hip surgery but those that cause no symptoms all lie distal to the vastus lateralis ridge and therefore do not encroach on the sliding, bursal surface of the trochanter.

3) Bolts and screws can resist abduction forces (especially if washers are used to spread the load) very powerfully but they are weak in resisting backward and forward shearing movements of the trochanter, especially if the thin cortical shell of the trochanter has been crushed. The hole through which the bolt passes in the thin cortex of the trochanter can enlarge in an antero-posterior direction, permitting the trochanter to move backwards and forwards.

To fix the trochanter with two or more ordinary bone screws is a popular method but it is by no means as simple as it sounds. With conventional designs of femoral prosthesis, with stems which are narrow in antero-posterior thickness, a layer

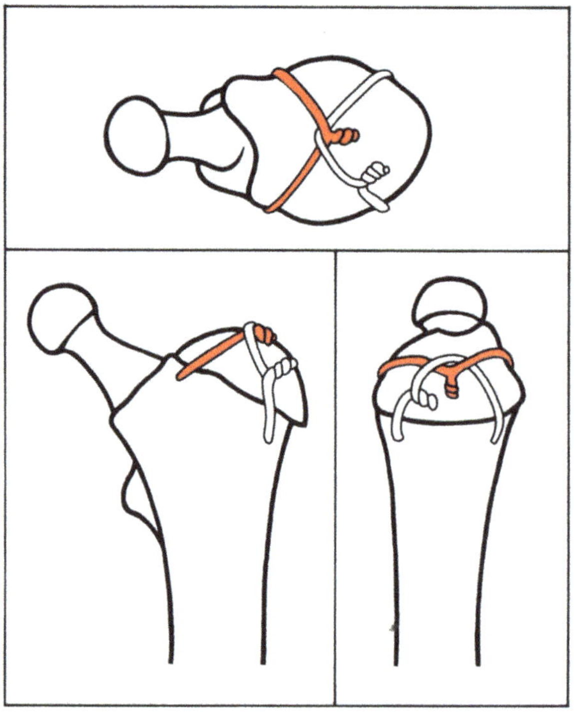

Fig. 12.4. The cruciate wire system. The red wire is the 'pulley'. For clarity the double vertical wire has not been included

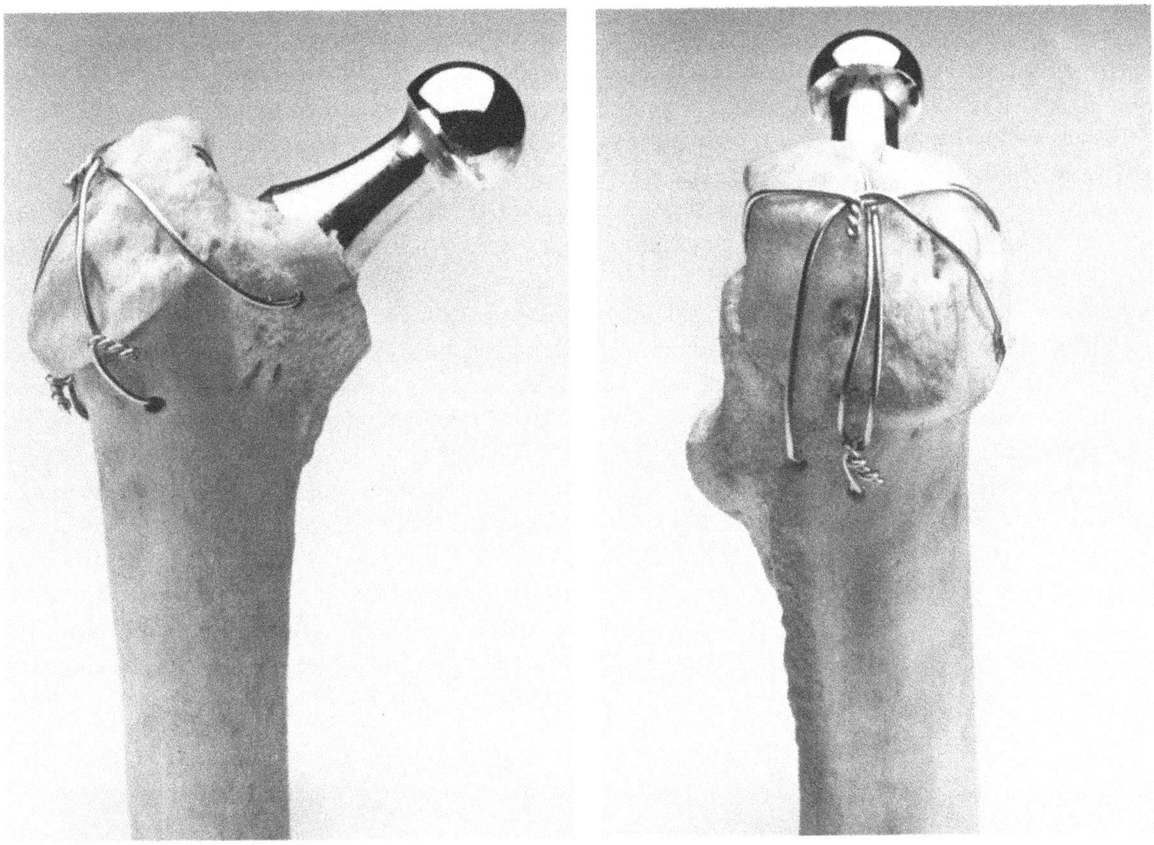

a b

Fig. 12.5a, b. Cruciate wiring system with vertical double wire. **a** Anterior view. **b** Lateral appearance

of cement can exist in front of and behind the stem and this can be drilled and tapped to receive the screws. But the flanged (Cobra) design of prosthesis occupies the full width of an enlarged medullary cavity and this technique with screws is not possible.

Cruciate Wiring System

The cruciate wiring system, with pulley component, is a very reliable technique (even without the staple-clamp) in the hands of surgeons who fully understand it. It is essential to appreciate how the cruciate system works because it is futile to use it without complete understanding. It is used always in conjunction with the vertical double loop of wire, though this latter is not truly part of the cruciate system. The vertical double loop offers a method of fixing the trochanter in the desired position while the cruciate system is being woven through the fibres of the abductor muscles close to the surface of the trochanter. For the sake of simplicity in the following description the vertical double loop will be ignored.

It will be seen (Fig. 12.4) that the cruciate wire is composed of two separate wires; the one indicated in red (the medial wire) will become the pulley and is completed first (but after the vertical double wire has been used to tack the trochanter in the desired position). The one indicated in white (the lateral wire) pulls round the completed pulley.

The special feature of the cruciate system is that by reason of the pulley the tightening of the last pair of wires is distributed to all four limbs of the cross simultaneously. Moreover, the pulley system tends to multiply the force and compensate for force lost in frictional resistance. The technique of using a spike or awl to centre the cruciate system on the trochanter and to initiate the uniform tightening of all four arms of the cross is very important (Chap. 15, stages 129 and 130).

Vertical, Double Wire Loop

The wire of the vertical double loop is not considered part of the cruciate system even though it contributes two more arms to give the final cross a total of six radial arms (Fig. 12.5a, b). The vertical double loop is prone to making a defective contribution in the final state of the fixation if it lies anterior to the centre of the trochanter. In this position it is lying 'on the side of a hill' and can easily slide forwards and lose all tension. Similarly if the vertical double loop does not achieve a stable purchase in a notch in the bone as it passes over the summit of the trochanter, the tension of tightening may be resisted merely by the tendinous fibres of the abductor muscles and when these have necrosed the loop will slide forwards and lose tension.

Wire Tighteners

There are many technical aspects in the tightening of wires which are surprisingly inefficient when tested away from the operating table. One common and serious defect is the failure to transmit tension caused by the very high frictional resistance of stainless steel sliding on stainless steel. For this reason no wire tightener should be used in which the two wires lie side by side in a steel tube, are both pulled **in the same direction**, and then diverge at 90° from each other. To change the direction of pull of the two stainless steel wires through 90° by friction round fixed points of small radius (also of stainless steel) can lose 75% of the force applied by the tightener.

The best wire tightener therefore must employ a spreading action pulling the wires **in opposite directions**. But even so the full tension will not reach the bone if it is applied through a half-hitch. The force lost in a stainless steel half-hitch is quite surprising. The best method is to tighten by pulling in opposite directions with the wires lying side by side; then, a mere 45° twist from the parallel alignment of the wires will lock the tension exerted on the bone, so great is the frictional resistance of stainless steel on stainless steel. Thereafter the tension generated by the tightener will not be lost when the tightener is relaxed **provided that traction is exerted on the holder** to keep the wires locked by friction in the 45° twisted position. Details of doing this are described (Chap. 15, stage 124).

The fastening of tensioned wires by twisting is preferred to the use of square knots; but it is essential that the wire should be not thinner than 18 s.w.g. if it is to be fastened by twisting. The fastening of wire by twisting can be disastrous if the operator does not understand what has to be done. Merely to go on twisting is to guarantee to cause the wire to break and to break exactly at the first twist, in contact with the bone, so that no fixation at all is left. It has to be understood that the tension on the bone is merely that applied by the wire tightener and no attempt must be made to raise it by twisting. The first 45° twist locks the tension applied by the tightener. Thereafter the wire tightener is slackened off as subsequent turns are applied distal to the first locking turn. It is easily possible to build up 1 cm of twisted

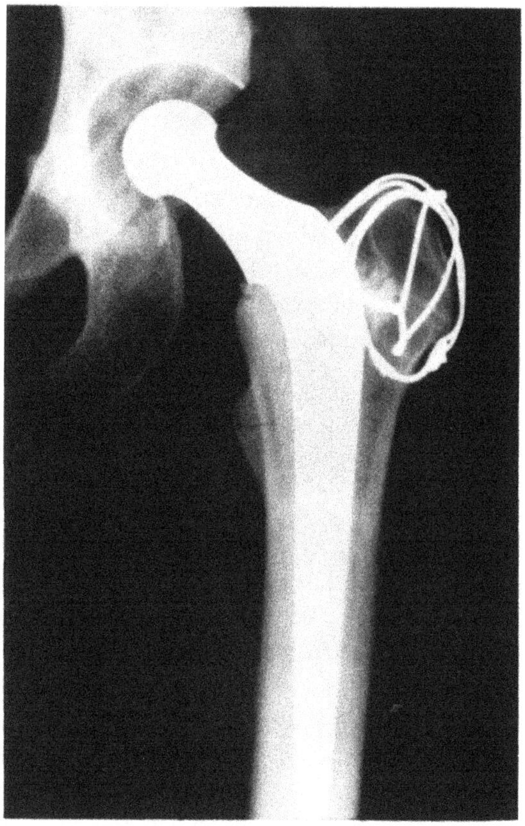

Fig. 12.6. X-ray appearance of complete cruciate wiring with double vertical wire. 35-mm-offset prosthesis

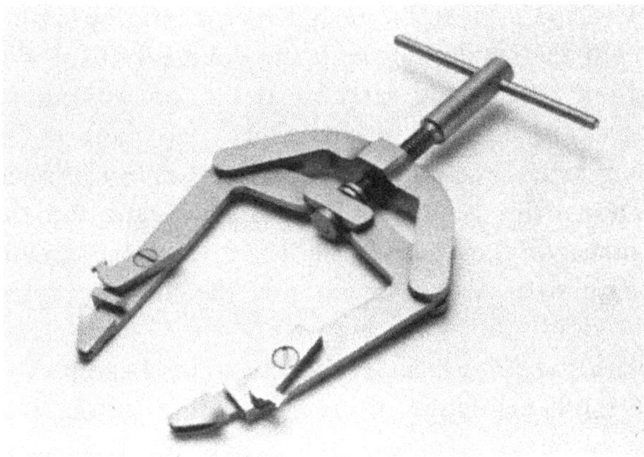

Fig. 12.7. Author's wire tighteners

wire distal to the first 45° twist without raising the tension in the essential part.

The use of a Kirschner wire tightener was our practice at Wrightington for many years but can no longer be recommended, for two reasons: First because the screw and its nut are made of stainless steel and after some years of use the frictional resistance under quite moderate tension is so great that the surgeon believes he is applying strong tension when in fact very little force is reaching the wire. Second, the Kirschner wire tightener employs a lever system where the mechanical advantage changes very markedly: the lever system is too advantageous when the jaws are wide apart. The surgeon therefore cannot assess the tension he is delivering to the bone.

The author considers that his design of tightener (Fig. 12.7) is a very important contribution to the successful reattachment of the trochanter. The mechanical advantage remains fairly constant for ordinary openings of the jaws. Because it is possible to take up slack in the process of inserting the wires into the jaws, full tightening can be obtained without the jaws having to separate very widely. This is convenient when working in a confined space. The method of locking the wires in the jaws employs a servo mechanism which eliminates slip and in addition makes it possible for the surgeon to apply the tightener without the skilled help of an assistant.

Wire Breakage During Tightening

Breakage of wire when tightening is always the operator's fault; it is impossible to break 18 s.w.g. stainless steel wire in pure tension under the highest forces likely to be used in surgery. The cause of a break is a kink (which may be out of sight under muscle) which shears the metal in torsion. Figure 12.7A shows how a kink (b) is formed if one continues to apply traction to a loop such as that in (a). At higher magnification (c) the surface of the metal can be seen showing the concentration of strain at the site where failure in torsion will occur. The only way to avoid this kink is not to permit a loop to form, or to unwind the loop before it gets to the state of (b).

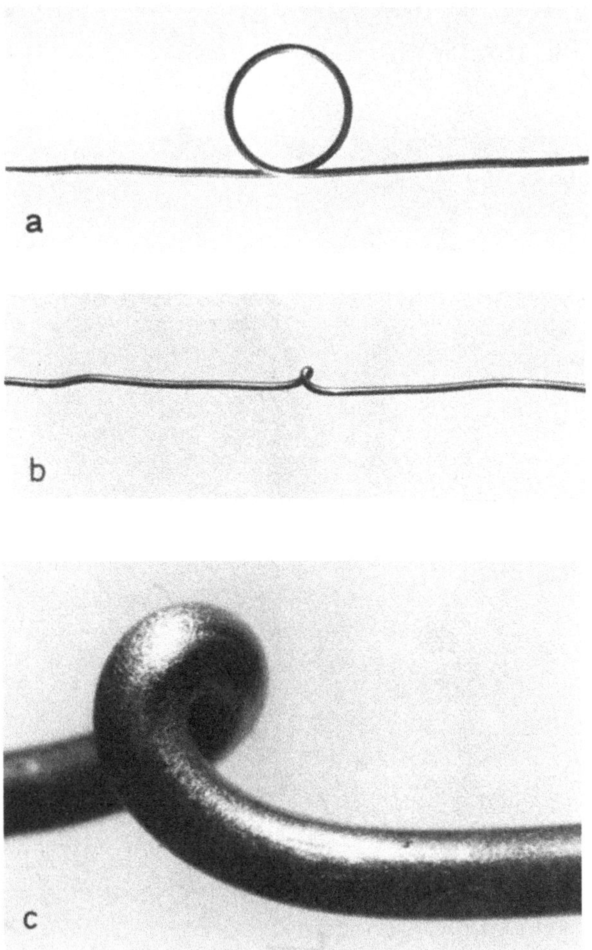

Fig. 12.7A. Mechanism of wire breakage during tightening. See text

Staple-Clamp

This device (Fig. 12.8) is designed **solely to resist backward and forward shearing motion** of the trochanter. It is **not** intended to resist the vertical pull of the abductors; this must be controlled by a wiring system. In early experiments the author used the staple-bolt with the double vertical wire alone, permitting early rehabilitation without restriction (Fig. 12.9a, b). Only two failures by complete detachment occurred in some 150 operations. But despite this low failure rate, the elegance of the X-ray (Fig. 12.10) and the greatly simplified surgical technique, the author prefers to go for 100% success by using the staple-clamp with the full cruciate wiring system. Examples of the full technique of cruciate wiring system plus staple-clamp show the appearance, Fig. 12.11 without lateral displacement of the trochanter and Fig. 12.12 with 1-cm lateral shift.

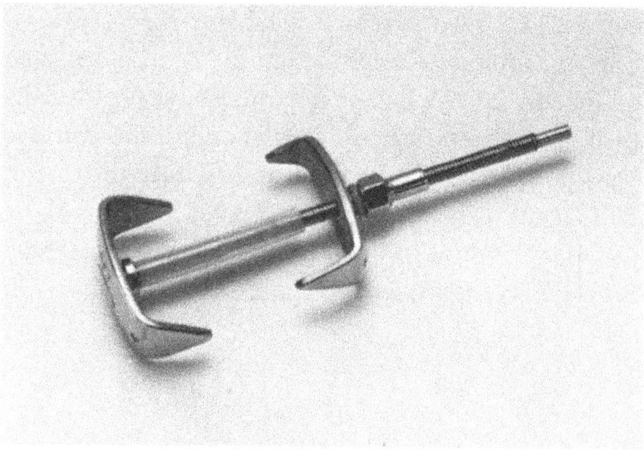

Fig. 12.8. The staple-clamp or staple-bolt

Fractures of Trochanter and Fractures of Upper End of Femur

An attractive feature of the staple-clamp is that if the trochanter should sustain a vertical split (as occasionally happens if it has been necessary to

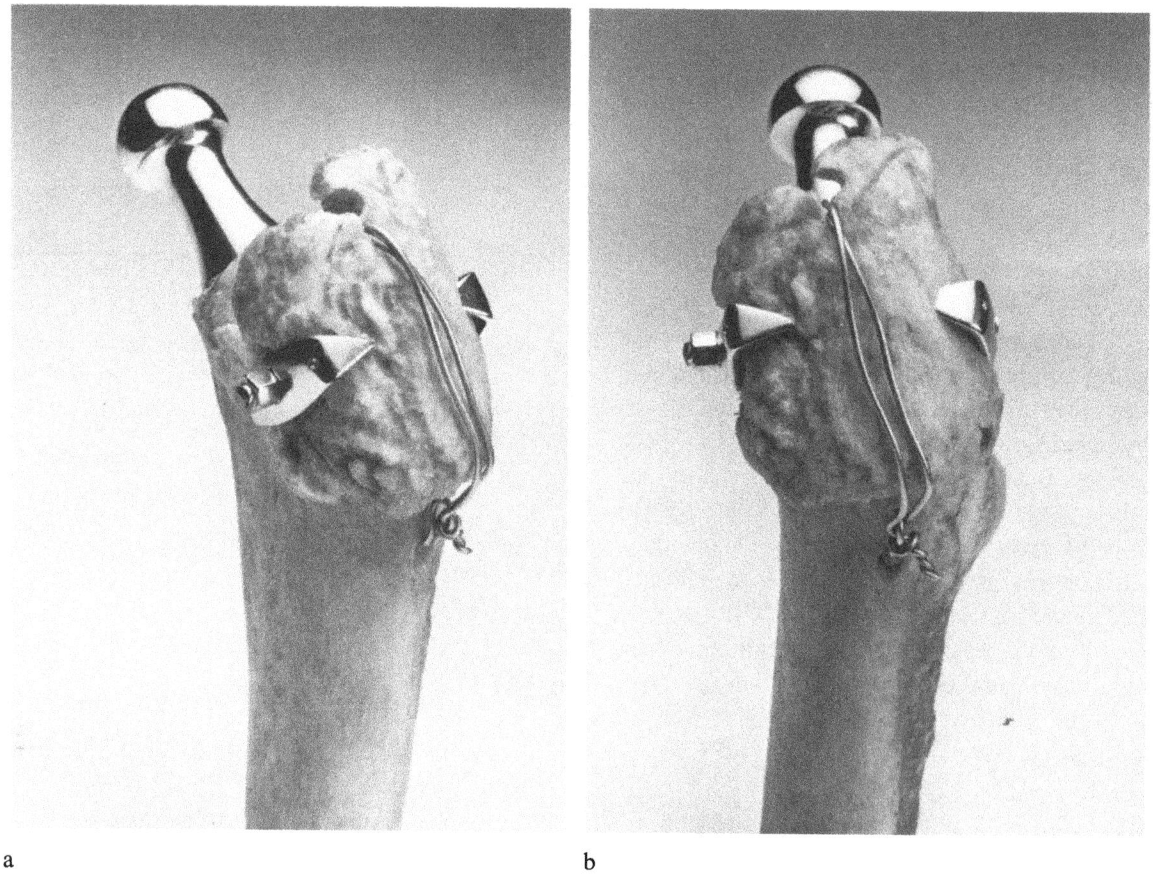

a b

Fig. 12.9a, b. Staple-clamp with double vertical wire alone. **a** Antero-lateral view. **b** Lateral view

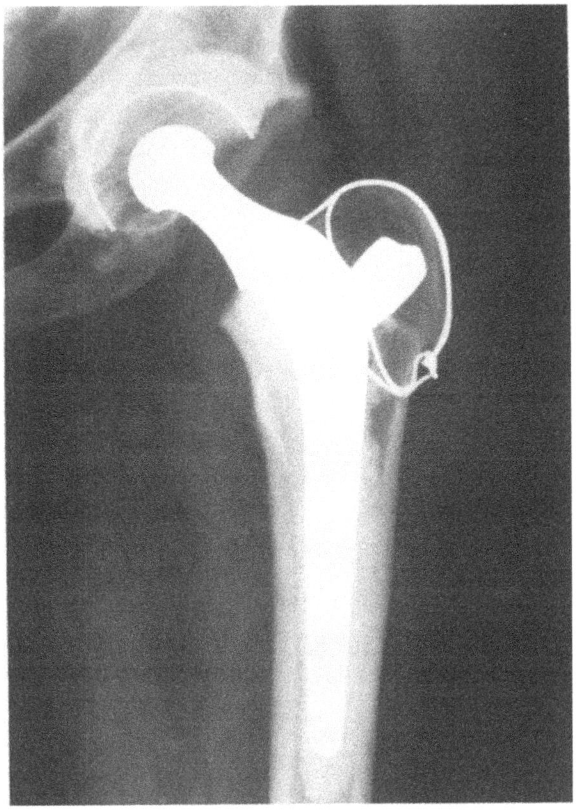

Fig. 12.10. X-ray appearance of staple-clamp with double vertical wire alone

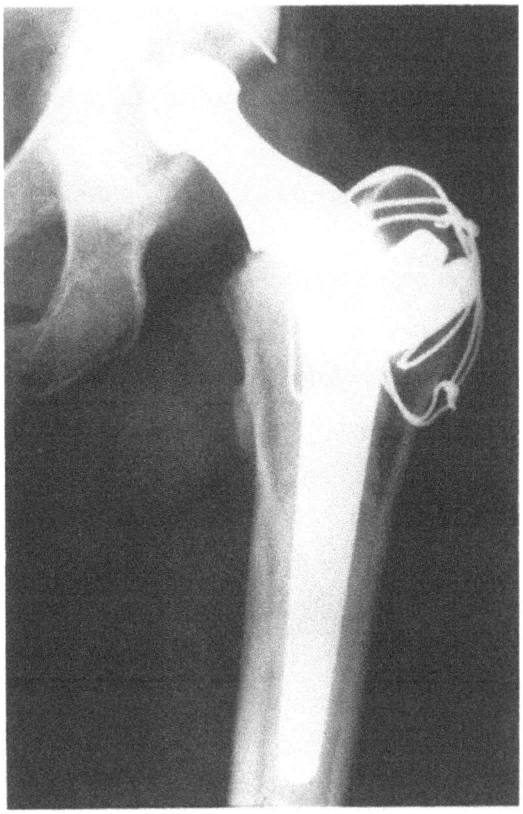

Fig. 12.11. X-ray appearance of 40-mm offset prosthesis with complete cruciate wiring system plus staple-bolt

detach the trochanter with an osteotome, or by over-tightening the vertical double wire in osteoporotic bone) the broken trochanter can be compressed in an antero-posterior direction by the staple-clamp, so achieving complete control of the situation and permitting rehabilitation at the ordinary rate. Similarly, if the anterior or the posterior cortex of the upper end of the medullary cavity of the femur is split away as a pedunculated flap (as can happen during the extraction of a Moore prosthesis) the trochanter staple-clamp applies a reassuring compressive force and early rehabilitation can be permitted as if no complication had been incurred.

Special Reattachment Problems

A method of using the staple-clamp in difficult reconstructions at secondary interventions is illustrated in Figs. 12.13 and 12.14. In this case the cut surface of the trochanter had to be applied to the lateral, cortical surface of the shaft of the femur. The deep surface of the trochanter was therefore hollowed in a roughly cylindrical fashion to fit approximately to the cylindrical lateral surface of the femur. A $^{1}/_{8}$-in. hole (3.2 mm) was drilled in an antero-posterior direction as superficially as possible under the lateral cortex of the femur and the staple-clamp was inserted from behind.

Speed of Recovery

It is not to be expected that the average show of early function, at 7–10 days after the operation with reattachment of the trochanter, will be quite as spectacular as can be the case when the trochanter has not been touched. Nevertheless, with efficient reattachment of the trochanter 50% of patients will equal the best performance of those without the trochanter having been touched, and in addition they can all be allowed to undertake activity without restraint.

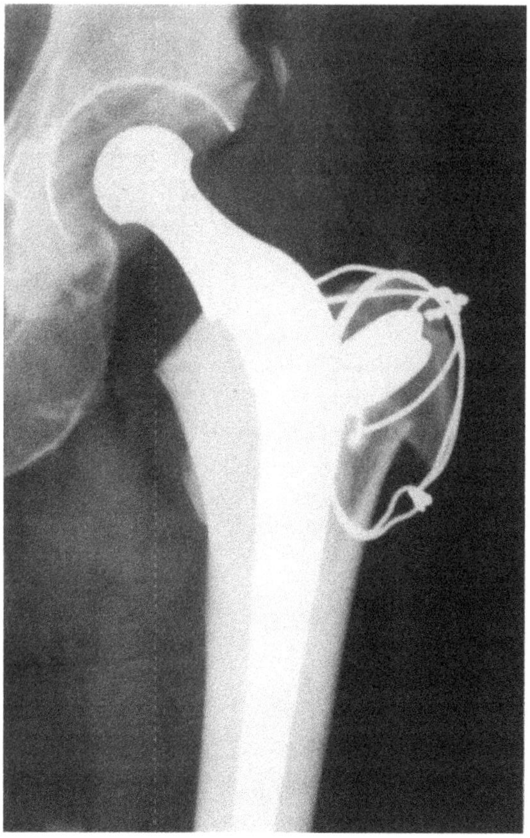

Fig. 12.12. X-ray appearance of 40-mm offset prosthesis and complete cruciate wiring system plus staple-bolt with 1-cm lateral displacement of trochanter

The object of total hip replacement is to build well for 20 years; it is not for sensational short-term results.

Discomfort over the Trochanter

Pain or discomfort over the trochanter, sometimes associated with clicking, can be a disadvantage of the lateral exposure. If the X-ray demonstrates an ugly arrangement of wires, and also perhaps broken wires, the patient cannot be blamed for attributing one to the other. The oblique incision centred on the trochanter as developed by Brady[32] was a landmark in the author's experience of access to the acetabulum by the lateral exposure, emphasizing as it did the extension of the proximal part of the incision in the direction of the fibres of gluteus maximus. But in the 2 years the author used this incision there was a noticeable increase in the frequency with which patients complained of pain and clicking and it seemed possible that this was caused by sutures in the ilio-tibial band passing over the bursal surface of the trochanter. It was for this reason that the author developed the current incision in the

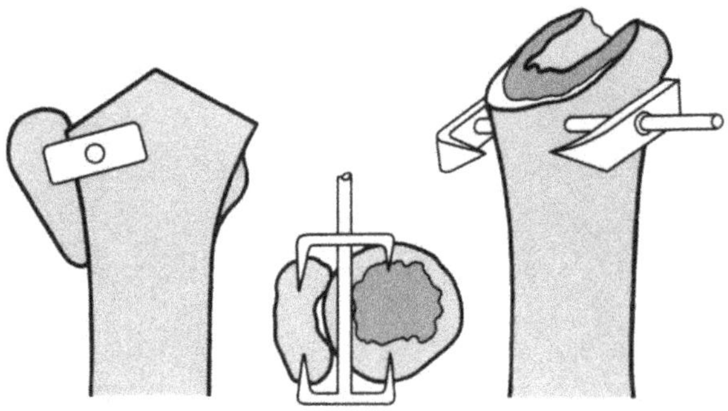

Fig. 12.13. Difficult problem solved in unusual way. (See text)

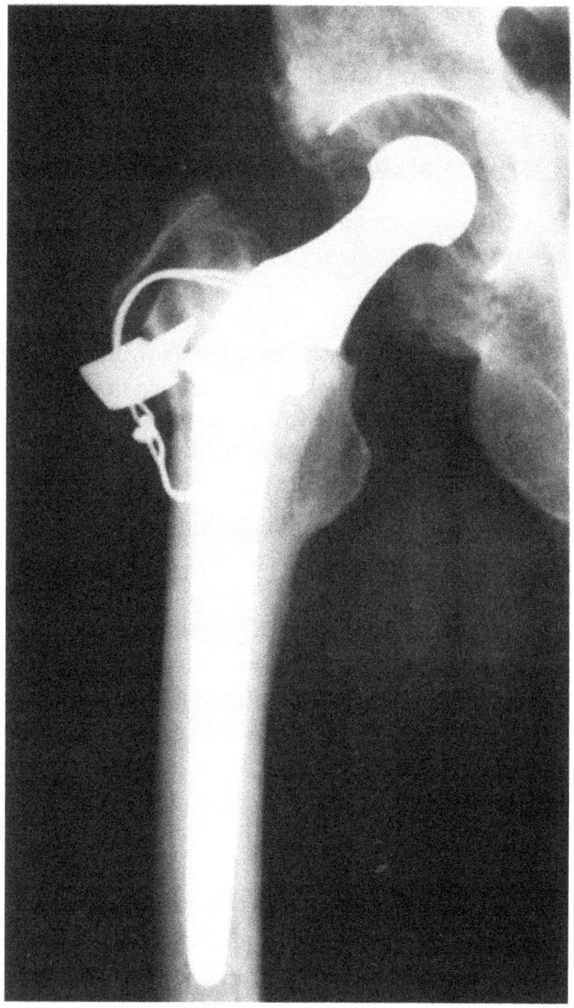

Fig. 12.14. X-ray appearance of Fig. 12.13

fascia lata which incorporates the improved access of Brady's exposure but permits the sutures to lie in front of the trochanter. It is now decidedly unusual for patients to make a volunteered remark about discomfort in this region.

As regards distaste for lying or sleeping on the operated trochanter it would not seem that this is confined only to trochanters which have been elevated in the course of the exposure. This complaint can be encountered when the trochanter has not been elevated, but how frequently one cannot judge.

Final Comments

The force generated by the abductor muscles, because of the well-known leverage systems in the hip joint, is among the highest muscle forces encountered in the body. In no other site of osteosynthesis do surgeons expect bones to unite within 3–4 weeks when exposed to distracting forces of such an order. If early rehabilitation is to be encouraged after total hip replacement conventional methods of reattachment of a trochanter are grossly inadequate.

When the trochanter is displaced laterally from its original site on the femur; and when the site of origin is encroached upon by reaming and by cement; it is all the more essential that a highly sophisticated method of reattachment should be used. Using the cruciate wire system plus the staple-clamp the author has had no problems when the prosthesis and cement have encroached on the area from which the trochanter was detached and when rehabilitation without restriction has been permitted from the third post-operative day.

The trochanter varies enormously in its mechanical strength in different diseases and any method of fixation must be able to cope with trochanters of osteoporotic or dense bone. No wiring system by itself can **maintain** perfect fixation, because of the intervention of necrosing soft tissues between wire and bone. It is therefore necessary to have an additional device which pierces the soft tissues to make direct contact with the bone of the two fragments. But no additional device can make direct contact with an area of cortical bone sufficient to resist by itself the enormous forces acting on the trochanter. The function of the cage of wire is to reduce the forces acting on the staple-clamp and permit it to continue to exercise its function of fixation against antero-posterior shearing movement.

The author's observations identify the antero-posterior direction of movement as the one which all other methods fail to control. Experience indicates that using these principles it is a practical possibility to achieve union of the trochanter in 3–4 weeks even with unrestricted rehabilitation.

A Technical Radiographic Detail

Post-operative external rotation distorts the antero-posterior X-ray appearances of a reattached trochanter; therefore the antero-posterior post-operative film should always be taken with the hip in internal rotation. Attempts to put the limb into internal rotation generally will only succeed in putting the upper end of the femur into neutral antero-posterior alignment.

Chapter 13

Clean Air Operating – Theory *

It is now 15 years since the author started to explore the effects of extreme aseptic precautions in the operating room in relation to post-operative infection after total hip replacement. We are still however a long way from agreement even on the most basic of all questions: whether post-operative infection is acquired in the operating room or not.

The classic attitude of the bacteriologist is against airborne infection in the operating room as a major factor in post-operative wound infection. This attitude probably derives from the dominant position occupied by **Staphylococcus aureus** in investigations of epidemics of post-operative infection and the rarity of this organism in the air of operating rooms. It is now becoming generally recognized that in infections after using acrylic cement, **Staph. aureus** is now responsible for less than half the infections; many of the organisms are of a type commonly found on the skin and not previously considered seriously as the cause of infection in surgery.

In this chapter experience with clean air and other aseptic precautions in the operating room is presented and especially experience subsequent to the author's paper of 1972(33) which was based on clinical data collected before the end of 1970. Since that time some 6000 more operations have been performed, with 2 years elapsing since the last operation, and in this new series there are none of the uncontrolled variables which were a serious defect of the previous published work.

Before presenting the evidence from Wrightington in favour of the 'ultra-clean' environment summaries will first be presented of two interesting recent studies of infection in total hip replacement where bacteriological contamination of the open wound is found to bear no relationship to the bacterial contamination of the surrounding air. What bearing these studies may have on the clinical situation will be considered in the discussion at the end of the chapter.

* This chapter incorporates material presented by the author in the Lister Oration of the Royal College of Surgeons of England, May 1976.

Bacteriological Studies Not Supporting 'Ultra-Clean' Air

1) McLauchlan, Logie, Smylie and Smith, 1976(34)

One-hundred and nine total hip operations were performed in a surgical isolator (Trexler) with 108 identical operations as controls in the same plenum-ventilated theatre without the isolator. The air inside the isolator was confirmed as being sterile by tests during each operation whereas the air of the open theatre had an average of 6.2 colony forming units per cubic foot of air (6.2 c.f.u./ft^3).

Bacteriological sampling of the wounds throughout the procedure revealed positive cultures in 36% of the isolator patients and 58% of the open theatre patients. Major wound contamination (defined as more than 100 colonies) was found in 12 of the isolator and 11 of the ordinary theatre cases. The contaminated wounds were found to be contaminated at an early stage of the operation. Of the 23 wounds with major contamination 17 were by coagulase-negative staphylococci and the remaining six by **Staph. pyogenes**. All wounds, including the six contaminated with **Staph. pyogenes** healed without infection (no prophylactic antibiotics being used in this study). Examples of heavy bacterial growth on culture media are illustrated in this paper showing colonies growing from a skin biopsy and from a knife blade in the isolator series. Bacteriological sampling of the exterior of the surgeon's gloves at the end of wound closure was positive in 18 of the isolator cases and 34 of the control cases.

In the open theatre the amount of contamination in the wound was considered to be 'far in excess of any possible contamination from airborne bacteria' and it is suggested that the bacteria which were recovered from the open wound during the operation derived from the cut skin edges. It is not stated whether skin-edge towels were used.

Two deep infections (1.8%) occurred in both the isolator and the control series (four infections or 1.8% in total). None of the deep infections could be attributed to bacteria grown from the wound and were attributed to cross-infection in the ward (open 'Nightingale-type' ward), because in all four instances of deep infection the wound dressings were so heavily soaked with exudate that they had to be changed within the first or second post-operative days.

2) Franco, Baer and Enneking, 1977[35]

Bacterial wound contamination in total hip replacement was estimated qualitatively and quantitatively using three types of wound environment:

1) LFS/AS (laminar air flow system with aspiration suits): 37 total hips
2) LFS (laminar air flow system with conventional operating room clothing): 41 total hips
3) Control: (surgery in the same enclosure but without the laminar air flow or the aspiration suits): 30 patients, all general orthopaedic operations

Airborne micro-organisms were monitored by slit-sampler. In the LFS/AS group 60% of cases, and in the LFS group 27%, had zero airborne organisms. In the control group 71% had airborne organisms in excess of 4 c.f.u./ft^3 air.

Slit-sampler tests in the control group showed 10 times higher counts than the LFS group and 25 times higher levels than the LFS/AS group. The LFS group had about twice as many airborne bacteria as the LFS/AS group. Wound contamination was monitored by specimens taken at 20-min intervals throughout the operation and expressed as the number of organisms recovered per wound culture.

Correlation air/wound contamination. Statistical analysis showed no correlation between the level of airborne microbial contamination in the air and contamination of the wound in any of the three groups.

Qualitative bacteriological studies. Staph. aureus was cultured from the air in seven cases and from the wound in three; in only one case was **Staph. aureus** recovered simultaneously from air and wound.

Post-operative infections. The organisms grown from the infected wounds in every case were different from those grown from the air or from the open wound at the operation.

Wound infections. There were four infections, but only one was a deep infection of a total hip. This was an infection of late onset with **Staph. aureus** and the operation had been performed in laminar air flow without aspiration suits. There was therefore one deep infection in 78 total hips = 1.3% (or 1 in 41 total hips in the LFS group = 2.5%).

Criteria for Diagnosing Post-operative Infection

In all studies of post-operative wound infection it is important to try to make some classification into types of post-operative infection, in the hope that this might help in deciding when and where the infection might have been acquired.

If sufficient time is allowed to elapse after the operation the **incidence** of deep infection is not difficult to decide after total hip replacement, because radiological and clinical proof can hardly ever be missed. In this respect acrylic cement can be regarded as a specially sensitive tool in the investigation of post-operative infection.

To classify types of infection, in the hope of casting light on the most likely time and place of acquiring the infection, has proved more difficult than we originally thought and an extended experience indicates that merely to classify as 'early' or 'late' manifestations is not very helpful.

The classification used by McLauchlan in the paper quoted above is that of Davidson et al. (1971) but this classification over-simplifies the situation after total hip replacement and is biased in favour of an assumption that cross-infection in the ward leading to deep infection is common.

Infections (Davidson et al., 1971[36]) were classified as:

Primary infections – Infection evident at the time of first inspection of the wound, there being no obvious contributing factor. By definition all primary infections were assumed to have resulted from contamination with organisms during the operative procedure, these organisms being endogenous or exogenous ('endogenous' here meaning, most particularly, from hollow viscera in general surgery).

Secondary infections – This group was made up from infections **'... which seemed to arise in the ward as a result of cross-infection'**. Four different ways of acquiring secondary infection were distinguished: (1) if at the time of the first inspection healing appeared satisfactory and no pathogens were grown from a wound swab, the development of infection later allowed it to be classified as secondary. (2) Ischaemic necrosis of wound edges, though the wound at first inspection was sterile. (3) Drain-site infection: if a precursor of the wound infection, then the same phage type of organism was cultured from both drain and wound. (4) A secondary staphylococcal infection was said to occur when initial cultures from an infected wound gave a growth of some other organism but subsequently **Staph. pyogenes** was isolated.

It is therefore desirable that the different patterns of infection encountered after total hip replacement should be described in some detail to show how complex this matter really is. Infections which are suspected or diagnosed in hospital are grouped as 'early' infections and those not diagnosed until weeks, or even months, after returning home are grouped as 'late' infections.

Early Infections

The problem with early infections is to decide whether the infection is localised to the superficial tissues or whether it is involving the deep tissues from the outset. In the end this distinction can only be partly decided **retrospectively.**

The two extreme patterns of early infection can be called (1) 'believed to be superficial only', and (2) 'suspected early deep'.

1) Believed to Be Superficial Only

Here an inflammatory blush extends a few centimetres from the edges of the sutured wound but the underlying tissues of the thigh remain soft. There may be some localisation of the redness in the sutured wound, suggesting superficial abscess formation or a localised haematoma which has become infected. There is little or no systemic reaction to suggest deep involvement.

The subsequent progress can be (a) uneventful healing, (b) spontaneous discharge of localised infected haematoma or abscess followed by healing or (c) surgical evacuation of an infected cavity apparently restricted to the fat. In the latter case the surgeon does not suspect infection deep to the fascia lata and the patient leaves hospital with a small dressing and without a continuous or voluminous discharge.

After a superficial infection, and especially after one requiring evacuation of a cavity in the superficial fat, a deep infection can manifest itself at a later date by the reappearance of a sinus and by the deep connection being demonstrated by sinogram. In these cases there is no way of deciding whether the deep infection was present from the beginning or whether it was secondary to the superficial infection. If a positive culture was obtained from the superficial wound and later a deep infection develops, not uncommonly the latter may grow a different organism.

2) Suspected Early Deep

The sutured wound shows no signs of redness or other clinical manifestations of superficial early inflammation. The thigh is rather more indurated and more swollen than is customary. In the absence of a marked systemic reaction and raised WBC count, this picture is consistent with a haematoma deep to the fascia lata and this is especially possible if anticoagulant prophylaxis is being used. If a systemic reaction is present and the WBC count is raised, the possibility of a deep infection is obvious. This type of infection, 'suspected early deep', usually subsides on antibiotic therapy and the patient returns home with the surgical staff optimistic. In this type of case material for early bacteriological examination is never available.

Combined 1 and 2

Obviously the two patterns of early infection just described are not always clear-cut and the two patterns may merge, so frustrating any attempt to estimate the origin of the organism responsible for a late-manifesting deep infection.

Significance of the Two Early Types

In the event of a deep infection manifesting at a later date the origin of the organism in the first type, (believed to be superficial only) is more likely to be from the patient's own skin, or from cross-infection in the ward, than from the operating room. In the second case infection acquired in the operating room seems to be the only possibility, though blood-borne infection is theoretically possible (see later).

Early 'Fulminating' Infection

This term is used to indicate a pattern of infection characterized by a very strong systemic reaction, with pain, swelling and induration of the thigh, culminating after 10–14 days in evacuation of a considerable volume of pus (300–400 ml) obviously coming from the deep implant. This pattern of early post-operative infection, though obviously the most serious, has been listed third, because it has completely disappeared at Wrightington in the 9000 LFA operations performed since 1968. Before this date, and therefore before all our aseptic precautions in the operating room were fully developed we had three examples of this type of infection in 2000 operations. All three were by **Staph. aureus**. The disappearance of this type of fulminating post-operative infection, in the absence of prophylactic antibiotics, is in itself a considerable matter. This important fact is not evident in the mere statistics of a reduction of the rate of post-operative infection.

Late Infections

Late infections can manifest at any time between 3 and 18 months after the operation and occasionally much longer delays are encountered. The author recognizes three patterns of late infection:

Pattern 1

This follows an early post-operative infection while in hospital (suspected or proved, superficial or deep).

Pattern 2

No early infection (not even suspected) but the clinical performance of the patient is disappointing at the early post-operative reviews without any obvious explanation. Only when deep infection manifests itself radiologically is the cause of the poor performance explained.

In the author's experience these are the two most common patterns of late-manifesting deep infection and both could have been present early (pattern 1 possibly acquired from the skin or by cross infection; pattern 2 from the operating room).

Pattern 3

No early infection (not even suspected) and the early post-operative rehabilitation normal. This is the pattern where bacteraemia can be advanced as the origin of the late infection. In the author's experience this is a rare pattern if good hospital records of the post-operative period are available.

Septicaemic Late Infection

This is a definite pattern of late infection. In our experience at Wrightington it is rare, accounting for not more than about 1 infection in 1500, or even more, patients. In this pattern no early infection was present or suspected, and rehabilitation was completely normal and occasionally above average. In our experience there has been a clear interval of 1 year or 18 months before the onset of the infection.

When the infection occurs it is sudden, with high temperatures, rigors and prostration. A positive blood culture may prove that the onset is part of a septicaemia. The source of the septicaemia is easily identified (such as a staphylococcal parotitis in one of the author's patients) or if the source is not obvious the septicaemic nature of the infection may be proved by the appearance of another site of infection (such as osteomyelitis of the spine developing simultaneously, in another of the author's patients). The author has the impression that the period of perfect recovery before the septicaemic episode occurs is longer than in cases where a bacteraemic origin is postulated.

Special Case of Acrylic Cement

The whole subject of the ultra-clean operating room environment has evolved from experience with acrylic cement. The implanting of any large foreign body always carries the risk of inviting infection, but when acrylic cement is implanted there are features which are quite different from the behaviour of infected metallic implants without cement.

The **special behaviour of acrylic cement in infection** is well seen after secondary hip replacements (such as after failed Moore and Thompson prostheses). In some of these cases at the secondary operation positive cultures of low-pathogenicity organisms are obtained even though no clinical or radiological evidence of infection of the previous operation was suspected (a total hip operation would never have been proposed if it had been). In the case of a femoral head prosthesis infected by mildly pathogenic organisms the only radiological suspicion of infection can be an unusual amount of 'boring' of the femoral head into the acetabulum or an unusual amount of loosening of the stem in a relatively short period of time (i.e. 18 months). The point at issue is that there will not be any radiological evidence of **osteitis** of the shaft of the femur to suggest infection. Following revision of such a case by a cemented total hip, in most cases the infection will become clearly evident by the appearance for the first time of radiological signs of osteitis.

At a secondary operation a negative bacteriological culture never proves a case to be sterile, but a successful revision with acrylic cement is proof that it was sterile. It can therefore be said that the radiological behaviour of bone after a secondary operation using cement is a more sensitive test for infection than any bacteriological test.

The characteristic behaviour of infected acrylic cement in bone can be summarized as:

1. Delay before diagnosis
2. For about 50% of the organisms to be of a type considered in the past to be non-pathogenic for surgical wounds
3. To be accompanied almost always by radiological signs of osteitis

Possible Explanation of Infections in Presence of Acrylic Cement

The fact that an implant such as a Moore prosthesis can harbour a mild infection without producing radiological signs of osteitis, might be explained by the fact that a smooth metallic implant lies in a track lined with strong collagenous tissue with this dense tissue presumably capable of preventing organisms of mild pathogenicity invading the cancellous bone of the medullary cavity. A rough surface of acrylic cement on the other hand does not evoke the same type of dense collagen response as does metal moving on bone. If sound fixation is achieved by cement the layer of tissue separating the cement surface from the marrow spaces can be so delicate as to be no more than a membrane two or three cells in thickness. The surface of the membrane in contact with cement always presents a layer of histiocytes and this is quite unlike the behaviour of a surface of fibrous tissue in contact with metal. It is postulated therefore that in some way the histiocyte layer modifies the reaction of the tissues to organisms of a type which normally have very low pathogenicity for ordinary surgical wounds.

There is no question that experience with acrylic cement has opened up a new field in bacteriology. When the author first encountered these complications using Teflon (PTFE) and acrylic cement (1958–1962) pathological material was repeatedly reported sterile even though the clinical picture seemed clearly to be one of infection. Such organisms as were recovered were often ignored and attributed to contamination. Nowadays, though infections occur 10 times less frequently than in the author's early experience it is becoming increasingly rare for a laboratory to fail to grow some type of organism when alerted to the special circumstances.

Experience with Clean Air at Wrightington

July 1960 to October 1967

In this first period we evolved, in four stages, from a primitive operating room with exhaust ventilation in the roof, to an operating enclosure with a vertical downflow of filtered air at a linear speed of approximately 1 ft/s (300 air changes/h). The data regarding infection rates in these four phases are given in Table 13.1.

It was on this experience that we decided that clean air **by itself** could not reduce the deep infection rate after total hip replacement below about 1.5%. We carried out experiments on the penetration of gown material by bacteria from the surgeon's body (Charnley and Eftekhar 1969[37]) and came to the conclusion that at least some of the 1.5% infection must be the result of direct contact contamination of the wound even in the presence of clean air. Not until the air of the environment could be considered sterile were cultures of any significance taken from the exterior of a surgeon's gown. In the LFA operation the surgeon has to use a brace-and-bit and to augment the force exerted by the gloved hand holding the brace it is customary for the surgeon to press against it with the front of his body. It seemed inevitable that the surgeon's glove must occasionally become contaminated in this way.

As an interim measure after the recognition of penetration of gown material by organisms, and

Table 13.1. Data July 60–Oct. 67

Operating room	Date	Air changes/h	No. of ops. LFA	% Infection
Exhaust ventilation	July 60–Oct. 61	–	190	>7
First enclosure	Nov. 61–June 62	10	108	3.5
First enclosure	June 62–May 66	130	1023	3.0
Second enclosure	June 66–Oct. 67	300	865	1.5
			2186	

Table 13.2. Data Nov. 67–Dec. 74

Operating room	Date	Air changes/h	No. of LFA operations	Total infection
Front aprons	Nov. 67–Dec. 69	300	1681	1.07%
Body exhaust	Jan. 70–Dec. 74	300	5405	0.61%
			7086	

during the time the 'body exhaust' system was being developed, we used an extra layer of ordinary gown material ('balloon' cloth) as an apron to cover the front of the surgeon's body. The effect on infection of the two precautions to prevent gown permeability is shown in the Table 13.2.

Diagnosis and Rate of Post-operative Infection

In the period January 1970 to December 1974, using the body exhaust system and with all ultraclean details finalized, there were sufficient cases to make it worth an attempt to assess infection rates for different diagnostic conditions. The data are presented in Table 13.3.

Table 13.3. Infection rates versus diagnoses

No. of LFA operations	Total	Primary LFA in osteoarthrosis	Rheumatoid arthritis	Failed previous surgery
	5405	4176	468	761
No. of infections	33	17	9	7
% infections	0.61	0.41	1.92	0.92

It is clear from this table that the infection rate for rheumatoid arthritis is over four times higher than that for a first intervention in degenerative osteoarthrosis. Infection also is rather more than twice as common after previous surgery on the hip.

Independent Check on Results of 1974 and 1975

As an independent check van Niekerk[38] working at Wrightington in 1977 studied independently the records of the operations performed during the

2 years January 1974 to January 1976 (the first of these 2 years overlapping with the last year of the series in Table 13.3. His results are shown in Table 13.4.

Table 13.4. Infection rates for 2 years 74 and 75

	Total	Osteo-arthrosis	Rheuma-toid arthritis	Secondary operations
No. of LFA operations	2154	1557	161	417
No. of infections (deep)	18	5	2	11
% infections	0.8	0.3	1.2	2.6

Again the incidence of infection in rheumatoid arthritis was four times higher than after primary operations for osteoarthrosis. There was a particularly high rate of infection after previous surgery in this group, over eight times that of LFA in primary osteoarthrosis.

Allowing for the overlap of the two studies in 1974 the number of arthroplasties involved in the whole study was over 6000 between January 1970 and January 1976.

Air Cleanliness

Settle-plate studies

In the early studies with settle-plates (blood agar 3.25-in., 8-cm, diameter) there was a special problem in estimating air contamination because in the first enclosure considerable air turbulence occurred when the air flow was raised from 10 changes/h to 130 in such a small space (6 × 6ft and only 6ft high). It was impossible to decide whether to choose the best figures or those which were about four times more dirty near the walls of the enclosure where it was thought that warm air was tending to rise. [Turbulence at 130 air changes/h in the very small first enclosure is held responsible for the infection rate falling only 0.5% (from 3.5% to 3.0%) as a result of raising the air flow from 10 changes to 130 changes/h, as seen in Table 13.1].

The Table 13.5 shows what, in the author's paper of 1972, were considered to be average settle-plate values for the various rates of airflow:

Table 13.5. Studies in air contamination

	Settle-plates c.f.u./8 cm plate/h	Slit-sampler c.f.u./ft^3/h
Exhaust ventilation (zero air changes)	70	18
1st Enclosure (10 changes)	10	2.5
2nd Enclosure (130 changes)	0.4–1.8	0.2
3rd Enclosure (300 changes)	0–0.2	0.1

In 1972, with the body exhaust system and 300 air changes in the enclosure, four settle-plates were put on the **floor** of the enclosure (one in each corner) and the average result from 277 operations was 0.92 c.f.u./plate/h (data collected by Dr. Terayama working in this unit). This can be regarded as a low count when one considers that the feet of one or other of the four persons of the operating team were only about 1 m from the settle-plates, the floor being swept by the air escaping below the walls of the enclosure.

Slit-sampler studies

On reviewing the slit-sampler studies quoted in the paper of 1972 the author now thinks that the figures of 0.2 to 0.1 c.f.u./ft^3 given in that paper must have been incorrect and that the air in fact was one order of magnitude cleaner. This change of opinion is because in 1972, with the same body exhaust system and the same 300 air changes in routine use, Dr. Terayama found the average of 15 studies to be 0.019 c.f.u./ft^3 (ranging from 0.005 to 0.07).

Some idea of the cleanliness of the air in the enclosure is seen in Fig. 13.1 which compares two slit-sampler plates (7 in., 17.5 cm, in diameter) making one rotation in 1 hour and exposed to 3/ft^3/min. The clean plate is from the interior of the operating room enclosure during an operation (with the team all wearing body exhaust clothing). The contaminated plate is from the anaesthetic

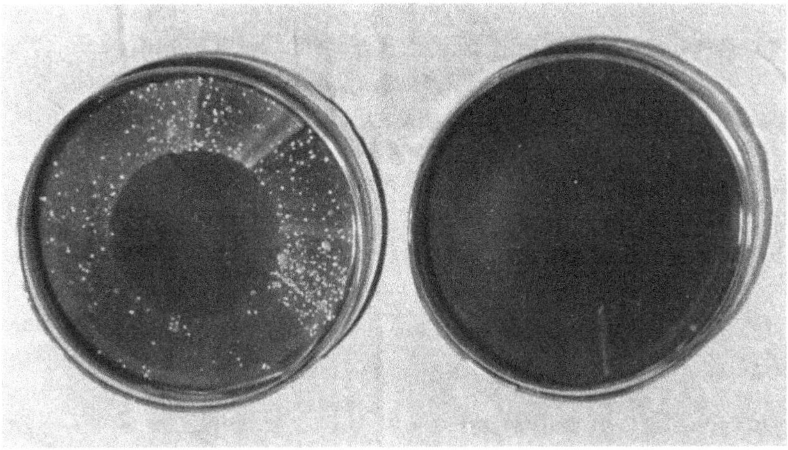

Fig. 13.1. Slit-sampler plates exposed for 1 h at 3 ft^3/min. On *left*, anaesthetic room at 5 c.f.u./ft^3. On *right*, clean air enclosure

room which is flushed with clean air escaping from the enclosure (because this particular enclosure is not a recirculation system and uses filtered fresh air at 4000 ft^3/min, 112 m^3/min). The contaminated plate corresponds to 5 colony-producing particles/ft^3, 180/^{3}. Generally, 5/c.p.p./ft^3 is accepted as indicating a high standard of air cleanliness in a conventional operating room and probably few conventional operating rooms achieve this level when a major operation is in progress with numerous personnel present.

Wound Swabs

The method used to detect (not estimate) bacterial contamination of the wound at the end of an operation consisted merely of passing four throat swabs over the wound just before closure and dropping each into a separate bottle of Robertson's cooked meat broth. We have not previously reported these tests because we realized that in very clean air one might expect, at the most, only 5–10 colony-producing particles in a wound measuring in area 41 in.^{2} (257 cm) and open for 1.25 h. The chance of 1 out of 4 swabs making contact with an infected particle therefore seemed infinitesmal. Since the work, quoted at the beginning of this chapter, reported 'heavy' bacterial contamination by the end of the operation in a significant number of operations, it now looks as though our simple swab test, used merely to detect rather than measure, might not have been quite as futile as we thought. As a rough check on the validity of using 4 swabs, 17 wounds were swabbed each with 12 swabs (each of the 12 swabs being dropped into a separate bottle of cooked broth medium), and in none (204 swabs) was a growth obtained. The result of these studies was that out of 492 operations (1968 swabs), positive cultures were obtained from 20 wounds (4%). Positive cultures were obtained from 1 of the 4 swabs in 16 operations (3.25%); from 2 of the 4 swabs in 3 operations (0.6%); and in all 4 swabs in 1 (0.2%).

A detail in using the 4 swabs was that the first pair of swabs were passed across the wound before the 'tetra' towels were removed from the skin edges, and the second pair of swabs after the tetra towels had been detached and after six deep tension-sutures had been inserted. During the passage of these sutures, a considerable amount of handling of the skin surface and the cut skin edges is inevitable, and this stage must be the most potentially dirty part of the whole operation. On the other hand, the exposed skin was routinely swabbed with 2% iodine in 70% alcohol immediately after removal of the tetra towels and before passing the deep tension sutures. The swabs did not touch the iodine. There was no difference in the contamination of swabs taken before and after removal of the tetra towels. Approximately 50% of the positive tests were positive before removing the skin towels and negative after; and vice versa.

Coagulase-negative cocci were recovered in 17 (85%) of the 20 positive operations and gram-negative bacilli in the remaining 3 (15%) (specified as coliforms in 2). As regards the number of positive swabs obtained per operation, and the nature of the organism, a rather surprising finding was that the contamination with gram-negative bacilli might be more profuse than with cocci. Thus bacilli were found in only 3 operations, but 2 of the 3 (66%) had 2 positive swabs, whereas the cocci encountered in 17 operations were found on more than 1 swab only three times (17.5%). None of the cases from which positive swabs were grown became infected nor did any where the wound swabs were sterile.

Bacteriology of Infection

The bacteriological statistics for the whole series are not materially different from the published experience of other hospitals performing large numbers of total hip replacements (i.e. Fitzgerald et al.[39]). For the present purpose the statistics from January 1974 to January 1976 (van Niekerk[38]) from 2136 operations performed in those recent 2 years are offered as typical.

Superficial Infection

In the superficial infections (see Table 13.6) **Staph. aureus** was cultured in 31 out of 73 patients (42.5%); coagulase-negative staphylococcus in 6 out of 73 (8%). In 19 out of 73 (26%) cultures no organisms were grown. Mixed cultures were obtained in 11 out of 73 (15%).

Table 13.6. Bacteriology of superficial infection (1974 and 1975)

	No. of patients
Staph. aureus	31 (42.5%)
No growth	19 (26%)
Coag.-neg. staph.	6 (8%)
Streptococcus faecalis	
Proteus	2 (2.7%)
Haemolytic strep.	1 (1.4%)
Coliform	1 (1.4%)
Mixed infections	
Staph. aureus	3 (4%)
Staph. faecalis	
Coag.-neg. staph.	2 (2.7%)
Coliform	
Staph. aureus	1 (1.4%)
Coliform	
Staph. aureus	1 (1.4%)
Coag.-neg. staph.	
Staph. aureus	1 (1.4%)
Strep. haemolyticus	

Deep Infection

Coagulase-negative staphylococci were cultured in 6 out of the 18 deep infections (33%) in this series and **Staph. aureus** and **Staph. pyogenes** in 4 (22%). The full picture of the organisms responsible for deep infections is shown in Table 13.7.

Table 13.7. Bacteriology of deep infection (1974 and 1975)

	No. of patients
Coag.-neg. staph.	6 (33%)
Staph. aureus	2 (11%)
Staph. pyogenes	2 (11%)
Not valid (late sinus)	2 (11%)
Sterile	2 (11%)
Haemolytic strep.	1 (5.5%)
Pseudomonas	1 (5.5%)
Propionibacterium	1 (5.5%)
Citrobacter freundii	1 (5.5%)
A. calcoaceticus	
Total	18

The possibility that superficial infection, arising from bacteria in or on the patient's skin, leads to deep infection is not supported by the bacteriology. Thus superficial infection was most commonly caused by **Staph. aureus** whereas deep infection by a coagulase-negative staphylococcus was more common.

Foam Pressure Pads; Fat Sutures

The use of sponge pressure-pads on the superficial wound, to prevent subcutaneous haematoma formation, was fully developed by the end of 1968 and has been employed routinely ever since. It is possible in theory that infection might be communicated from the skin down to the deep fascia, but experience suggests that this is a less serious risk than to have a haematoma involving the deep fascia and for this to be in danger of communicating with the skin (stages 146–149 Chap. 15).

Ward Procedure and Post-operative Infection

It is important to emphasize that the progressive fall in infection rate extending over a period of 10 years at Wrightington has been achieved without any change in ward routine. The vast majority of patients at Wrightington are nursed in wards of 20–35 beds. There has never been any attempt to isolate new patients from the pre-existing ward population prior to operation. Nor has there been any attempt to isolate patients who have developed post-operative infections from the rest of the patients in the ward. Because of the success of this policy over many years patients with old infections, and even with a sinus, are often admitted to such wards, many of these coming from other hospitals.

Skin preparation is started in the ward 24 h before operation and consists of washes with hibitane soap and in male patients shaving of the operation site with an electric razor (**never with a sharp razor**). On the morning of operation the patient is transferred from the ward to the operating room with the hip for operation wrapped in sterile drapes (including the foot) after the last skin preparation.

In the anaesthetic room, as part of the immediate pre-operative preparation when the patient is under anaesthesia, one of the first tasks is to isolate the patient's perineum by sterile adhesive drapes. The skin is degreased with commercial ether and painted with 2% iodine in 7% spirit (sensitivity having been tested 48 h previously by painting the skin with iodine on admission and covering with a plastic spray).

On admission to the clean-air operating enclosure the skin is again painted with 2% iodine in spirit, this time by the operating surgeon prior to draping the wound; 2% iodine in spirit is used a third time after completion of the operation and immediately prior to suturing the skin. (Iodine is not used if skin sensitivity is proved or if the patient alleges sensitivity; but this in fact is a rare occurrence.)

McLauchlan et al.[34] postulate that cross-infection in their four infections was by cross-infection in the ward, because all the wounds were heavily soaked with blood and required to be redressed within 24–48 h. It is our experience at Wrightington that extra absorbent packing on the exterior of the dressing is needed in the majority of cases and frequently saturation with blood is so heavy that all the external dressings have to be removed and changed (despite three suction drains).

Prophylactic Antibiotics

It is important to emphasize that in this 15-year study of post-operative wound infection after total hip replacement, prophylactic antibiotics have not been used. This was a deliberate policy in an attempt to assess the contribution of blood-borne infection to the total infection rate by not preventing it. A fall in infection rate when antibiotics are not used must surely be the result of reducing contamination from the environment.

Late Infection with Special Reference to Bacteraemia

Undoubtedly there must exist cases of late infection of bacteraemic origin, but the author believes these to be very rare. The fact that the infection rate has been reduced from the 7%, 5% and 3% levels to the region of 0.5% after first interventions in osteoarthrosis, by measures directed solely at improving asepsis in the operating room, and in the absence of antibiotic prophylaxis, supports this. When an infection rate is at, say, the 5.0% level it is 'anyone's guess' whether a bacteraemic contribution might be 50% (in this case 2.5%); but if the total infection rate is only 0.5% then a 50% bacteraemic contribution becomes very small indeed.

In rheumatoid arthritis the relatively high infection rate might be evidence of bacteraemic infection but also, and probably more likely, it could be the result of bacteria being present in the joint from some previous bacteraemic process and as part of the disease.

In the early days of our experience not infrequently we attributed late infections, especially of **Bacillus coli** and **Bacillus proteus**, to a urinary tract origin, but precautions in the operating room have reduced the general infection rate; yet the frequency of urinary infection in our elderly female patients is almost certainly as high as ever it was. When bacteraemic infection is postulated the organism ought to be consistent with this route; thus it seems unlikely that a dental extraction would cause a total hip to acquire a deep infection by **Staph. epidermidis** (Creuss et al.[40]).

Total Hip Replacement with Sepsis Elsewhere in the Patient

Over the last 11 years it has been our policy at Wrightington to perform total hip replacement on a second hip even if infection had occurred after the first hip and we have no instance of infection occurring in the second hip.

The results of 43 such operations have been reported (Del Sel and Charnley[41]). In 23 patients the infected hip had already been made into a pseudarthrosis by the time the operation on the clean side was performed, and four of these had draining sinuses. In 20 patients the clean side was operated on with the infected arthroplasty or the infected osteotomy plate still in situ in the opposite hip. Four of these had draining sinuses at the time of the operation on the clean side. One patient had had a biopsy of a radiological cavity at the tip of a femoral prosthesis on the other side only 2 months previously and **Staph. aureus** had been cultured from it.

In 23 patients the clean side was operated on under 2 years (averaging 9 months) since the previous operation and in 20 over 2 years after the infected side (1 of these was a veteran of the 1918 war still draining from a sinus 55 years later). Twenty-four patients were followed 2–10 years (average 50 months after the second operation); and 19 were followed 3–20 months (average 11.7 months). These experiences are quoted to support the idea that bacteraemic infection of total hips, even in the presence of acrylic cement, is not common.

That there is no irresponsibility in this surgical policy is based on the fact that a pseudarthrosis on the side opposite a painful, unoperated, arthrosic hip is a very serious handicap for any patient and especially in the elderly. A pseudarthrosis of the hip is only tolerable if the patient has a very good hip on the other side, which can take more than the ordinary share of load-bearing and gymnastic activity when sitting down and standing up, etc. Therefore when there is a painful arthrosic hip on the side opposite a pseudarthrosis performed for a previous infection, it is more than ever important to have a good total replacement to offset the handicap of the pseudarthrosis and also because the old infected side probably will never be tried again with another total hip.

The ultimate in this policy is seen where a patient has a total hip showing evidence, or a suspicion, of late infection (say about a year after the operation) with an unoperated and painful arthrosis on the other side. By operating on the second arthrosic hip, with the infected hip in situ, the patient will be ready to face up to whatever may have to be done to the infected side and so avoid a phase of serious disability and alarm.

Skill and Post-operative Infection

It is sometimes advanced as an argument against the ultra-clean environment that the wide range of rates of post-operative infection in different hospitals (1%–10%) is more likely to be from variations in surgical skill than from an order of magnitude difference in the air cleanliness between modern operating rooms. However it is well recognized with us at Wrightington that new surgical residents (five every 6 months) do not have a significantly higher infection rate than the permanent staff, and this despite the fact that the majority of new postgraduates have not had much previous personal responsibility for major surgery.

In the 5 years 1970 through 1974, over 4000 primary interventions for osteoarthrosis were performed at Wrightington and the residents had an infection rate (assessed more than 18 months from the operation) of 0.5% and the permanent consultant staff 0.4%. The residents performed more than twice the number of operations performed by the consultants though the consultants generally performed more difficult operations. If this very low rate of infection for our residents were not indeed a fact, Wrightington, as a postgraduate unit for the teaching of surgical technique, would have had to close down many years ago. It is possible that this evidence for clean air operating room conditions could be one of the most impressive of all the arguments.

It is admitted that in the training programme at Wrightington new residents are graded into the operation and they have standards set for them which make it normal to complete a primary operation within 1.5 h. In surgical units where standards such as this are not set the same residents might operate for 2–3 h. Nevertheless, if a wound does not receive contamination from the environment the duration of an operation ought not to matter and exposure time theoretically should be important only when the air is contaminated.

Last 0.5% of the Infection Rate

In attempts to trace the cause of the 0.5% of deep infection after primary operations for osteoarthrosis which so far has defied the clean environment precautions in the operating room, the author continues in his belief that the most likely source of organisms is still the four human beings for an hour or more in close proximity to the open wound. All the different organisms which have been grown from deep infections of total implants at some time or another have been found on human skin in the various tests we have made. Because transfer of bacteria through the medium of the air from the operating team to the open wound is out of the question in the clean air environment, we must continue to look for some pathway of direct contact responsible for the 'last 0.5%'.

1) Cuffs of the Gown

One possibility might be the sweat which can saturate the cuffs of a surgeon's gown as a result of being prevented from evaporating by the rubber cuff of the glove.

When surgeons wear two pairs of gloves it is not unusual to change the outer pair repeatedly if the slightest suspicion of contamination is thought to have been incurred. If the surgeon changes the outer gloves himself one or more digits of the new pair may be contaminated by contact with the damp textile of the cuff previously covered by the rubber cuff. **Even if sweat is harmless this is a failure of asepsis because the sweat has not been sterilised.**

This mechanism makes possible direct contamination of the **exterior** of the fingers of the new gloves and therefore **direct contamination of the implant or the cement.** This type of contamination is unique, because it is 100% certain to enter the wound.

To investigate this matter the author and his colleagues encircled their bare wrists with short lengths of sterile stockinette (2 in. diameter and 2 in. long) immediately before applying the first pair of gloves.

Thirty-nine tests were carried out in which the test cuff was put into a dry, sterile container and sent to the laboratory for the making of viable counts by shaking in a known volume of fluid. The limit of sensitivity of the test was about 40 organisms per cuff. Out of 39 tests 5 (13%) indicated some 300 coagulase-negative staphylococci per cuff; 3 (7.7%), about 900 coagulase-negative staphylococci per cuff; and 1 (2.5%), about 300 aerobic spore-bearing bacilli.

In one test the author refrained from applying bactericidal cream before the first pair of gloves; the two cuffs were estimated as holding 12,300 and 66,600 organisms of coagulase-negative staphylococci; for obvious reasons this test was not repeated.[1])

In view of the ease with which this breach of asepsis can be closed the author now routinely takes precautions and the method which has been found simple and satisfactory (Charnley 1976)[(41 a)] is as follows:

Cylindrical cuffs (Fig. 13.2a) are made of two layers of towelling material, about 6 in. (15 cm) long and of a circumference just large enough to permit the surgeon to insert the widest part of his hand (heads of the metacarpals). The surgeon puts these cuffs on as the first act and the first pair of gloves is then pulled on, taking care that the rubber cuffs overlap the distal ends of the absorbent cuffs (Fig. 13.2b). The gown is then put on, (Fig. 13.2c) followed by the second pair of gloves (Fig. 13.2d). The pulling on of the second pair of gloves is delayed till the draping has been completed and the operation is about to start.

The mechanism of this arrangement is that movements of the surgeon's wrists exert a pumping action on the voluminous porous mass of the towel material and so ventilate away the humid air before it can condense as moisture. This results in the exterior of the textile cuff of the gown remaining perfectly dry.

---

[1]) The author is indebted to Miss Carol MacKenzie, Senior Laboratory Technician, Wrightington Hospital, for advising on and carrying out these tests.

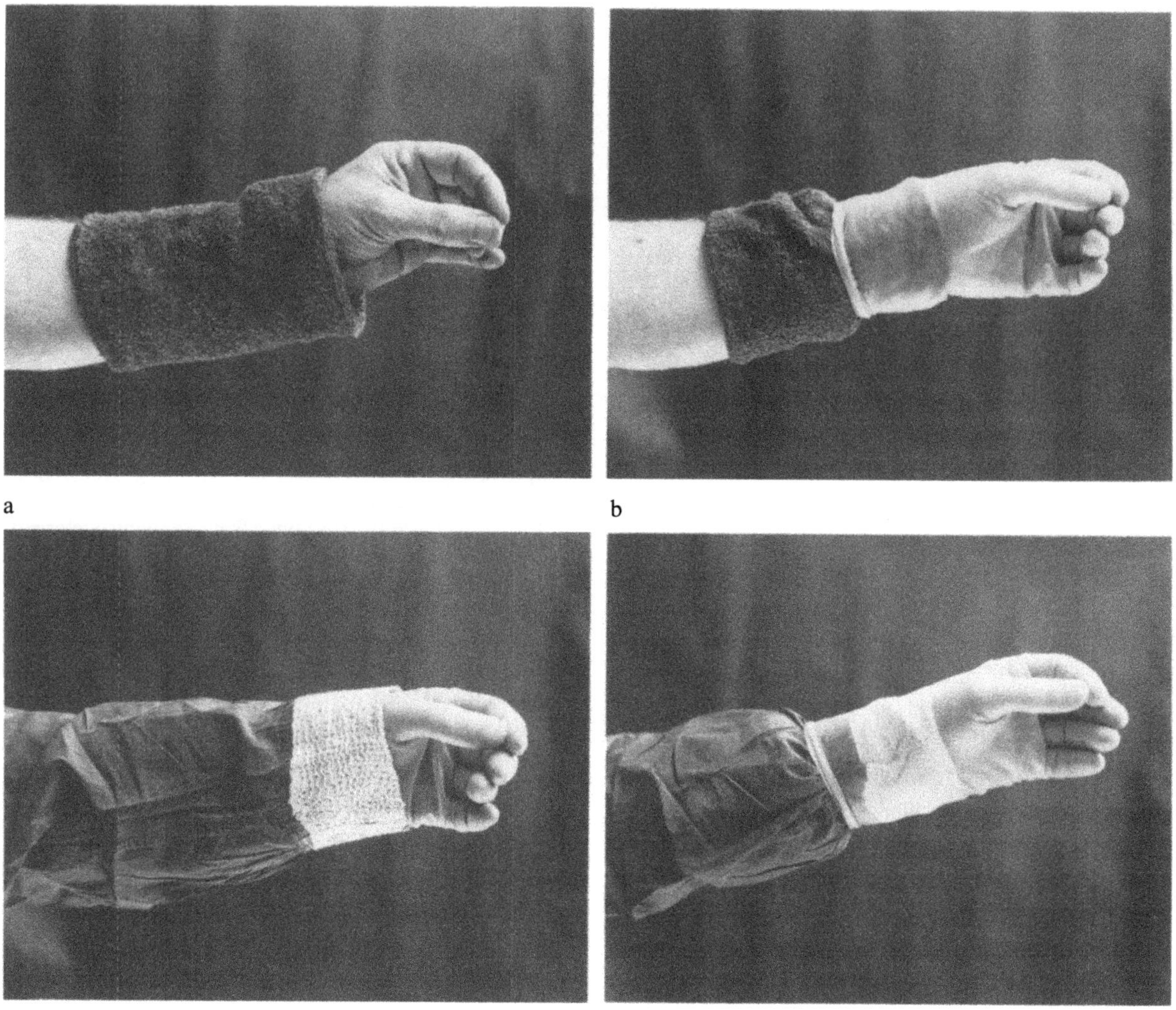

a b c d

Fig. 13.2a–d. Cuffs to prevent sweating under rubber of gloves. **a** Cuff of towelling material in position. **b** First pair of rubber gloves. **c** Gown in position. **d** Second pair of rubber gloves

2) Residual Porosity of the Gown

Hamilton et al. [42] have suggested that the 'Ventile' cloth used in the body exhaust system despite the greatly improved resistance to penetration by bacteria from the surgeon's body compared with ordinary gown material, is still not absolutely impermeable. They have recovered organisms from the surface of gowns made of this type of material at the end of total hip operations when tests have shown the air in the laminar flow enclosure to be so clean that their presence could only be explained by penetration from the interior. It is true that after the original tests which demonstrated penetration of balloon cloth gown material (Charnley and Eftekhar 1969[37]) we were so confident that this could not happen with 'Ventile' cloth that we did not pursue this matter. This is a possibility which Hamilton has only just brought to the author's attention and it merits further study.

Discussion

It is necessary to attempt to comment on the two papers quoted at the beginning of this chapter, which both show no correlation between contamination in the environment and the open wound, in view of the author's opposite opinion that the reduction of the infection rate at Wrightington followed mechanical measures to protect the wound from the environment of the operating room. Two quite different aspects of the problem are involved: (1) the significance of the design of the investigations, in relation to clinical results and (2) the significance of the bacteriological observations.

An unavoidable difficulty in the design of the reported investigations is the lack of contrast between the experimental and the control environments. The bacterial contamination of the control environments averaged only 4–6.2 c.f.u./ft^3, which on general standards are still very clean environments. Because the ultra-clean test environment produced the same infection rate as the controls this must have resulted from some factor common to both. (Infection in the post-operative phase through dressings wet with soakage was suggested.) But though no differences were found in the reported series this does not exclude the possibility that **if a very large number of operations** had been performed the control environments might then have shown a higher rate of infection than the 1.5%–2% level. Similarly the high rate of infection following operations in the enclosure is curious and might not be typical of a very much larger series.

In the isolator the air of the wound environment certainly would be cleaner than that in the author's routine; does this suggest therefore that the author's lower infection rate was merely the result of preventing infection from the skin in the post-operative period by, let us say, the pressure-pads on the deep fat sutures preventing haematomata? The author believes the pressure-pad dressing to be an important element in attacking this multi-factorial problem, but it is doubtful whether many surgeons would be happy to depend merely on post-operative pressure dressings (even with the isolation of patients in separately ventilated rooms) after performing the operation in a second-class operating room environment.

Because this problem **is** multi-factorial; with some factors more important than others; with all the factors relatively rare; and perhaps with some factors as yet unknown; it is quite possible that we shall never be able to identify the size of the contributions made by all the individual factors, for statistical reasons. Even if we were to be on the right track an isolated 'accidental' infection – e.g. an undetected furuncle in the skin incision – could mask the basic truth. Therefore we must abandon that attitude, so deeply engrained in the medical profession, which is to look for one answer to solve all problems. In this multifactorial subject there is no future for comparing infection rates in circumstances with only one variable: the only hope is to adopt protective measures against every conceivable route of infection and then see if we can achieve very low levels of infection and **hold these low levels over large numbers of operations**. By striving in this direction the author has achieved an infection rate of slightly under 0.5% in primary operations for osteoarthrosis over an experience of the order of 6000 operations, whereas in the investigations under discussion an infection rate touching 2% has resulted from not more than about 300 operations. The author remains optimistic that in his methods of mechanical protection a loophole still must exist which is responsible for the 0.5% of infection, and efforts to find and close it must still be pursued.

The **bacteriological observations** in the reported investigations are of great importance if only to remind us of our abysmal ignorance of many fundamental matters in bacteriology. It is agreed by both investigating groups that the wound contamination they encountered must have come from the cut edges of the patient's skin. The fact that the contamination was overwhelmingly by relatively innocuous organisms (such as coagulase-negative staphylococci) does not explain why deep infection did not ensue because coagulase-negative cocci are responsible for at least one-third of all deep infections after total hip replacement. It seems unreasonable to postulate some route for infection by skin-borne cocci other than via the open wound at the time of the operation.

There seems no way to explain this behaviour other than by postulating the existence of pathogenic strains among these common and generally non-pathogenic species. In the paper by McLauchlan et al., [34] **Staph. pyogenes** was grown from six wounds but the wounds healed uneventfully without deep infection. This fact raises no special comment because we are all now aware of the existence of non-pathogenic strains in this much-studied staphylococcus responsible for nosocomial infections. But the idea that highly pathogenic strains of organisms such as **Staph. albus** might exist is something we do not seem seriously to envisage. Is it possible that cocci saprophytic on a particular individual's skin are non-pathogenic for that person's deep tissues whereas cocci of the same species acquired from other persons could be pathogenic?

When discussing high pathogenicity in relation to common skin organisms some readjustment of our conventional thinking might be necessary. Virulence in an organism is usually manifested by the classic signs of acute inflammation (rubor, calor, tumor, dolor) which are signs of a rapid invasion of the tissues, but when **Staph. albus** infects a cemented implant it produces none of these signs. Though the ESR is usually raised, there is no pus; there is merely some slimy granulation tissue and signs of bone necrosis. This type of chronic inflammation is caused by an organism which behaves with great tenacity; though the invasion is slow, it is relentless. In the bone-cement junction **Staph. albus** is as aggressive as any **Staph. aureus**.

The possibility postulated, that highly pathogenic strains of 'saprophytic' skin cocci exist but are very rare, might explain why in 1960–1961 the author's exhaust-ventilated operating room, with air contamination almost as heavy as in a hospital ward, produced only 7%–8% of deep infections. Only about 50% of these infections were **Staph. aureus**. Because deep infections by **Staph. aureus** and coagulase-negative staphylococci occur with not very dissimilar frequency this could indicate (if we postulate air-borne infection) that the pathogenic strains of organisms such as coagulase-negative staphylococci have the same rarity in the air of an operating room as **Staph. aureus**, irrespective of the myriads of non-pathogenic members of the same species from which they cannot be identified by laboratory tests.

Even if we are prepared to accept the hypothesis of rare but very active pathogenic strains of skin commensals, the dosage needed to produce an infection is yet another problem. Dosage has always been a factor against the theory of air-borne infection in the operating room because of a widespread belief that it requires considerably more than one or two cocci to produce an infection. The author's

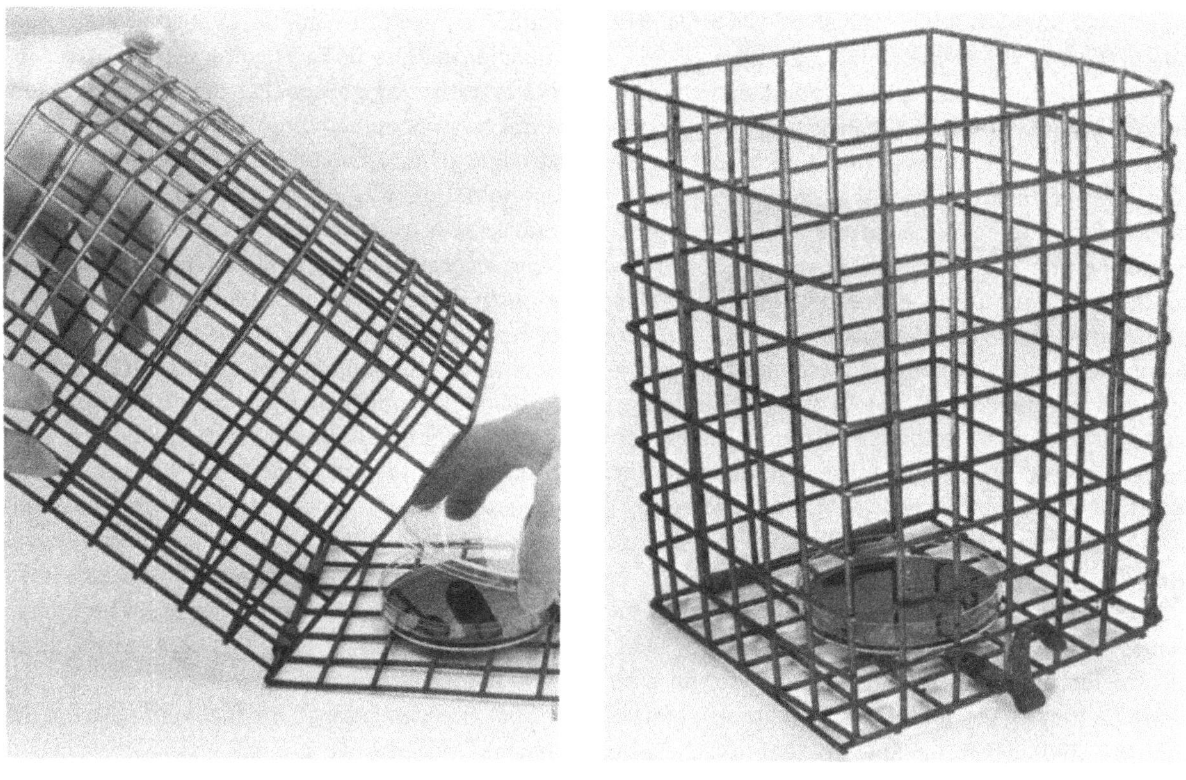

a b

Fig. 13.3. a 'Lobster pot' offered by sterile member of team to receive Petri dish from circulating nurse. **b** 'Lobster pot' closed with Petri dish in situ experience in attempting to close all routes of contamination in the operating room indicates an exponential pattern. The fall from the 7%–8% level to 1.5% demanded increasing attempts at perfection, but we are now stuck at the 0.5% level. This suggests, if these infections come from the environment of the operating room by any route, that the number of pathogenic organisms needed to establish a deep infection in a cemented implant is very small indeed.

Routine Settle-Plate Monitoring

To monitor air contamination close to the operation site by means of settle-plates can be hazardous because of the difficulty of producing, for routine use, Petri dishes sterile on the outside to a degree to satisfy surgical criteria. This is especially the case when the culture medium is blood-agar. The following technique, in which ordinary Petri dishes (not sterile on the outside) are used, has proved efficacious:

A box made of coarse wire mesh (1 in., 2.5 cm.), is open at the top and provided with a hinged bottom and spring catch (Fig. 13.3a). This 'bird-cage' or 'lobster-pot' is autoclaved and therefore can be handled by a sterile member of the operating team. The hinged bottom is opened and presented at the 'service hatch' of the operating enclosure as in Fig. 13.3a. A circulating nurse deposits a Petri dish on the hinged bottom and takes away the cover plate to be retained inside a folded, sterile towel or drape. The 'lobster-pot' is closed and can be attached to drapes on the sides of the operating table with towel clips or be placed on top of the operating table. When the exposure is to be terminated the procedure is reversed: the lobster pot is opened at the service hatch and the original lid of the Petri dish is dropped over the exposed plate by the circulating nurse who then takes the whole unit away.

Some observations are here reported. These were made in the vertical downflow enclosure, with the team wearing the body-exhaust clothing of Ventile material, and with the lobster-pot attached to the surgeon's side of the operating table at about the level of the patient's knee. In this position the Petri dish would be swept by air leaving the table top not far from the surgeon's elbow and in many movements the surgeon's arm is vertically above the sampling surface.

Between February 1974 and May 1975, 197 operations were monitored with zero growth in 76.7%. In the 46 positive results (23.3%) the average number of c.f.u. per plate was 2.7. The average number of c.f.u. for all 197 plates was 0.62 and this was higher than the 0.1–0.2 obtained previously at table-top level. There seems no doubt therefore that some emission of organisms occasionally can take place in the vicinity of the operating site.

The wide variations in the number of c.f.u.s obtained at different operations is seen in Table 13.8.

Table 13.8. Scatter of settle-plate contamination

No. of operations	No. of c.f.u./plate	% of total (197 ops.)
151	0	76.7
24	1	12.2
11	2	5.6
3	3	1.5
2	4	1.0
3	5	1.5
1	10	0.5
1	13	0.5
1	22	0.5
197		

Whereas only 5.5% of the positive plates had more than 2 c.f.u. per plate the fact is that 1.5% had contamination of more than 10 c.f.u. At the moment no explanation can be offered for these examples presumably of heavy emission from the region of the operation site.

Observations such as these suggest that we still do not have grounds for complacency and that the unexplained last 0.5% of infection still might be acquired from the environment.

Expense and Clean Air Systems

A number of factors are tending to increase the running costs of clean air operating room systems and perhaps we are in danger of overlooking methods of economising. The lowest running costs are those incurred by the author's three prototype installations which are still running effectively (the first, at the present moment, after 12 years and the other two after 8 years) and they are capable of going on for many years to come. It is to be emphasized that the 6000 total hip operations performed since 1969, which produced the data for the author's studies of infection reported in this chapter, were all carried out under the simple and relatively inexpensive conditions described below.

Air Filtration

The air is filtered only at the 1–2-μm level, using cloth 'pocket' filters. The filtered air is in fact merely 'dust-free' air rather than sterile air. This policy was adopted because it is generally considered that bacteria are not free in the air but are carried as clusters of many organisms on particulate matter such as dry epithelial scales.

The air in the three prototype enclosures is not recycled; it is taken from outside the hospital and spills to waste through the operating room block. With a 10–12-μm pre-filter (automatically changing the filter element as resistance rises) the 1–2-μm cloth pocket filters have lasted as long as 6 years. They are initially cheaper than an equivalent battery of absolute filters. If used for about 2 years these pocket filters can be replaced by new filters and the dirty pockets laundered and re-used later. Laundering and labour costs for changing are about £300 every 2 years at 1977 rates. Much higher charges have been suggested for changing the same capacity of filter when of the disposable, 0.3-μm type.

The question whether heat loss in winter (even during the limited hours during which the full purge of 4000 ft^3/min is in use) would be too expensive, especially in certain climates, has to be balanced against the cost of cooling the air for the rest of the year. Cooling costs can be just as expensive as heating costs and it is essential to get rid of a considerable amount of heat generated in the enclosure throughout the year and not in summer alone.

Regulations in some hospitals permit only recirculation. Because recirculated hospital air is at high risk of contamination from pathogenic human sources (which is not the case with primary air from outside the hospital) absolute filters are essential. Absolute filters offer greater resistance to airflow than do 1–2-μm filters so that there is an increase of heat production from this cause when the electric motors are in the operating room. Designs using fresh air from the environment have the disadvantage of needing expensive external building programmes, and this is of course not possible in multi-story hospitals.

In none of the three prototype installations used by the author has a true 'laminar flow' system been used. 'Bulk downward flow', using cloth diffuser bags in the ceiling, has proved adequate because the body-exhaust system eliminates the emission of organisms at source. The diffuser bags are changed once per month, being autoclaved after ordinary hospital laundering. To place newly cleaned diffuser bags in position takes only about an hour, with the operating room staff wearing ordinary, unsterile operating room clothes.

Body Exhaust

It has always been recognized that even a single laundering of the Ventile textile would destroy the chemical waterproofing necessary when it is used for raincoats. We have always considered that in its surgical application the close weave of this material is its most important characteristic and not its success as a waterproof. A really effective air vacuum source, maintaining a depression of 1 cm of water-gauge inside the head part of the gown, is increasingly important if doubts exist about the permeability of the textile to bacteria. Until the author has had more information on the results of tests for bacteriological permeability he is considering the use of an additional gown, of ordinary balloon cloth, external to the body exhaust gown and involving only the surgeon in the team. With a vigorous airflow inside the gown this extra layer does not noticeably raise the internal temperature in the gown.

Chapter 14

Clean Air Operating – Practice

This chapter describes details of the Wrightington aseptic operating room routine as used in practice.

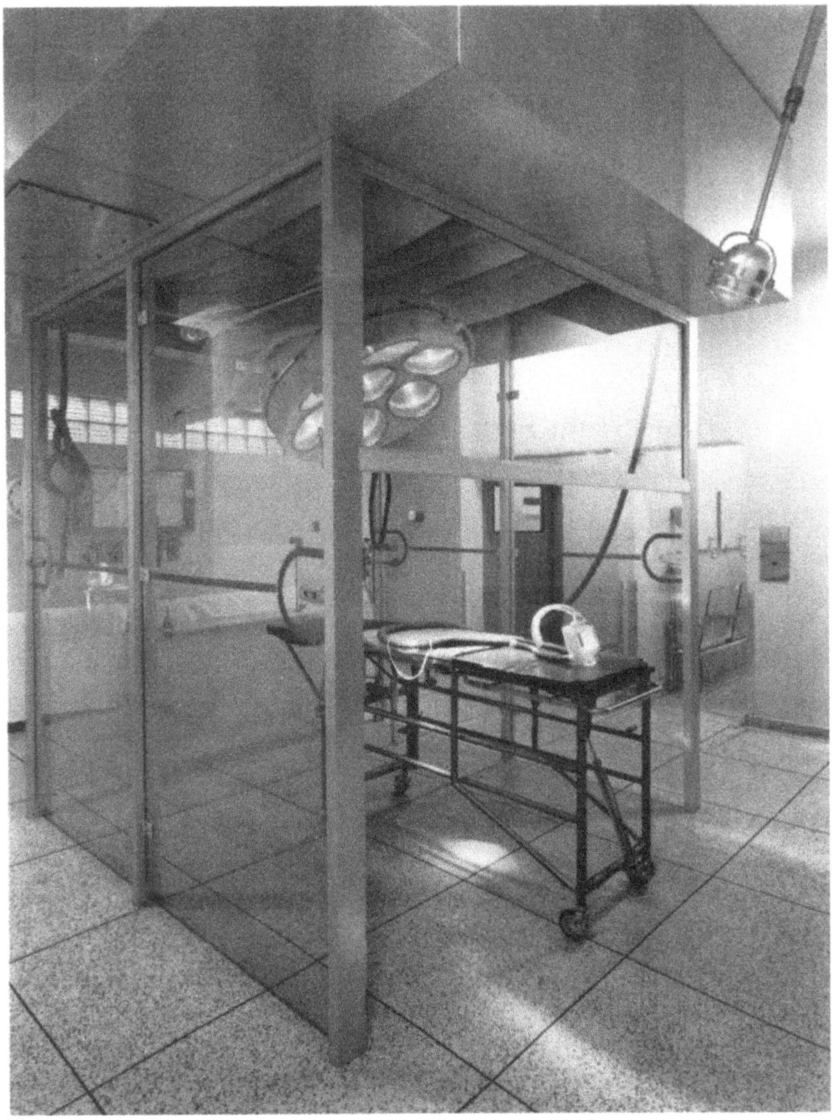

Fig. 14.1. The downflow clean air enclosure (1970) at Wrightington

Clean Air Operating Rooms

'Downflow' air systems, with walls which separate the operating team from the rest of the room, have psychological features which enhance aseptic thinking more than horizontal flow systems. However, when the 'scrub-nurse' is incarcerated inside a sterile enclosure the circulating personnel outside the enclosure must be well trained in their duties. Surgery in ultra-clean conditions demands adequate staffing but, as will be shown, it can also be economical in staff.

The downflow clean-air enclosure at Wrightington (Fig. 14.1) has three walls extending from the ceiling to within 10 cm of the floor; the fourth wall extends from the ceiling to about 6 ft from the ground. The opening produced by the short wall allows the surgical team and the lower half of the patient to enter. The foot-end of the enclosure has a service opening provided with a shelf. The outwards flow of air through this service opening makes it unnecessary to use doors. The instruments are autoclaved in trays, wrapped in special bags, so that they can be delivered to the team inside the enclosure against the air stream. The autoclave thus becomes a 'diverticulum' of the sterile enclosure and contamination of instruments in passage from autoclave to wound, as by crossing of clean and dirty pathways, is impossible.

Tray System and the Surgical Team

As developed at Wrightington the tray system of handling of instruments has an important bearing on the discipline of the surgical team and it simplifies the work of the nursing staff. The surgical operation is divided into seven convenient stages and the instruments for each stage are kept permanently in separate trays. Each tray contains the special instruments for that particular phase of the operation. The ordinary instruments (i.e. haemostats, retractors, dissecting forceps, etc.) are reduplicated in each tray. Therefore the surgeon might use five or six different dissecting forceps, etc. during the whole operation.

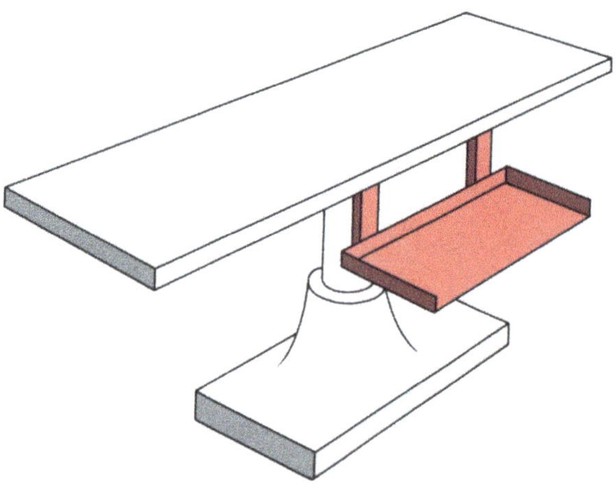

Fig. 14.2. Shelf attached to surgeon's side of operating table

The operating table is provided with a shelf (under the drapes) at such a height that it will be above the surgeon's knees when he is sitting and which can be changed from left to right sides (Fig. 14.2). The instrument trays are placed on this shelf, in sequence, and the surgeon picks out the instrument he needs and drops it back when he has finished with it. The scrub-nurse does not lay out instruments on a table-top and she does not have to hand instruments to the surgeon. This enhances asepsis and simplifies the nurse's task.

At the end of each phase of the operation the used tray is handed out of the sterile enclosure and is replaced by a new tray with the instruments for the next phase. Outside the enclosure the contents of each used tray are washed and the tray is recycled through the autoclave and can be waiting in its sterile bag ready for the next operation, even before the one in progress has been completed. To achieve the most efficient recycling, so that one set of the expensive special instruments can be used for a series of operations with intervals of not more than about 20 min between each, it is necessary to duplicate (1) the set of 18 Moynihan skin-edge towel forceps, (2) the initial wound retractor and (3) the serrated and angulated femur lever, because these are retained in the wound from beginning to end leaving no time to wash and resterilize before the next case.

The seven trays are shown in Fig. 14.3 with the heavy, double-thickness cloth bags in which they are wrapped for autoclaving in Fig. 14.4. The bags are longer than the trays, so permitting the mouths to be folded in such a way that the sterile trays can be extruded into the scrub-nurse's hands without being soiled by contact with the exterior of the bag (Fig. 14.5).

Contents of Trays

The contents of the trays are listed below. Instruments special to each stage of the operation are marked with asterisks. In the preparation room of the operating suite a list of contents of each tray is on a permanent wall display; therefore the

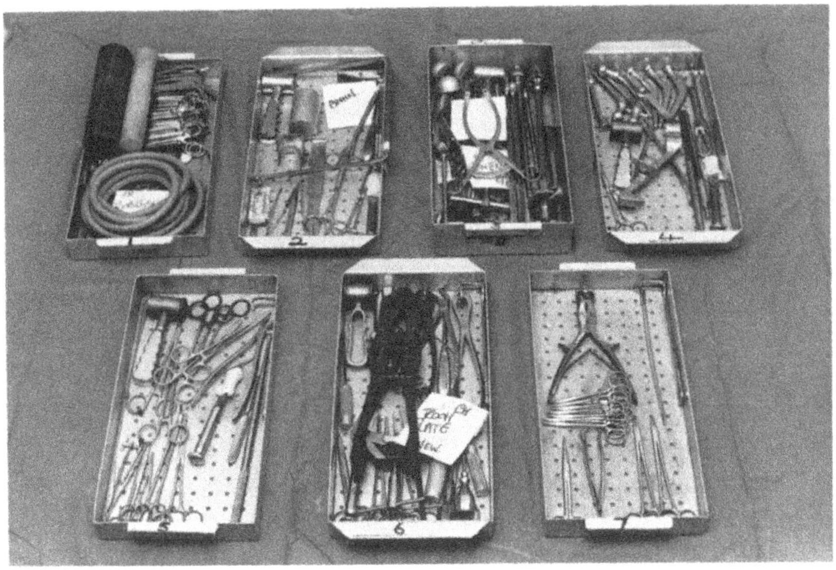

Fig. 14.3. The seven trays containing the instruments for individual, progressive phases of the operation

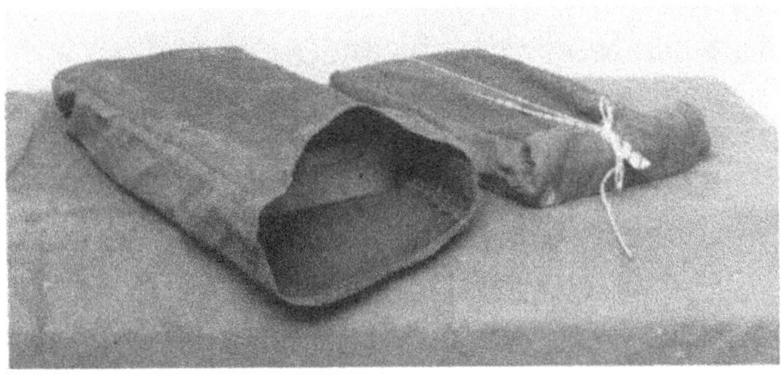

Fig. 14.4. Cloth bags in which the trays are autoclaved

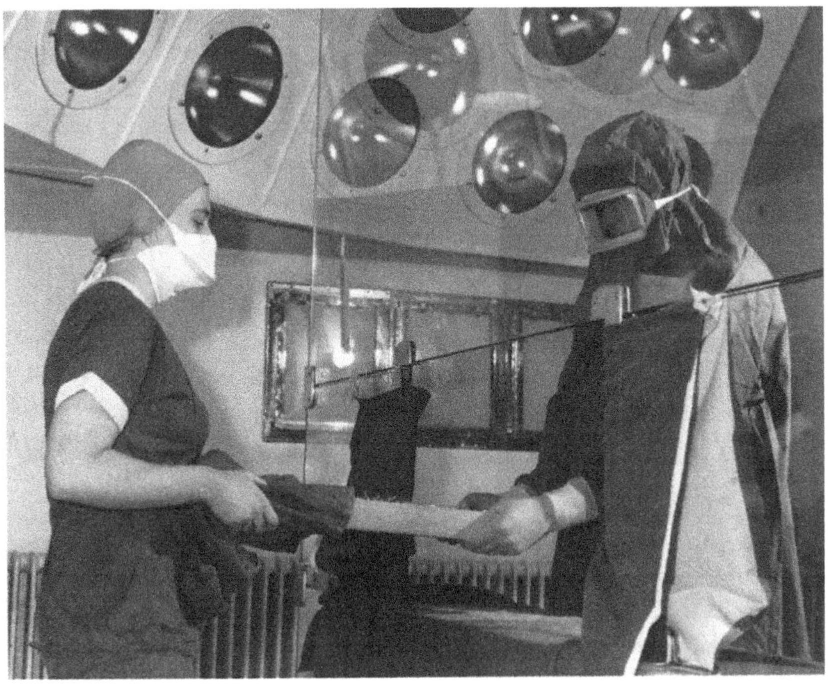

Fig. 14.5. Circulating nurse offering sterile contents of unsterile bag to scrub nurse inside the sterile enclosure

nurses can check the contents of each tray prior to sealing the appropriate bag for transmission to the autoclave.

Tray 1. Skin Incision

5 Mayo towel clips with ball-guarded points
1 Lane's dissecting forceps
1 Knife handle with blade
18 Moynihan skin-towel clips
6 Heavy rubber bands for skin-towel clips
1 Diathermy forceps (Richies)
2 Long diathermy leads
1 Diathermy cutting needle
2 Clips for diathermy leads
1 Sucker
1 Sucker tubing
(18 Moynihan skin-towel clips to Sucker tubing: all retained on table until end of tray 6)

Tray 2. Exposure of Acetabulum

1 Knife handle with blade
1 Lane's dissecting forceps
1 Mayo straight scissors ($6^{1}/_{2}$ in.)
2 Kocher's Artery Forceps (8 in.)
1 Durham retractor
*1 Morris retractor
1 Cholecystectomy forceps
1 Langenbech sharp bone hook
1 Chisel ($^{1}/_{2}$ in.)
1 Mallet
2 Gigli saws with pair of handles
*1 Initial incision retractor
1 Weight and chain
1 Watson-Jones gouge
*1 Serrated and angulated femur lever
(Initial incision retractor to femur lever: Retained on table till end of tray 6)

Tray 3. Cementing Hip Socket

1 Long knife handle with blade
2 Kocher's forceps
*1 Nail retractor and introducer
1 Hohman retractor
*1 Hohman retractor angulated 45°
*1 Small weight and chain for use with 45° angulated Hohman retractor
*1 Horizontal retractor
*1 Retractor screw-jack
*2 Double-handed Volkmann spoons (large and small)
*1 Serrated ring curette double-handed
1 Mallet
*3 Socket size gauges
*1 12.5-mm pilot hole drill with centring disc
*1 Deepening reamer
*1 Expanding reamer
*1 Heavy brace handle
*1 6-mm drill with collar
*1 Rotary acetabulum nylon brush
*1 Cement restrictor and introducer
*1 Self-ejecting socket-holder
*1 Socket pusher
*1 Socket trimming scissors with serrated blades

Tray 4. Preparation of Femur—Test Reduction

1 Trotters bone rongeur
*1 Taper reamer with T-handle
*2 Rotary taper femoral reamers, brace driven (large and small)
*1 Heavy brace handle
1 Ollier retractor
2 Kocher's forceps (8 in.)
1 Chisel (1 in.)
1 Mallet
*1 Femoral prosthesis holder (hold over to next tray)
*1 Set of test prostheses

(If neck-length jig used it is introduced at end of this stage plus additional tools (Chap. 16). The neck-length jig makes the set of test prostheses redundant.)

Tray 5. Wires in Femur: Cement Femoral Prosthesis

1 Lane's dissecting forceps
1 Mayo scissors
2 Kocher's artery forceps (8 in.)
1 Ollier retractor
1 Chisel ($^{1}/_{2}$ in.)
1 Mallet
*1 Long-handled small curette
1 Short Volkmann spoon
*6 Wire-holding forceps
*1 Set of wires 18 s.w.g. 1 double, 2 single
1 Narrow bone rongeur (6 mm)
*1 Trochanter staple-bolt length measuring device
*1 3.2-mm drill and drill stock
*1 Femoral prosthesis holder (held over from previous tray)
*1 Small fish-tailed wire pusher

Tray 6. Reattachment of Trochanter

2 Kocher's forceps (8 in.)
1 Mayo scissors
2 Ollier retractors
1 Chisel (1 in.)
1 Mallet
*1 Trochanter-holding forceps
*1 Wire passer ($^1/_4$ circle)
*1 Narrow bone awl
*1 Large bone awl
*1 Trochanter staple-bolt forceps
*1 Trochanter staple-bolt anterior holding device
*1 Wire tightener
*1 Wire-cutting forceps
*1 Heavy trochanter punch
*1 Small, fish-tailed wire punch
*1 Bolt cropper (12 in.)
*1 Fine-toothed metal file

Tray 7. Wound Closure

2 Needle holders
1 Mayo scissors
2 Dissecting forceps ($5^3/_4$ in. and 7 in.)
1 Ollier retractor
7 Haemostats (for fat suture)
1 Pkt. 12 suture buttons (aluminium)
1 Pkt. 12 plastic foam pressure-pads
3 Drainage tubes with trocars
*1 Button crusher

Surgical Team

In addition to the surgeon and scrub nurse it is customary at Wrightington to have: a first assistant on the same side as (and standing headward of) the surgeon; and a surgical technician (male) to manipulate the lower extremity on the side opposite from the surgeon. The first assistant is the least essential and is usually a postgraduate under instruction. The team therefore can be reduced to three. The surgical technician ('leg-holder') is an essential member of the team and the operation is enormously facilitated when he is familiar with the procedure. Most female nurses would be unable to control the leg in all its necessary positions when the patient is a heavy male if having to act as leg-holder and even if standing on a platform. Therefore if only one male assistant is available it can be better for him to take charge of manipulating the leg rather than be first assistant on the same side of the table as the surgeon. In the text describing the operation the attitude of the leg at each stage in the operation is indicated diagrammatically.

Anaesthetic Room

The patient must be anaesthetised outside the sterile enclosure and brought to the enclosure only when the sterile team is ready to receive the patient.

Final Pre-operative Skin Preparation

If it is necessary that the surgeon or his first assistant should perform the final skin preparation on the anaesthetised patient this must be done outside the clean air enclosure. A U-shaped adhesive plastic drape is essential for isolation of the perineum and this is applied in the anaesthetic room as part of the final skin preparation. Having completed the final skin preparation the prepared limb must be temporarily covered with a sterile drape and the patient must stay outside the enclosure until the four (or three) persons of the sterile team have assembled inside the enclosure and are ready to receive the patient.

Body Exhaust System

The body exhaust system designed by the author is illustrated in Figs. 14.6, 14.7 and 14.8. The headpiece carries wide-bore exhaust tubes which evacuate air from the region of the face. The replaceable window of transparent plastic film and the headpiece do not need to be sterile. The gown, of a textile (Ventile) almost impermeable to air, is of one-piece construction without a back opening. It is donned over the head using a simple folding technique to be described. The head part of the gown has a rectangular aperture which registers with four pegs projecting from the corners of the transparent window of the head-piece.

It is an **essential part of the design of the body exhaust gown** that there is **no constriction at the neck** and that there is **no belt at the waist**, because both these would restrict the upward flow of air over the surgeon's body. The heat of the body

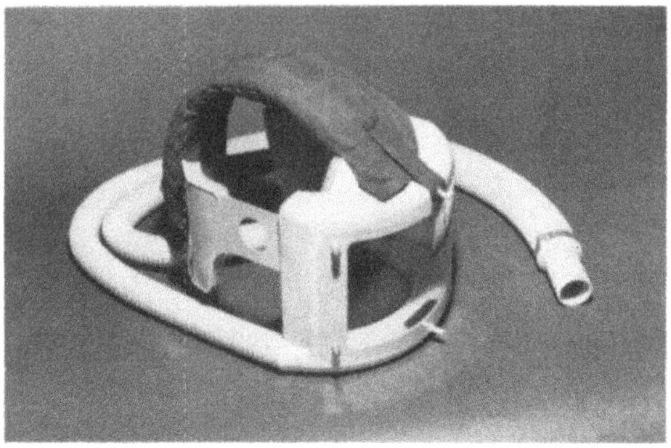

Fig. 14.6. Head-piece of Charnley body exhaust system

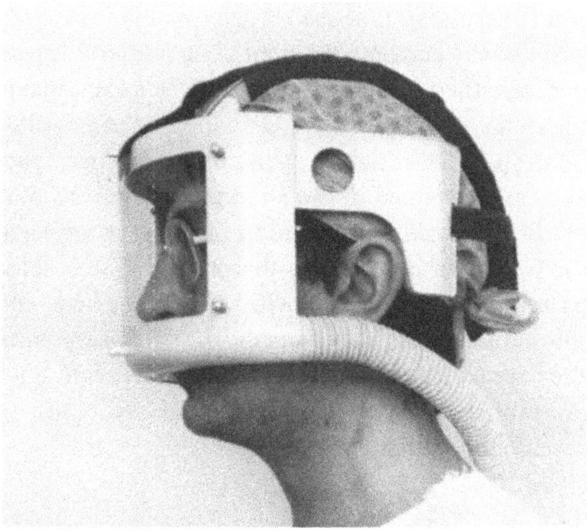

Fig. 14.7. Head-piece as worn

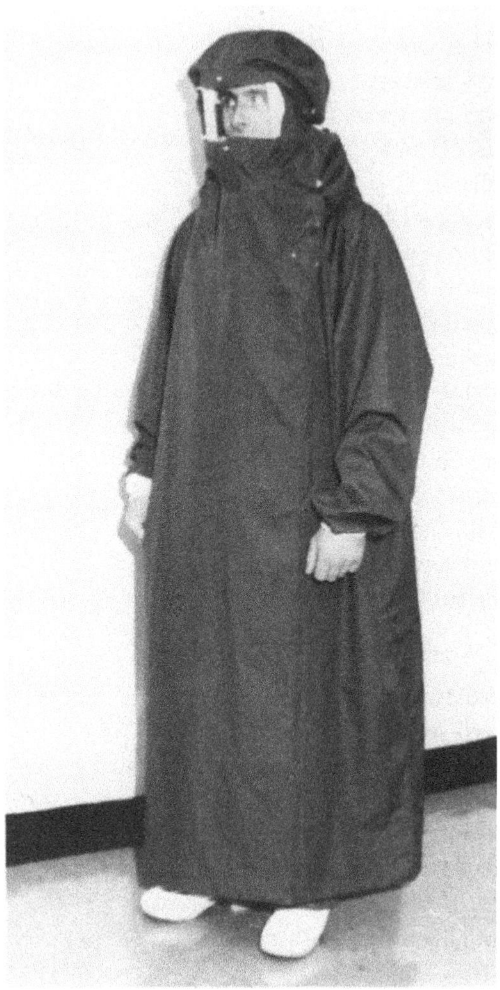

Fig. 14.8. Gown applied over the head-piece

assists the upward airflow to the point where the exhaust tubes extract it near the face (Fig. 14.9).

The body exhaust system serves four functions:

1) Above waist level the bodies of the surgical team are at a slight sub-atmospheric pressure. Therefore the 'bellows action' of a gown as for instance when the arms are raised and lowered, cannot pump air contaminated with epithelial scales into the operating atmospheric environment of the open wound.

2) For the interior of the gown to be held at sub-atmospheric pressure the material of the gown must be relatively impervious to air. This makes it likely that it is absolutely impervious to penetration by bacteria from the wearer's body.

The cotton material used for the gown has a weave known as 'Ventile', as used for raincoats and by mountaineers as protection against wind. When fresh from the weaver it is chemically waterproofed but repeated washing and autoclaving does not seem to impair its surgical function (though the manufacturers do not guarantee it to be waterproof after washing and autoclaving).

3) The flow of air over the body removes body heat which otherwise would become intolerable inside an impervious gown. A surgeon can emit heat at the rate of a 250 watt electric light bulb and 30 s of failure of the exhaust source can produce an intolerable situation. From an ordinary gown, epithelial scales are carried in rising convection currents of warm air, thereafter to be deposited at a distance.

4) Sub-atmospheric pressure inside the gown makes for a 'fail-safe' situation; this will be very

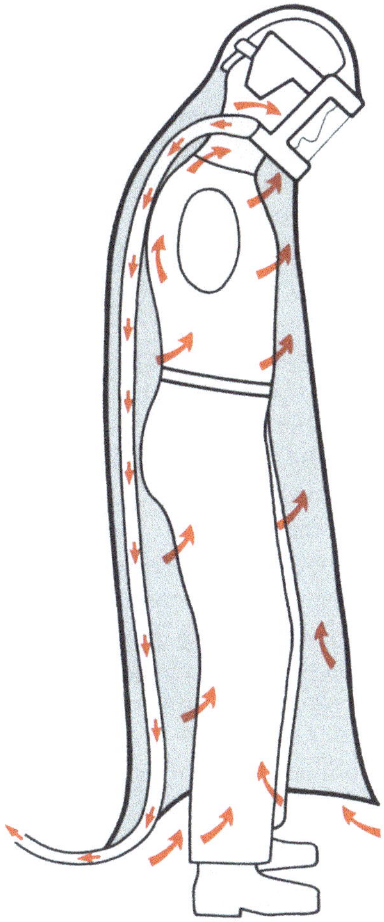

Fig. 14.9. Path of air-flow to point of extraction near the mouth. Note absence of constriction at the neck or at the waist (i.e. no belt or wrap-around design)

important if paper gowns ever become popular in this application.

Rate of Air Extraction from Body Exhaust

Measurements of rates of air-flow can be made only with special apparatus and even then there are many snags of interpretation which can be quite unexpected.

The author likes to estimate the vigour of the suction by the level of sub-atmospheric pressure inside the head and neck part of the gown and prefers that this should be about 1.0 cm water. This produces a tendency for the gown to close down on to the wearer's head and chest. At this pressure the air-flow is noisy; conversation without an intercom system is practically impossible but like noise in a light aeroplane one soon becomes accustomed to it and in routine hip surgery there is no need for true conversation. If the team is experienced occasional shouted instructions or requests are all that is needed.

The level of sub-atmospheric pressure can be very easily tested (at the end of an operation) by pushing a rubber tube inside the cuff of the gown, passing it up the sleeve and into the head-piece, and connecting the outer end to a water manometer. A straight length of glass tube dipped vertically under the surface of water in any sort of beaker will suffice as a manometer; water should rise in the tube about 1 cm above the general water level in the beaker.

If the clean air system uses **recirculating** air **it is essential that refrigeration should be incorporated to extract the heat generated by the electric motors driving the fans, the surgical lights and the body heat of the four persons in the surgical team**. If the body exhaust is delivering only a modest suction (rather than the noisy and powerful suction advocated by the author) the surgeon can sweat intolerably, even being unable to see the wound for sweat running into his eyes.

When the atmospheric conditions inside the body exhaust system are correct the ambience is delightful and makes for better surgery than in a conventional theatre. With air at 68°–70° F (20°–21° C) flowing over the body it is possible to perform four total hip replacements in one day without feeling more tired than after an equivalent period of exercise out of doors and with none of the enervated feeling experienced after a day in a hot, conventional operating room. In the author's experience the body exhaust system is worthwhile for this alone.

Other Air-Flow Systems

Horizontal air-flow systems have obvious disadvantages when the surgical team is wearing ordinary operating room clothing if the wound cannot be sited 'upstream'. In these circumstances the body exhaust system ought to make an important contribution.

The Allender system is theoretically sound but the operating team must be rigidly grouped in the centre of the room and the periphery of the room must be empty and devoid of persons or all other obstructions to the air-flow. A body exhaust system would enable the team to wear impermeable clothing.

The Howorth Exponential air-flow system has a pattern of air-flow which renders it unnecessary to have a central enclosure or to keep the periphery of the room free of persons or obstructions. For those who prefer the isolation provided by an enclosure it is said that half-length walls can be used with this system.

Monitoring of Air-Flow

All clean air systems should have the rate of air-flow monitored to make sure that the filters are not offering too much resistance as they accumulate airborne particles. Routine periodic servicing should be arranged. In years gone by it has been known for pigeons, etc. to be nesting in the air-intake ducts of operating suites: it is easy for these matters to become 'out of sight, out of mind'.

Gowning the Surgical Team (Body Exhaust)

The surgical team of four persons in the Wrightington system (surgeon and first assistant; scrub nurse and surgical technician) enter the enclosure from the open end, with hands scrubbed, and wearing their body exhaust head-pieces. On entering the enclosure a circulating nurse connects them to the tubes of the exhaust system on the walls

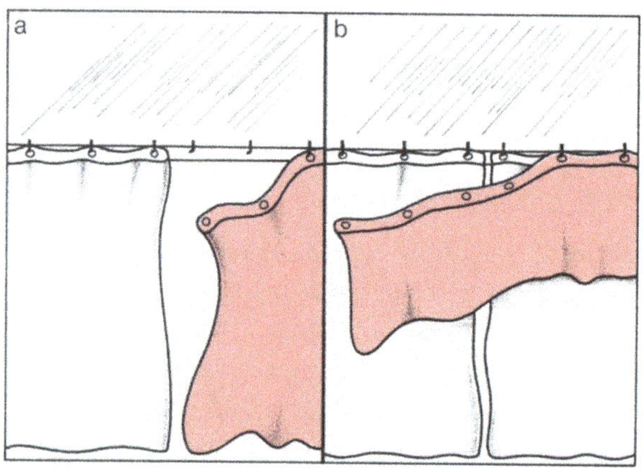

Fig. 14.10. Sterile curtains applied from within the enclosure to close the entrance. *a* two vertical curtains; *b* a single, short transverse curtain

of the enclosure. Inside the enclosure the team finds a sterile pack waiting on a small mobile table in the centre of the enclosure. The external layer of the double-wrap of this pack has already been opened by the circulating nurse. The surgical team opens the internal pack with scrubbed hands.
The sterile pack contains:
3 sterile curtains and 2 towel forceps
1 sterile cover for the surgeon's stool
4 surgical gowns

With bare hands the surgeon drapes his stool with the sterile cover taken from the pack. The surgeon and the scrub nurse who have entered first stand near the service opening. The assistant and surgical technician who enter second stand near the entrance to the enclosure. The assistant and surgical technician close the entrance by hanging the sterile curtains with bare hands. This limits the free excape of air, raises the air-pressure inside the enclosure and increases the airflow from the service aperture, which remains open throughout the operation.

The curtains are provided with holes (Fig. 14.10) to engage with hooks (non-sterile) spaced across the top of the entrance to the enclosure. Two curtains (one right and one left) hang the length of the open end. Finally a third curtain, which extends the width of the enclosure but hangs down only to table-top level, is superimposed from the inside of the enclosure. The outer edges of the right and left curtains are clipped to the vertical, unsterile edges of the side walls of the enclosure with large paper-clips (also non-sterile) applied from outside by a circulating nurse. All four members of the team now put on their first pairs of gloves which are handed in through the service aperture.

The four members of the team now gown each other, working in pairs. In this design of body exhaust system it is emphasized that the gowns have no back openings so that it is unnecessary to be helped by unsterile personnel when putting on the gowns. Only the four sterile persons of the operating team touch the gowns and they do this with gloved hands. Because no back aperture has to be closed there is no possibility of the back of one of the gowns or of one of the gloves becoming accidentally contaminated. The gowns are folded (see below) so that only the inside of the gown presents to the person about to put it on. Thereafter the exterior of the gown emerges, progressively presenting itself to the sterile gloves of the person helping to put it on.

Folding and Putting on Gowns

The method of folding the body-exhaust gown before autoclaving is indicated in Fig. 14.11 a, b, c). An essential feature is that three cloth tabs, coloured to distinguish them from the rest of the gown, are stitched to the **inner surface** of the gown: one tab is at the level of the middle of the back of the gown on the inside, and the other two are on **the back of the inside of the sleeves** at about the middle of their length.

To fold the gown for packing and autoclaving it is first turned inside out, at half length, to expose the tab at the middle of the back. The sleeves are then invaginated inside the gown till their tabs are exposed as in Fig. 14.11 b, which is the 'first folding position'. The gown is now folded again twice, to a quarter its size, for convenience of packing.

When unpacked and ready for putting on, the gown is unfolded to the first folding position on the mobile table in the centre of the clean air enclosure. It is important that **the position of the tabs should indicate that the back of the gown is uppermost** (and therefore that the opening for the face is underneath). The person who is to wear the gown and the one who helps him put it on have already put on their first pair of sterile gloves. The assistant takes hold of the tab on the back of the gown with one hand and the tab on the nearest sleeve with the other (Fig. 14.11 c). The person who is to wear the gown takes hold of the tab on the sleeve nearest him with the hand which will **not** be inserted into the sleeve (i.e. for a left sleeve he holds the tab with his right hand). Exerting counter-traction on the tab he insinuates

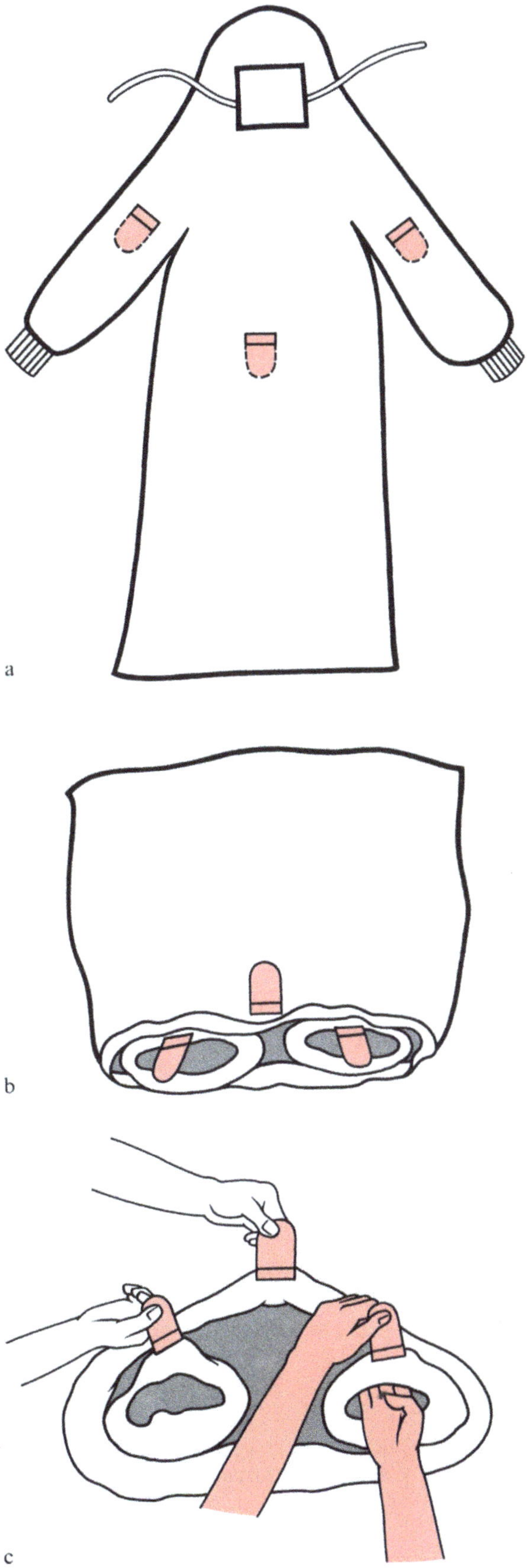

Fig. 14.11 a–c. Method of folding gown. **a** shows sites of the three tabs (but on the inner surface of the back of the gown); **b** 'first folding position' – or 'last unfolding position' before putting on. **c** shows method of putting on; white, assistants hands; red, wearer's hands

the other hand into the sleeve until it enters the elasticated cuff. He now has to put into the other sleeve the hand he used for exerting counter-traction on the first sleeve. For this the assistant exerts the counter-traction. When the hand has entered the elasticated cuff the assistant lifts the back of the gown and the wearer 'dives' his head into the interior of the gown. The rest of the procedure is simply that of straightening up from the stooping position and having the assistant pull the gown downwards over the wearer's body.

The stage of helping the wearer to get his head-piece into the head part of the gown is obvious but the next step, pulling down the body of the gown, can be awkward unless the assistant goes straightway to **freeing the wearer's elbows**; when this is done the rest follows easily.

The last step, tying the tapes behind the head, is done by the wearer himself; this is critical in achieving comfort because **up to this moment the head-piece will be unstable on the wearer's head.** The tying of the tapes at the back of the head (1) pulls the face piece against the forehead, (2) pulls the two padded earpieces against the sides of the head behind the ears and (3) pulls the curved component on the top of the head against the occipital region. **Not until this moment does the head-piece take a firm location on the head.** When tied, the head-piece and the head part of the gown become a single unit which moves with the head. Because the material of the gown is impermeable it is permitted to readjust the tension with which the tapes are tied during the operation. The wearer will find that if he lifts the back of the gown upwards by taking hold of the cloth over the back of his neck, this will remove a feeling of tension at the back of the neck and if negative pressure is in action inside the gown, the gown will tend to hold in the new position by friction against the underclothing.

The mobile table, with the now-empty remains of the sterile pack, is pushed out of the enclosure between the curtains.

Supporting Weight of Exhaust Tubing

For comfort and maximum efficiency it is necessary that the surgeon's body should take the weight of the exhaust tubing rather than that this should pull on the head-piece. Different wearers have their own favourite methods. The commonest method is to have tapes attached to the tube at waist level and tie these in front of the body like a belt.

The author prefers the following method (Fig. 14.11 A); two long tapes are attached to the tube (very much longer than needed for tying like a belt) and the two ends are passed one over each shoulder and crossed in front of the chest (a). The crossed tapes are then pulled to take the weight of the tube and to lift it till the two smaller tubes from the bifurcation bulge backwards (b). The tapes are then passed under each arm, crossed behind the body, and brought forward to be tied in front of the chest. By tying high on the chest, the total length of the tapes can be kept to a reasonable length (otherwise they have to be so long they trail on the floor when first putting on the head-piece). The cavity inside the head part of the gown produced by the bulging of the tubes is advantageous to the air-flow and tends to reduce noise.

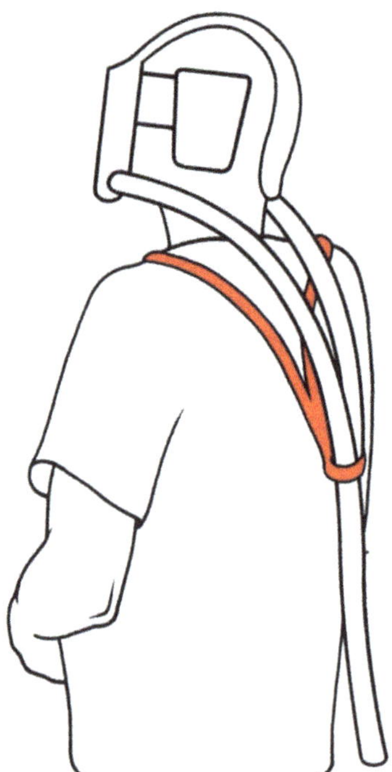

a

Fig. 14.11 A. a Two tapes supporting the weight of the tubing of the body-exhaust head-piece. **b** Pulling on tapes to lift the tubes and take weight off the head-piece. **c** Frontal view of **b**. **d** Tapes passed round the body under the axillae. **e** Tapes being tied in front of the body

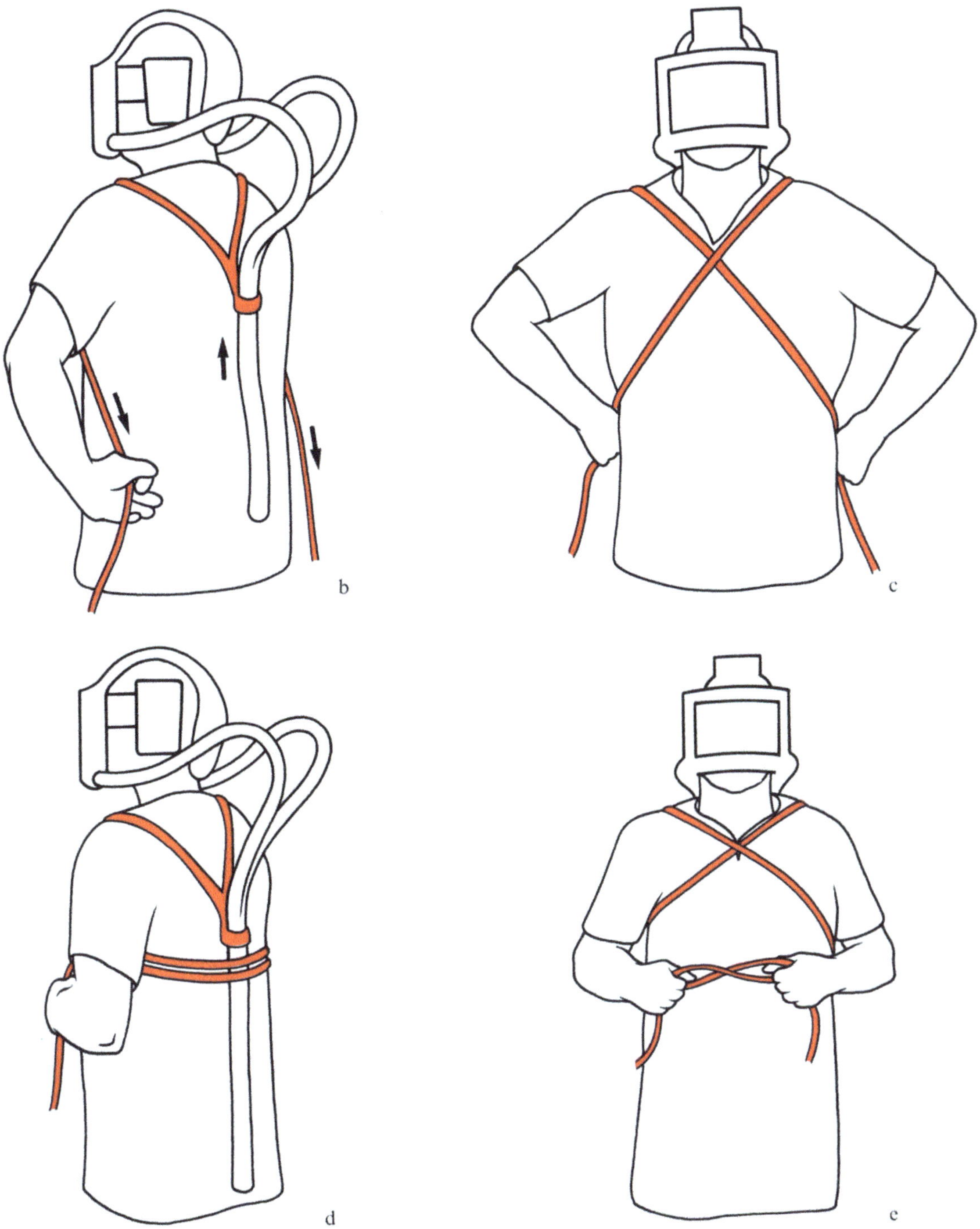

b c d e

Preparation of Service Aperture

The scrub nurse turns her attention to double-wrapped packs outside the service aperture which are opened for her on mobile tables. From these she extracts sterile drapes to cover the working surface of the shelf of the service aperture and also a specially shaped sterile cover to protect the right and left vertical edges of the service aperture. A sketch of this specially shaped drape is shown in Fig. 14.12. Sterile packs of drapes are opened and their contents stacked on the shelf of the service aperture in preparation for the entry of the patient.

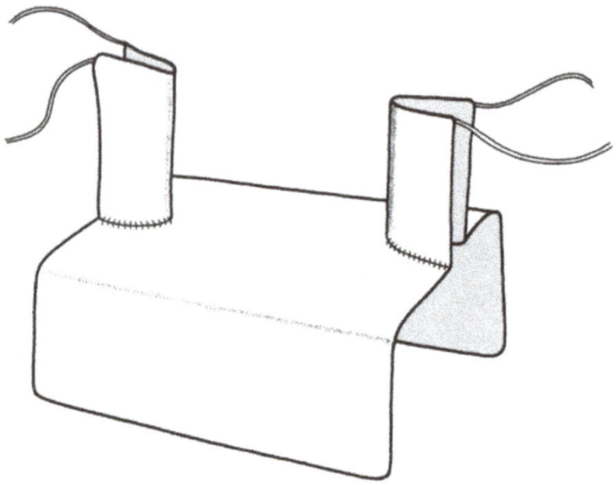

Fig. 14.12. Special drape for protecting service hatch

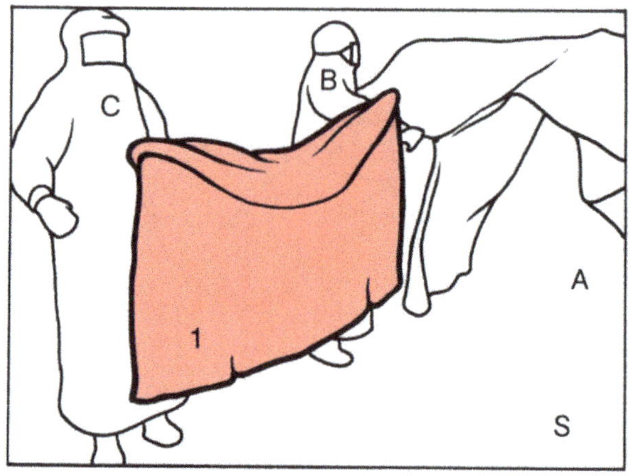

Fig. 14.13. Drape 1, 47 × 70 in. (118 cm × 175 cm). Positions of the four persons of the surgical team denoted by *S* (surgeon); *A* (first assistant); *B* (surgical technician or 'leg holder'); *C* scrub nurse

Entry of the Patient

The first assistant and the surgical technician (the leg-holder) take hold of the inner edges of the right and left curtains, using towel clips, and draw them apart for the entry of the foot end of the operating table. As the foot of the table starts to enter the enclosure, the sterile drape, which was used to cover the prepared lower extremity while waiting in the anaesthetic area, is pulled out by a member of the anaesthetics team from the head end of the table. There is a danger at this stage that the technician and the scrub nurse might have their gowns soiled by contact with the operating table as it enters the enclosure. To avoid this source of contamination they hold between and in front of themselves (Fig. 14.13) a large sterile drape (drape 1) while waiting for the patient to enter. When the table has penetrated fully into the enclosure drape 1 is deposited on their side of the operating table (Fig. 14.14).

Drape 1 is further important in protecting the front of the technician's gown as he leans forward to pick up the patient's foot in the roll of sterile stockinette (Fig. 14.15).

With the surgical technician strongly adducting the limb and lifting the buttock off the table (Fig. 14.16) drape 2 is inserted (preceded by an impervious paper drape) and the buttock is allowed to fall back on to the table to trap it against the table top.

Drape 3 is now applied to cover the whole of the lower end of the table (Fig. 14.17).

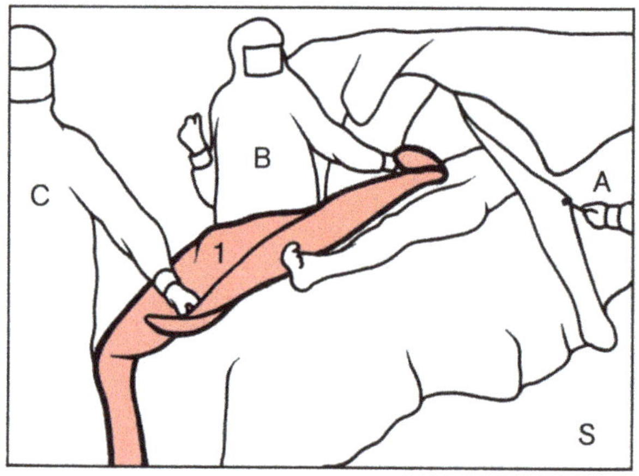

Fig. 14.14. Drape 1 deposited on table as patient enters

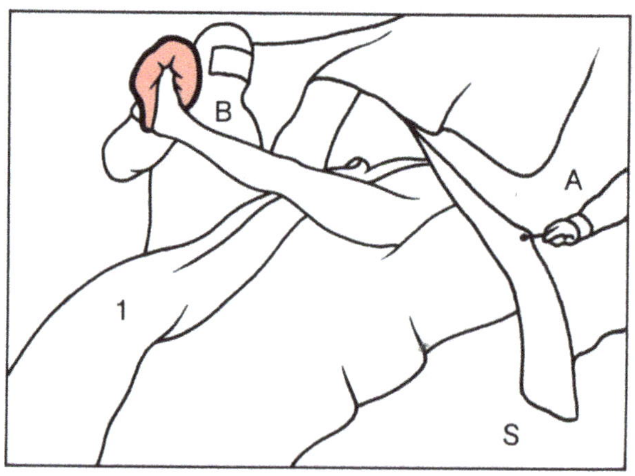

Fig. 14.15. Surgical technician (*B*) picks up foot in rolled stockinette

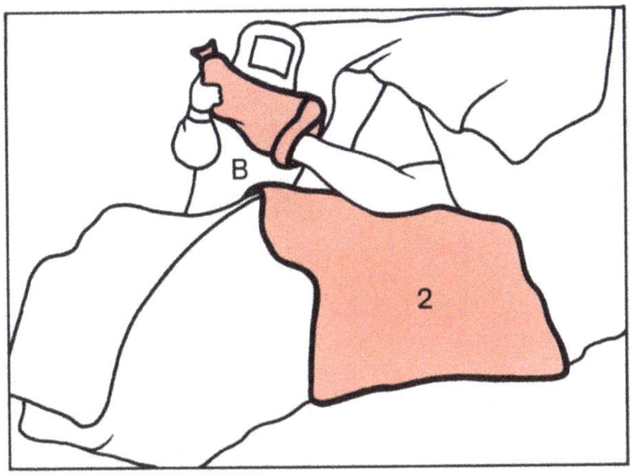

Fig. 14.16. Drape 2, 34 × 39 in. (85 × 98 cm)

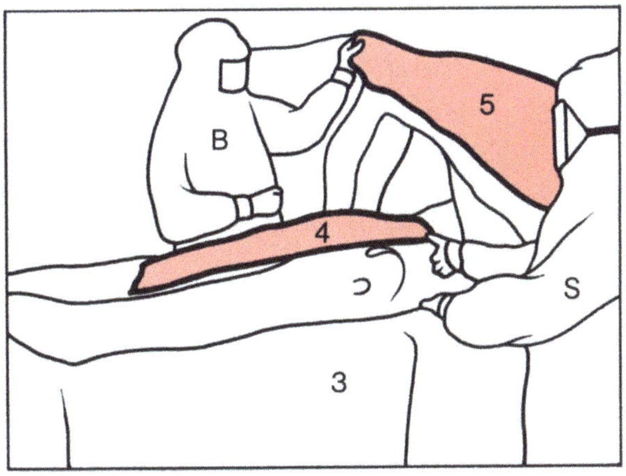

Fig. 14.19. Drape 4, 34 × 39 in. (85 × 98 cm) is folded longitudinally with fold near the surgeon. Drape 5 is a large sheet 47 × 70 in. (118 × 175 cm). The first assistant (*B*) is not visible in this picture but he is holding the near end of drape 5

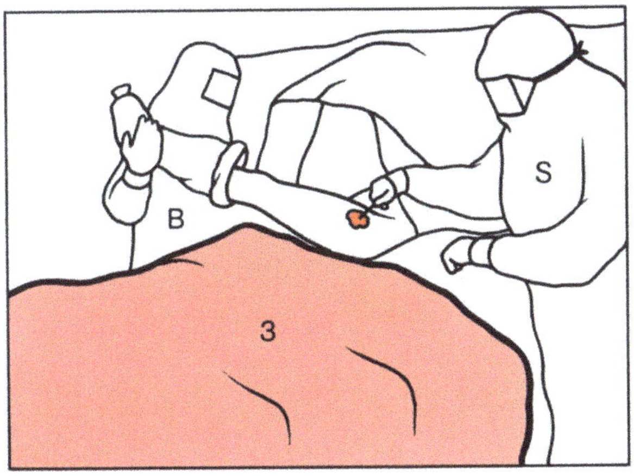

Fig. 14.17. Drape 3, 47 × 70 in. (118 × 175 cm)

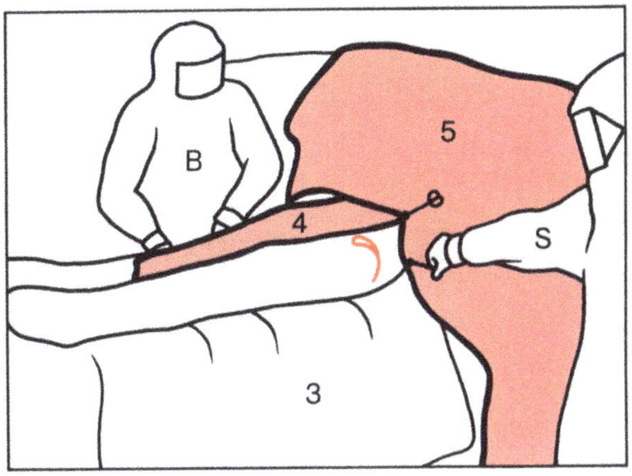

Fig. 14.20. Drapes 4 and 5 and upper end of stockinette clipped, as high as possible on patient's rib-cage, as indicated by space above iliac crest

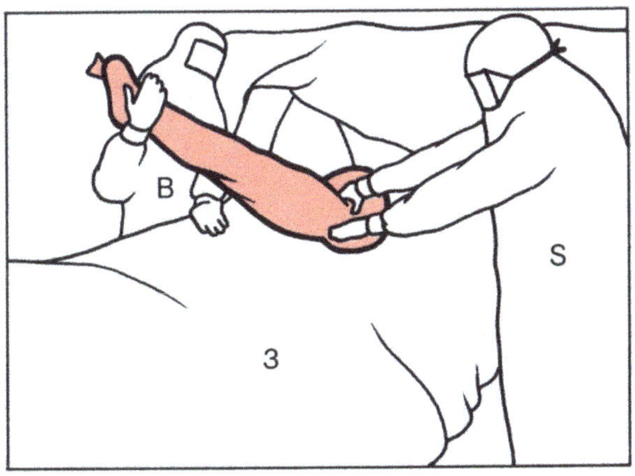

Fig. 14.18. Stockinette (170 cm long, 30 cm wide) must unroll to reach the patient's rib-cage

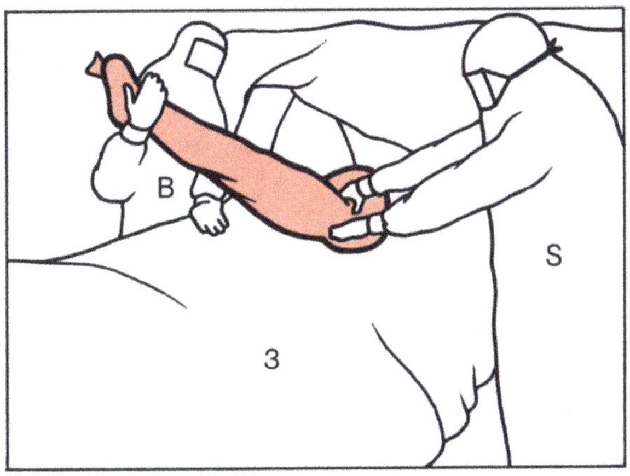

Fig. 14.21. Distal end of drape 4 pulled round buttock and clipped as high as possible above iliac crest

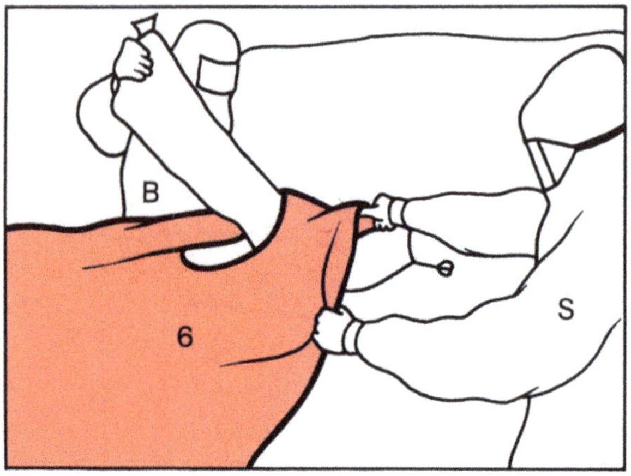

Fig. 14.22. Drape 6 with hole. This is the largest drape, 80 × 93 in. (200 × 233 cm). The hole is offset from the centre to give more drape on the surgeon's side (so that it will hang down over the surgeon's shelf) and more drape below the hole than above it

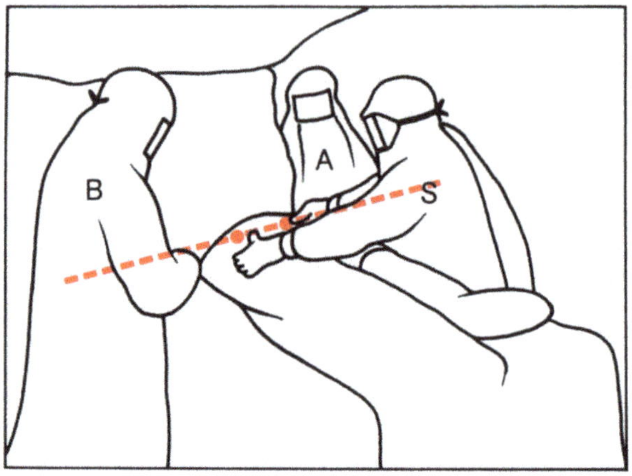

Fig. 14.25. Surgeon assessing transverse lie of the pelvis

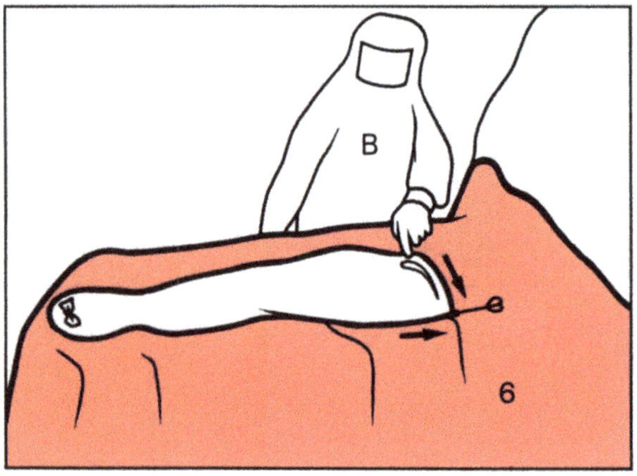

Fig. 14.23. Showing how the hole in drape 6 is pulled round the iliac crest and pinched to the lower part as close to the table top as possible

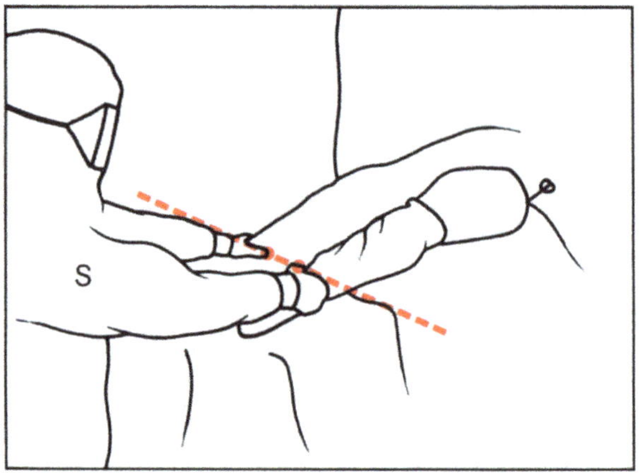

Fig. 14.26. Surgeon assessing length of legs

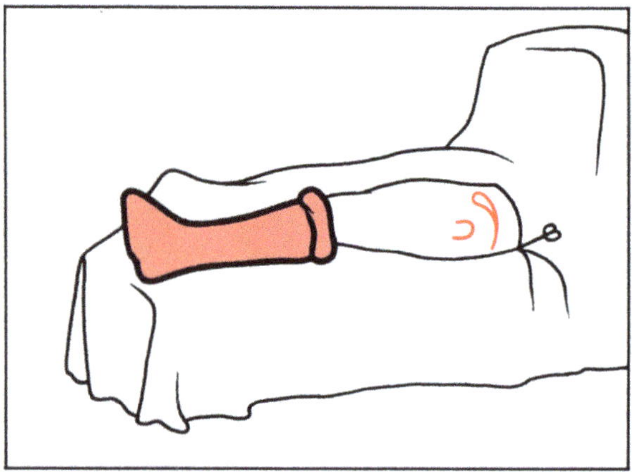

Fig. 14.24. The stockinette over the foot is enclosed in a cloth bag held by Velcro just below the knee

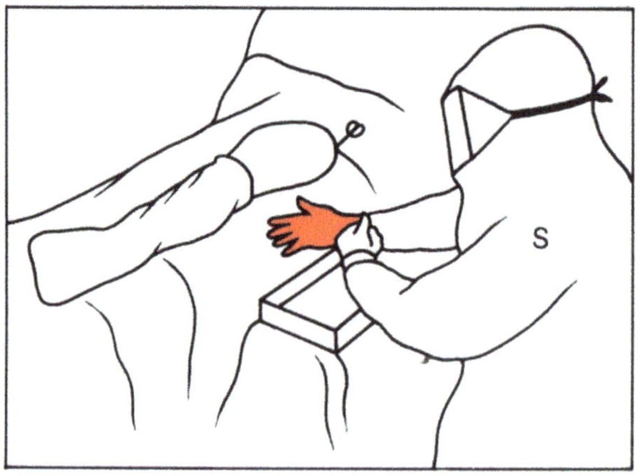

Fig. 14.27. Surgeon sitting and pulling on second pair of gloves immediately before starting to operate. Note tray 1 on shelf attached to table

The stockinette (170 cm long, 30 cm wide) is unrolled, with the leg adducted, to permit the stockinette to be trapped under the buttock (Fig. 14.18).

The stockinette is further unrolled by the surgeon to reach as high as possible over the patient's lower ribs. Failure to get as high as this can result in the iliac crest being obscured under several layers of drapes with a very real danger of the exposure being hampered in the upper end of the wound.

Two drapes (drape 4 and drape 5) are placed simultaneously (Fig. 14.19). Drape 4 is a small drape folded longitudinally with the folded edge near the surgeon; it covers the genitalia and the top is pulled up to rib level by the surgeon. In this diagram the surgeon's right index finger is holding simultaneously drape 4 in contact with the lower ribs and the upper edge of the stockinette. Drape 5, held between the technician and the first assistant (the latter not seen here because in this view he is obscured by the surgeon), is being spread between them across the upper end of the table.

In Fig. 14.20, drapes 4 and 5 and the stockinette have been clipped together by a towel clip taking also the skin over the patient's ribs. A second towel clip takes drape 5, the upper edge of drape 3, and skin as high as possible over the posterior region of the chest or loin. By striving to clip these first drapes at the level of the ribs, space is made available above the iliac crests; without this precaution the further drapes which have yet to be applied will overlie the iliac crest and restrict the surgical exposure.

In Fig. 14.21, the lower end of drape 4 is pulled tightly against the perineum, with the hip flexed, and is attached with a towel clip high in the region of the ribs.

In Fig. 14.22, the large drape 6, with central hole, is pulled over the lower extremity and the lower edge of the aperture adjusted to the patient's perineum.

An attempt is made in Fig. 14.23 to illustrate the two directions, one headwards and one vertically backwards, by which tension is applied when closing the upper end of the aperture in drape 6. By pulling in the directions indicated by the arrows, and by applying the towel clip as near as possible to the table top, the iliac crest can be made to project. This detail can almost always be achieved in females though not in males. This detail is not possible unless drapes 4 and 5 have been attached at rib level.

The open texture of stockinette should be reinforced against danger of penetration by bacteria from the foot (during manipulation by the second assistant) in a bag of the same material as the drapes (Fig. 14.24). This is conveniently closed round the knee, without causing constriction, by a band of velcro.

Figure 14.25 shows the surgeon assessing the transverse alignment of the pelvis in relation to the operating table.

In Fig. 14.26 he is assessing the length of the lower extremities by palpating the medial malleoli while standing at the foot of the table.

Figure 14.27 shows application of the second pair of gloves (by all members of the team). The surgeon is sitting with the position of a tray on the shelf demonstrated.

Towel Clips

Towel clips of the type 'Mayo with ball-guarded points' are immeasurably superior to ordinary towel clips because the towels do not slide along the jaws. They are easily made by having $^{1}/_{4}$-in. (6.4-mm) diameter discs brazed to the jaws 0.5 in. (12.5 mm) from the points [Appendix C (1)].

Chapter 15

Technique of Low Friction Arthroplasty of the Hip

1

Vastus Lateralis Ridge

The vastus lateralis ridge is best palpated with finger tips acting from below upwards. The vastus lateralis ridge is nearly 5 cm distal to the upper level of the trochanter. The skin incision is centred on the vastus lateralis ridge.

2

Skin Incision

The skin incision is 20–25 cm long (8–10 in.) and is centred on the vastus lateralis ridge of the trochanter. The distal half of the incision is at the level of the anterior margin of the trochanter; the proximal half inclines backwards as in the diagram. The upper limit of the incision is about 2.5 cm headward of a perpendicular through the antero-superior iliac spine. The incision is made with the thigh and pelvis flat on the table and not tilted with sand bags. This ensures that skin and subcutaneous tissues are incised in the position they will occupy in bed.

3

Skin-Edge Towels

Skin-edge towels are of thick turkish towelling. Nine Moynihan forceps are used per side (total of 18). The catches on Moynihan forceps tend to unfasten; rubber bands are used to stop this, grouping the forceps in threes. The best end-clips are Mayo's with ball-guarded points; these are immeasurably better than plain towel clips (see Appendix C.). Even if the surface of the skin is isolated with adhesive plastic film, skin-edge towels will still be used to protect instruments from contact with cut glands, hair follicles, etc. in the skin edges.

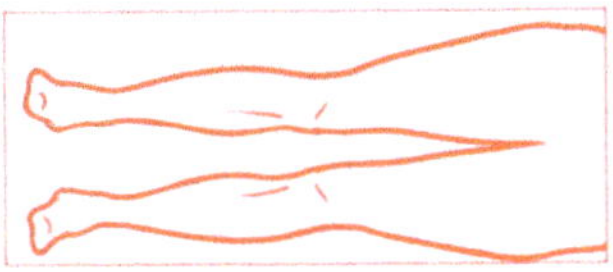

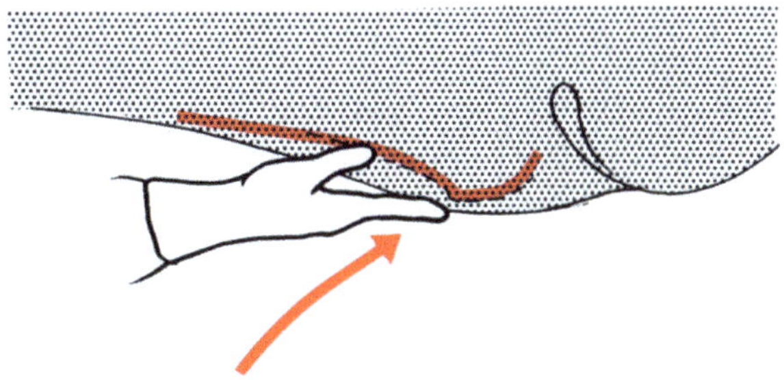

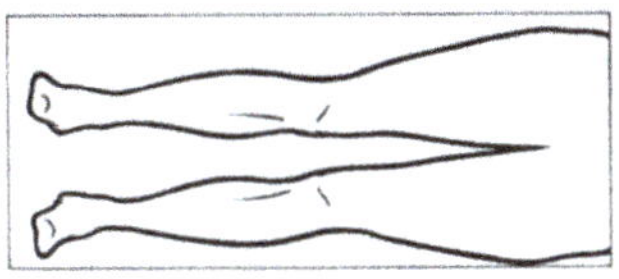

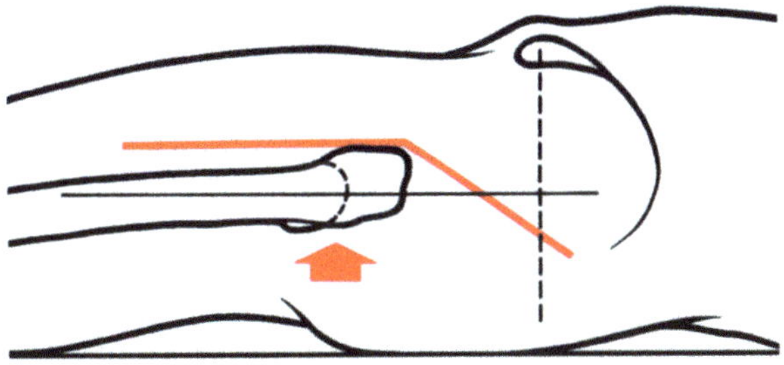

Time: 0 min

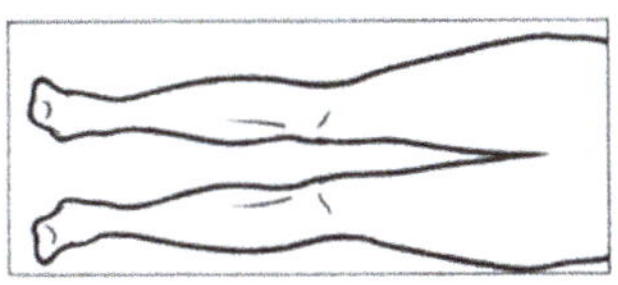

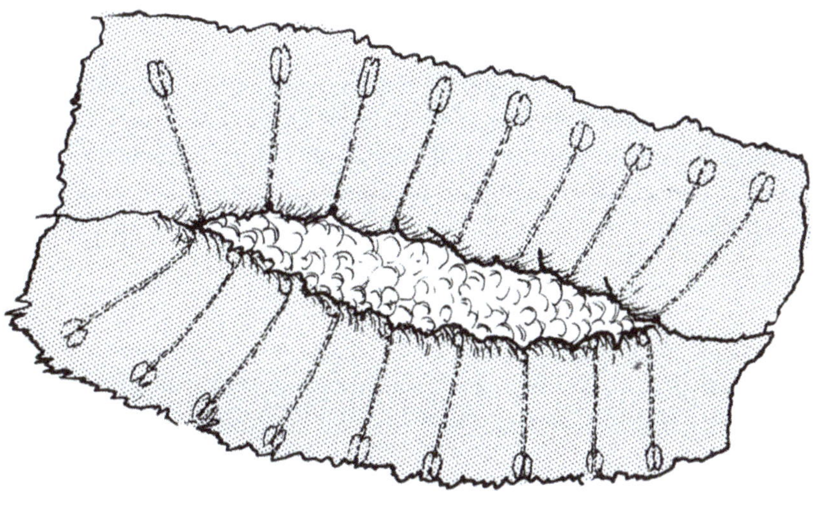

4

Incision of Deep Fascia – Central Part

The incision in the deep fascia starts anterior to the trochanter and rather headward of its upper level. The fascia is very thin at this point and quite unlike the dense ilio-tibial band over the trochanter. This central part of the incision is about 2.0 cm long. This incision should be made cautiously because the gluteus medius muscle may bulge out and be accidentally cut. The position of tensor fasciae femoris (TFF) muscle is indicated in the diagram and is often visible through the fat. The fat should be scraped away to reveal the posterior margin of the TFF.

5

Incision of Deep Fascia – Distal Extension

An index finger is inserted under the deep fascia in a distal and posterior direction to enter the space between deep fascia and lateral surface of vastus lateralis. The finger follows the posterior edge of the tensor fasciae femoris muscle.

6

Incision of Deep Fascia – Distal Extension

Cutting from inside outwards is helpful because the incision in the fascia at this point lies posterior to the skin incision (*a*) and passes obliquely through fat to emerge at (*b*). It is difficult to find the posterior margin of the tensor fasciae femoris if incising from outside and obliquely through fat.

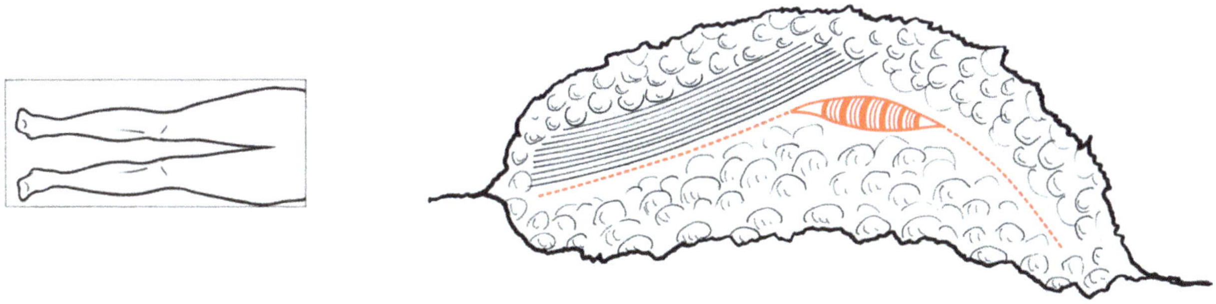

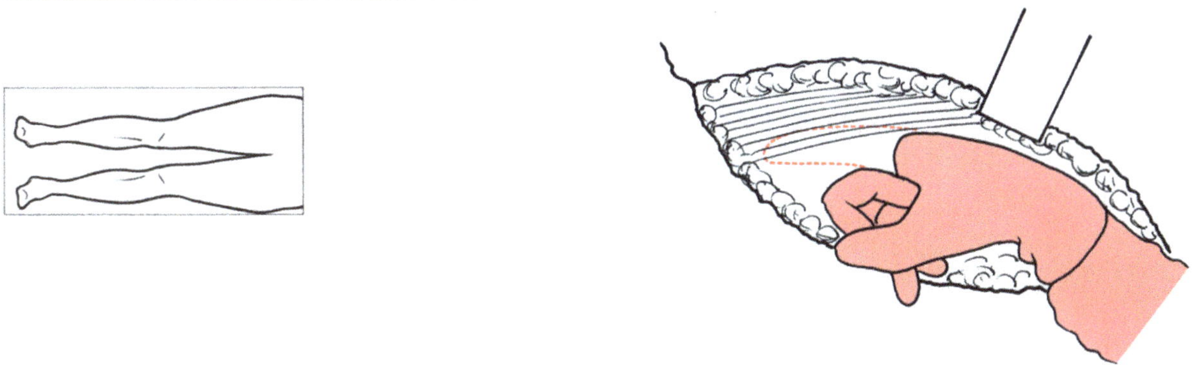

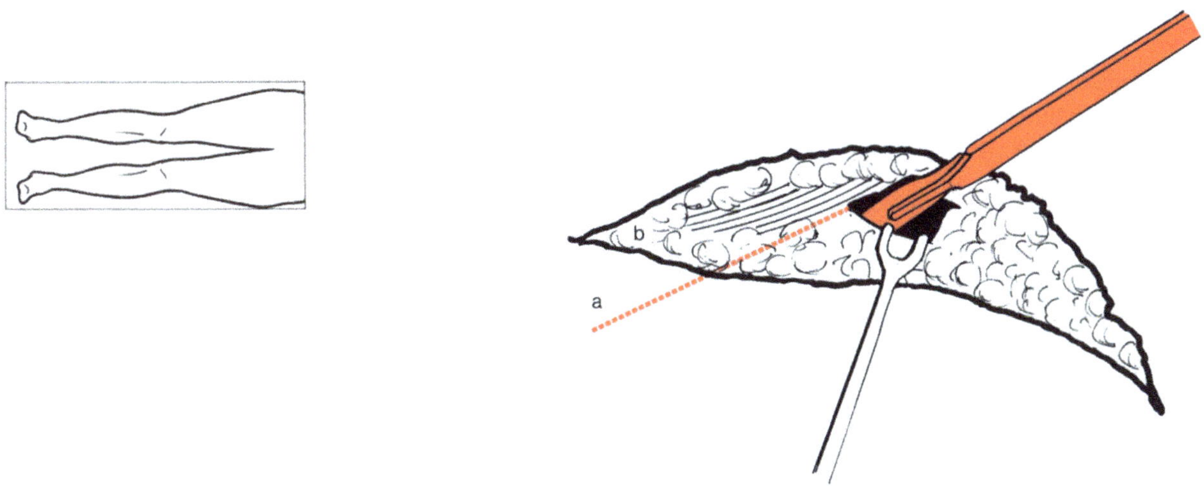
b
a

7

Incision of Deep Fascia – Distal Extension

This diagram explains the direction of the incision when made from within outwards. The knife starts in the space between the lateral aspect of vastus lateralis and the deep fascia and cuts obliquely forwards and laterally through the fat.

8

Incision of Deep Fascia – Distal Extension

Two points of brisk haemorrhage are always encountered at the posterior edge of the tensor fasciae femoris and two corresponding points on the opposite edge of the incision in the deep fascia. Coagulate with diathermy forceps.

9

Incision of Deep Fascia – Proximal Extension

The index finger is inserted under the deep fascia in a headward direction and inclined posteriorly at about 45°. The finger can scrape away fibres of gluteus medius taking origin from the deep surface at this point.

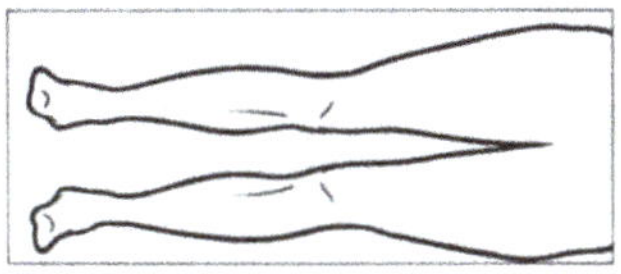

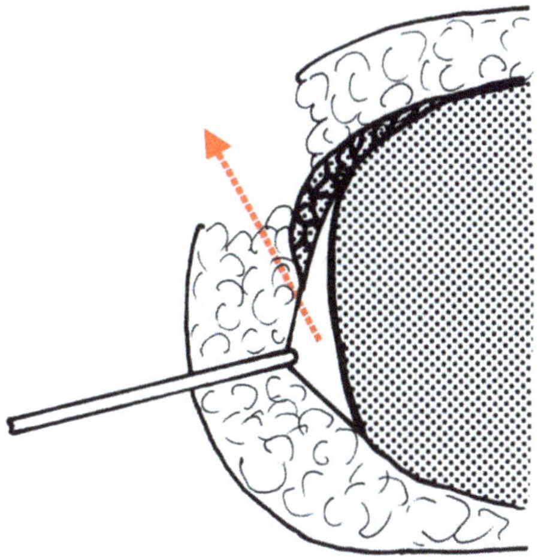

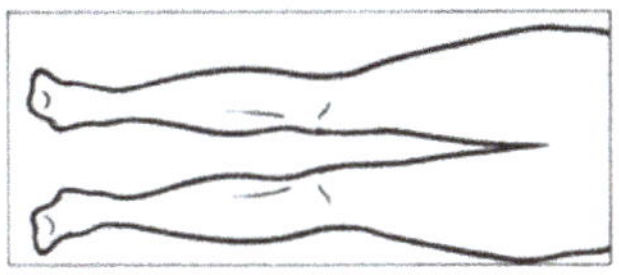

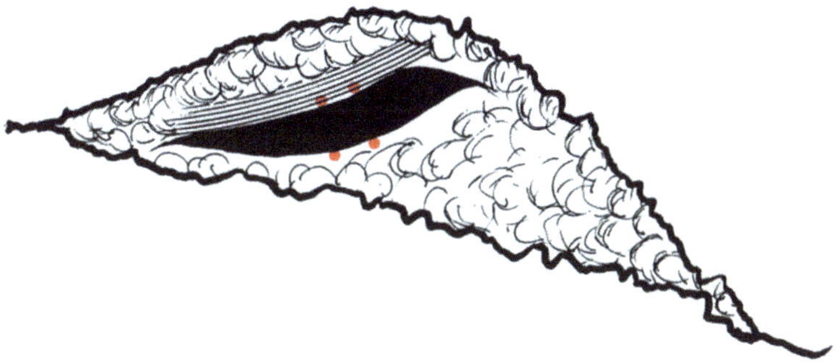

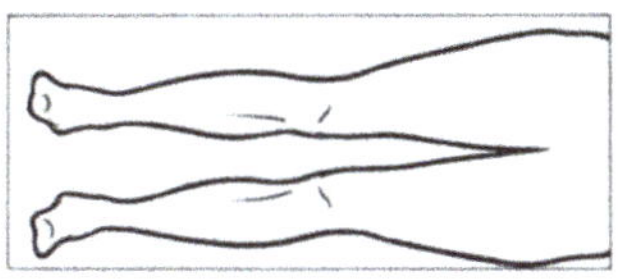

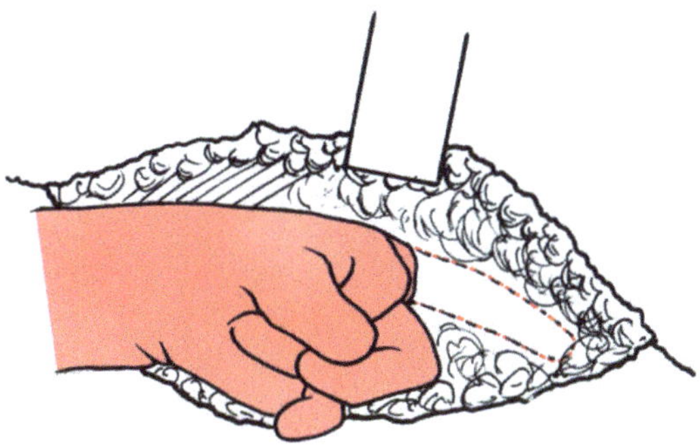

10

Incision of Deep Fascia — Proximal Extension

The strong fascia covering the gluteus medius muscle, and more proximally the gluteus maximus, is incised without cutting muscle fibres.

11

Incision of Deep Fascia — Proximal Extension

Access in the headward direction is completed by splitting the muscle fibres of gluteus maximus with the thumb.

12

Exposure of Trochanter

Free access to the posterior surface of the upper end of the femur is important.

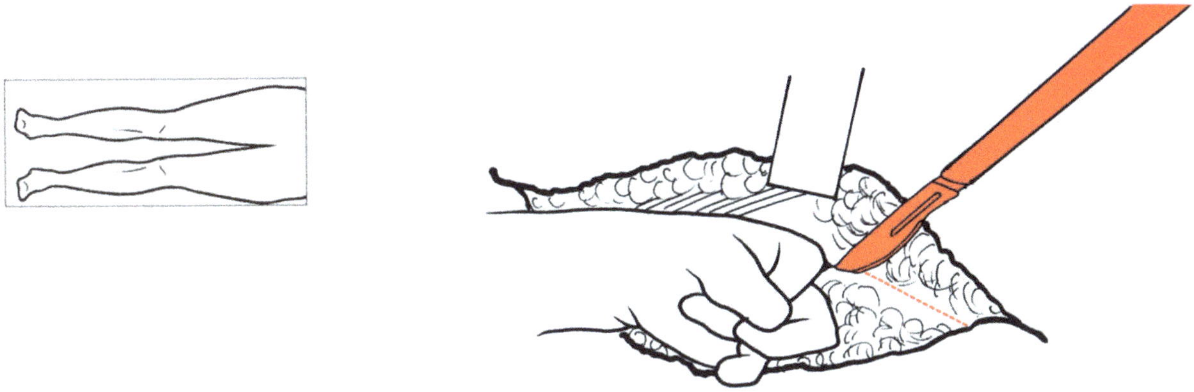

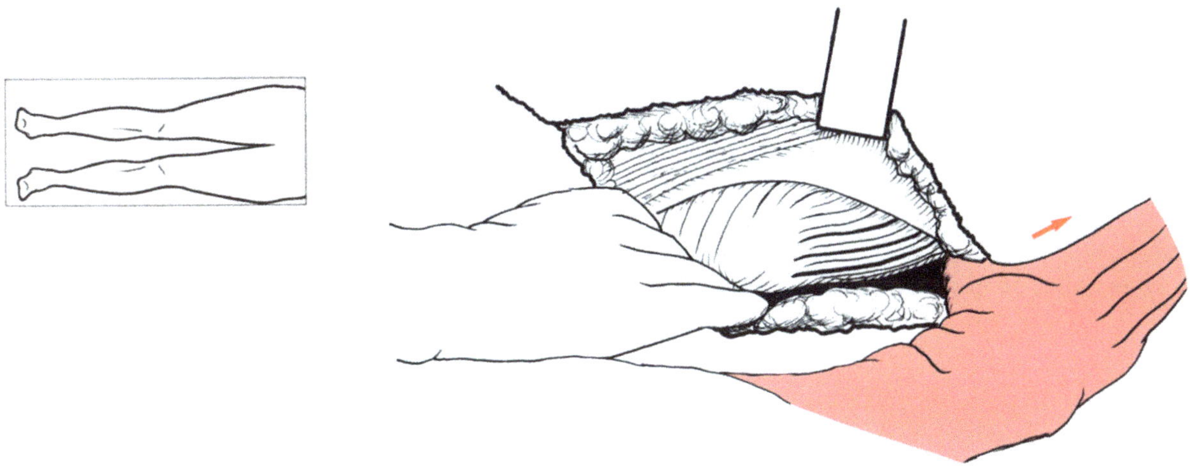

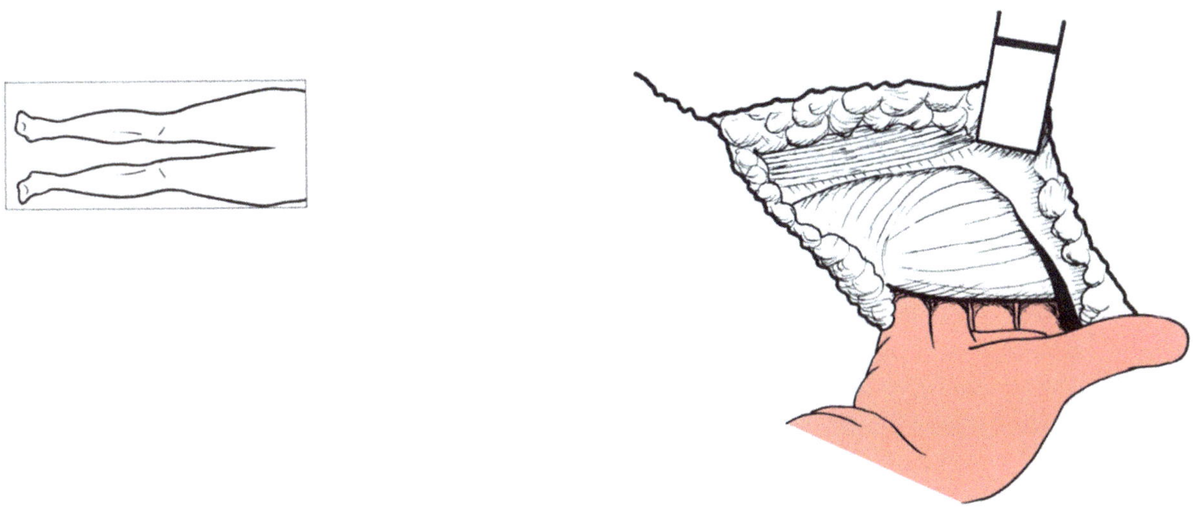

13

Exposure of Trochanter

The membranous and semi-translucent tissues of the trochanteric bursa are stripped from the trochanter in a headward direction. Stripping is best started at the vastus lateralis ridge.

14

Exposure of Gluteus Medius

A thumb is inserted under the anterior edge of the deep fascia and an attempt is made to strip it medially in the direction of the fibres of gluteus medius. Often this will complete the exposure of gluteus medius without any bleeding. Sometimes stripping to expose the anterior edge of the gluteus medius is resisted by an arcuate fold of dense fibrous tissue, as in this diagram. This fold must be nicked transversely with a knife and stripping then becomes possible.

15

Exposure of Gluteus Medius

To complete the bloodless stripping of the anterior margin of the gluteus medius both thumbs are now inserted under the anterior edge of the deep fascia as in the diagram.

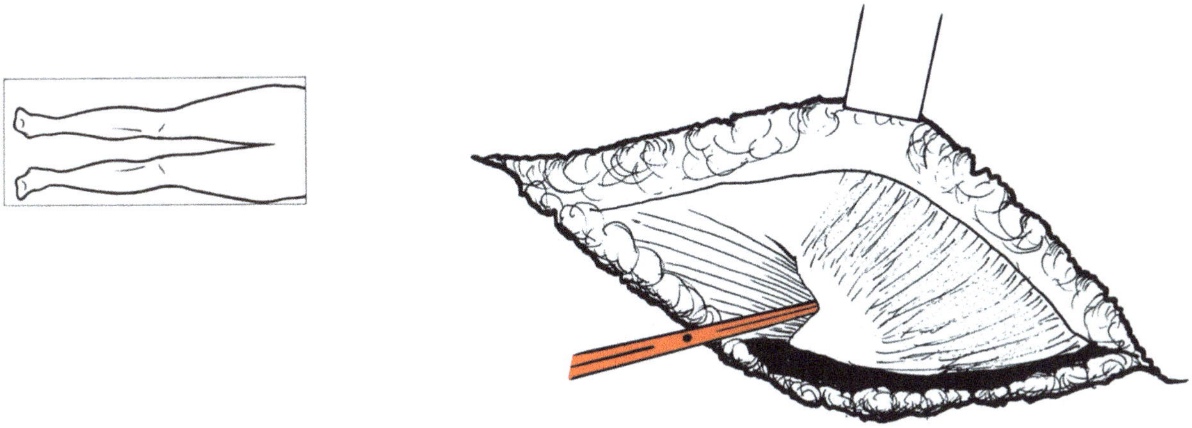

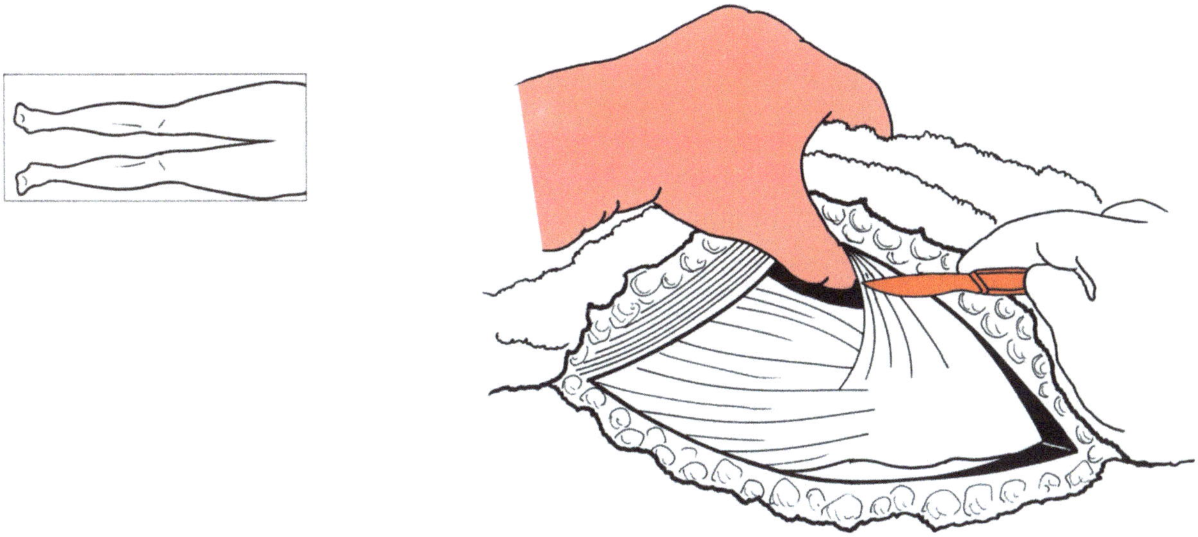

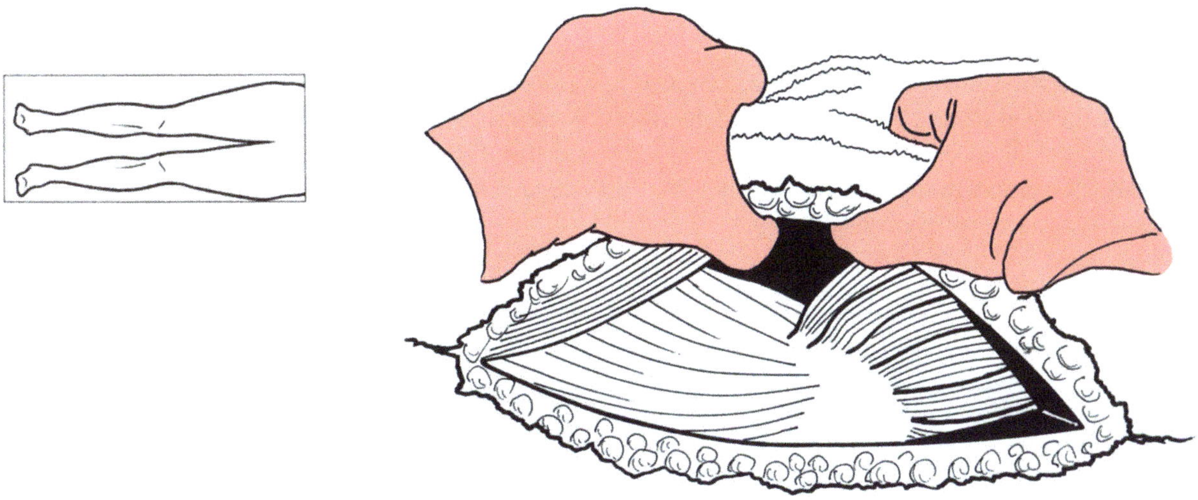

16

Initial Retractor

The weight and chain used with this retractor on the opposite side of the table tilts the plane of the retractor away from the surgeon. The **vertical arrow** indicates how the tilt of the initial retractor permits vertical access to the neck of the femur. The curved incision in the fascia (4–11) greatly helps in this anterior access by removing any overhang of anterior fascia.

17

Initial Retractor

Fig. 1 shows how restricted the exposure of the front of the neck of the femur can be if the incision in the fascia lata is straight and centred over the trochanter. Fig. 2 shows how the curved incision in the fascia lata, convex anteriorly, centred anterior to the trochanter, makes for easy access to the front of the neck of the femur.

18

Gluteus Medius Retracted

External rotation of the femur is important at this stage to stretch the front of the capsule and enlarge the available space. When there is fixed external rotation in osteoarthrosis this detail looks after itself, but **failure to remember to externally rotate** a mobile hip at this stage can hamper the surgeon's access very considerably.

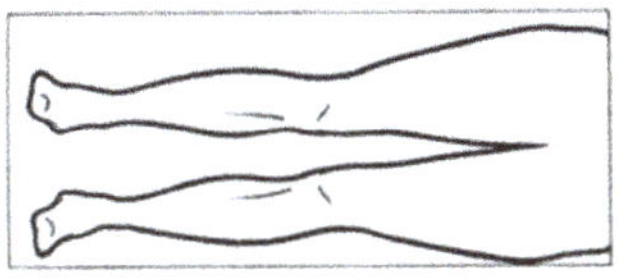

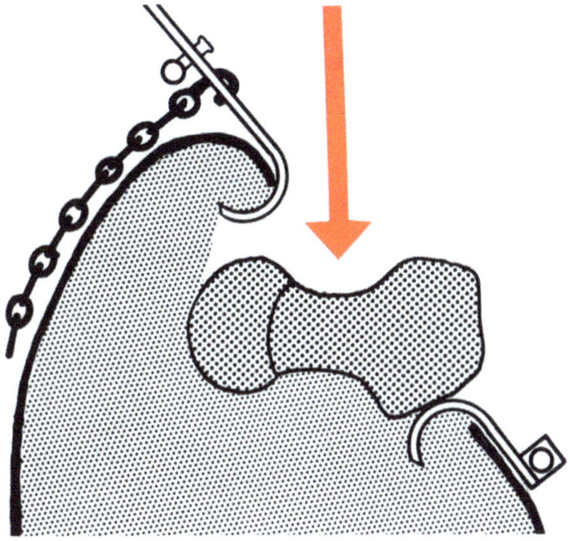

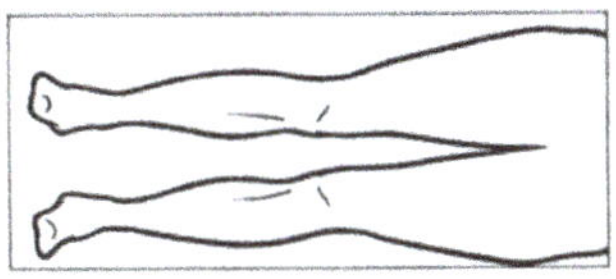

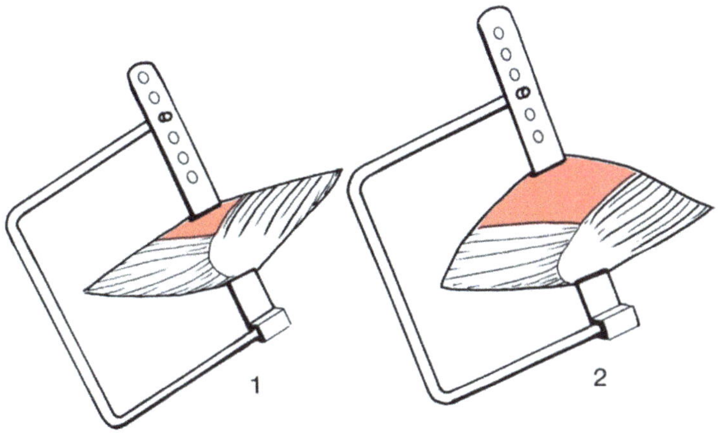
1
2

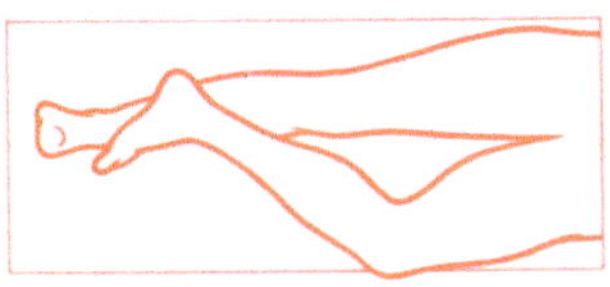

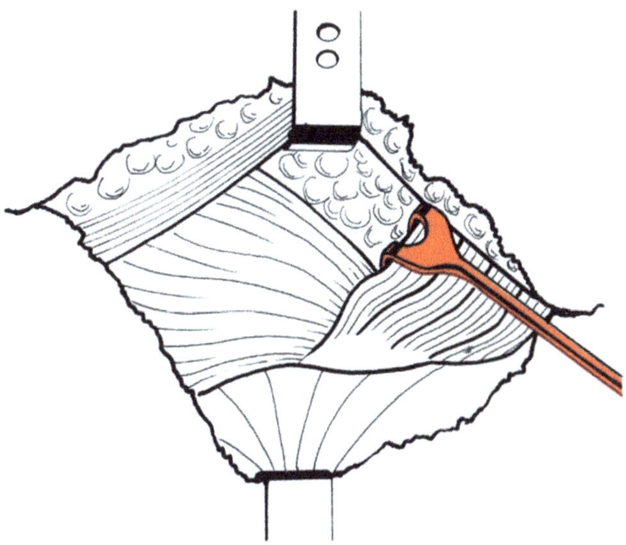

19

Exposure of Capsule of Joint

Fat over the front of the hip joint capsule is scraped in a medial direction to reveal the capsule of the joint. The scalpel in this diagram is not cutting; it is merely scraping the fatty tissue medially.

20

Deep Retraction Headwards and Medially

The blade of this important retractor should be about 8 cm deep and about 3 cm wide. Get the assistant to lift the handle of this retractor so that the tip of the blade retracts under the overhanging tissue till the rim of the acetabulum is reached. Two vessels on the surface of the capsule often can be cauterised before cutting.

21

Exposure of Vastus Lateralis Ridge

Internal rotation of the femur helps access to the posterior region of the vastus lateralis ridge. A diathermy needle is advantageous here. The incision is sited **exactly on the summit of vastus lateralis ridge**. Silvery fibres of the aponeurosis of vastus lateralis will be seen on the headward side of this incision [**see** later (115)]. The incision goes down to bone and the ascending branch of the circumflex artery will be divided at the most distal level of the anterior fibres of gluteus medius.

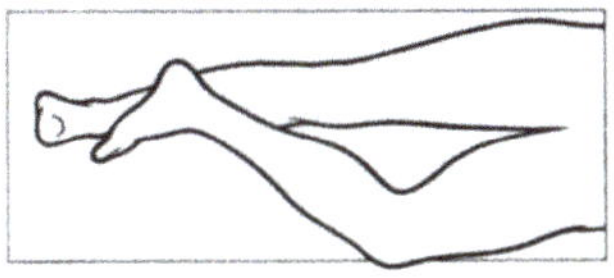
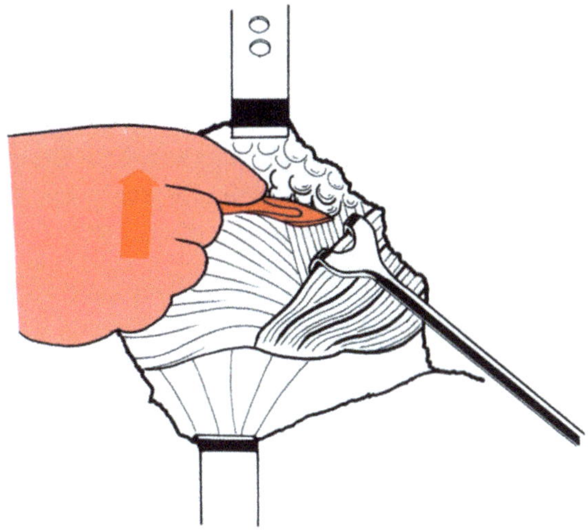

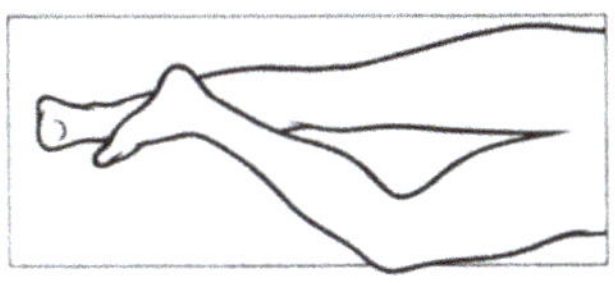
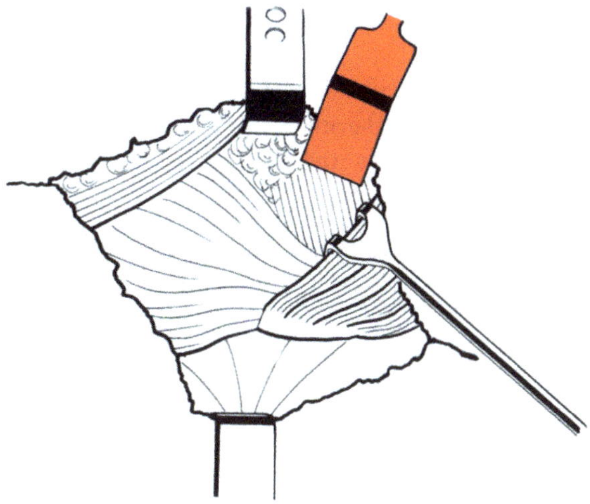

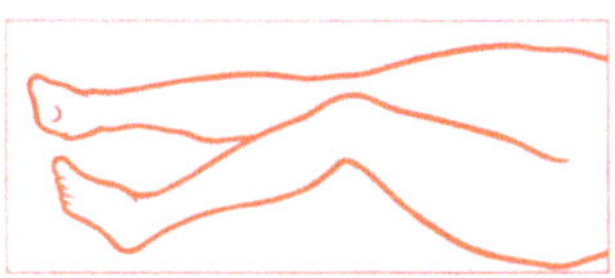
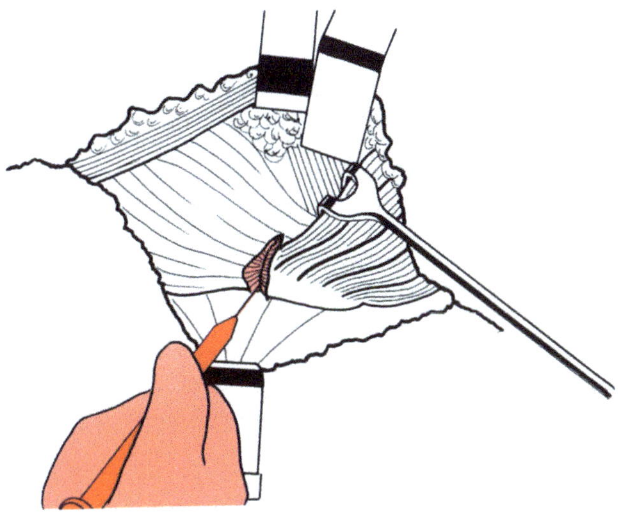

22

Palpation of Neck of Femur

The femur is externally rotated again. The index finger palpates to locate the **inferior** level of the neck of the femur (**not** the centre of the neck of the femur, as was previously taught). The inferior level of the femoral neck is located by running the finger tip distally from the highest convexity, which indicates the centre of the neck.

23

Incision in Capsule

Incision of the capsule with the diathermy needle reduces bleeding. The handle of the diathermy needle is inclined away from the vertical to avoid passing below the neck of the femur. Note how the new incision lies distal to the old incision (*dotted line*) which previously was centred over the middle of the femoral neck.

24

Low Capsular, Incision

The low incision lies in the pubo-capsular ligament. This incision is **almost** horizontal at the level of the vastus lateralis ridge. This illustration shows the ligaments in the anterior capsule in external rotation.

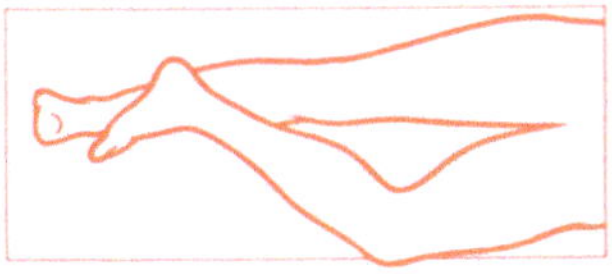

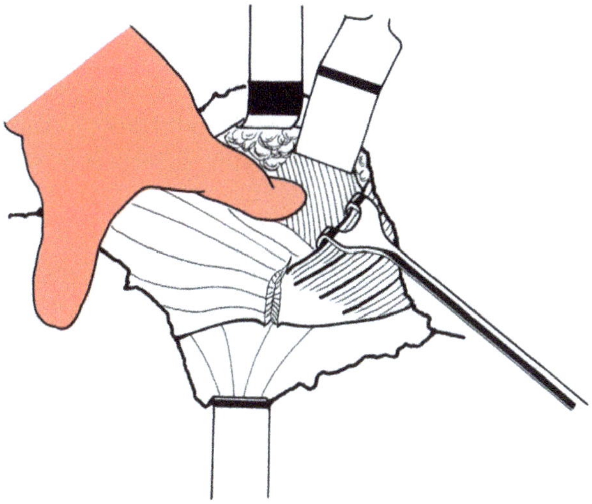

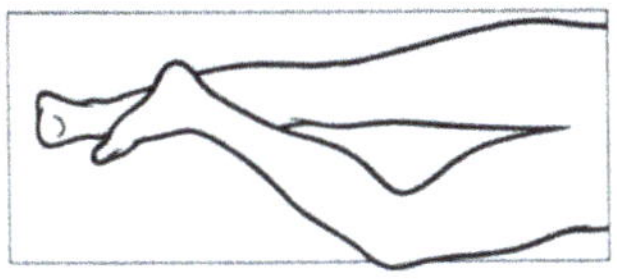

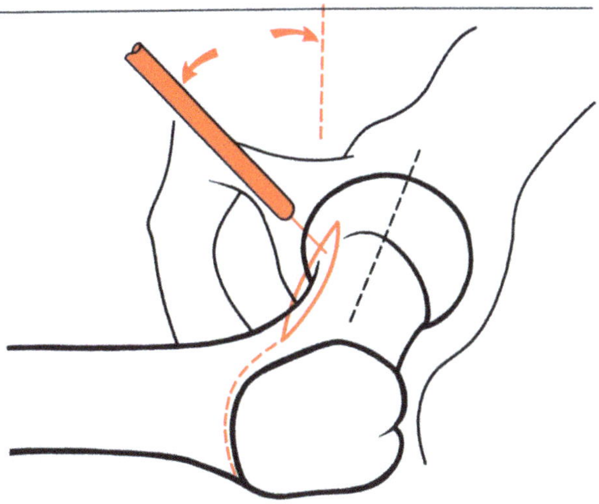

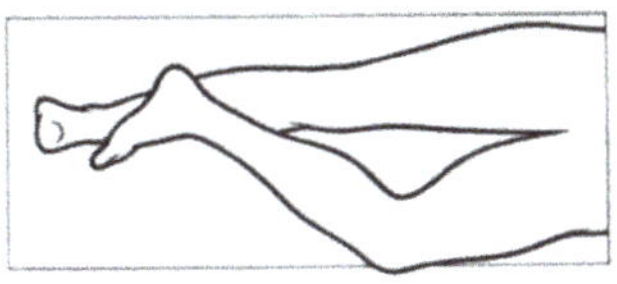

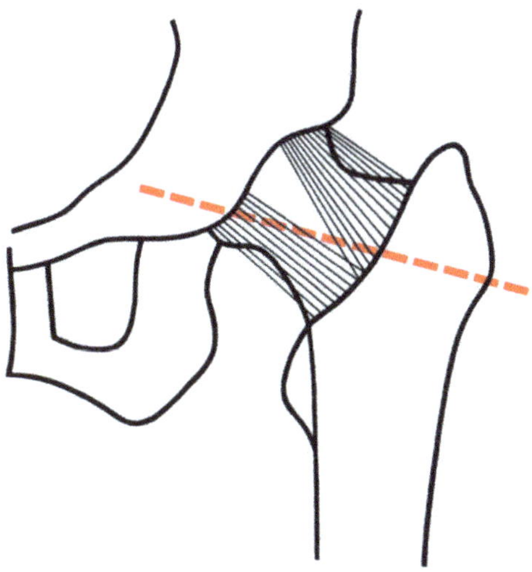

25

Incision in Capsule

The incision in the capsule joins the incision already made over the summit of the vastus lateralis ridge. Some muscle fibres of the vasti will be transected in the centre of the incision and are indicated diagrammatically here.

26

Cholecystectomy Forceps

It is important to see clearly the interior of the synovial cavity before inserting forceps. Some time spent doing this facilitates passage of the forceps and avoids passing outside the capsule.

27

Piercing Posterior Capsule

Thigh back to neutral to relax the superior capsule and make room for passage of the cholecystectomy forceps. The handles of the forceps are brought to the vertical. This procedure is greatly facilitated by the curved incision in the deep fascia lying anterior to the trochanter (6–18). If the hip is in fixed external rotation the direction of the cholecystectomy forceps may have to be inclined so that jaws emerge from the back of the joint more medially than is normally the case. This is a very important detail (see 28).

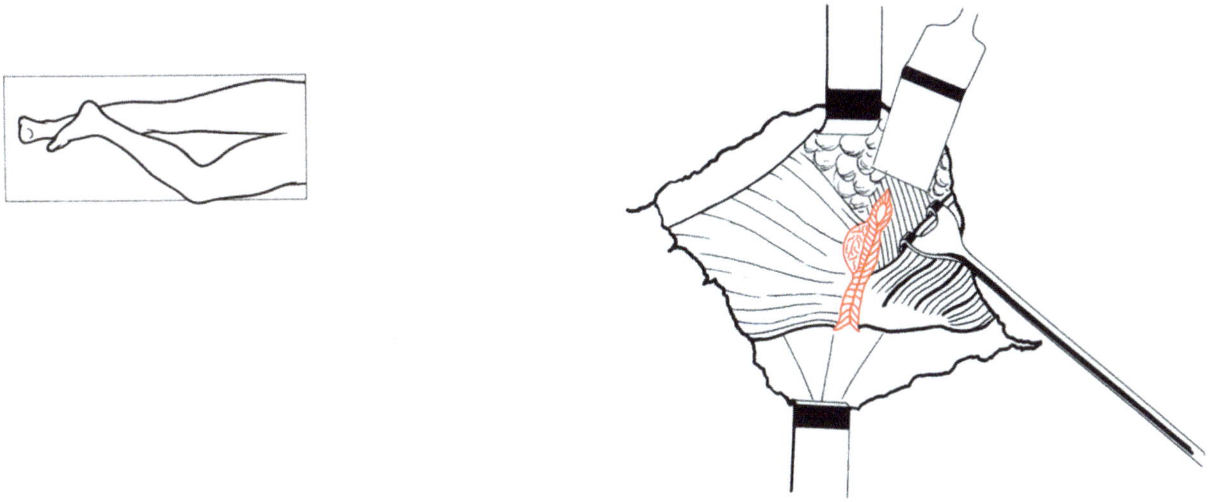

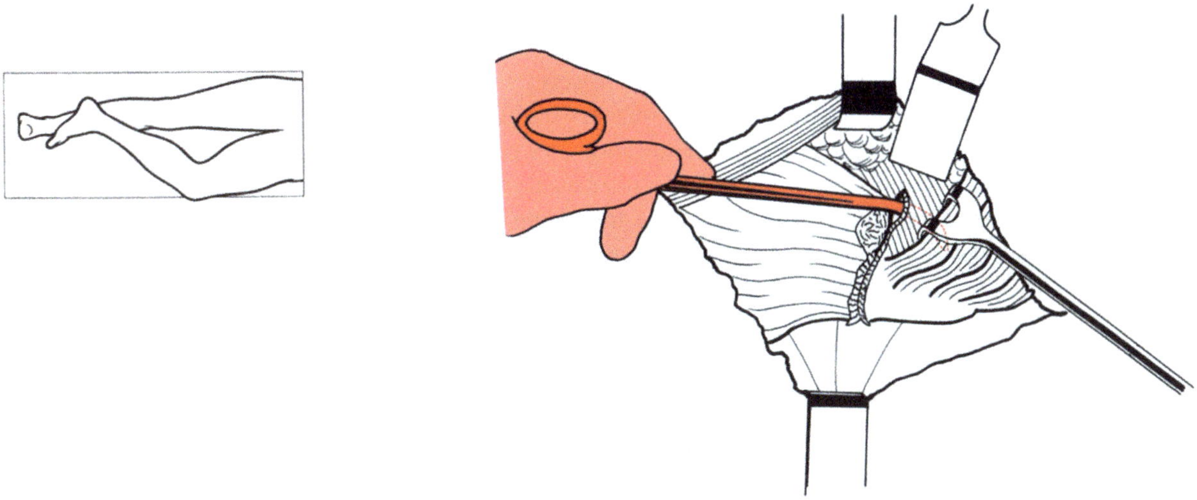

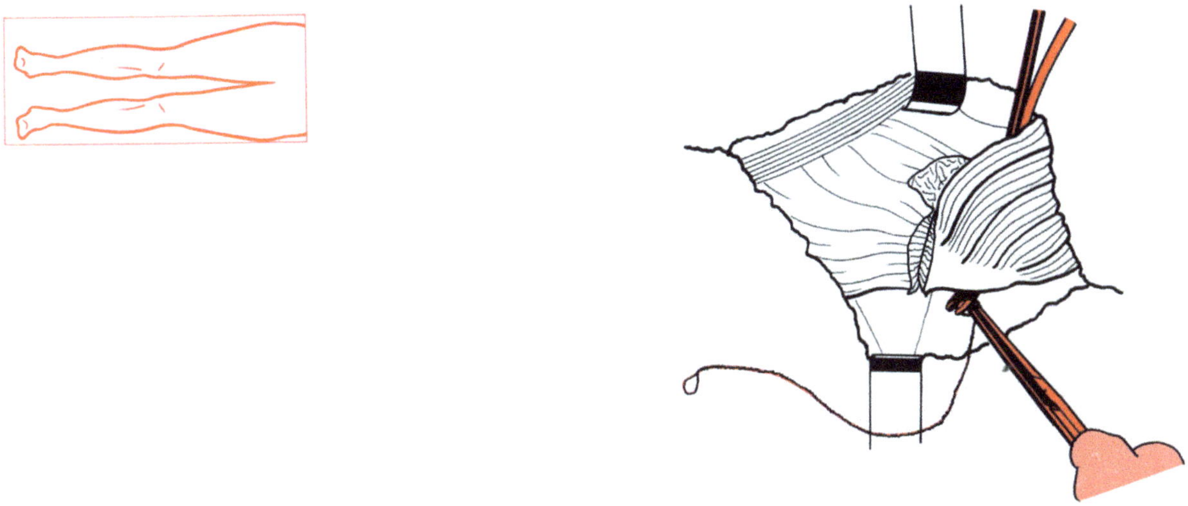

28

Tubercle on Trochanter

Adduction and internal rotation of the femur brings the trochanter to the surface of the wound and facilitates use of the saw. Even when the hip is in **fixed** external rotation to attempt this movement still helps (in this case by tilting the pelvis and allowing the buttock to fall away from the trochanter, so removing the pressure of the table). Palpate for the tubercle on the postero-superior surface of the trochanter and make sure that the Gigli saw lies deep to it. When the hip is in strong fixed external rotation the Gigli saw can be superficial to this tubercle unless special care is taken. The tip of the cholecystectomy forceps (29) also should be passed deep to this tubercle. Failure to observe this can result in detaching a very small trochanter causing difficulty in reattachment.

29

Cutting Trochanter

Note the small retractor to protect the skin-edge towels and to prevent bacterial contamination of the saw if these towels are cut. Operate the Gigli saw slowly. Watch the advance of the anterior and posterior ends alternately at each traction stroke. There is no need to watch the end not under traction. **Successful reattachment of a trochanter demands that the detached trochanter be of correct size and shape (neither too large nor too small)**. The Gigli saw should emerge through the middle of the vastus lateralis ridge: if it emerges above the ridge the trochanter will be too small; if it emerges below the ridge, the femoral prosthesis will project above the cut surface of the femur and make the staple-clamp (if used) more difficult to site.

30

Haemostasis

The femur is adducted. Retract the trochanter with a hook. There are only four important sites of bleeding: (*1*) The digital fossa of the femur. (*2*) A branch of the posterior circumflex artery on the posterior margin of the detached trochanter. (*3*) A branch of the anterior circumflex artery on antero-lateral edge of the femur. (*4*) A branch of the anterior circumflex artery halfway along anterior edge of the femur.

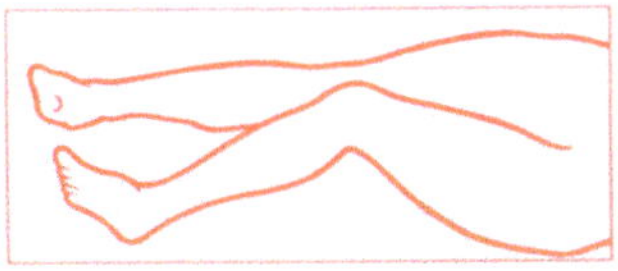

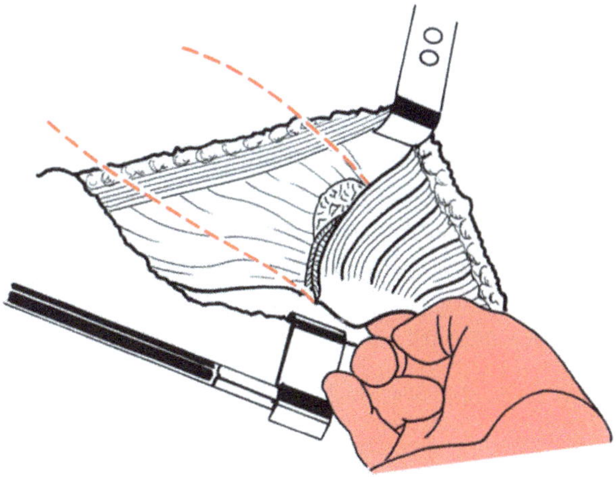

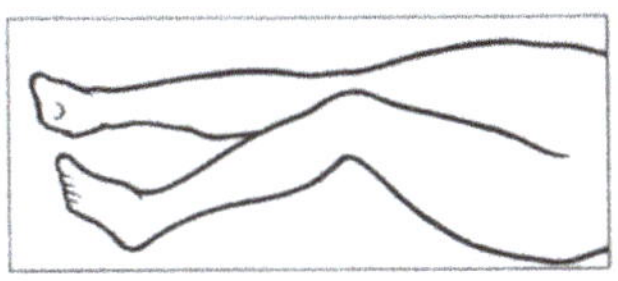

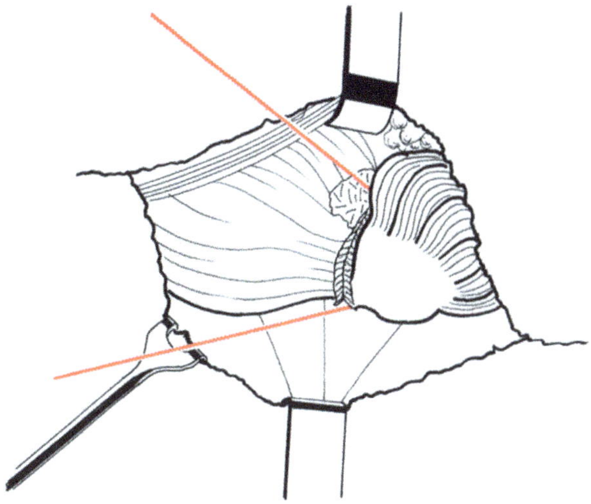

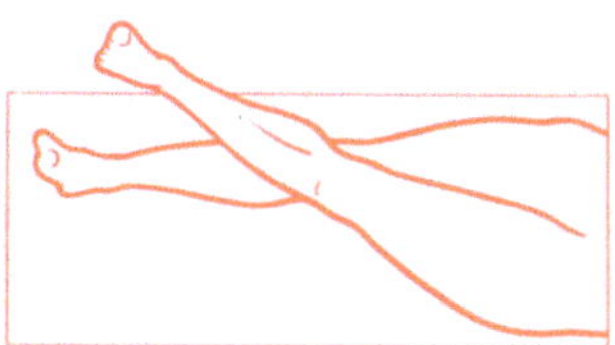

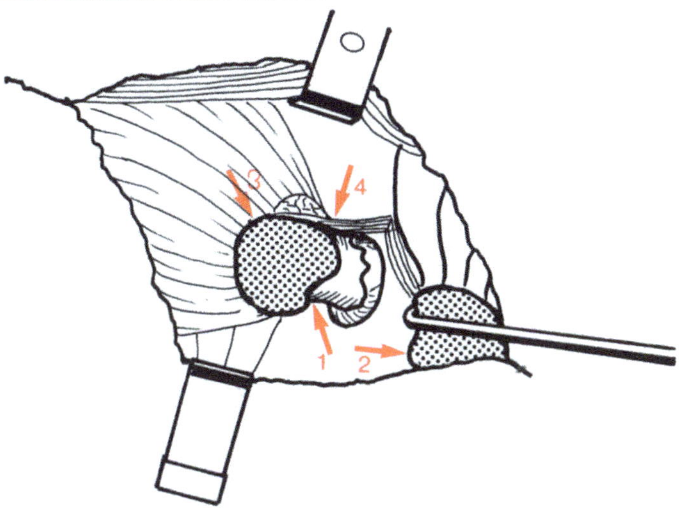
3
4
1
2

31

Division of Glenoid Labrum

The femur is adducted. Divide the glenoid labrum at 5 o'clock position for left hip and 7 o'clock for right. Division of the external rotators is **no longer advised as routine**; it can release the trochanter too much. It is never needed in rheumatoid arthritis or in post-traumatic arthritis. Medial displacement of the shaft of the femur (the combination of deepening the acetabulum and the 40-mm offset prosthesis) usually permits the trochanter to rotate forwards into a good position even if the posterior attachments are short.

32

Start of Dislocation

The femur is adducted. A Watson-Jones gouge, useful for its long leverage, is inserted between the capsule and the femoral head to assist dislocation if dislocation is not spontaneous on adduction. External rotation of the femur must be avoided before the head of the femur is well out of the acetabulum. Forced external rotation can cause spiral fractures of the femur, especially if weakened by screws (as in secondary surgery after femoral osteotomy). Detachment of the trochanter in the lateral exposure permits dislocation by pure adduction. A tubular bone is very strong against the bending forces of adduction, but it is not strong against the torsion forces of external rotation.

33

Serrated and Angulated Femur Lever

The femur is in strong adduction with the foot over the opposite side of the table. This simple lever is essential in several applications: (1) to complete the exposure of the upper end of the femur, (2) throughout the later stages of reaming the medullary cavity and (3) reattaching the trochanter (**see** Appendix C). In this diagram the serrated and angulated femur lever is about to be inserted behind the upper end of the femur to depress the fascia lata and to elevate the femur out of the wound.

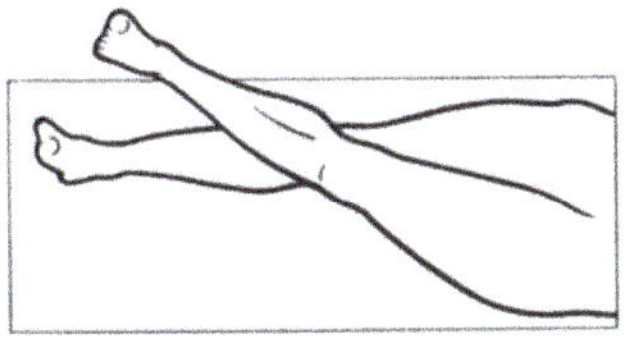

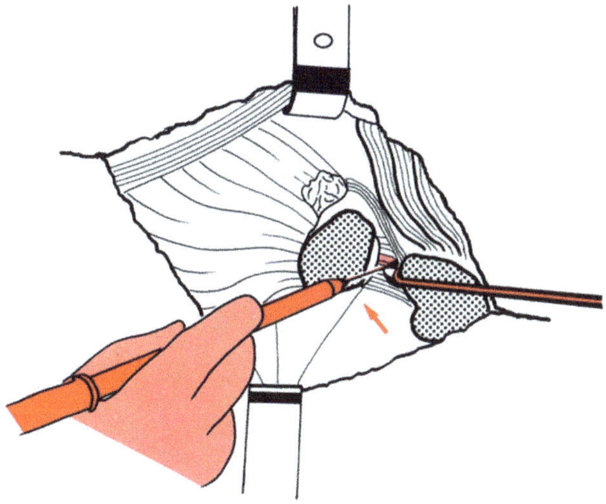

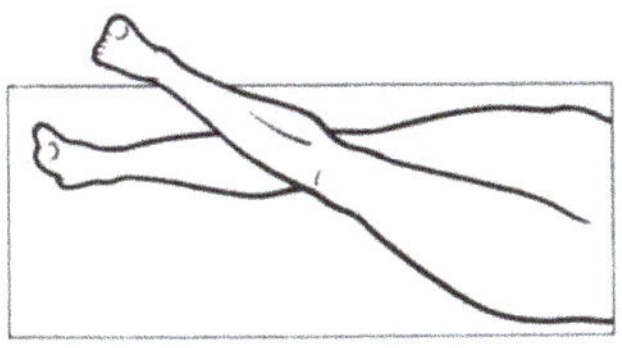

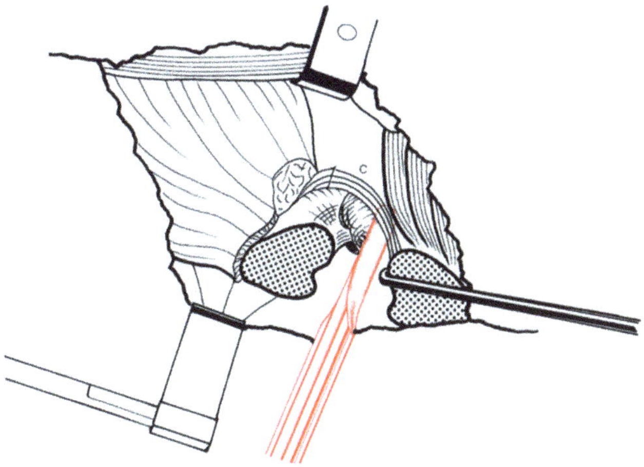

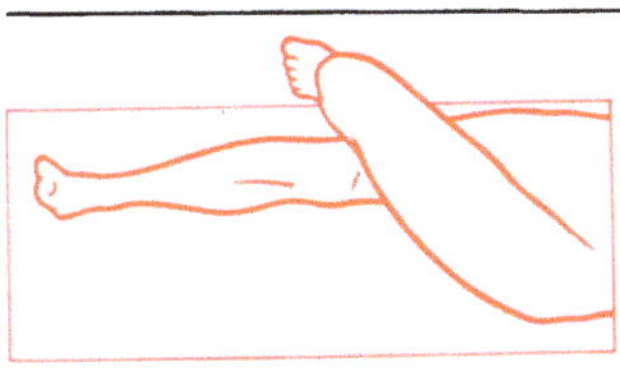

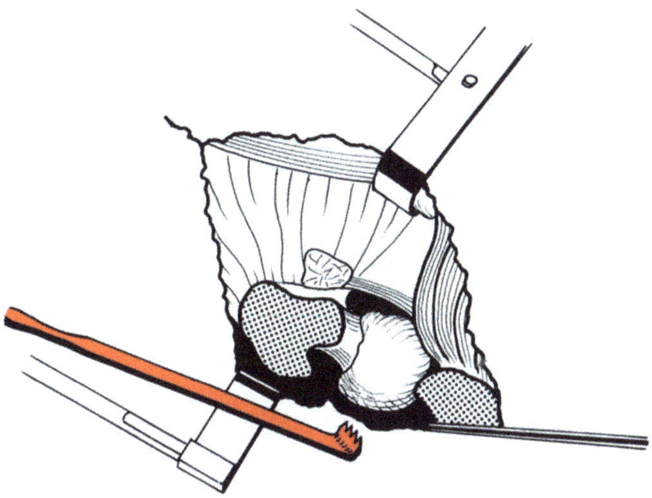

34

Resection of Femoral Head

Serrated and angulated femur lever is in position. The femur is adducted to become almost transverse to the operating table. The Gigli saw is in position round the neck of the femur.

35

Sagittal Plane of Femur

This diagram shows how the sagittal plane of the femur can be recognized as the same plane which contains the tibia when the knee is flexed. The assistant on the opposite side of the table holds the tibia vertical, with the knee flexed at 90°, to help the surgeon to estimate this plane. The neck of femur should be transected without anteversion. When the neck of the femur is anteverted or retroverted in the pre-operative condition, the plane of section should ignore the axis of the neck and relate only to the sagittal plane of the femur. This diagram shows how the plane of section of the neck without anteversion is about 45° to the sagittal plane of the femur.

36

Resection of Head

The femur is in strong adduction; the serrated and angulated femur lever is in position. The plane of the Gigli saw is vertical irrespective of the axis of the neck. The assistant presses on the head with a swab to resist the pull of the saw. Without this sometimes the pull of the saw can avulse the pubo-femoral ligament, especially in osteoporotic conditions.

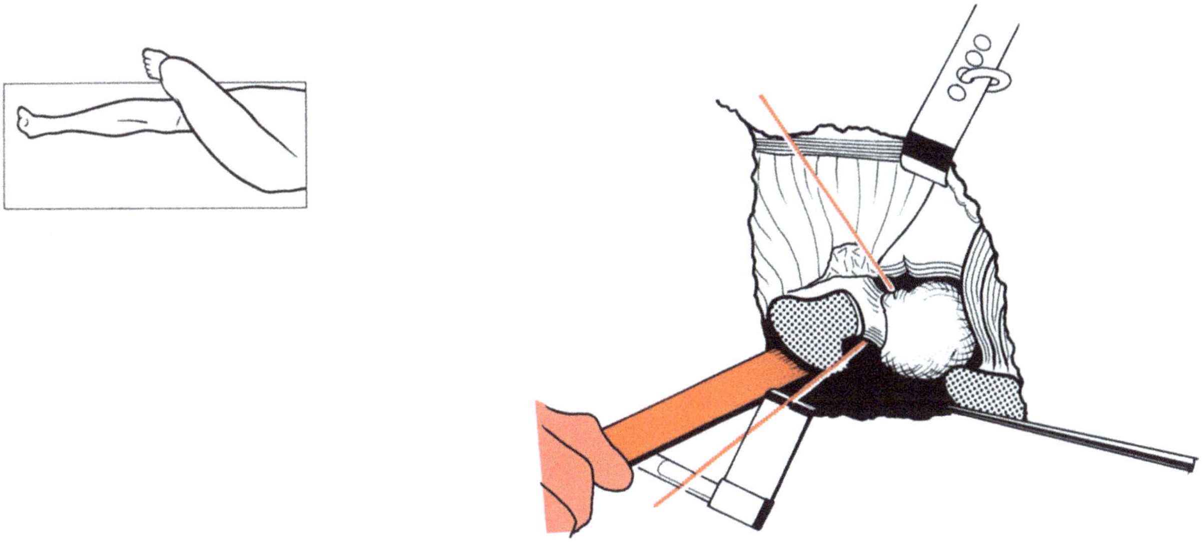

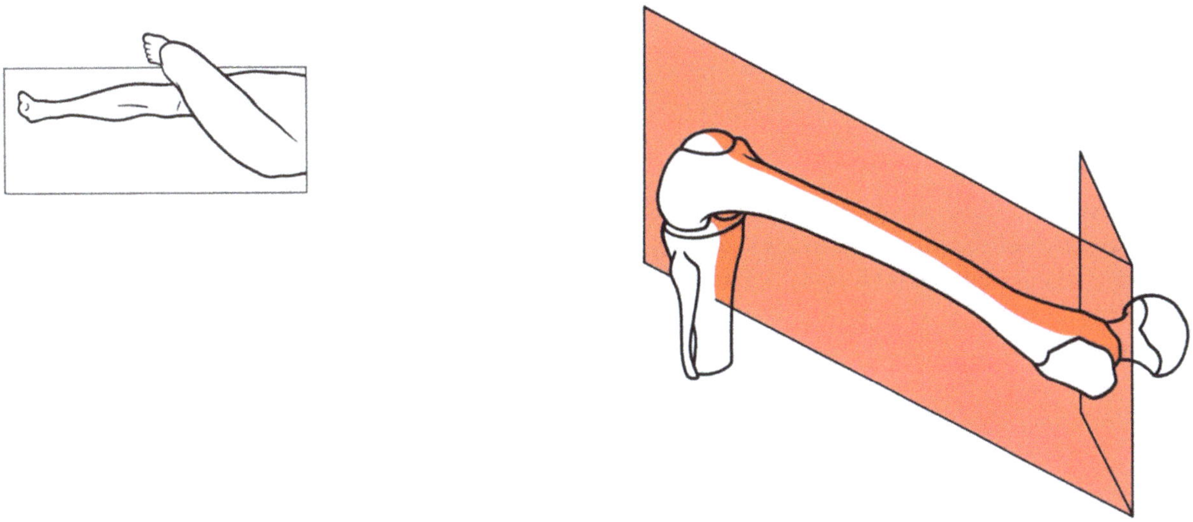

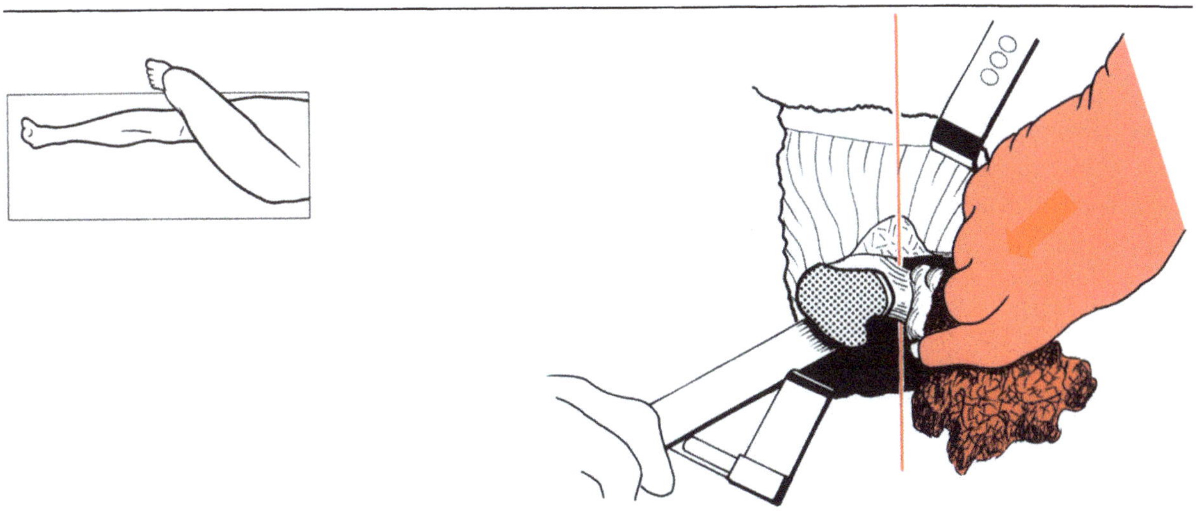

37

Geometry of Head and Neck of Femur

The line *X Y* is transverse to the long axis of the femur at the level of the vastus lateralis ridge. (**see** p. 139: the datum for lowest part of neck of femoral prosthesis is about 1 cm headwards of *X Y*.) Inspect to confirm that the saw is starting on the medial femoral neck at the same level as the vastus lateralis ridge. The saw is made to emerge at *Z*, with about 1.0 cm of cortex separating it from the cut surface of the trochanter. Too much cortex at this point is better than too little; it can always be cut back later.

38

Head of Femur Resected

The femur is in strong adduction. Note the bridge of cortex of the femoral neck. Note also that **no capsulectomy is performed in this operation**. The femur is tethered to the pelvis by the pubo-femoral ligament. The capsule is not usually seen as clearly as in this diagram but it is always there. The pubo-femoral ligament can always be demonstrated but the headward part of the anterior capsule has been stretched by the cholecystectomy forceps and is out of sight. To achieve exposure by resecting the anterior capsule is a frequent source of post-operative haematoma because of the vascular nature of the capsule.

39

Horizontal Retractor

The femur is in strong adduction. The horizontal retractor carries L-shaped jaws each with two spikes. The jaws can be turned up or down according to the situation (**see** Appendix C). The distal jaw engages one spike inside the cut surface of the femoral neck.

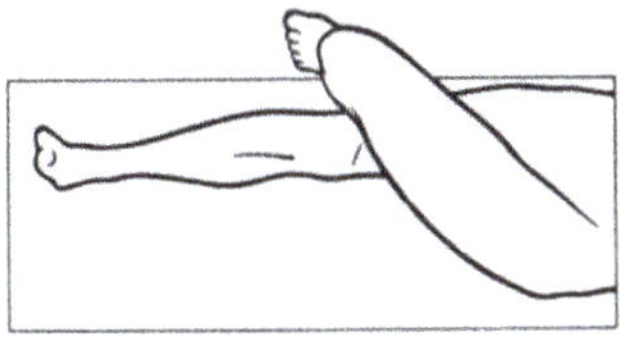

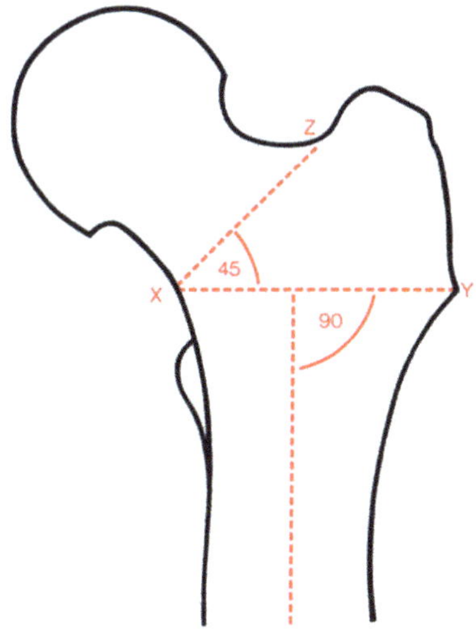
Z
45
X
Y
90

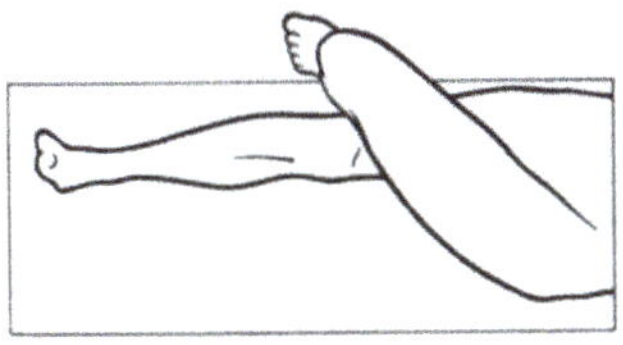

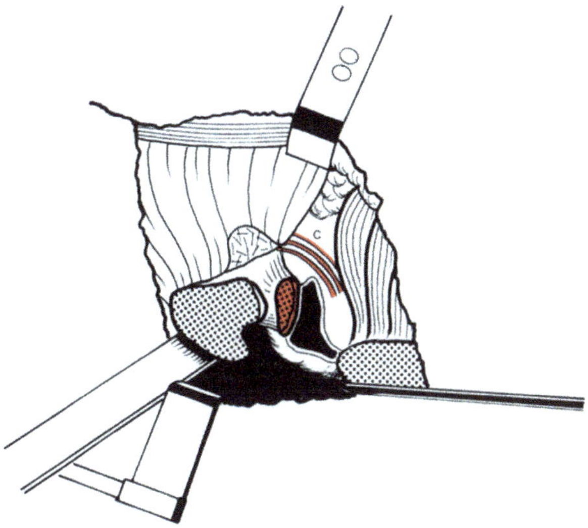
C

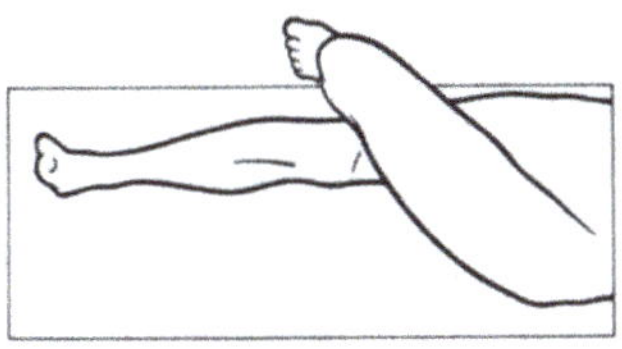

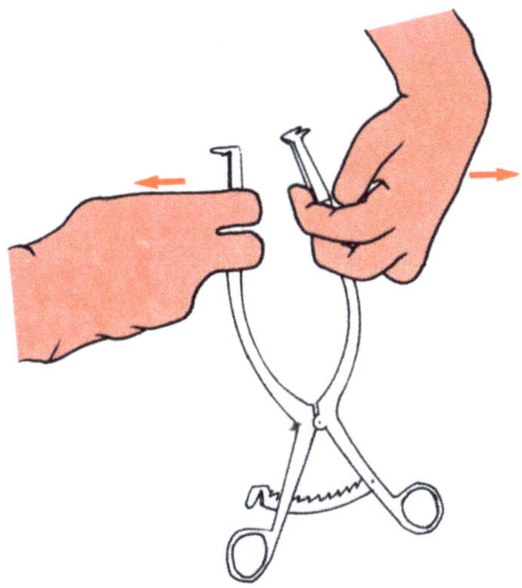

40

Horizontal Retractor

The two spikes in the headward jaw are placed **to straddle the upper edge of the trochanter**. This is not well shown in all diagrams and the present diagram is to illustrate this important detail. Jaws can be turned down (*a*) or turned up (*b*). The **posterior spike is in the capsular tissue above the trochanter**; the anterior spike enters the cancellous bone of the cut surface of the trochanter.

41

Full Retraction: The Screw-Jack

The surgeon cannot exert sufficient force on the handles of this retractor to achieve full distraction. The screw-jack is essential. This has a rapid-action screw; and is 'jacked' open in 90° turns by using Kocher's forceps in the holes of the drum (see Appendix C).

42

Division of Glenoid Labrum

The glenoid labrum is divided down to the bone of the rim of the acetabulum in the 5 o'clock or 7 o'clock position, as before.

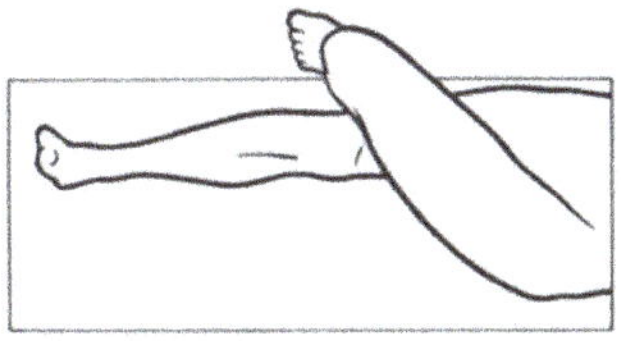

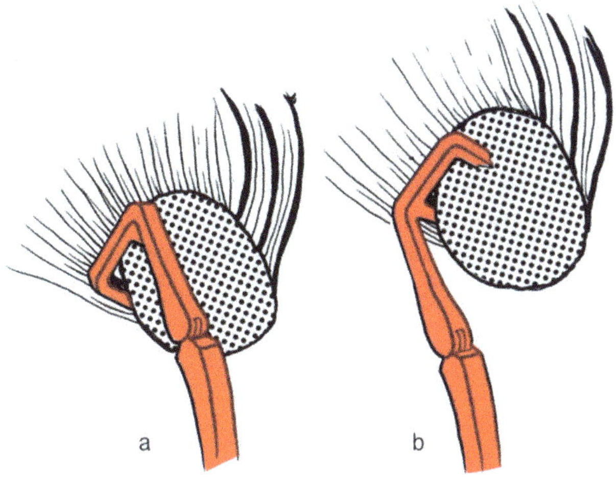
a
b

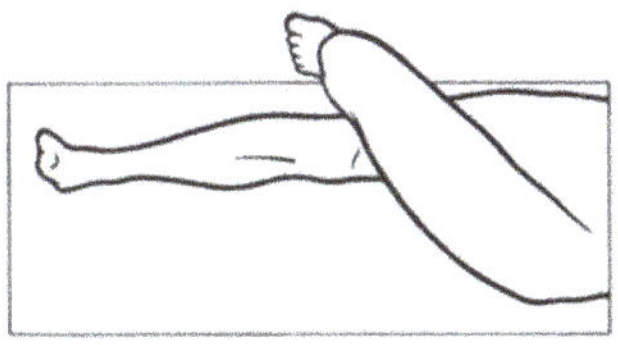

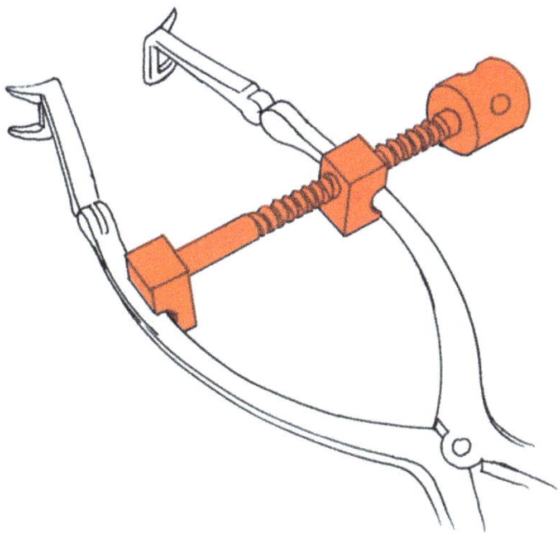

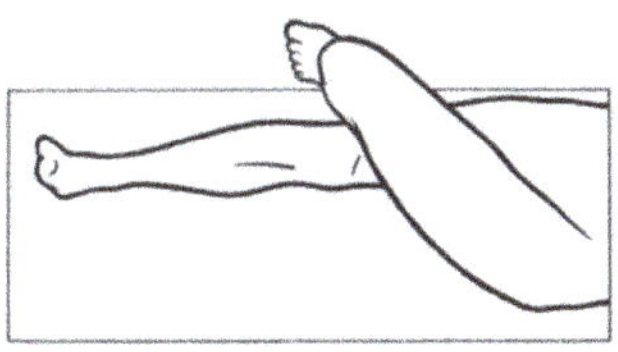

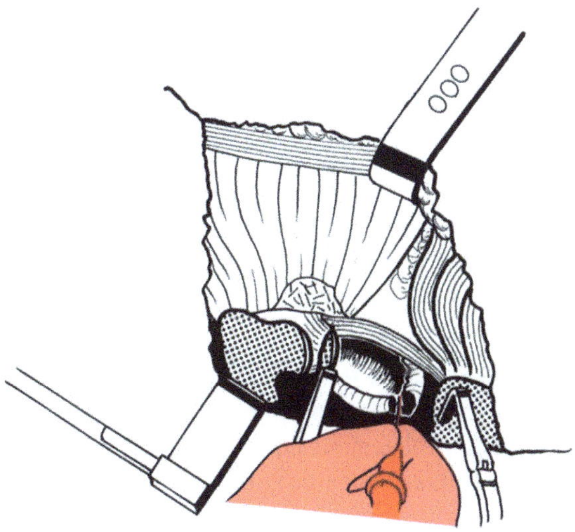

43

Nail Retractor

First position. The nail retractor is used to expose the superior lip of the acetabulum. It is imperative that the superior lip of the acetabulum should be made clearly visible (**see** Appendix C). Usually one nail is sufficient but two can be used if desired. The chain prevents the nail or nails being accidentally left in the wound. The nail is introduced under the glenoid labrum in a headward direction, at the 2 o'clock position for left hip and the 10 o'clock for the right hip.

44

Nail Retractor

Final position. The nail is levered, bit by bit, to the transverse position. To reach the transverse position the nail must be drawn back in steps, because in the first position the point of the nail is usually too high on the ilium. The next diagram explains this.

45

Mechanics of Nail Retractor

In position (*1*) the nail is directed too much in the headward direction: the leverage is disadvantageous and the nail will bend if strained too far. (*2*) The nail is withdrawn a little and again an attempt is made to lever in a headward direction. The leverage is still insufficient to stretch the tissues to reach the transverse position without bending the nail. (*3*) The nail is withdrawn yet again and now it can be levered to the transverse position. It is essential to reach the transverse position because otherwise the nail will obstruct access to the acetabulum. **The key to exposure of the acetabulum lies in upward retraction of the trochanter, NOT in downward mobilisation of the femur**. The pubo-femoral ligament holding the femur to the pelvis never need be cut in a primary intervention.

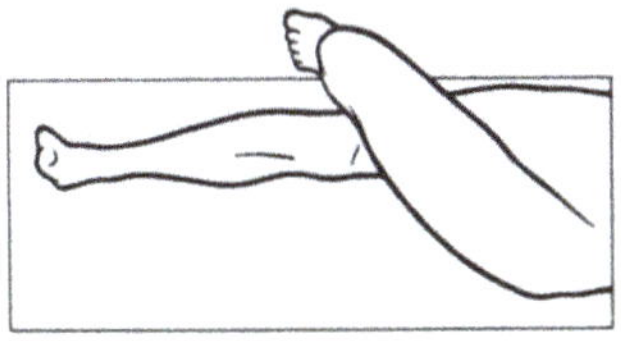

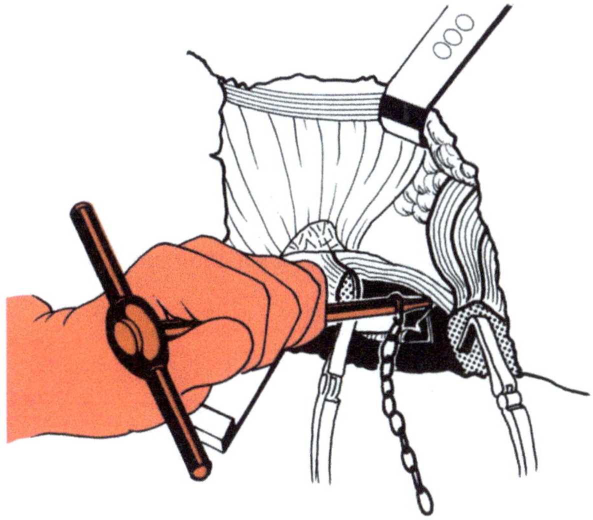

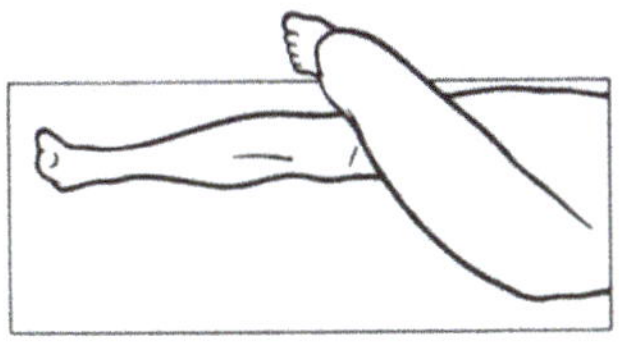

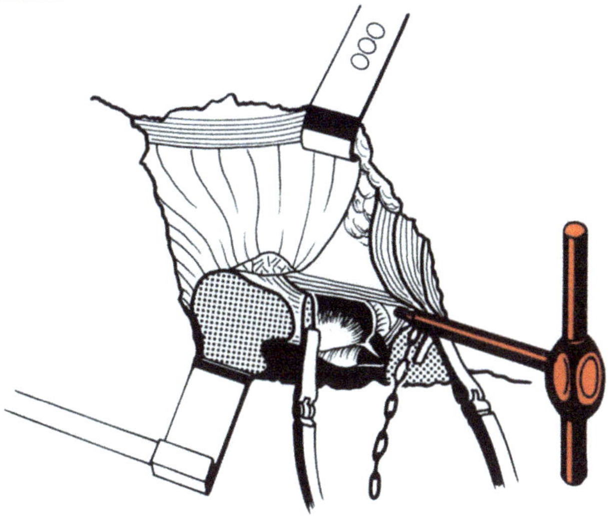

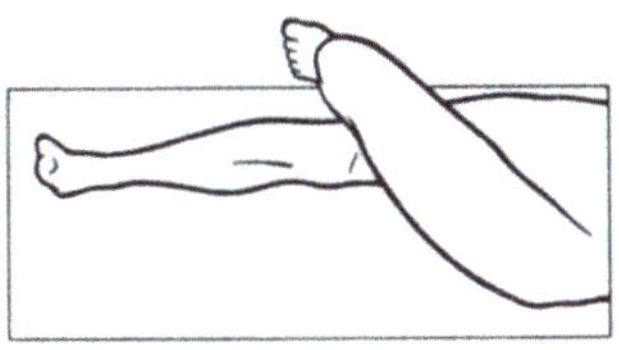

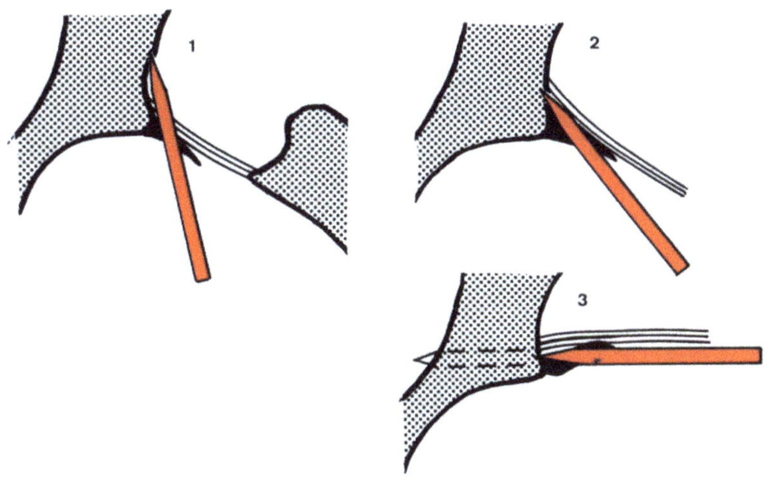
1
2
3

46

Nail Retractor

The holder is detached. The nail retractor should be driven to full depth so that it does not obstruct access to the acetabulum. When extracting these nails, note that the bayonet catch on the holder permits the nail to be oscillated in clockwise-anticlockwise rotation. If traction is maintained on the holder while oscillating the holder clockwise-anticlockwise this makes extraction much quicker than rotating in one direction while applying traction.

47

Hohman Retractors

The anterior and posterior lips of the acetabulum are exposed with Hohman retractors, which take a purchase on bone and reveal the acetabulum perfectly.

48

Self-Retaining Anterior Hohman Retractor

The handle of the anterior Hohman retractor is bent 45° away from the working surface to be out of the surgeon's way (**see** Appendix C). A short length of chain with a hook can be hitched over the finger-guard on the initial retractor to make a self-retaining arrangement.

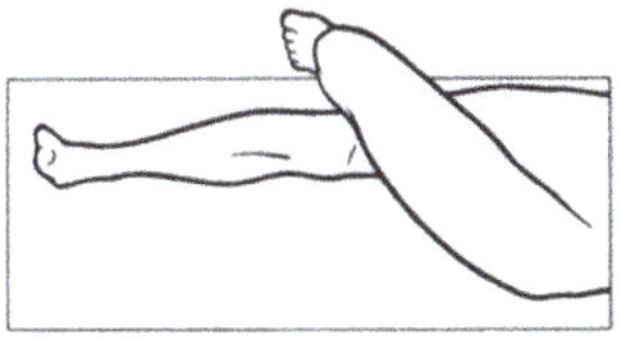

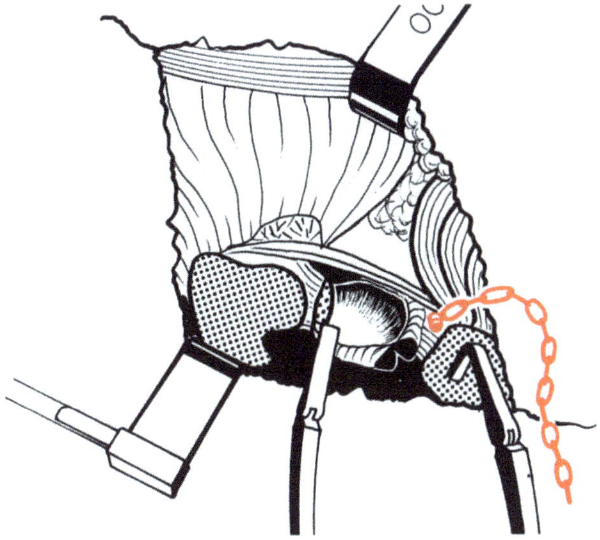

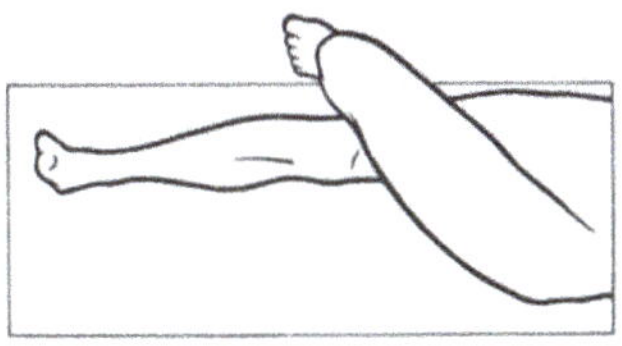

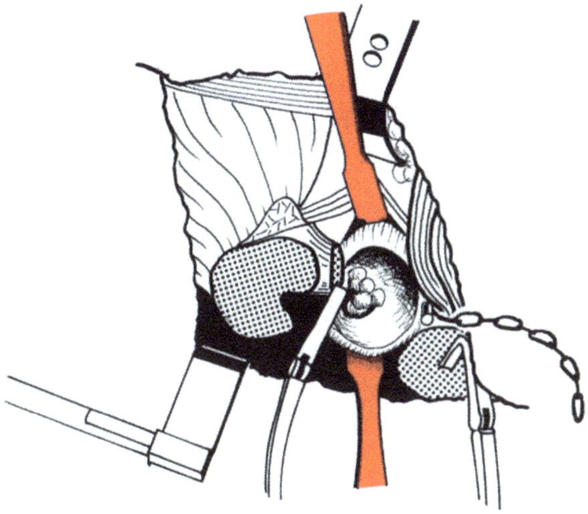

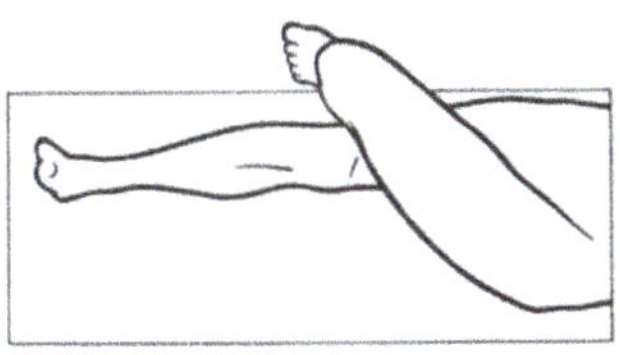

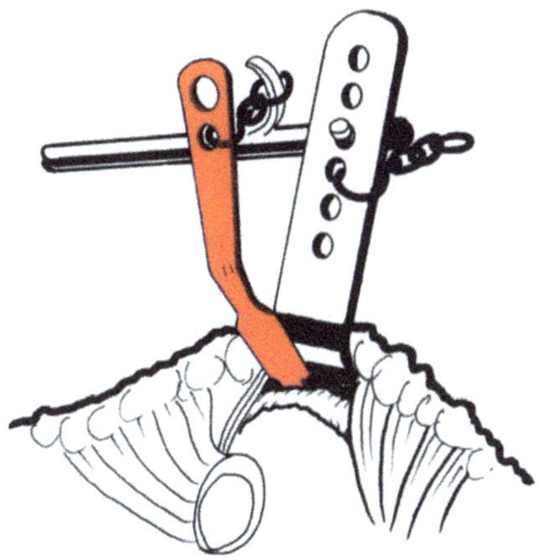

49

Excising Ligamentum Teres

The floor of the acetabular fossa is the key to the deepening of the acetabulum. '**Deepening by eye**' is now preferred to deepening by palpating the thickness of the floor through the pilot hole. When the acetabulum contains a ligamentum teres it can be excised with the diathermy neadle at this stage to reveal the floor of the acetabular fossa. Equally well the pilot drill can be inserted into ligamentum teres without excising it.

50

Normal Acetabular Fossa

After removal of the ligamentum teres the surface of the cortical bone (*A*) in the floor of the acetabular fossa is revealed.

51

Buried Acetabular Fossa

In advanced osteoarthrosis no acetabular fossa and no ligamentum teres is visible. In these cases the floor of the acetabulum is merely a smooth hemispherical surface. The buried acetabular fossa in osteoarthrosis is the result of osteophytes growing away from the edges of the acetabular fossa and fusing together (*c*). It is not generally realized that the acetabular fossa is still present, containing relics of the original ligamentum teres, but roofed over by new bone (*d*).

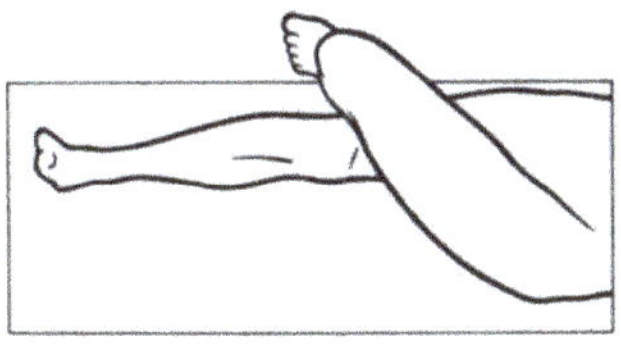

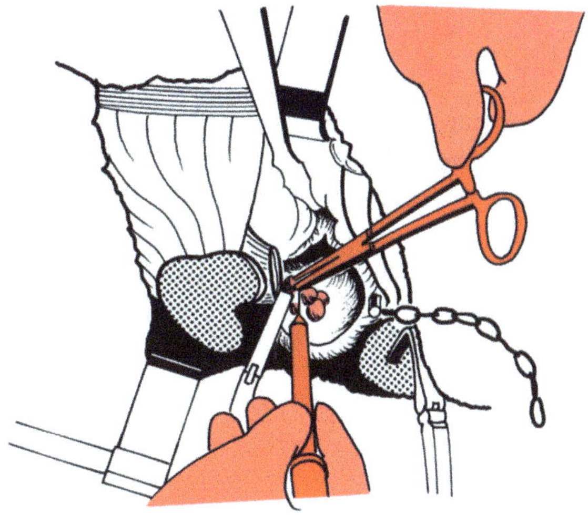

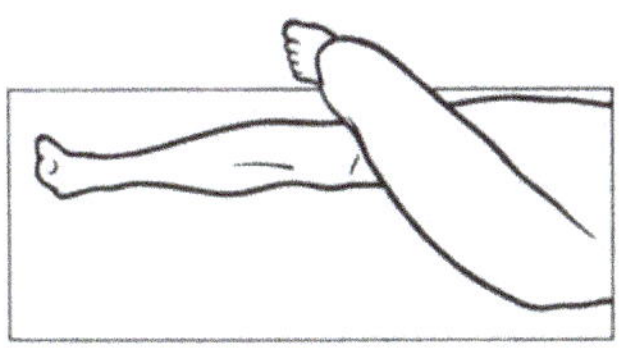

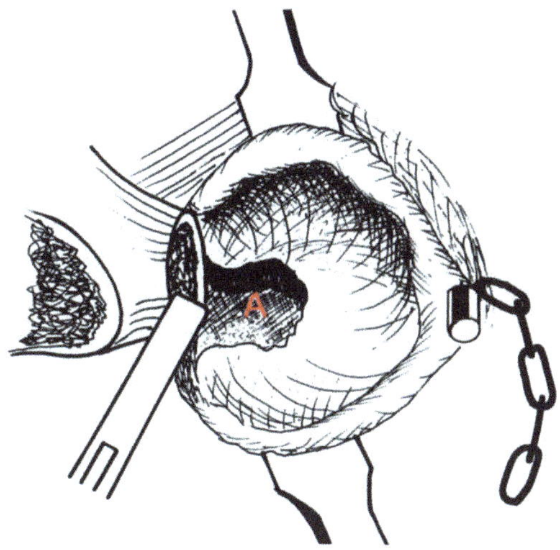
A

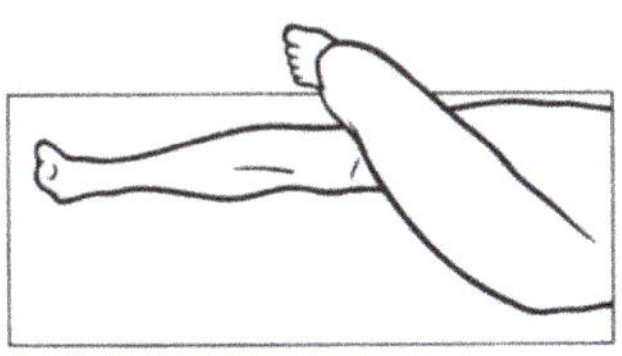

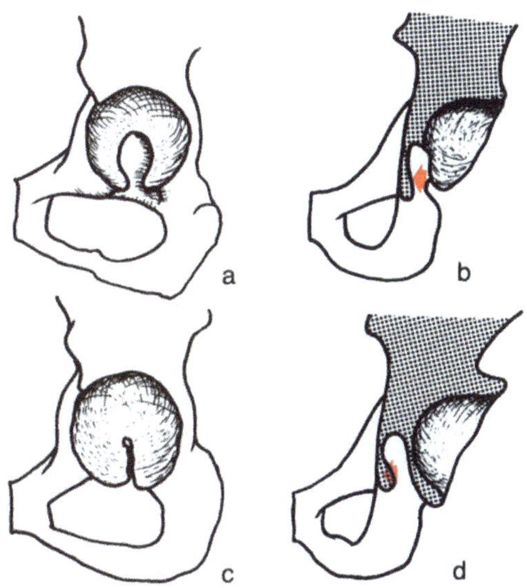
a
b
c
d

52

Centring Ring

When the acetabular fossa is not visible, as a result of being roofed over by new bone, the centring ring used with the pilot drill will find the true centre of the acetabulum. The centring ring must be pressed to the floor of the acetabulum to find the correct centre.

53

Tranverse Drilling of Pilot Hole

(*a*) Normal and (*b*) adducted hip. The line joining the antero-superior iliac spines determines the transverse direction of the pilot drill and of all subsequent reaming tools. The tilt of the pelvis in Fig. 2 is exaggerated and is greater than anything likely to be encountered in practice. There is much less subtlety, and more latitude for error, in assessing the transverse lie of the pelvis than newcomers to this operation tend to think. Pelvic tilt has to be very marked to require that the pilot drill and reamers be operated other than transverse to the operating table.

54

Lateral Tilt of Pelvis

When the lower extremity is strongly adducted over the opposite side of the table the pelvis tends to be tilted away from the surgeon. The pilot drill therefore should be elevated about 10° above the horizontal.

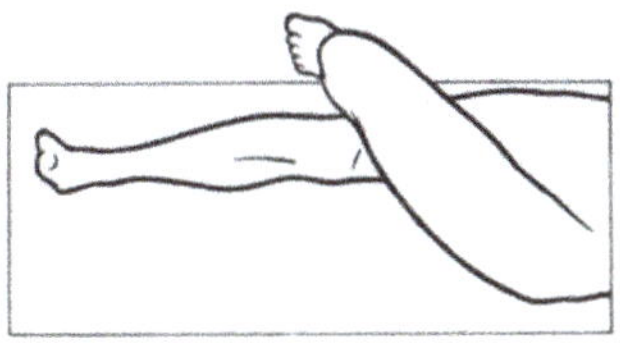

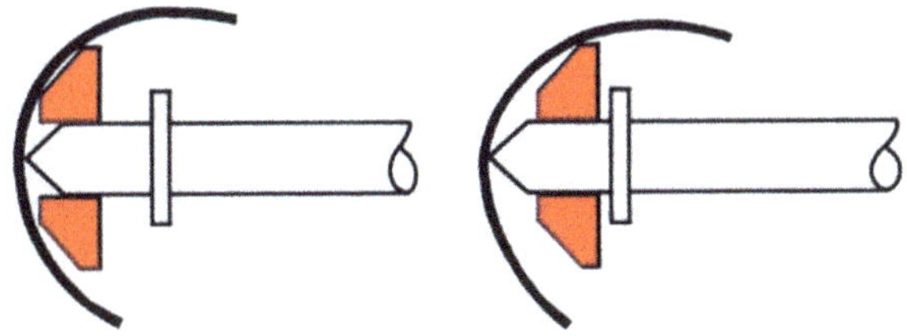

Time: 12 min

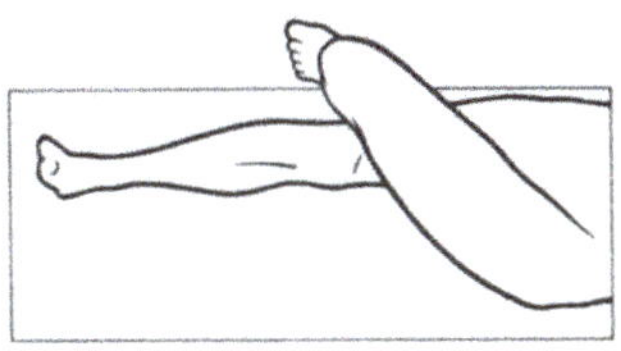

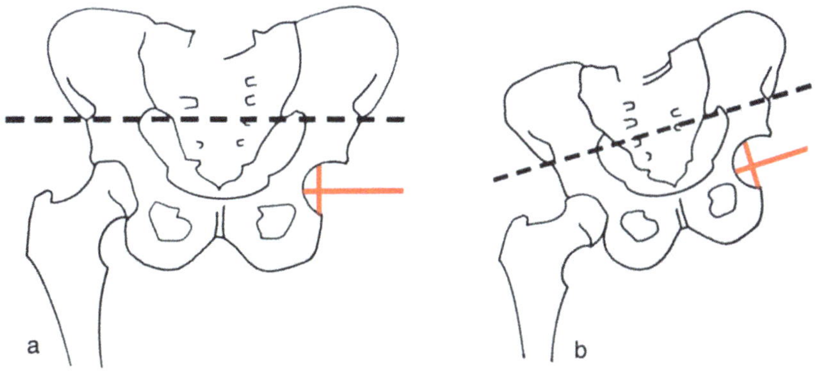

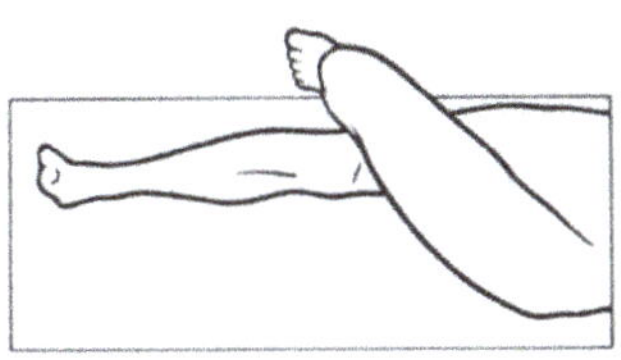

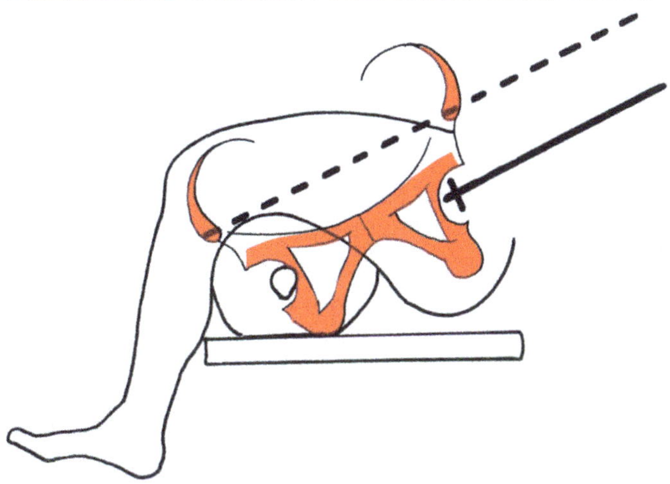

55

Deepening Acetabulum — Large Acetabulum — Thick Floor

In this case the siting of the pilot hole is important. Inclining the pilot drill in a headward direction, followed by deepening in the same direction, will place the centre of the socket too high (*a* and *b*).

The transverse direction of the pilot drill, followed by transverse deepening, will keep the centre of the socket at the anatomical ('low') level (*c* and *d*).

56

Centring Ring and Pilot Drill

The **site of the pilot hole** in the floor of the acetabulum **determines the level of the socket**. This can be decided pre-operatively. The pilot hole, 12.5-mm diameter, permits palpation of the thickness of the floor. When cutting against eburnated bone, the large-diameter spigot of the expanding reamer does not break the hole in the floor of the acetabulum in a distal direction, as would happen with a narrow spigot. In this diagram the centring drill, with the centring ring, is being withdrawn, It demonstrates how the pilot hole lies at the top of the acetabular fossa.

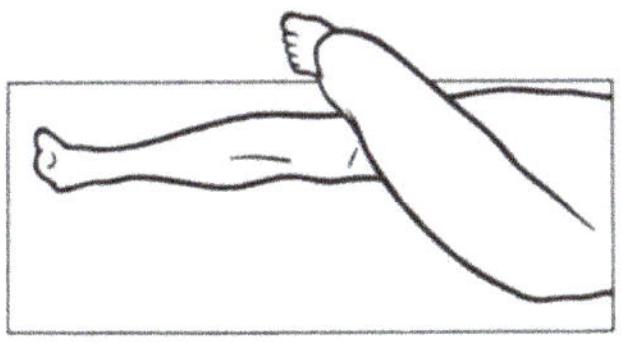

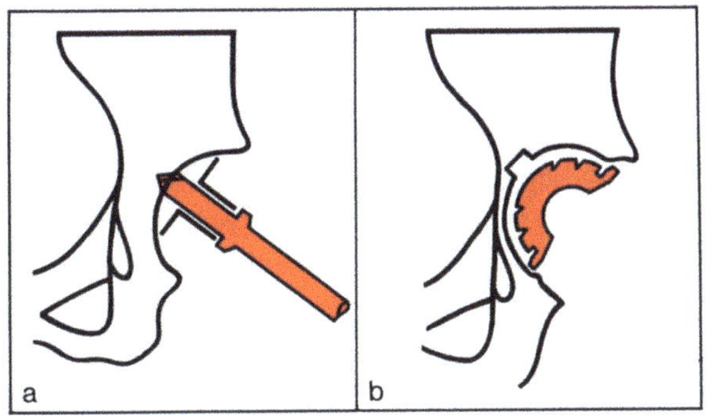
a
b

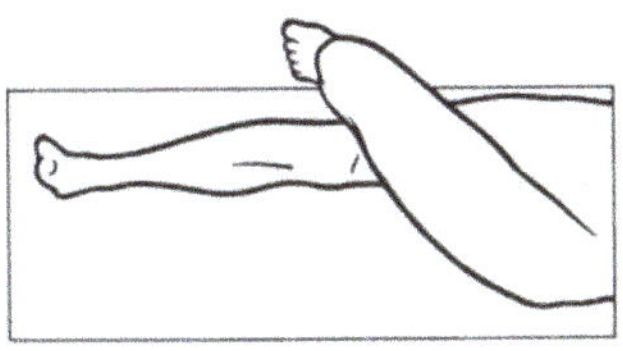

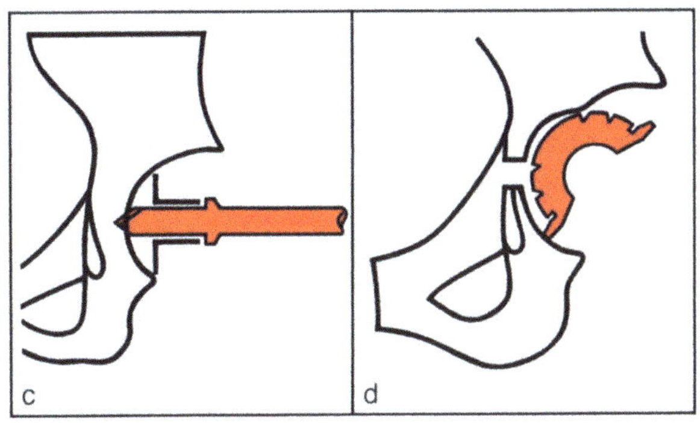
c
d

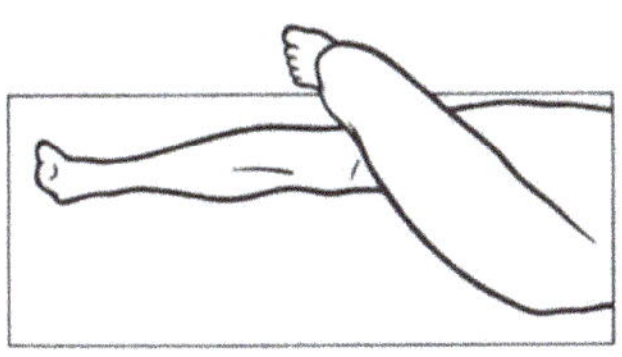

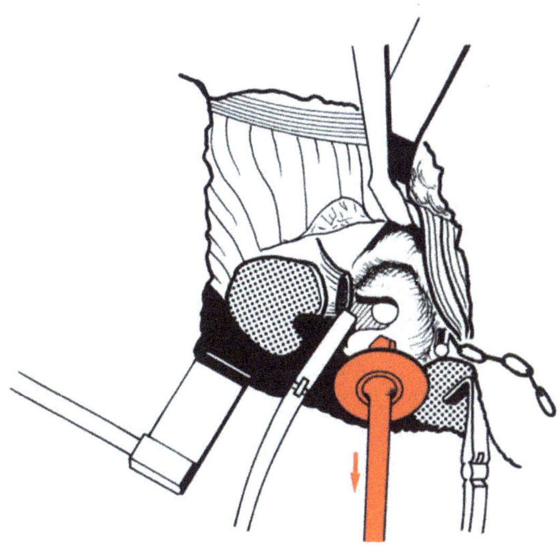

57

Unroofing Buried Acetabular Fossa

(*a*) The pilot hole has been made using the transverse drill and the centring ring as above. (*b*) The two-handed Volkmann spoon (see Appendix C) is inserted; directed towards the patient's feet and the roof broken out. This process should be continued till all the overhanging osteophytes have been removed and the acetabular fossa is fully demonstrated as far down as site of original acetabular notch.

58

First Insertion of Deepening Reamer

The first insertion of the deepening reamer merely skims the bottom of the acetabulum without removing much bone. If access is cramped do not forget to make extra turns, at this stage, on the screw-jack (stage 41).

59

Result of First Deepening

This is merely a skimming of the floor of the acetabulum.

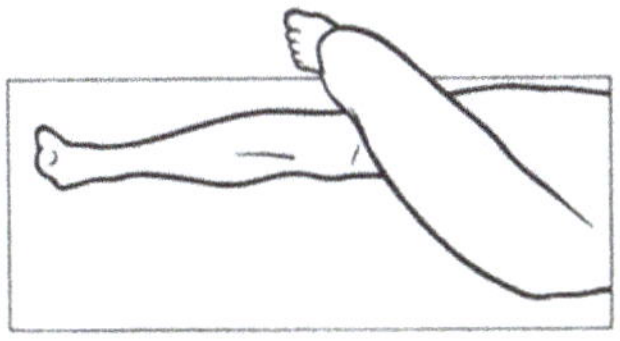

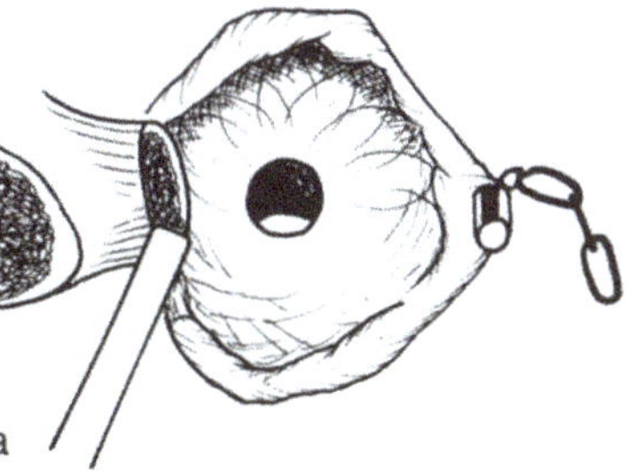

a

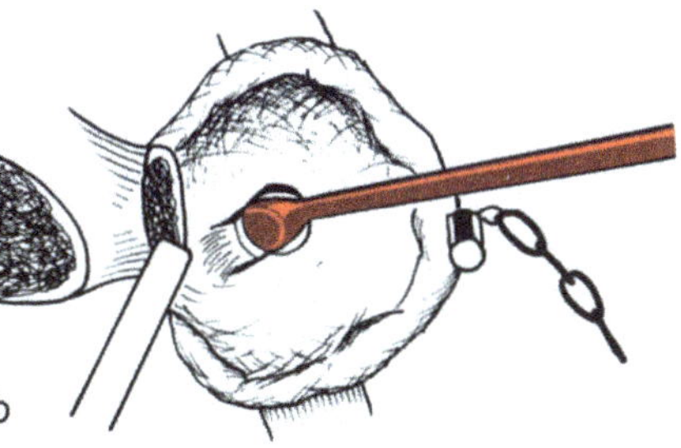

b

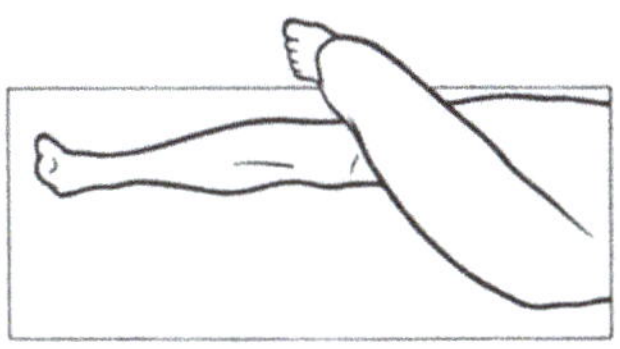

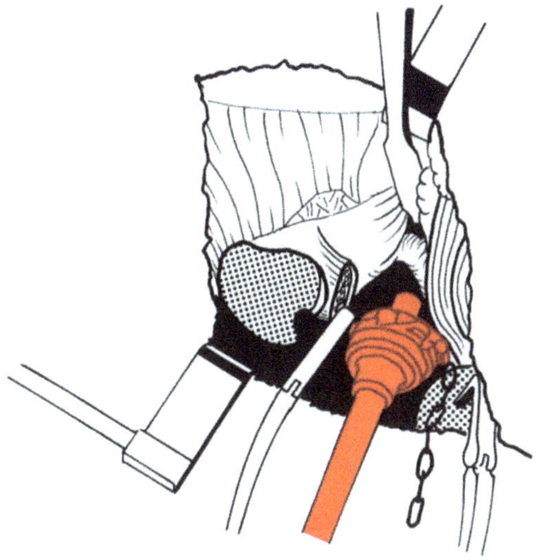

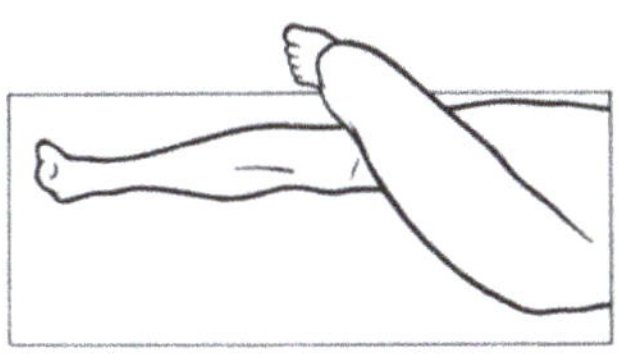

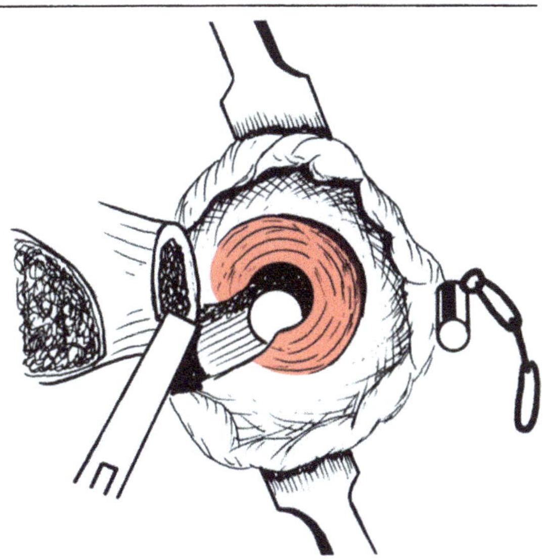

60

First Insertion of Expanding Reamer

Once again do not forget extra turns on the screw-jack if access is at all cramped.

61

Result of First Insertion of Expanding Reamer

The mouth of the acetabulum is reamed to size; the cutters work superficially because the floor has not yet been fully deepened. If the acetabulum is small, the small socket size-gauge is used to test its size and the expanding reamer is opened only as far as the small socket size-gauge indicates.

62

Final Deepening

The acetabulum is deepened until the reamed cancellous surface is level with the cortical surface of the floor of the acetabular fossa (the lateral surface of the tear drop). The tip of the index finger can be used to check the thickness of the walls of the pilot hole if there is any doubt. Two to six insertions of the deepening reamer may be needed to reach the desired depth if proceeding cautiously.

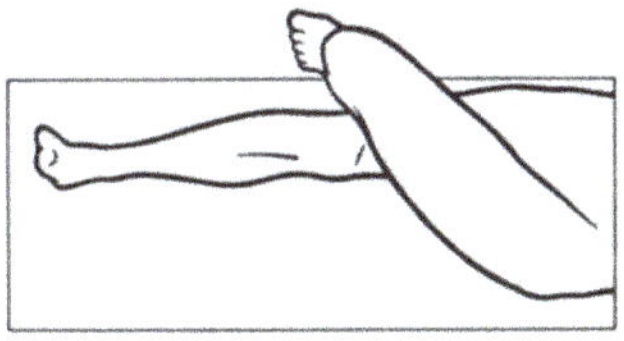

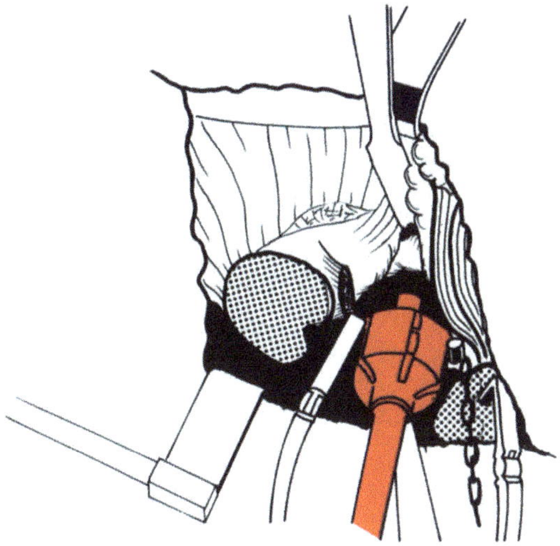

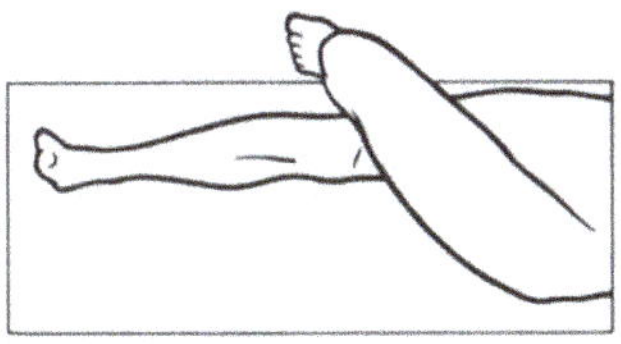

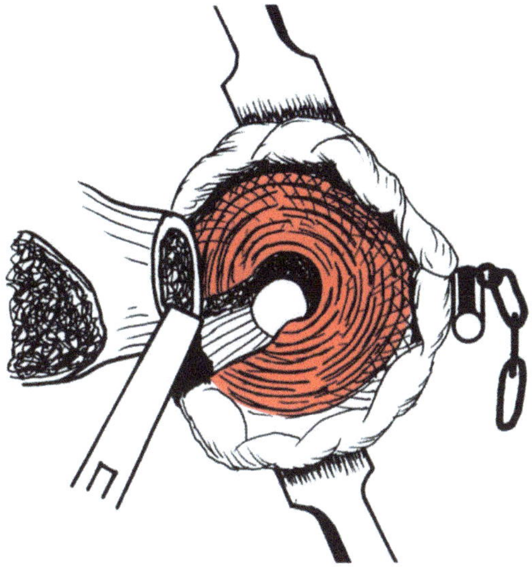

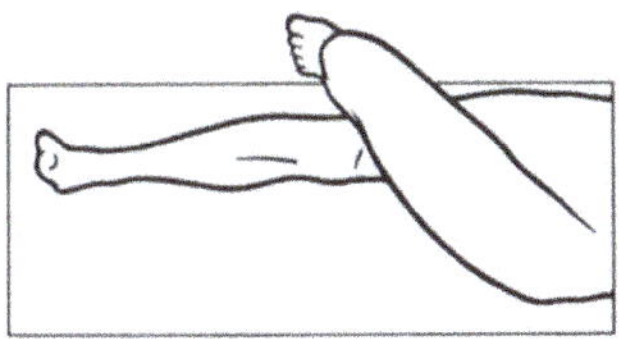

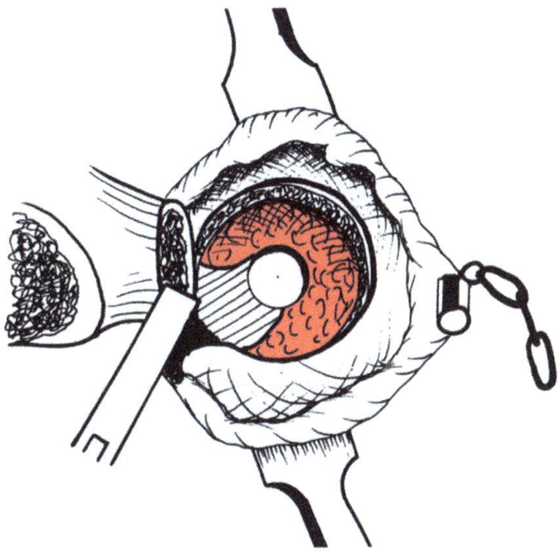

63

Result of Final Insertion of Expanding Reamer

If the socket size-gauge indicates the need for a small socket then the expanding reamer is not opened fully. After the final reaming the cancellous surface of the acetabulum will be flush with the cortical surface of the acetabular fossa (the lateral surface of the tear drop).

64

Very Large Acetabulum

In a very large acetabulum, with low siting of the pilot hole to keep the socket at anatomical level, the expanding reamer may not reach the eburnated roof of the acetabulum. It is usually possible to reach some of the eburnated surface by angulating the expanding reamer in a headward direction. No attempt is made to cut out the eburnated roof to reach cancellous bone. Mere scraping of eburnated surface is adequate.

65

Scraping of Eburnated Bone

The eburnated bone left after the completion of reaming must be vigorously scraped in an endeavour to roughen it. The two-handed, serrated acetabular scraper is valuable for this. This scraper is useful also in finding and opening up cystic cavities in the roof of the acetabulum (**see** Appendix C). Two-handed Volkmann's spoons are also effective in scraping the acetabulum and should be maintained in a sharp condition. Large cysts in the roof of the acetabulum are very easily evacuated with a sharp two-handed Volkmann spoon. Rotation of the sharp spoon on its long axis will enlarge the aperture and scoop out the cyst contents in one movement.

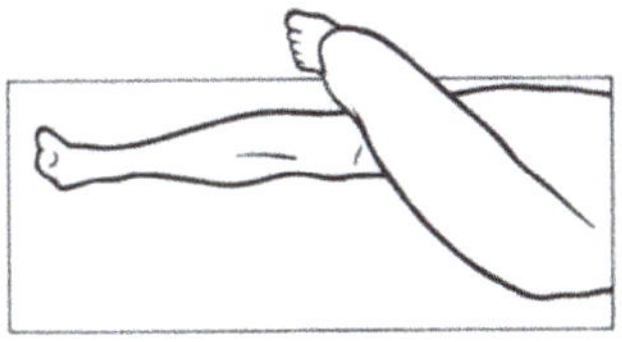

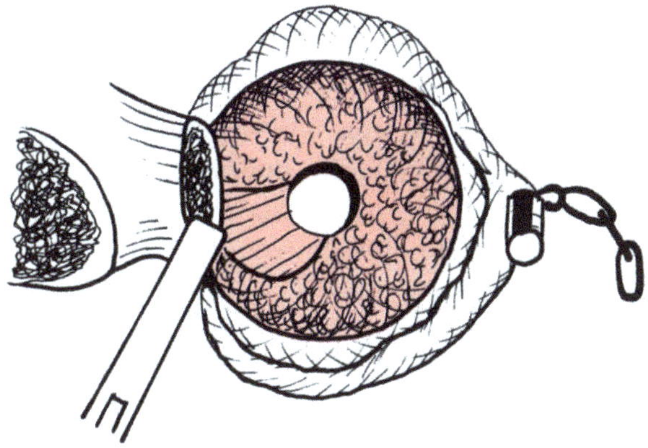

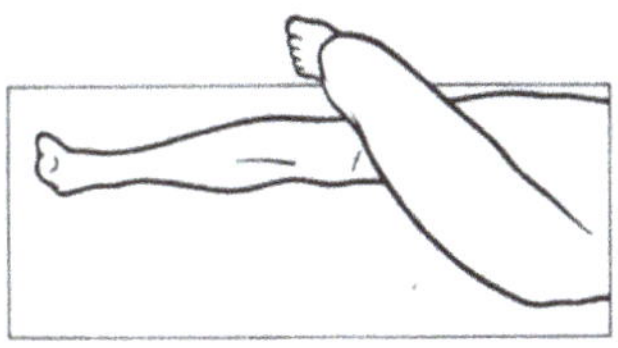

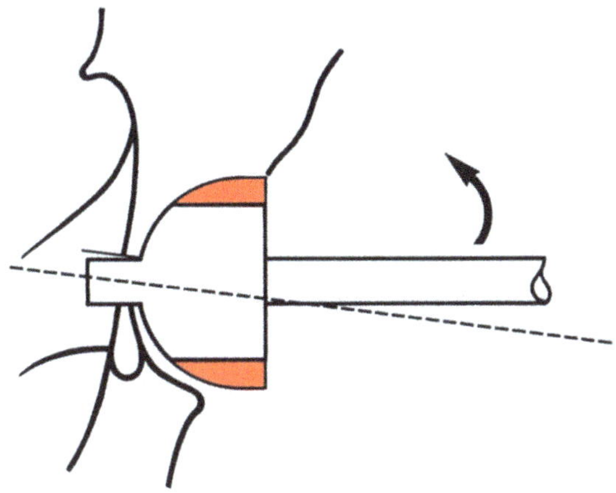

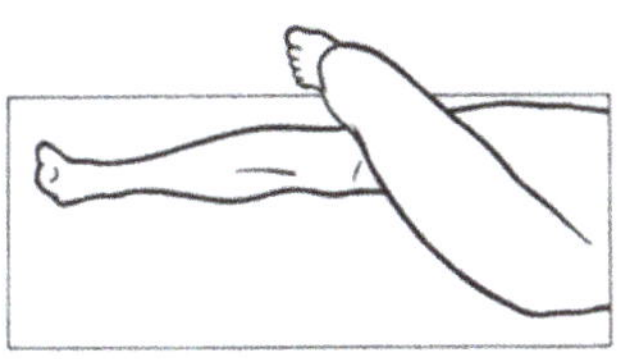

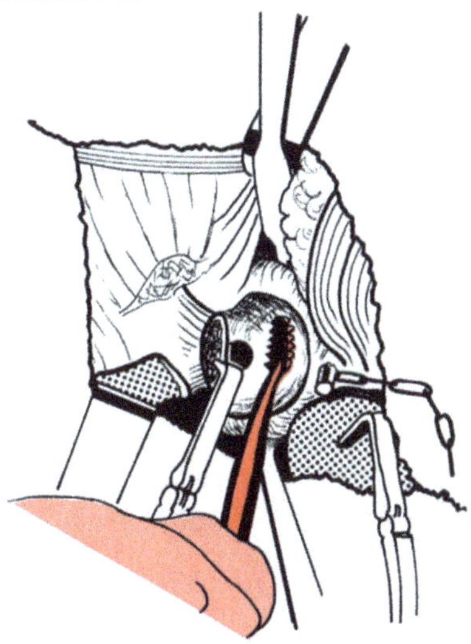

66

Superior Cement Anchorage Hole

The pilot drill (12.5-mm diameter) is convenient for this purpose. It is not necessary to pierce bone for more than about 1 cm (i.e. half-way to the collar of the drill). Endeavour to avoid damage to the anterior circumflex vessels, by contact with the shaft of the drill, when this is in the angulated position required to reach the roof of the acetabulum.

67

Ischial Cement Anchorage Hole

The ischial bone is usually very soft and often the drill will pierce without rotation. Enter between 7 and 8 o'clock (right hip) and between 4 and 5 o'clock (left hip) in relation to the central pilot hole. Note the 45° angulation towards the patient's feet. Avoid the vertical position because this would pierce the thin posterior wall of the acetabulum and theoretically could permit cement to reach the sciatic nerve.

68

Pubic Cement Anchorage Hole

At the 10 o'clock position for the left hip, or the 2 o'clock for the right hip, in relation to the pilot hole, and aim for the symphysis pubis. Pierce only for 1 cm and do not breach the deep cortex.

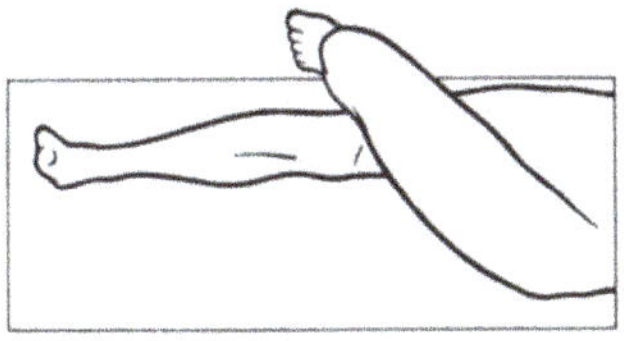

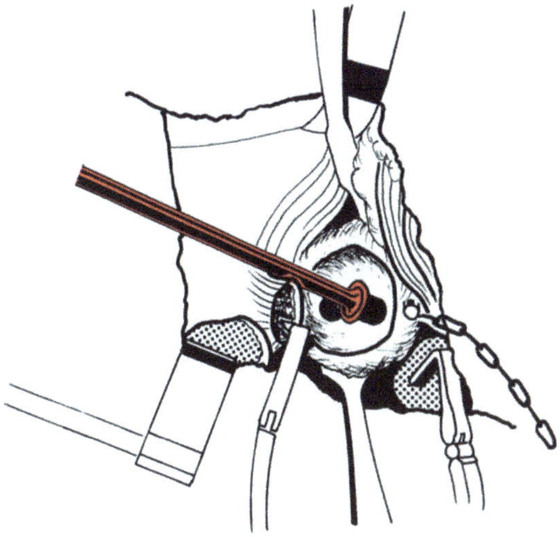

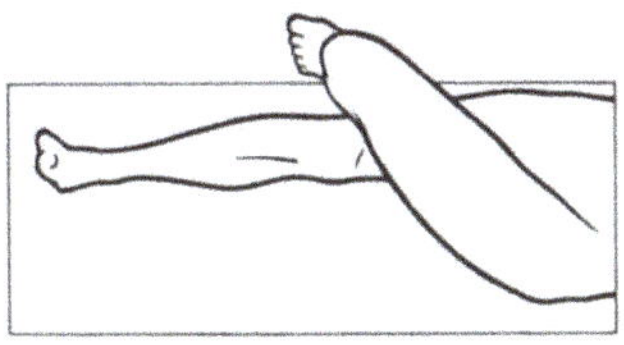

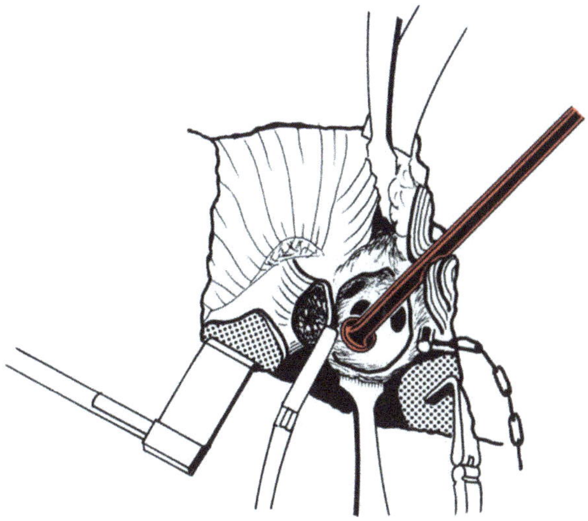

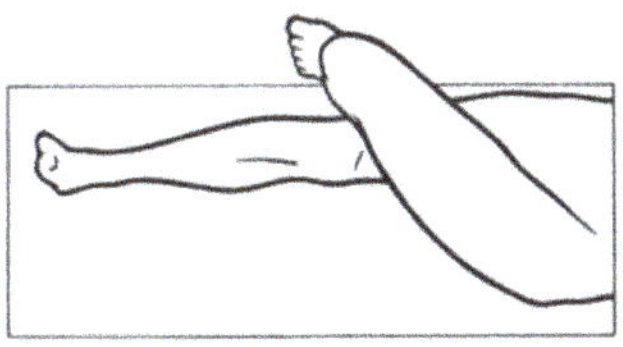

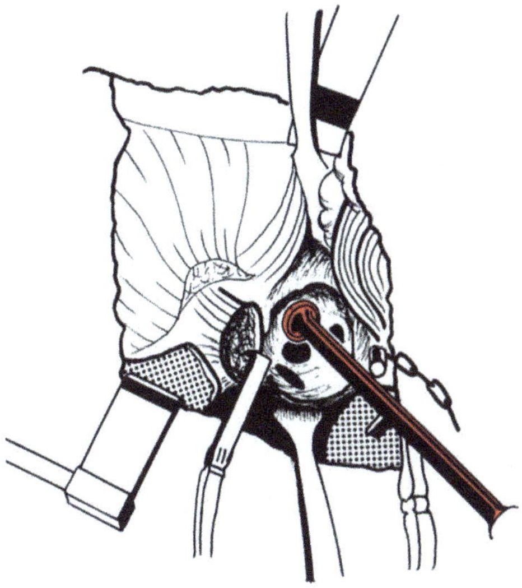

69

Multiple Small Cement Anchorage Holes

Between the three large cement anchor holes the remaining bone surfaces should be opened up with multiple 6-mm holes ($^1/_4$ in.). This drill must have a collar to prevent accidentally penetrating more than about 9 mm ($^3/_8$ in.). Up to 10 holes often can be made. It is best operated by a power source because of the eburnated bone. This is the point where **a rotary nylon brush** can be used in a power tool.

70

Cement Restrictor

The edges of the wire mesh are 'dished' to present vertically to the cancellous bone of the acetabulum. The punch has a circular flange by which the dished edge of the restrictor can be hammered into the bone. This prevents the restrictor being accidentally pulled out if a gauze swab catches on the cut edge of the wire mesh (**see** Appendix C). An extra-wide cement restrictor (about 4-cm diameter) is available if the pilot hole in a thin floor has become unduly large. The acetabulum should be kept irrigated with water or saline till the last second before inserting cement. Water or saline is more readily displaced into cancellous trabeculae by pressure of cement than is blood, which is more viscous.

71

Irrigation

Irrigation to remove bone detritus is **most important**. A sucker in conjunction with an irrigation syringe is essential. Irrigation reveals adherent fibrous tissue which would not have been detected if dry gauze alone were used. It also reveals many sites where the 6-mm drill can be used which would have been overlooked with dry swabbing alone. Hydrogen peroxide, 10 vols, is often useful to help stop bleeding.

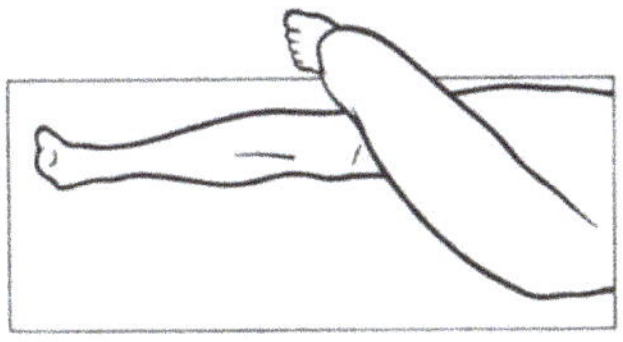

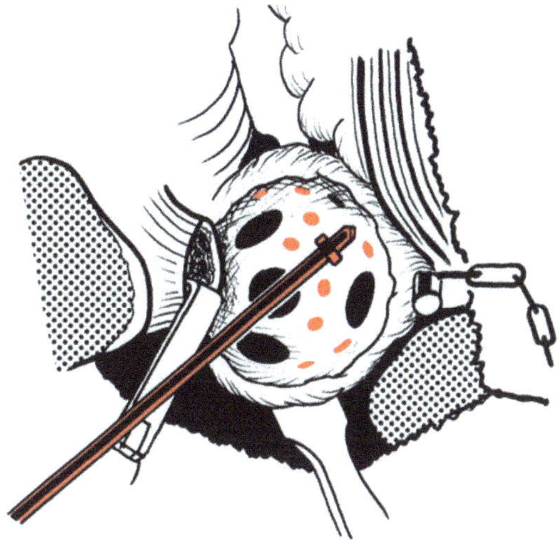

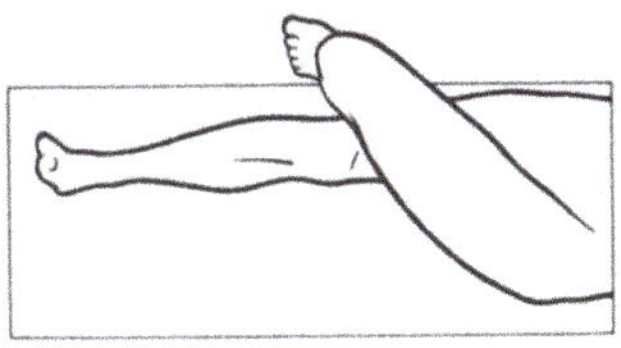

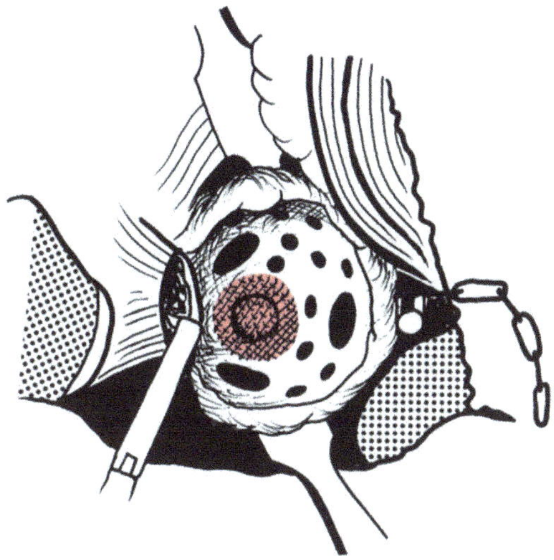

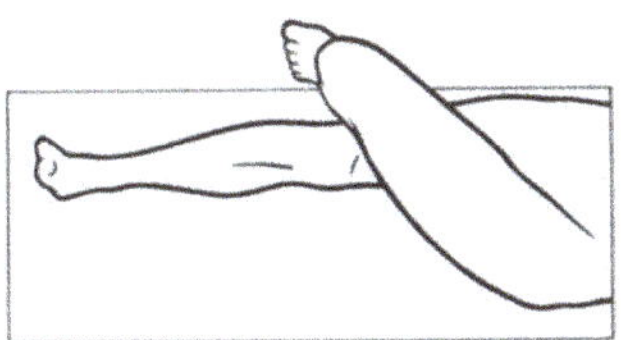

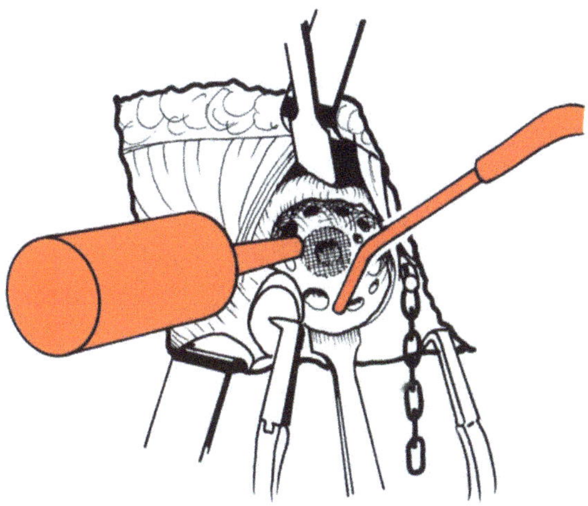

72

Socket Size-Gauges

It is useful to have socket-size-gauges of 52 and 54 mm diameter for use with the PIJ sockets because this design of socket is specially valuable in large acetabula. Standard Thackray socket size-gauges are 47 and 50 mm in. diameter. Socket size-gauges are circular. The essence of a PIJ socket is that it has an oval face. Circular-faced socket size-gauges are used to estimate the antero-posterior diameter of the reamed acetabulum.

73

Trimming the PIJ Socket

(*a*) Cutting the antero-posterior dimensions of the socket to the antero-posterior dimensions of the acetabulum as estimated from the fit of the socket size-gauges. (*b*) Cutting the distal radius to the appropriate inscribed circle. Advise to leave this a little longer than antero-posterior radius. (*c*) Trimming the superior, oval radius to fit the roof to the acetabulum. (*d*) The end result.

74

Trimming PIJ – LPW Socket

(*a*) This socket is held with the LPW feature below. For a left-sided acetabulum, as in this case, the inferior lobe is removed as indicated. (*b*) Completing the trimming of the antero-posterior dimension, on the socket-holder, to fit the antero-posterior dimension of the acetabulum.

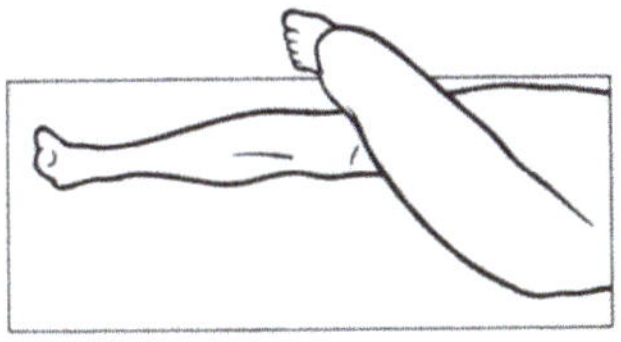

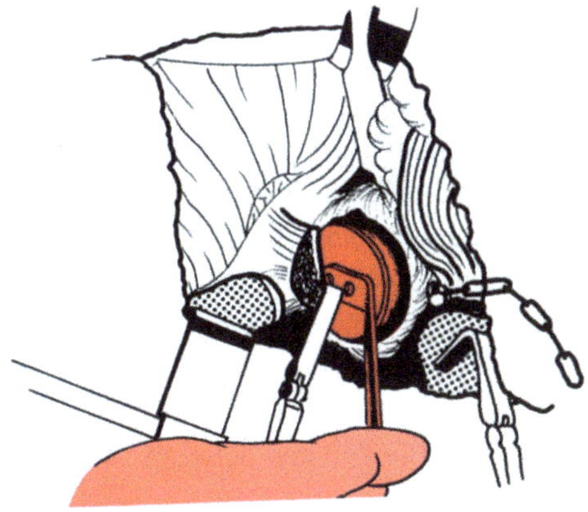

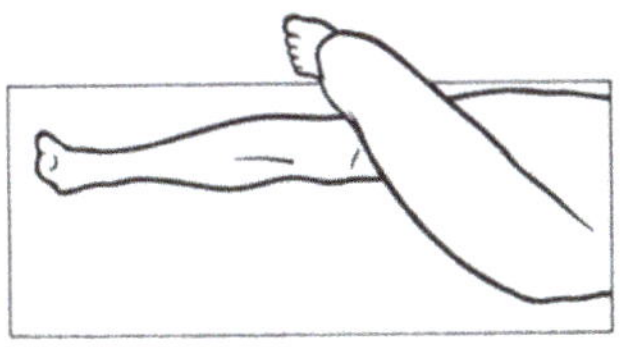

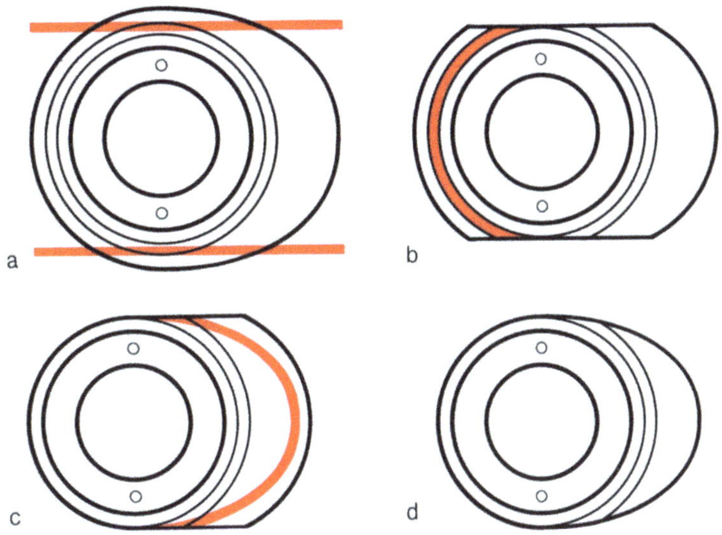
a
b
c
d

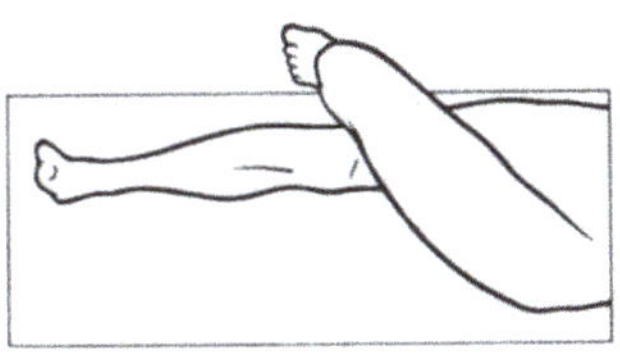

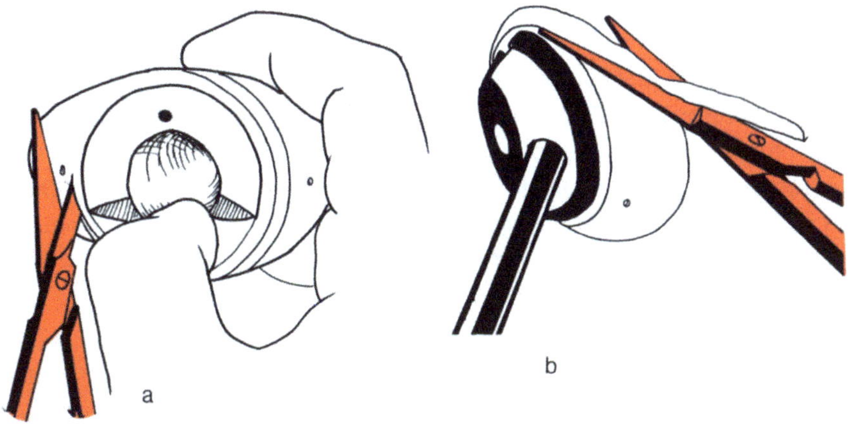
a
b

75

Final Trimming of Superior Lobe

The final length of the superior lobe is judged by the ability to bring the handle of the socket-holder to the transverse position. The superior lobe ideally (but not imperatively) should make contact with the roof of the acetabulum just before the socket-holder reaches the transverse position. This will be shown by the superior lobe deflecting to show slight lateral concavity. It is essential to maintain full pressure with the pusher at this stage, otherwise the socket-holder will detach itself from the socket. The ideal end result is when, under full force of the pusher (*arrow A*) the friction between the rim of the socket and the acetabulum will sustain the weight of the handle of the socket-holder (*arrow B*).

76

Cementing the Socket

Before inserting the cement and the prosthesis check that full retraction by the horizontal retractor is holding the stump of the neck of the femur out of the way and that this will not obstruct easy access at the critical moment. **A few more turns on the screw-jack at this point are useful.** See Chap. 7, pp. 98 and 99 for special details.The handle of the pusher is usually at a higher level than the tip on the face of the socket-holder, and because it rests on the neck of the femur this acts as a fulcrum; **raising or lowering the handle of the pusher can therefore change the orientation of the face of the socket.**

77

Pelvic Obliquity and Socket Alignment

If the hip is strongly adducted (*b*) and the pelvis oblique on the table, the transverse limb of the socket-holder may need to be moved towards the patient's head rather than be merely transverse to the table. The datum line is the line connecting the anterior superior iliac spines. There is considerable latitude here and special alignment of the socket-holder from the ordinary position (i.e. transverse to the table) only very rarely is needed.

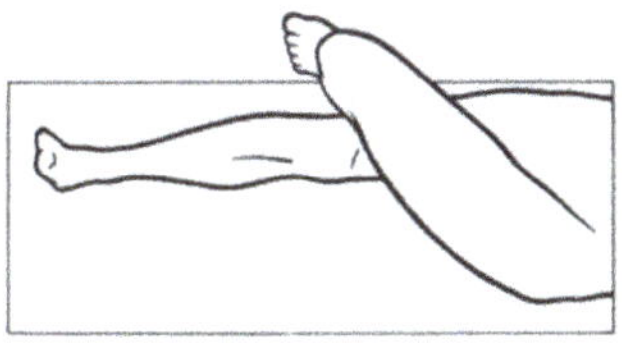

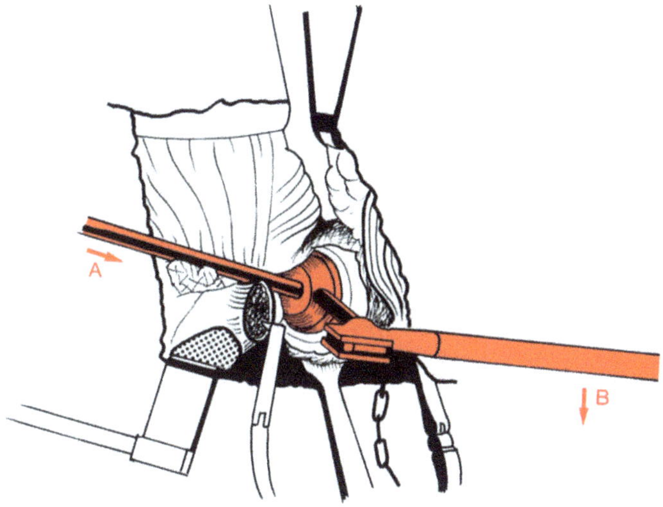

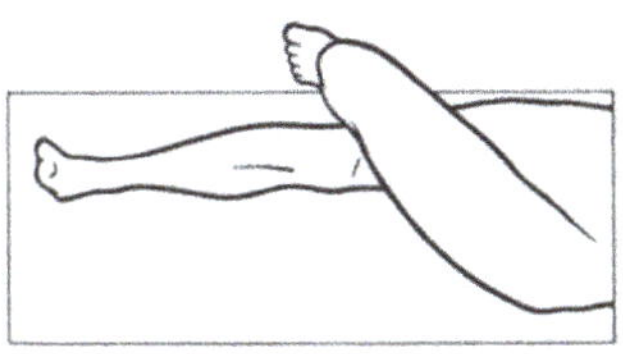

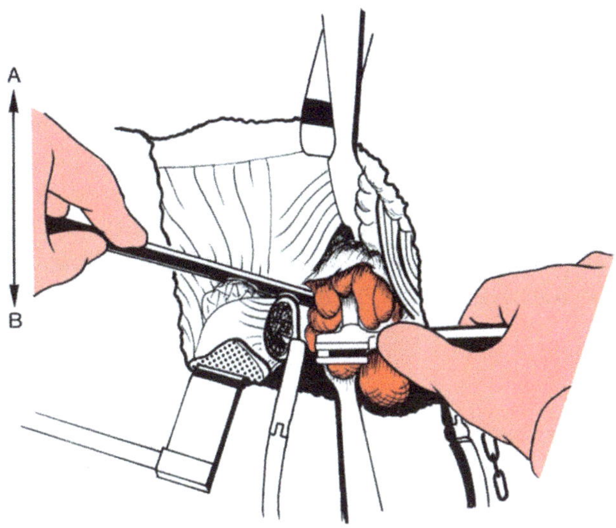

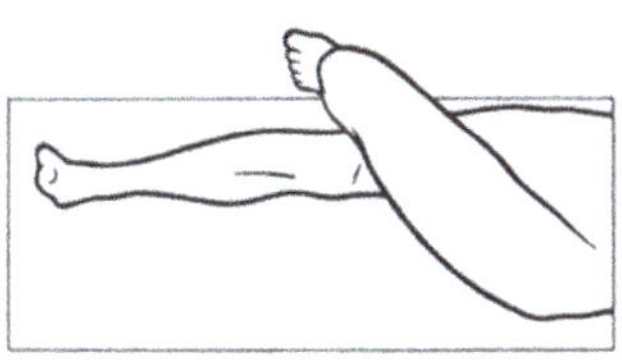

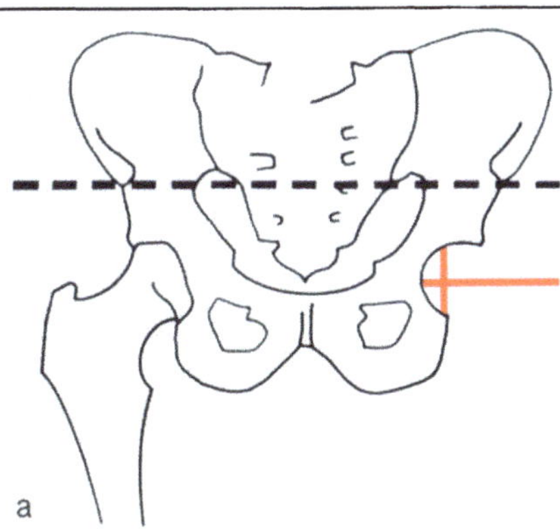

a

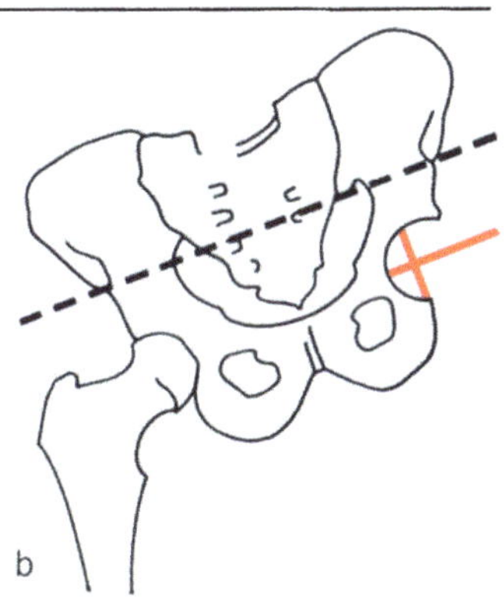

b

78

Tilt of the Pelvis

The pelvis is always tilted 10° (rolled away from the surgeon) so that the handle of the socket-holder must always be held 10° above the horizontal plane.

79

Absence of Anteversion of Socket

A long-established feature of this operation is that the socket should not be anteverted. Lack of anteversion does not prevent the hip flexing beyond 90°, because this is achieved by a combination of abduction and external rotation. The absence of anteversion is shown by the horizontal limb of the socket-holder being parallel with the floor (*1*). If the horizontal limb of the socket-holder is inclined, with the free end lower than the transverse limb (*2*) then the face of the socket will be anteverted (and vice versa).

80

Waiting for Final Polymerisation

It is important to remove the socket-holder while the cement is still truly plastic and long before it is in the rubbery phase before hardening. This is to minimise accidental movements of the socket-holder pulling the cement away from the moist bone surface which is more likely when cement is rubbery than when still truly plastic. The enhanced mechanical stability of the PIJ socket in the acetabulum in comparison with conventional designs, protects it against accidental movement. This is very important with cements that take a long time to set.

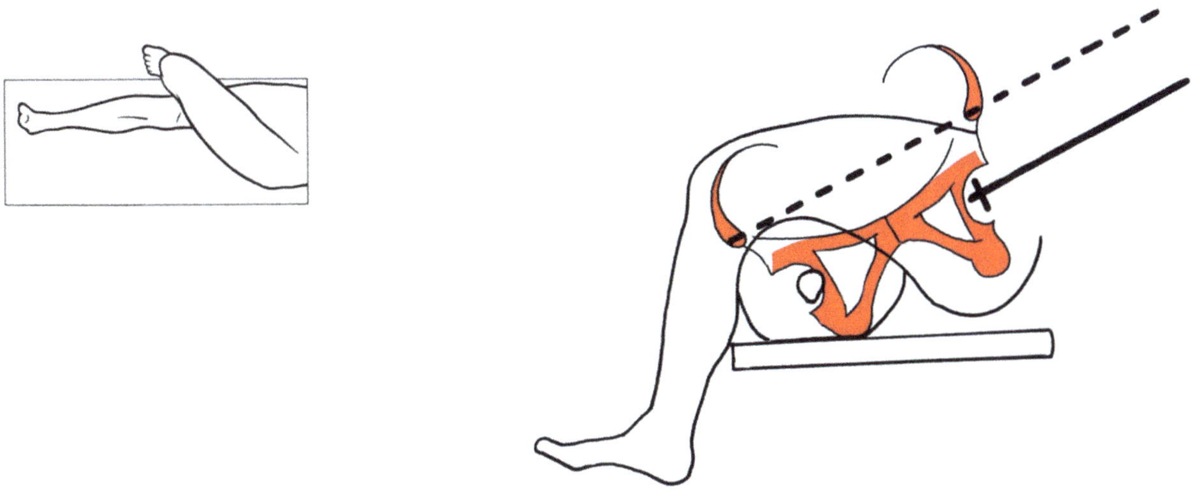

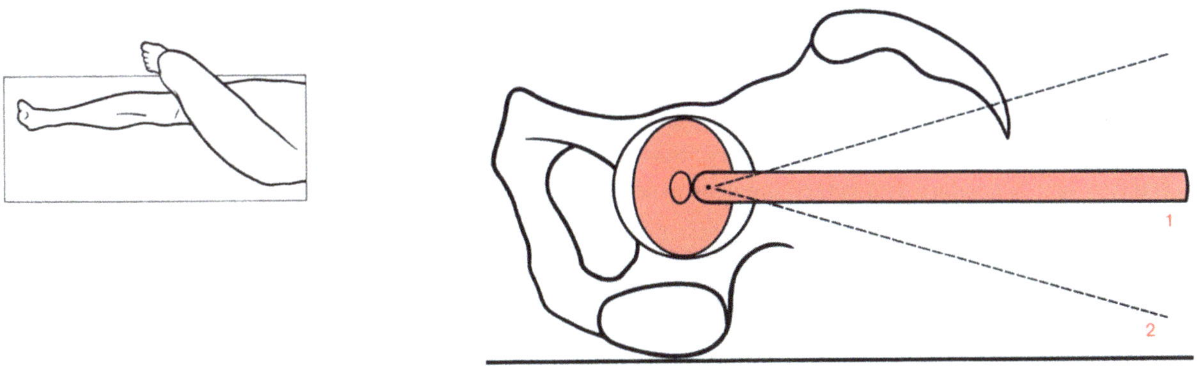
1
2

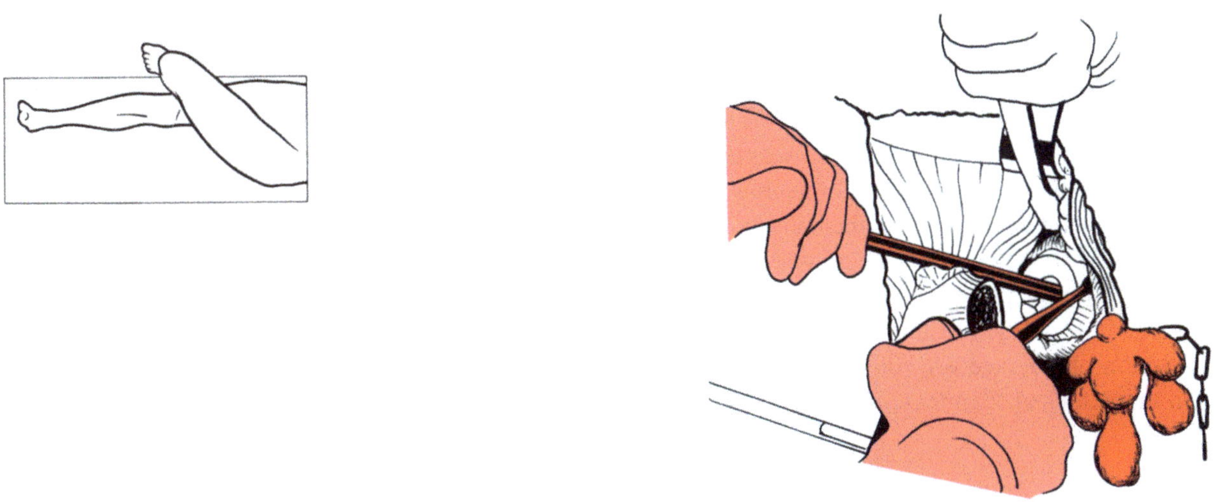

81

Removing Socket-Holder

The rim of the PIJ socket severs connection between the deep cement and the superficial excess. The self-ejecting socket-holder is lifted from the face of the socket by pressing the operating lever, **while maintaining full force of the pusher on the face of the holder.** If the socket-holder is now **pulled sharply away** from the socket it will usually bring the excess cement with it in one piece.

As soon as the socket-holder is detached the superior lobe of the PIJ socket may tilt away from close contact with the roof of the acetabulum. This must be counteracted **immediately** by **applying pressure with the thumb on the superior lobe. Keep pressure of thumb until cement has set—this detail is of extreme importance.**

82

Resection of Osteophytes from Acetabulum

Resection of inferior osteophytes is simple and safe (no serious haemorrhage; no damage to sciatic nerve). The surgeon should not hesitate if osteophytes project more than 0.5 cm. It is best to resect, **while all the retractors are in position and before the cemented femoral prosthesis becomes an obstruction** (see Chap. 21).

The projecting bone can be nibbled away with bone rongeurs, cut away with a chisel. A chisel (not an osteotome) is important. The first stage is to pass a Watson-Jones gouge below the inferior rim and hammer it in the direction of the base of the ischium. Osteophytes are inside the capsule at this site so there is no danger to the sciatic nerve.

83

Cutting Osteophytes with Chisel

The chisel, 2 cm wide, is applied to the internal surface of the rim of the acetabulum **with the bevel facing the socket**. This will cause the chisel to cut parallel with the face of the socket and **not** in the direction of the axis of the chisel. An osteotome cuts in the direction of the axis of the instrument; this could be dangerous in this situation. Four or five cuts distributed over 4–6 cm will detach the rim en bloc. The Watson-Jones lever protects soft parts posteriorly. When detachment is almost complete the last tetherings of fibrous tissue can be torn by a combination of leverage with the lever and traction with a Kocher's forceps on the detached fragment.

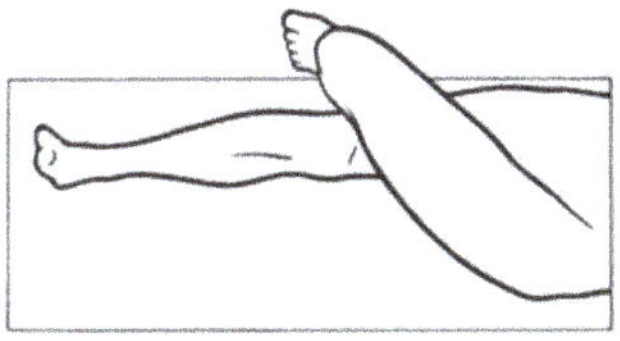

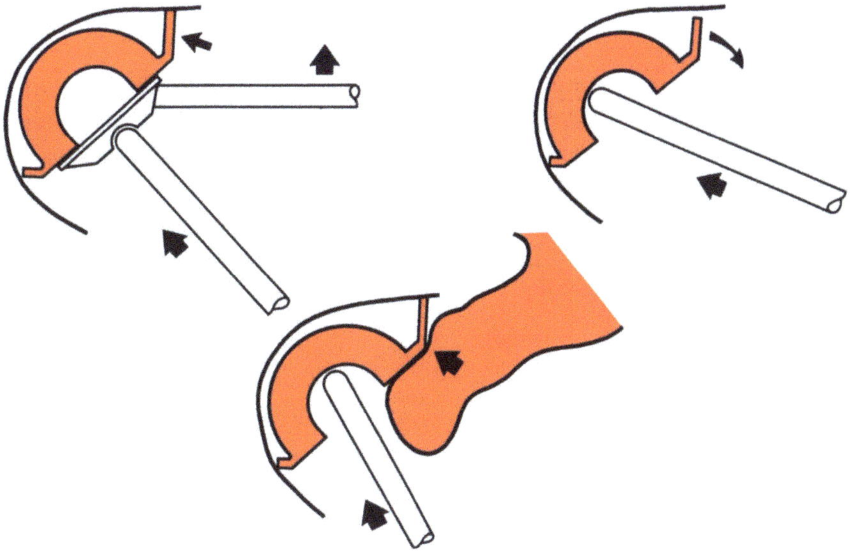

Time: 28.5 min

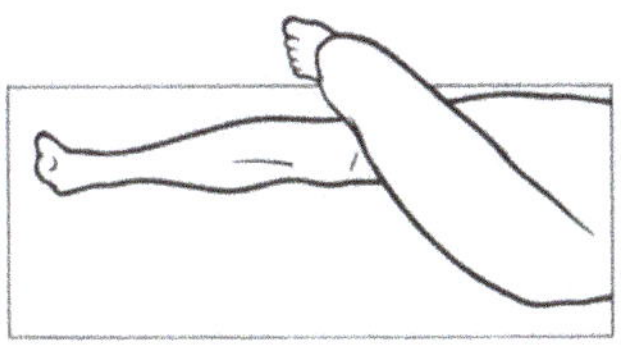

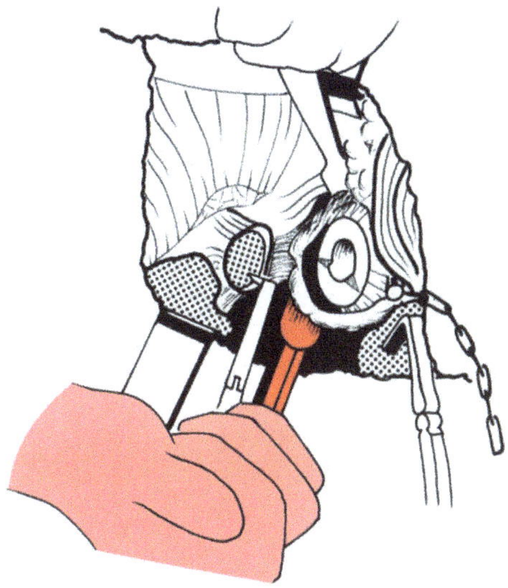

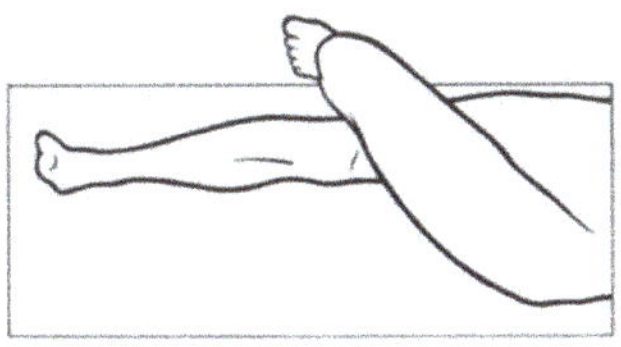

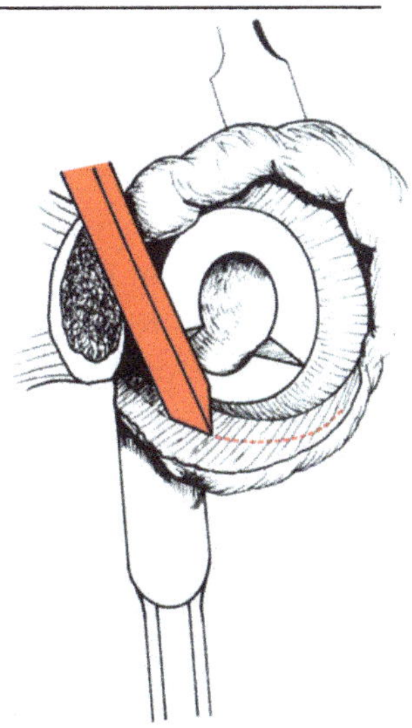

84

End of Socket Implantation

This diagram shows the PIJ socket in situ without anteversion and with a typical area of cancellous bone exposed after removal of osteophytes from inferior rim. Resection of osteophytes does not increase the tendency to new bone formation. New bone in this region (DeLee and Charnley)[67] occurred in only 1% of post-operative results though resection of osteophytes might be performed in 30% of cases (Appendix A).

85

Bridge of Cortical Bone

The Femoral Prosthesis

For latitude in the length of the stump of the femoral neck it is better that error should favour too wide rather than too narrow a bridge of bone. The bone rongeur is useful to remove the bone bridge and to reveal the maximum antero-posterior width of the medullary cavity in the neck of the femur.

86

Finding Axis of Femoral Medulla

The hand-operated taper reamer is inserted, just lateral to the cut surface of the neck and therefore in the most medial part of the cancellous surface left after detachment of the trochanter. It is impossible to wander from the axis of the femur and emerge through the lateral cortex of the femur. **Note. It is important** at this stage to pack gauze below and on each side of the upper end of the femur to prevent marrow tissue running out of the femur and depositing itself in the lower part of the wound. **It is possible that marrow tissue is more responsible for causing ectopic bone formation than detritus of cancellous bone produced by reaming the acetabulum.**

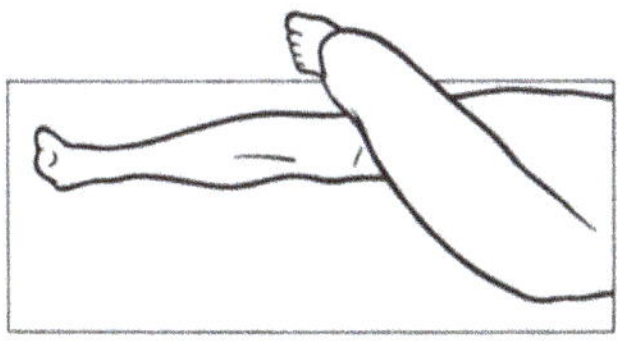

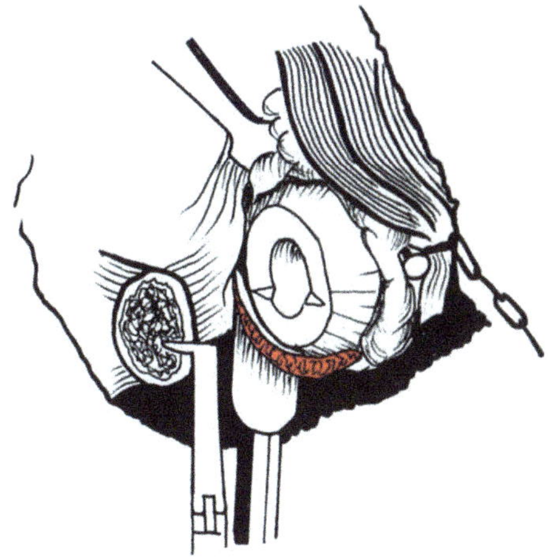

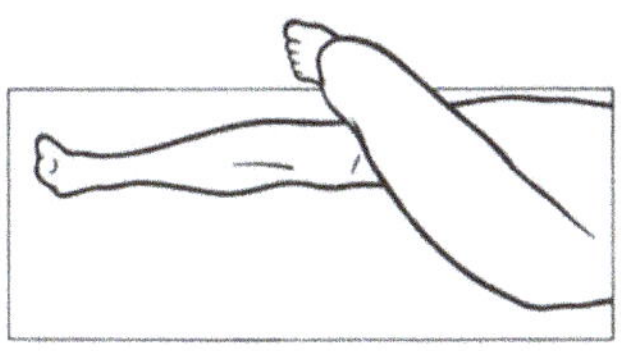

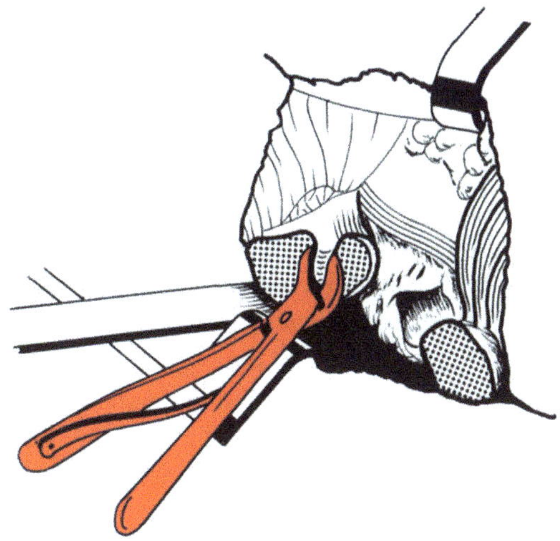

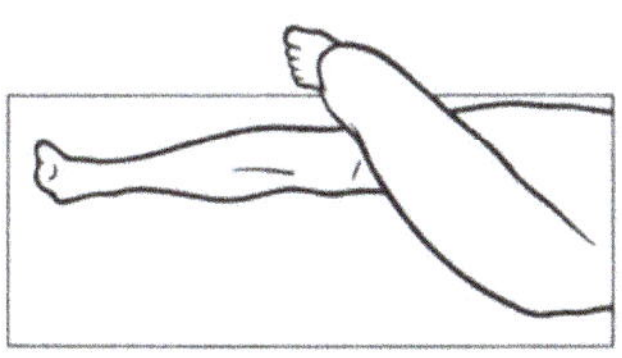

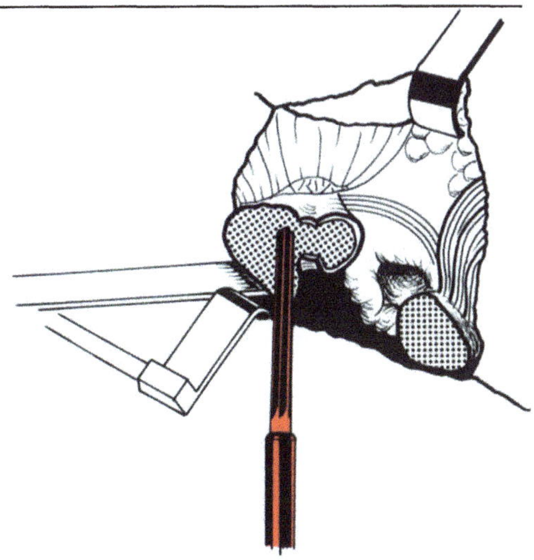

87

External Check on Alignment

Should there be any doubt whether the taper reamer is correctly in the femoral cavity (as in difficult secondary operations with displaced osteotomies of femur) inspection of alignment of the axis of the reamer in two planes in relation to the knee (frontal and lateral) is reassuring.

88

Rotary Femoral Reamers

Rotary reaming is absolutely essential with the flanged, Cobra prostheses. Only one size of rotary reamer [95 mm $^{3}/_{8}''$ at tip] is required to enlarge the track made by the hand-operated reamer. The rotary reamer is operated in a hand-brace or by a slow-speed power source. Ream from valgus to varus at the **full depth of the reamer.** Ream the medial femoral neck while withdrawing rotating reamer in varus, *C*. Do **not** ream down to cortical bone on endosteal surface of the medial femoral neck. Try to leave 2–3 mm of cancellous bone.

With the flanged designs of prostheses the medullary cavity must be enlarged in antero-posterior diameter to accept the width of the flange. The widest part of flange corresponds to the central part of cancellous bone in the neck (i.e. where the trochanteric surface meets the cut surface of the neck).

89

Antero-posterior Dimension of Medullary Cavity in Neck

The flange of the Cobra prosthesis must fit **inside** the medullary cavity and **not** on the cut edge of the cortex of the neck of the femur. When the flange is properly inside the medullary cavity: (*a*) It centralizes the prosthetic stem in the cement, and so avoids a source of fracture of cement, caused by an eccentric position allowed by conventional designs. (*b*) It is capable of acting somewhat as a piston to help in generating pressure on the soft cement. (*c*) It transmits load when the cement is hard.

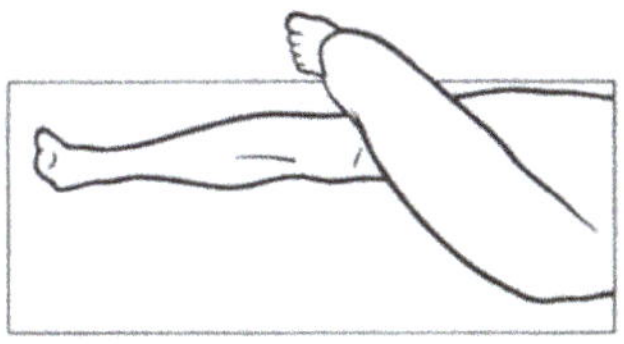

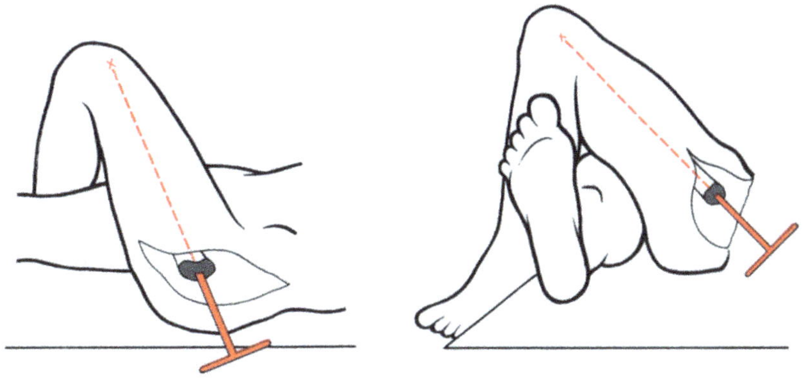

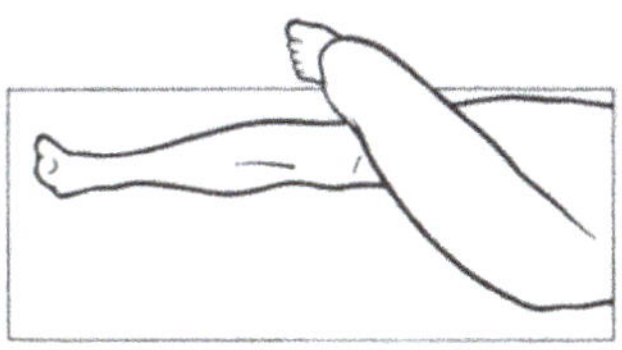

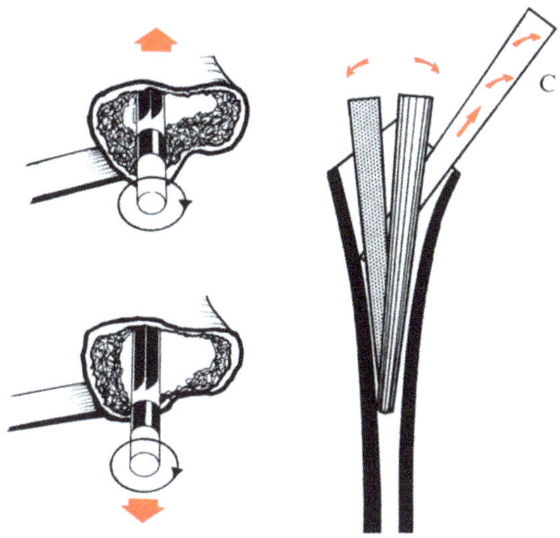
c

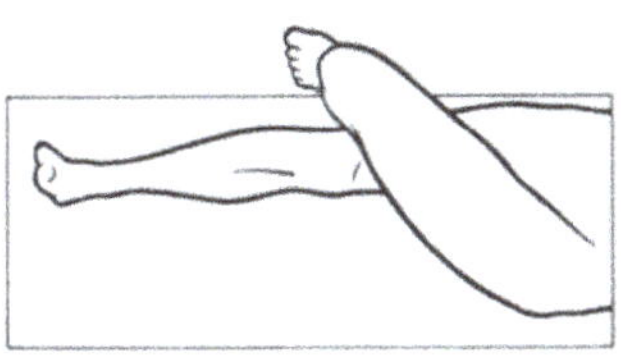

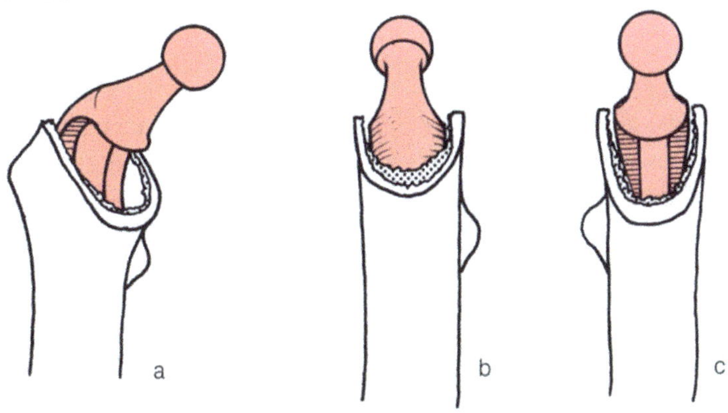
a
b
c

90

Antero-posterior Reaming of Neck Cavity

The *lower diagram* shows the type of asymmetry to be avoided. Antero-posterior reaming has been concentrated asymmetrically at upper level. The *upper diagram* shows the desired symmetry. This is achieved by keeping the reamer deep inside the femur when enlarging the medullary cavity in the anterior and posterior directions. The stem of the femoral prosthesis is not held rigidly in the axis of the distal femur because the length of the medullary cavity, *A*, is short. It must be emphasized that maximum enlargement in the antero-posterior direction, for the flange of the Cobra prosthesis, is needed only in the centre of the neck where trochanteric and neck surfaces meet. This will be the site of the widest part of the flange.

91

Avoiding Anteversion

Reaming with the rotary reamers in a varus direction, with a little posterior inclination, will reduce an unacceptable degree of anteversion; 5° of anteversion is the preferred maximum but 10° can be accepted if unavoidable.

92

Test Reduction – Long Axis Traction

At the test reduction in the absence of cement, the Cobra design of prosthesis does not fall into the varus position under axial load as much as conventional designs because the edges of the flange engage the antero-posterior diameter of the medullary cavity. The lengths of the extremities are compared by palpating the medial malleoli through the drapes. Apply long-axis traction to the lower extremity at the knee. Ideally the prosthetic head should not distract from the acetabulum, but if distraction is not possible the limb could be too long. If the prosthetic femoral head distracts 2–3 mm from the socket this can just be accepted because it will become accepted because it stable when the trochanter is reattached.

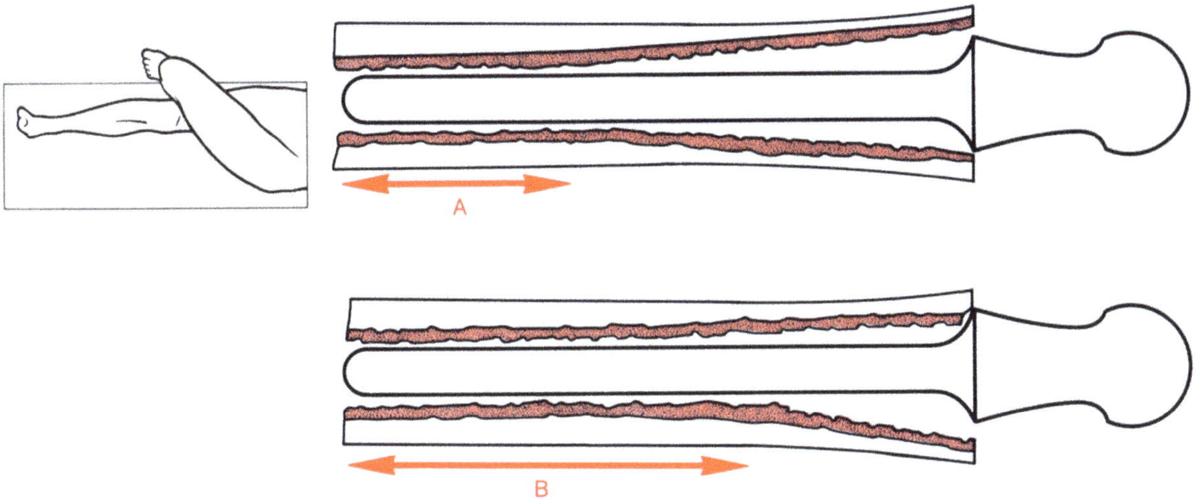
A
B

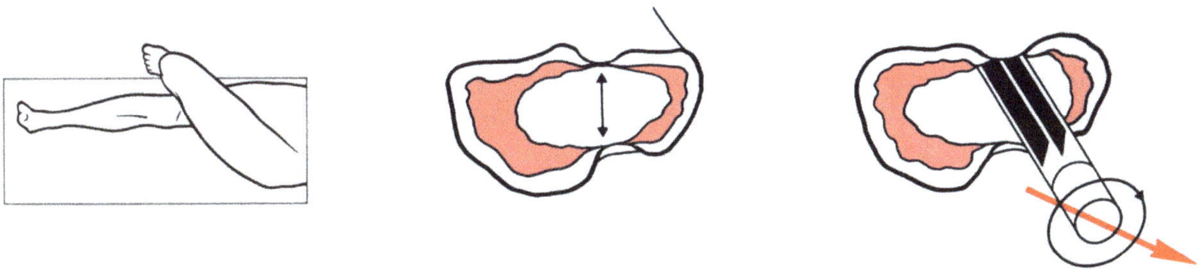

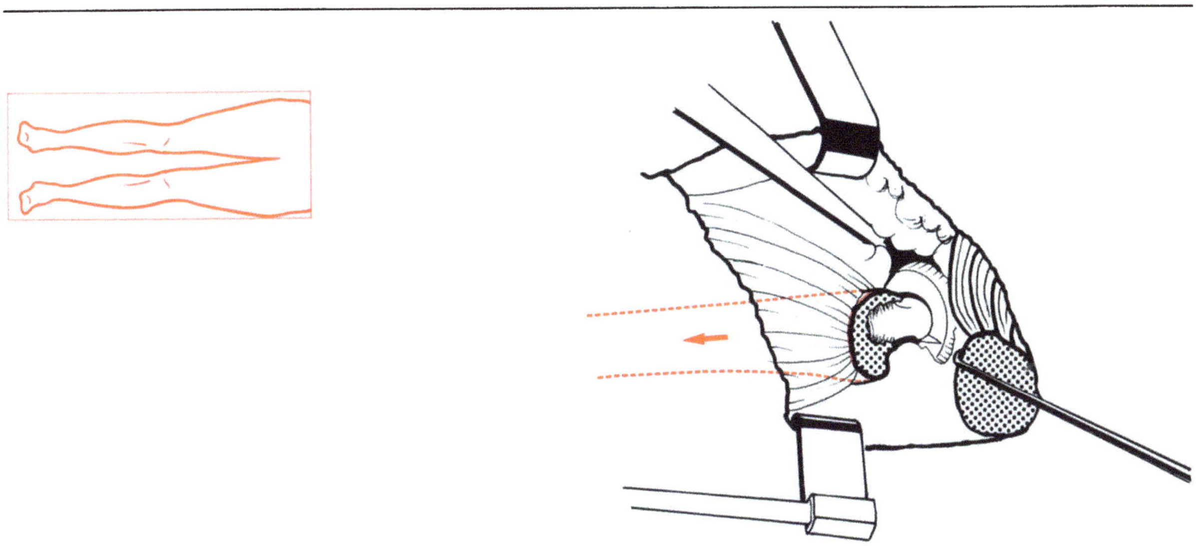

93

Adduction—Test Reduction

Ideally the thigh should reach 40° of adduction before the femoral head dislocates. If there was no distraction of the femoral head when tested by long-axis traction, dislocation will frequently be resisted even at 40° of adduction. If dislocation occurs at 20° a search should be made for a bony fulcrum (osteophyte not removed from the acetabulum).

94

External Rotation—Test Reduction

Stability to external rotation **is the most important of all test ranges.** If a hip is stable to external rotation, slight laxity under long-axis traction and instability at 20° of adduction can be ignored because reattachment of the trochanter has yet to be performed and this will add considerably to total stability. It is not safe to rely on reattachment of the trochanter alone if the hip is unstable to external rotation at the test reduction. Testing for stability to **flexion** is unnecessary. Indeed it is inadvisable because strong flexion can disturb the bacteriological seal of the drapes round the perineum. It is unnecessary to test stability in flexion because it is not reasonable to expect stability beyond 90° of flexion before the trochanter is reattached.

95

Position of Detached Trochanter

With the limb in neutral position, approximate the detached trochanter to the cut surface on the femur. If the trochanter does not slightly overlap check again whether limb has been over-lengthened.

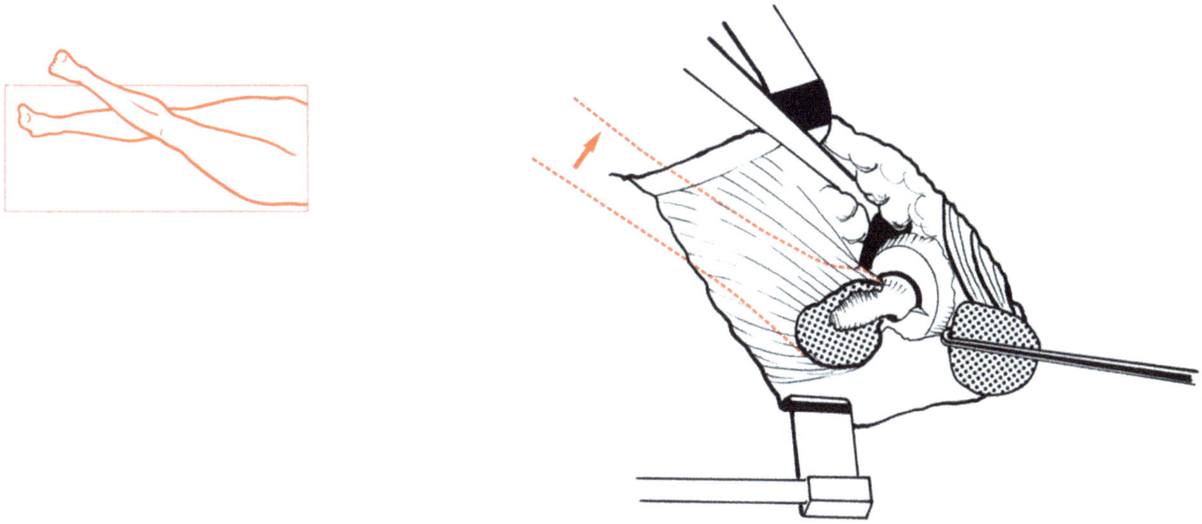

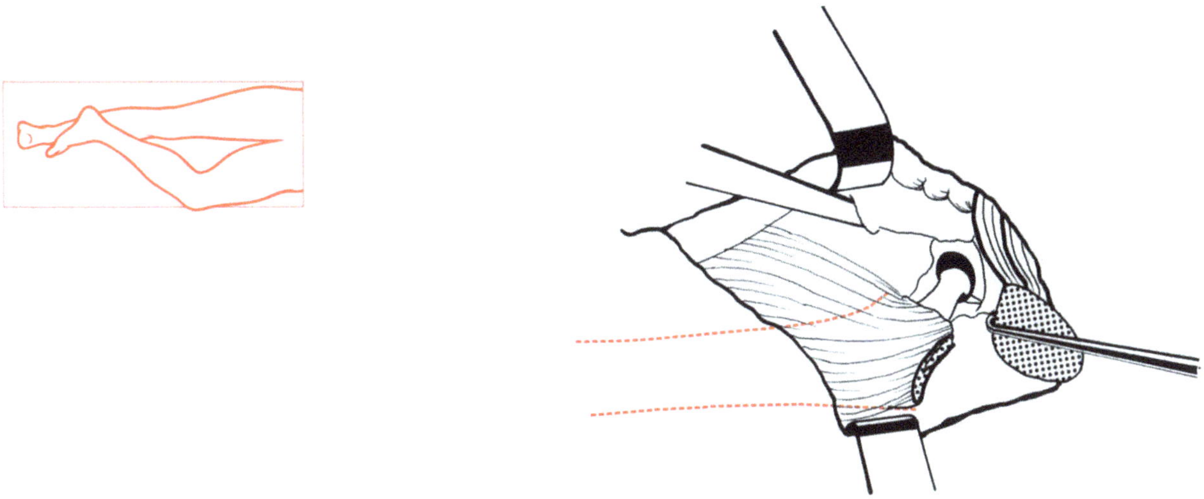

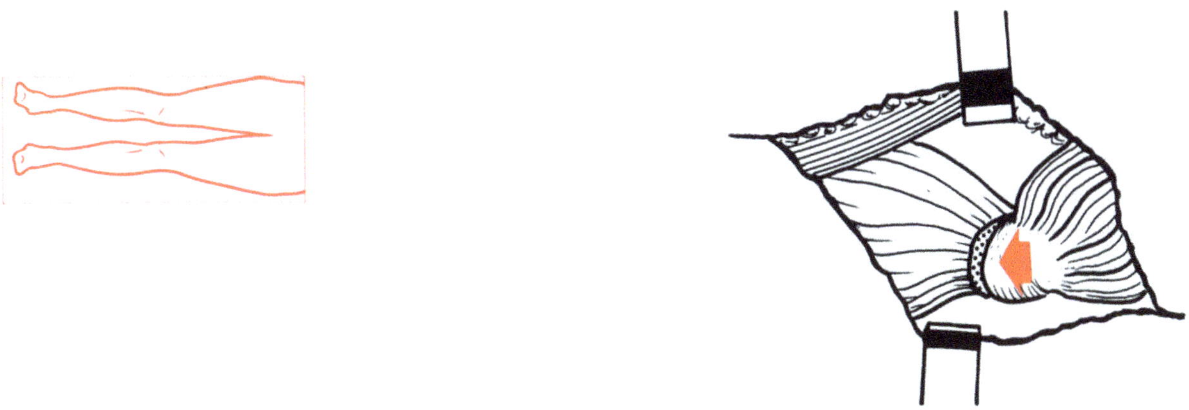

96

Anteversion and/or Neck Stump too long

Excessive anteversion of the prosthesis (more than about 5°) may be caused by the neck of the femur having been sectioned obliquely at stage 36. The posterior cortex of the neck can be shortened by nibbling with rongeur. If test reductions have shown the limb to be too long the stump of the neck should be shortened by nibbling with bone rongeurs.

Insertion of Wires for Trochanter Fixation

The wires for fixation of the trochanter must now be inserted before cementing the femoral prosthesis. In this section the practical details of using the vertical double loop plus the cruciate wire system are described.

97

Drilling Lateral Femoral Cortex

The femur is in internal rotation and adduction. It is unnecessary to strip the vastus lateralis muscle to expose the lateral cortex of the femur. An $^1/_8$-in. (3.2-mm) drill is used 3 cm below the cut trochanteric surface on the femur. The drill is centred in the middle of the lateral surface of the femur and directed towards the medullary cavity under direct vision. To prevent the drill picking up fibrous tissue a cholecystectomy forceps, open, is pressed hard on the muscle. This marks the site of the hole into which the double wire must be inserted.

98

Vertical Double Loop

The vertical double wire (18 s.w.g.) is inserted. The opposite end of the double wire is a loop. The overall length of the double wire is 76 cm (i.e. single and before being doubled to 38 cm). To identify the ends of the double wire a pair of wire-holding forceps with colour-coded handles are used. Mulier (personal communication) has the two ends soldered side by side to facilitate passage through the hole and later cuts the end off; this is a very useful idea.

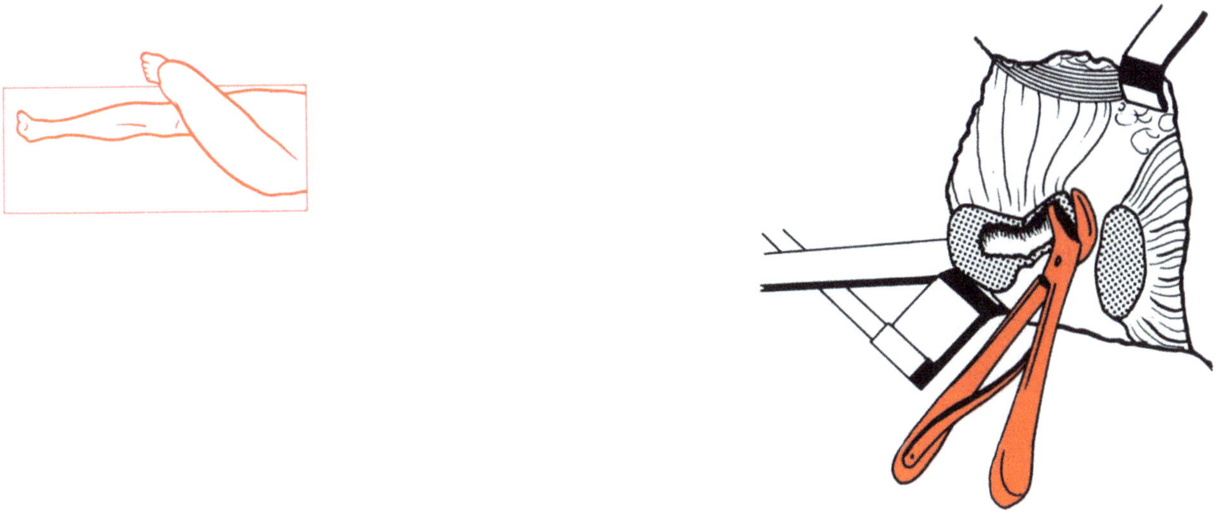

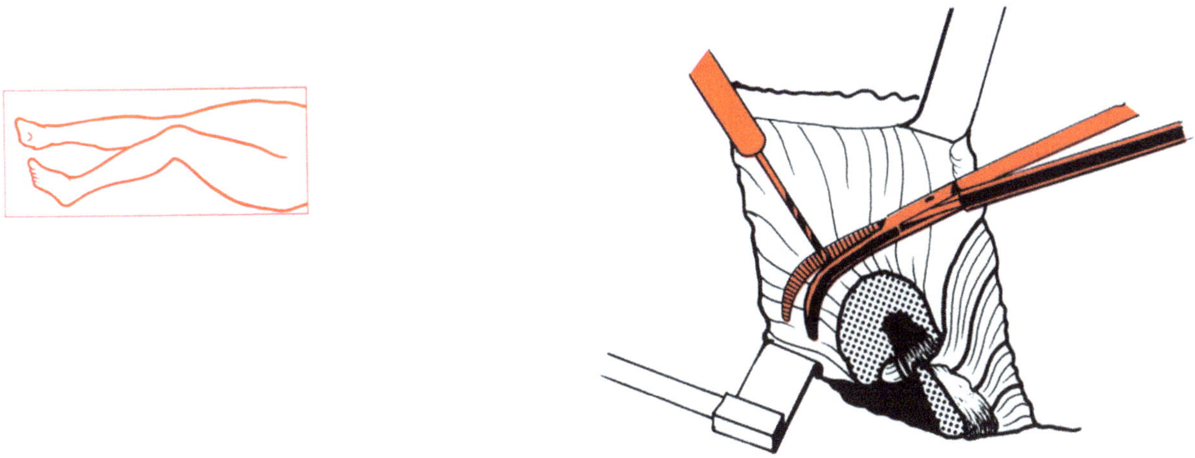

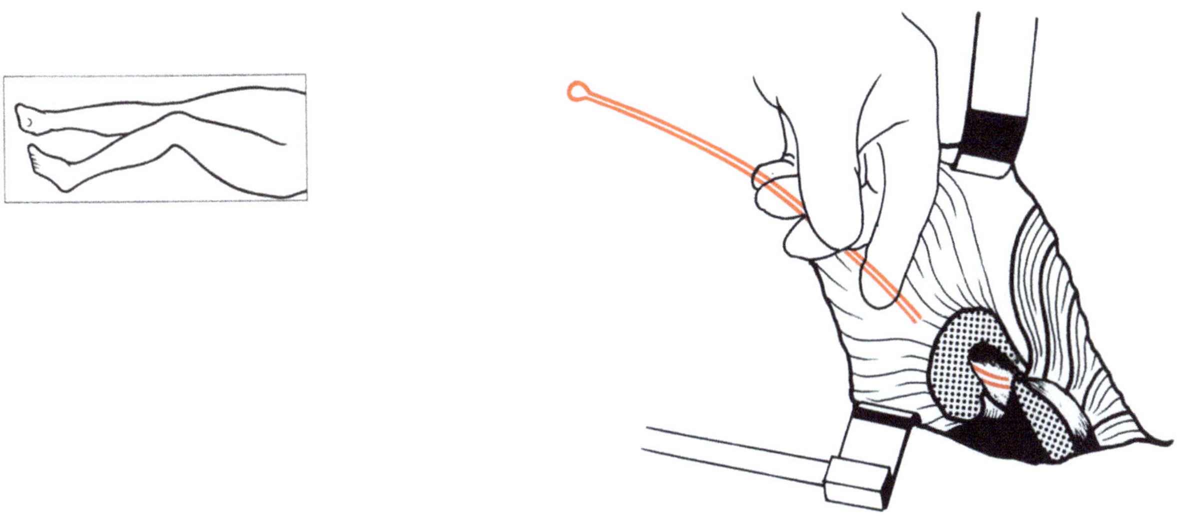

99

Vertical Double Loop

The loop is held in a small haemostat because otherwise the loop can be lost by being accidentally pulled inside the medullary cavity. This haemostat is retained till stage 122 though not illustrated in subsequent diagrams. Avoid the loop projecting too far out of the cortex of the femur in order to avoid the final twisted end of wire lying in the trochanteric bursa on the lateral surface of the trochanter.

100

Drilling for Medial Wire of Cruciate System

The femur is in full adduction. The serrated and angulated femur lever is in situ. This lever is essential to facilitate access to the posterior surface of the femur. The drill is sited about 1 cm from the cut edges of the femur. The medial wire will not cut out of the bone because later it is buried in the cement.

101

Medial Wire of Cruciate System

The femur is in full adduction. This single wire is 45 cm long. Identify both ends with a pair of wire-holding forceps with colour-coded handles.

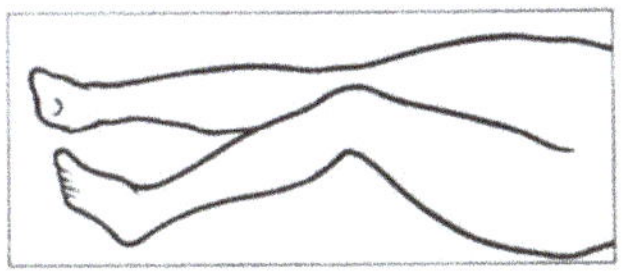

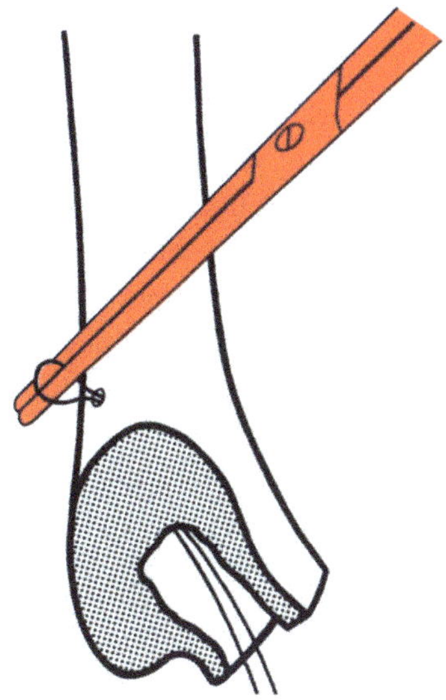

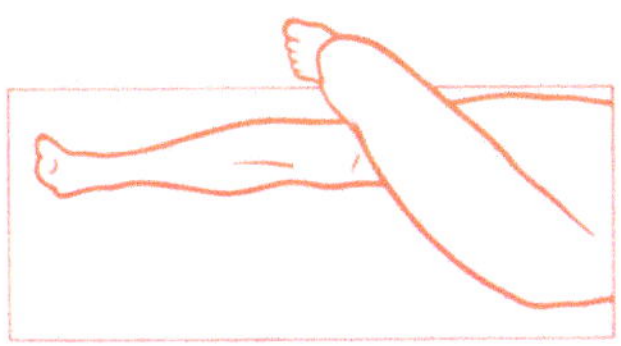

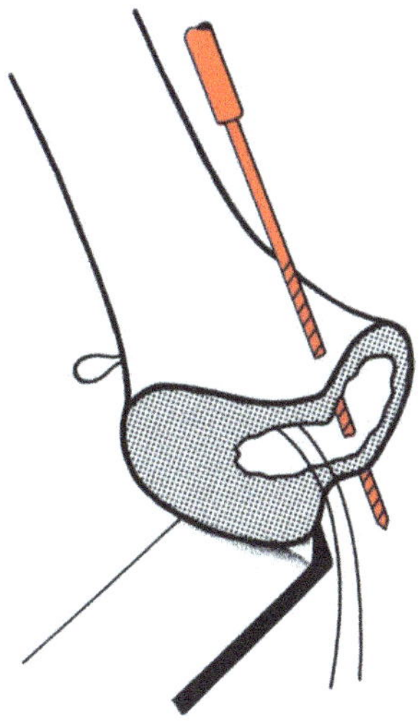

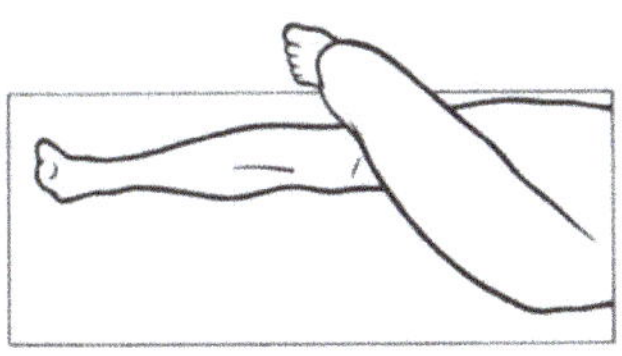

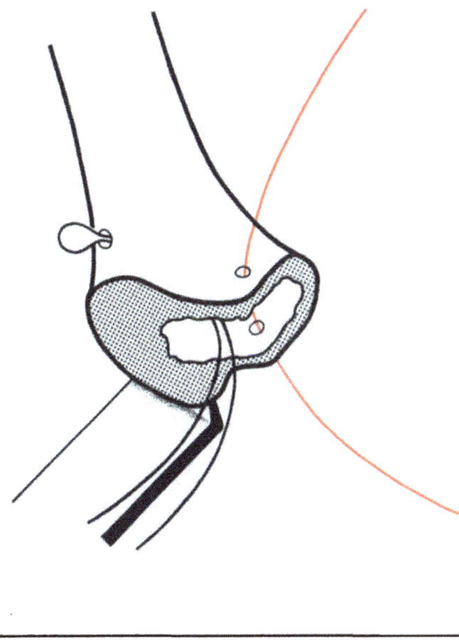

102

Lateral Displacement of Medial Wire

The femur is in full adduction. To prevent the medial wire obstructing the stem of the prosthesis where it crosses the medullary cavity, it must be displaced by a test entry of the prosthesis. It is preferable to displace the medial wire laterally in the medullary cavity, because lateral displacement leaves the medial femoral neck free for final curettage and for packing with gauze immediately prior to inserting cement. The wire is displaced using the stem of the **final prosthesis held in the prosthesis-holder**. If it is proposed to use the staple-clamp, the laterally displaced loop of the medial wire must be pushed into the medullary cavity to lie well below the cut trochanteric surface. The fish-tail punch (Appendix C) is useful for this.

103

Drilling for Lateral Wire

The femur is in full adduction. The serrated and angulated femur lever is even more essential for the lateral wire than for the medial wire. Make sure this lever is placed laterally under the cut trochanteric surface of the femur. The lateral drill should be directed parallel with the direction of the previous medial drill, so that both drill holes on the posterior surface of the femur are about the same distance apart as at the points of entry on the anterior surface. The lateral drill does not transfix the medullary cavity.

104

Lateral Wire Inserted

The femur is in full adduction. The serrated and angulated lever is essential at this stage. Identify the two ends of the lateral wire with colour-coded wire-holding forceps to identify the pair when tightening all the wires.

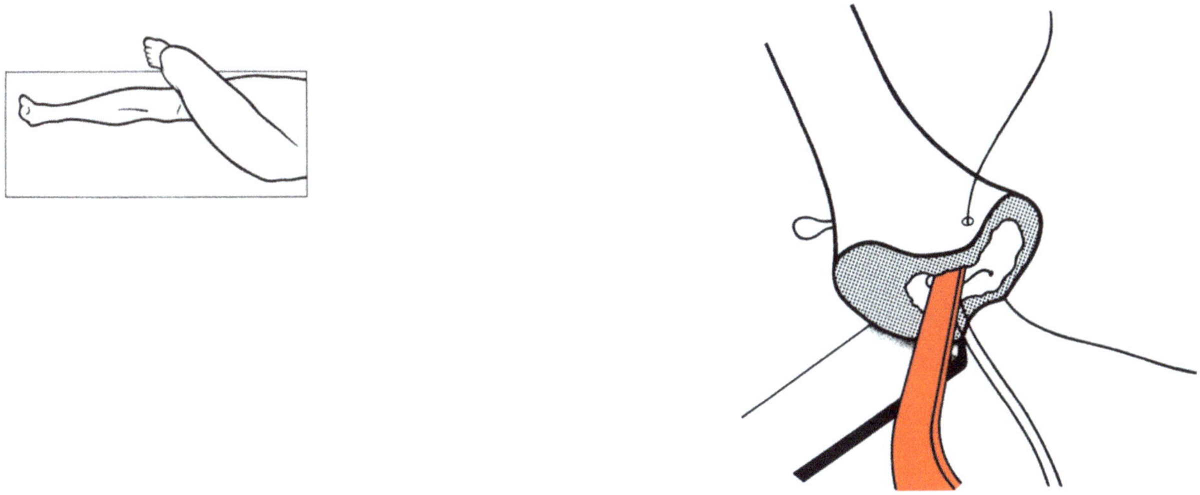

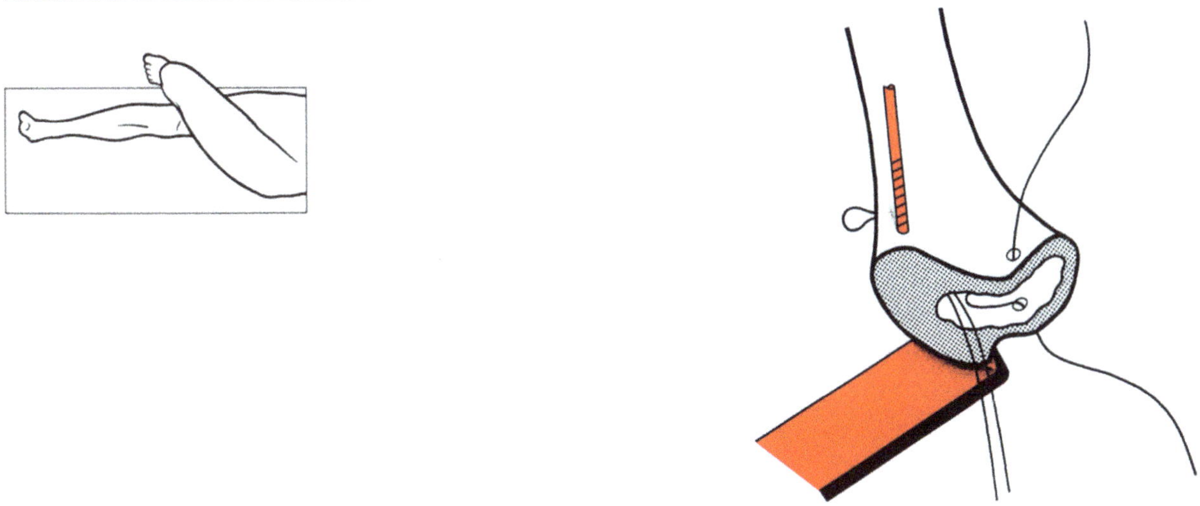

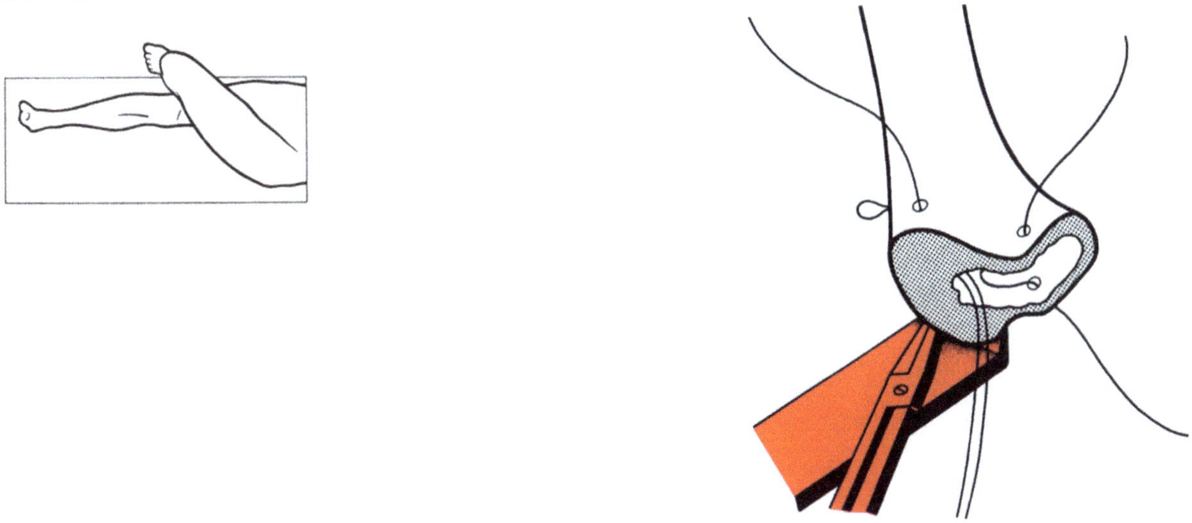

105

Access to Posterior End of Lateral Wire

This diagram shows how the angulated element of the femur lever affords access to the posterior end of the lateral wire.

106

Final Curettage of Medullary Cavity

Cementing of Femoral Prosthesis

The femur is in full adduction. The serrated and angulated lever is still in situ. Curettage of the medullary cavity should be performed quite lightly to remove osteoporotic cancellous bone and loose fatty marrow. No attempt should be made to curette vigorously down to the smooth cortical bone; this might remove all asperities capable of locking cement.

107

Rehearsal of Insertion of Prosthesis

The femur is in full adduction. The serrated and angulated lever is still in situ. Check that there is parallel alignment of the stem of the femoral prosthesis with the handle of the prosthesis holder. If there is any error in alignment make a note to allow for this. The axis of the handle of the prosthesis holder should be parallel with the axis of the femur and directed to the medial side of the patella, **P**. **Rehearsal of the insertion** will make sure that nothing will obstruct the insertion of the prosthesis in a straight line to its final **seating**. Identify landmarks to guide insertion when the medullary cavity of the femur is concealed by excess cement.

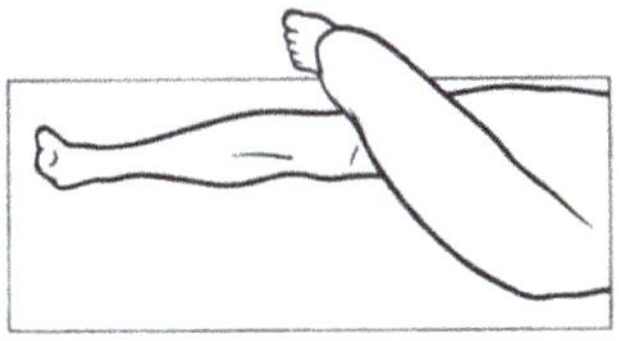

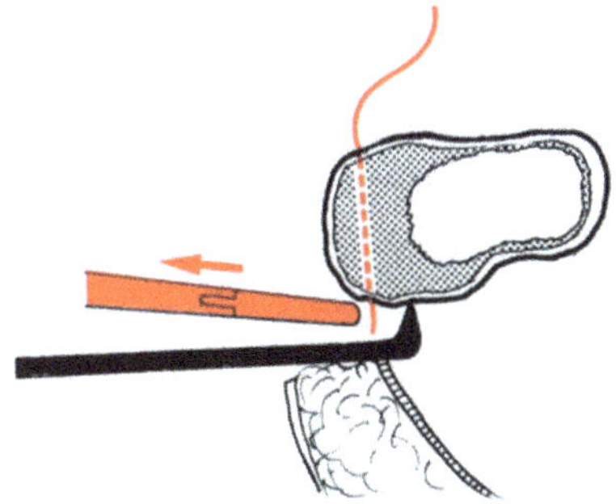

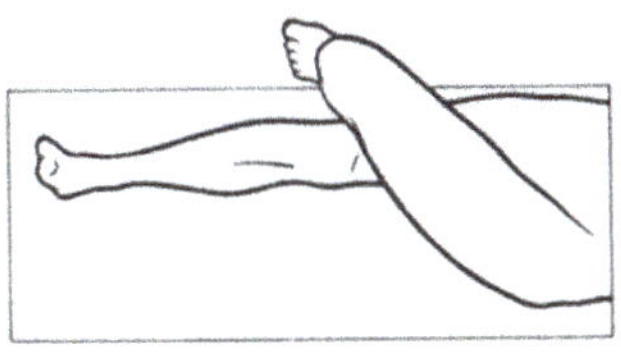

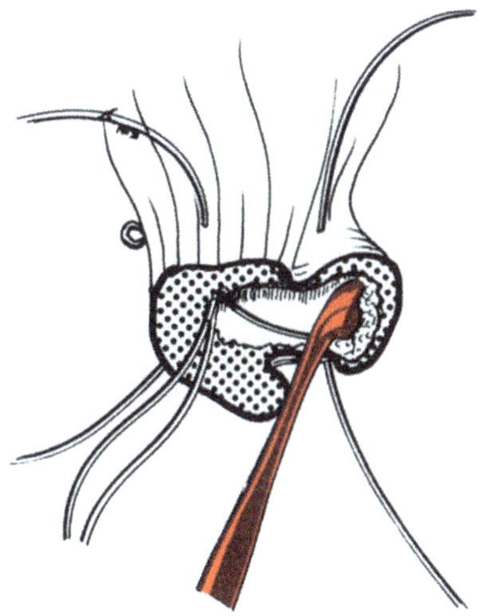

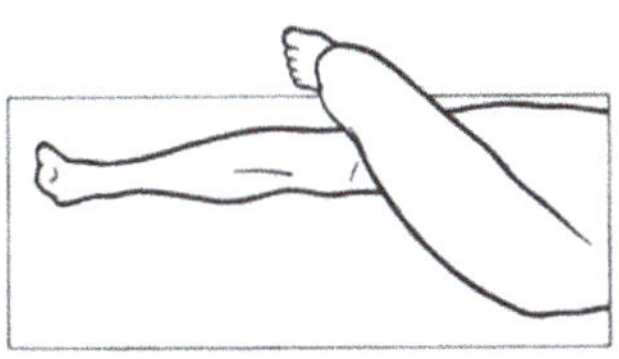

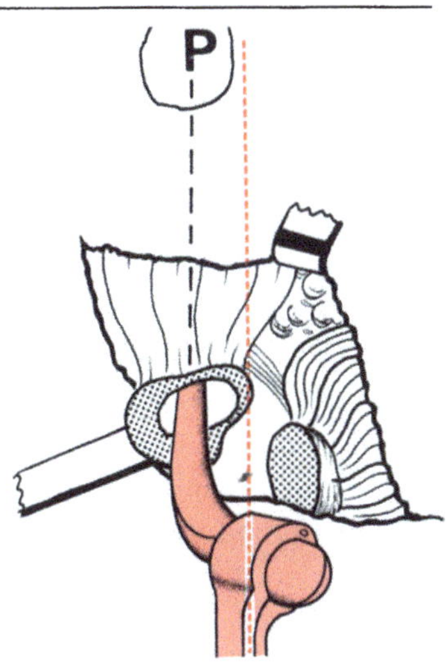
P

108

Packing Medullary Cavity with Dry Gauze

The femur is in full adduction. The medullary cavity is packed with dry gauze. There is a subtle detail in doing this effectively: when a **corner** of the gauze swab has been pushed to the furthest depth, withdraw the forceps only 1–2 cm and then grip the medial side of the gauze and push it again to full depth. Repeating this process will cause the swab to be pulled into the medullary cavity **from the depths. If pushed from the open mouth of the cavity** the gauze will impact and will not go to full depth. In reverse, when wishing to extract the gauze quickly, before inserting the cement, start by pulling out the last part of the gauze to be inserted and then it will all come out very easily.

109

Isolating Cement from Contamination with Blood

Pack dry gauze swabs behind and at sides of the upper end of the femur to prevent blood becoming mixed in with the cement. These gauze swabs should be new and not previously wetted with blood.

110

Insertion of Cement

The thumbs fit the medullary cavity like pistons. The thumb applied to the trochanter (*T*) blocks the escape of cement from this part of the open medullary cavity. The full power of insertion is generated by the 'femoral neck thumb' (*FN*) acting against the relatively passive *T* thumb.
It is important that blood should not be mixed in the cement. The last thrusts of cement are most likely to be mixed with blood unless precautions are taken against this. The last thrusts of cement occupy the most heavily stressed site, i.e. the medial femoral neck region and fragmentation of cement in the medial femoral neck region could be caused by admixed blood weakening cement at this most critical point.

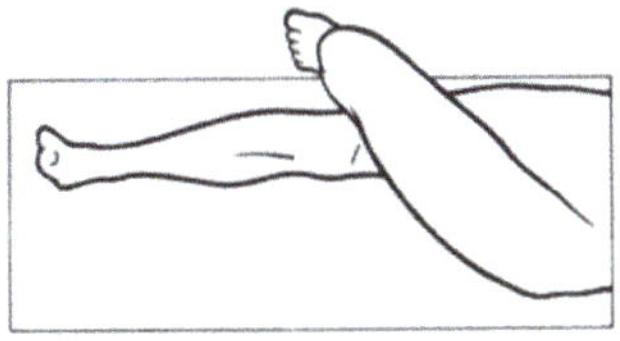

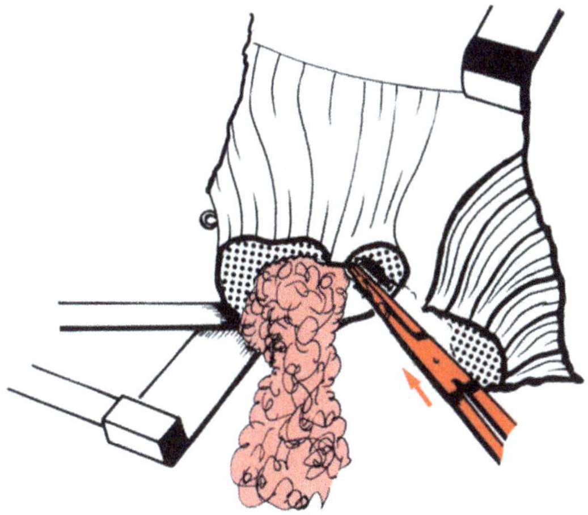

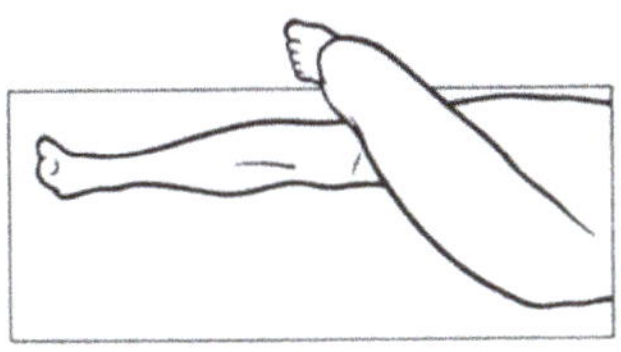

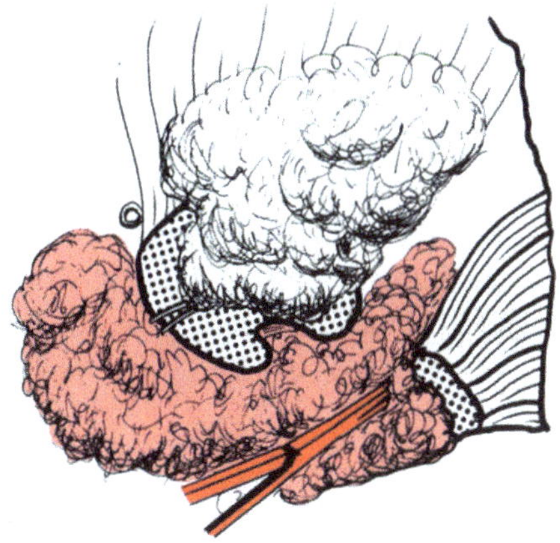

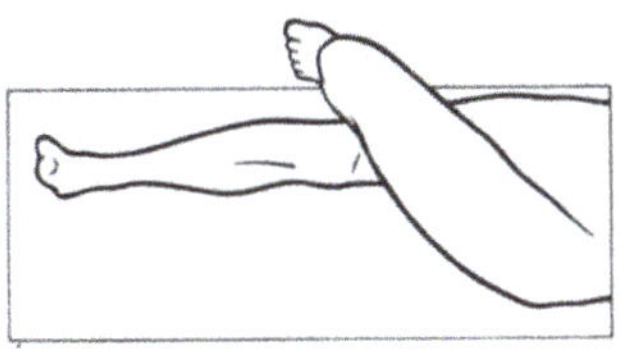

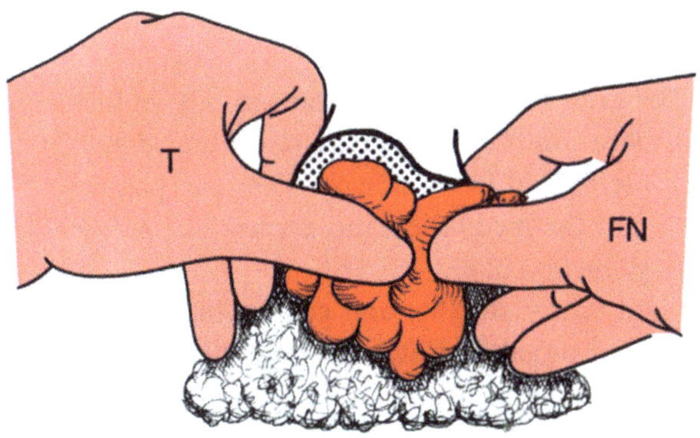

Time: 49 min

111

Insertion of Prosthesis

The prosthesis, held in the prosthesis-holder, is inserted into the cement taking alignment from the landmarks noted at the previous rehearsal (107). Insertion should be in a straight line from the point of entry of the tip of the stem, to the settling of the dorsal flange of the prosthesis in the medullary cavity. There must be no changing of direction because of unrehearsed obstacles lying in the way.

112

Packing Cement into Flanges of Prosthesis

Before the last 1–2 cm of the stem sink into the medullary cavity, pack the flanges on the front and back surfaces of the prosthesis with cement. As insertion proceeds, and as the aperture between the bone and the flange diminishes, the escape of cement as viscous dough is increasingly resisted and pressure rises. The flange reduces free escape of cement posteriorly and directs it towards the medial femoral neck.

113

Digital Pressure on Medial Femoral Neck Cement

The prosthesis-holder is removed before the cement is set to permit final application of thumb pressure on the cement in the important region of the medial femoral neck. The final packing of cement by thumb pressure at the medial femoral neck is not possible if the prosthesis has a large metal collar.

Final test of stability and general inspection after reduction of the cemented prosthesis into the socket: very occasionally a little fixed flexion with the popliteal surface of the knee failing to lie flat on the table will be found. Palpate for a tight anterior capsule with a finger in the joint. If present it can be nicked with a knife or scissors, and the leg will then lie flat. This does not impair stability or post-operative routine.

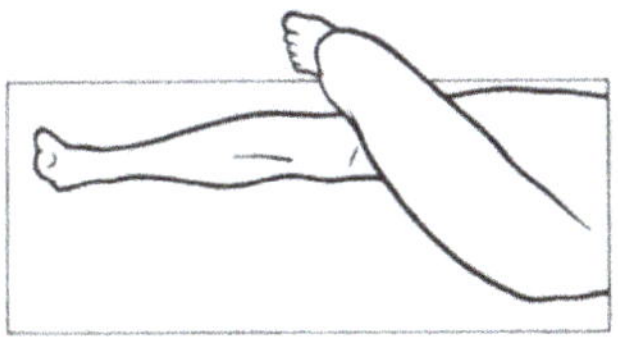

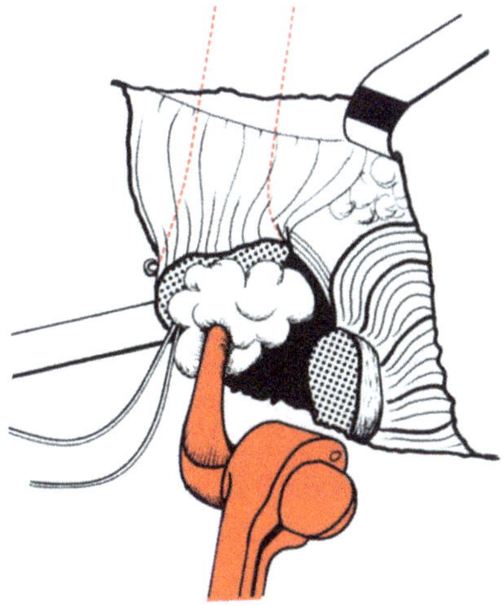

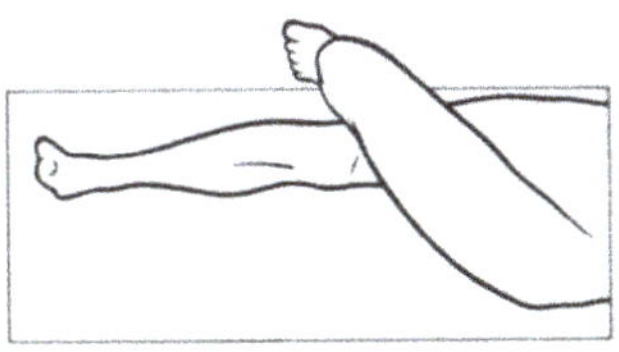

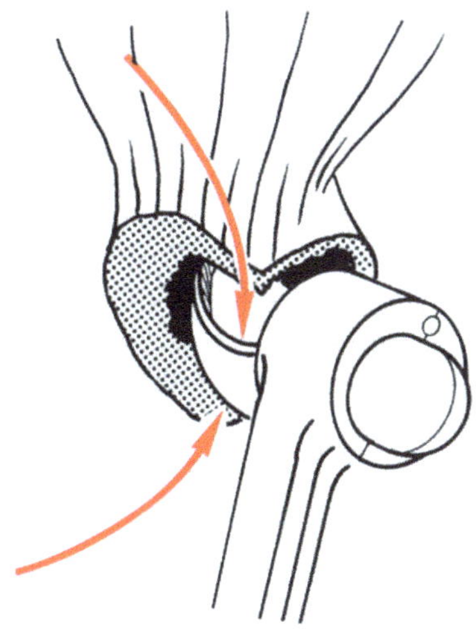

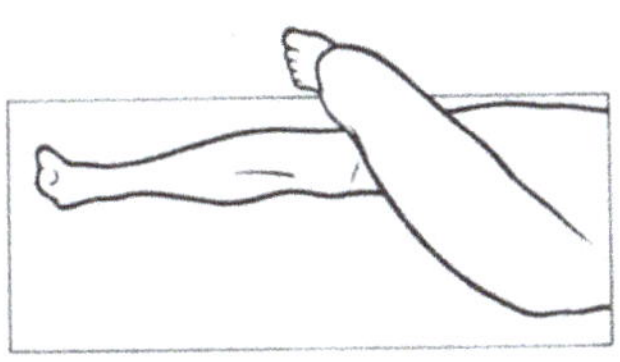

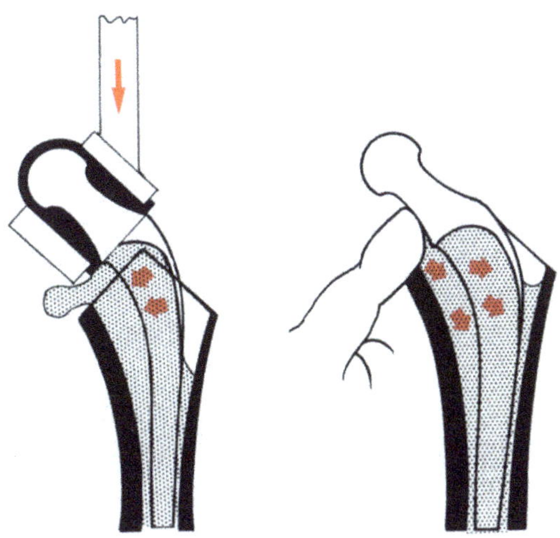

114

Position of Vertical Double Wire

Reattachment of Trochanter by Cruciate System

Before introducing the cement the double wire should be arranged to emerge from the medullary cavity **posterior to the femoral prosthesis.** If the medial wire emerges laterally, and in line with the axis of the prosthesis, there is a tendency for it to lie anterior to the centre of the trochanter and so slip forward when tightening. A useful detail is to make a 3-mm notch in the cut edge of the posterior cortex of the neck of the femur in which to locate the double wire as it emerges from the medullary canal, particularly if it is proposed to use the trochanter staple-clamp (**see** inset diagram).

115

Trochanter-Holding Forceps

The femur is in neutral position. The detached trochanter tends to lie with its distal end tilted forwards. If this is not recognized the trochanter could be reattached incorrectly and it would then seem to be wider than the surface from which it was detached. The distal end of the detached trochanter can be recognized by the cut aponeurotic fibres of vastus lateralis: if the diathermy needle was used to expose the vastus lateralis ridge a cauterised section through these fibres about 1.5 cm long will be recognizable. The trochanter-holding forceps should be applied with the handle inclined 45° higher than the jaws so as to align correctly with the forward tilted trochanter.

116

Groove for Vertical Double Wire

A large awl (6-mm diameter) with a triangular cutting, trocar point is used (Appendix C). The point of the large awl pierces the soft tissues on the lateral surface of the trochanter about one-third of the length of the trochanter from its superior margin. The awl burrows under the soft tissues keeping close to the bone and then the handle is raised to make it pierce the abductor insertion at the top of the trochanter. It is important to cut a groove in the bone of the upper margin so that the vertical double wire will lodge in it and not slip forwards or backwards. A common error is to be anterior to the mid-point of the trochanter. Check this and make a second passage of the awl if the first is not quite in the centre.

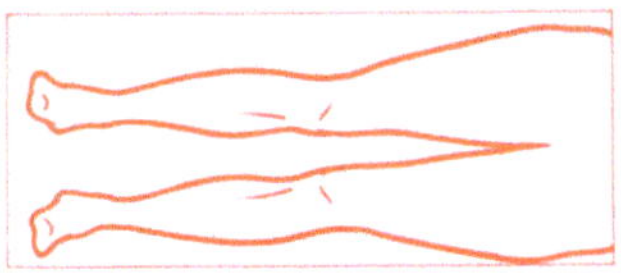

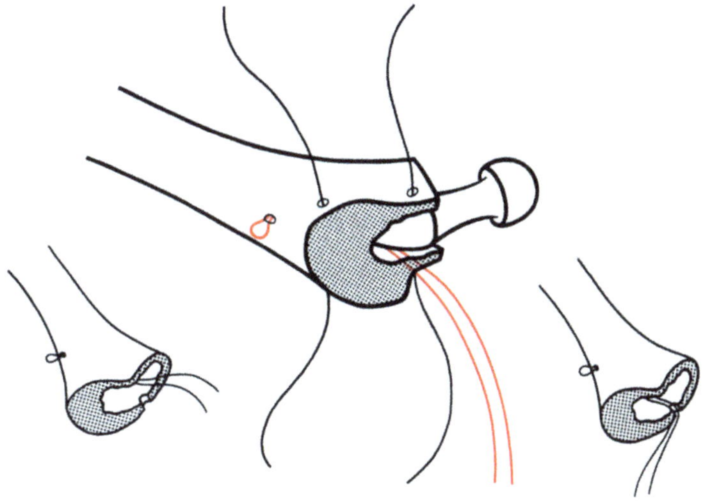

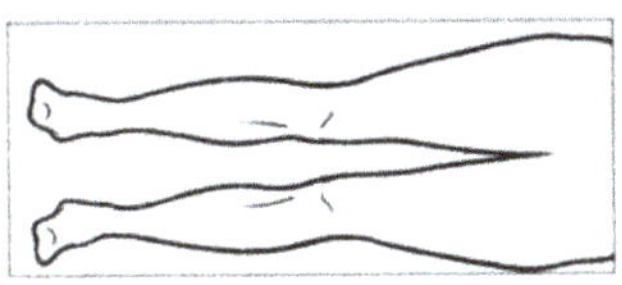

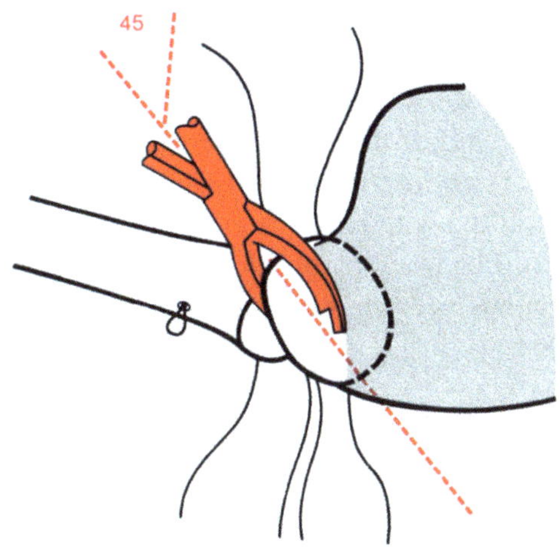

Time: 56.5 min

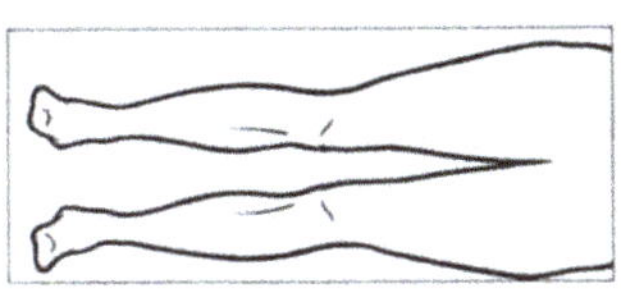

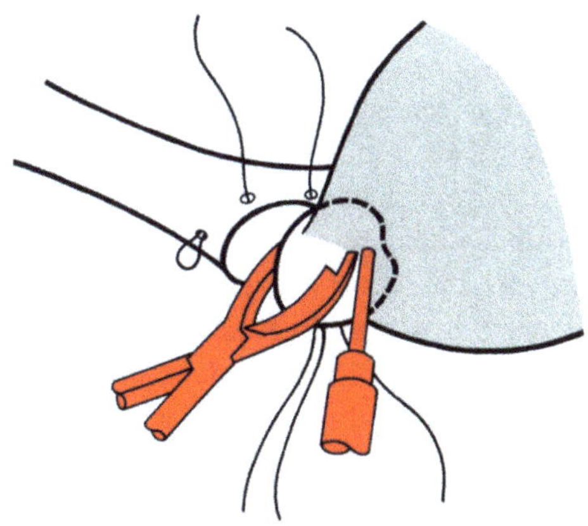

117

Quarter-Circle Wire-Passer

Still holding the trochanter in the trochanter-holding forceps the large awl is extracted and the quarter-circle wire-passer is passed in the same track. The wire-passer emerges on the deep surface as close as possible to the bone of the trochanter. The quarter-circle wire-passer (*A*) is much easier to use than the original half-circle pattern (*B*).

118

Passing Double Wire Above Trochanter

The two ends of the double wire are pushed, side by side, into the hollow end of the wire-passer. Having the two ends soldered side by side is a very useful detail. The trick of using this wire-passer is **never to pull** the wire-passer. Let the wire-passer lie passive and push it back into its track by pushing with the wires. If the wires are kept **strictly in line with the wire-passer** the stiff 18-s.w.g. material will not buckle.

119

Traction on Vertical Double Wire

Reapply the colour-coded wire-forceps to the ends of the vertical double wire. Always make sure that all ends of wire are entirely inside the jaws of the forceps to avoid the hazard of glove puncture. Make sure the double wires are not kinked as they cross the short distance between leaving the femur and entering the deep surface of the trochanter. Loops of wire crossing this zone must be carefully straightened while applying traction, and all hidden slack must be taken up. The diagram shows how traction on the double wire tends to rotate the trochanter offering a new threat that it might be reattached incorrectly.

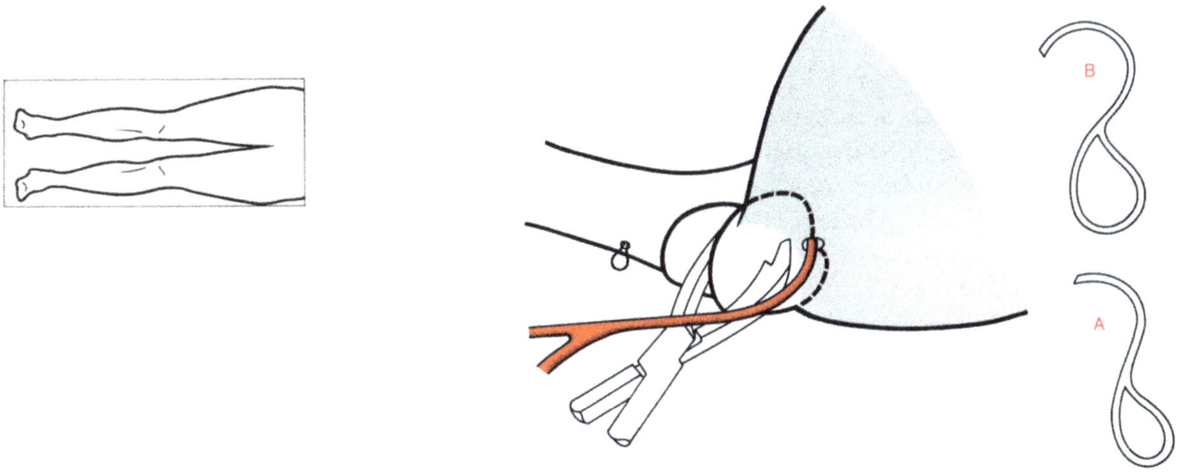
B
A

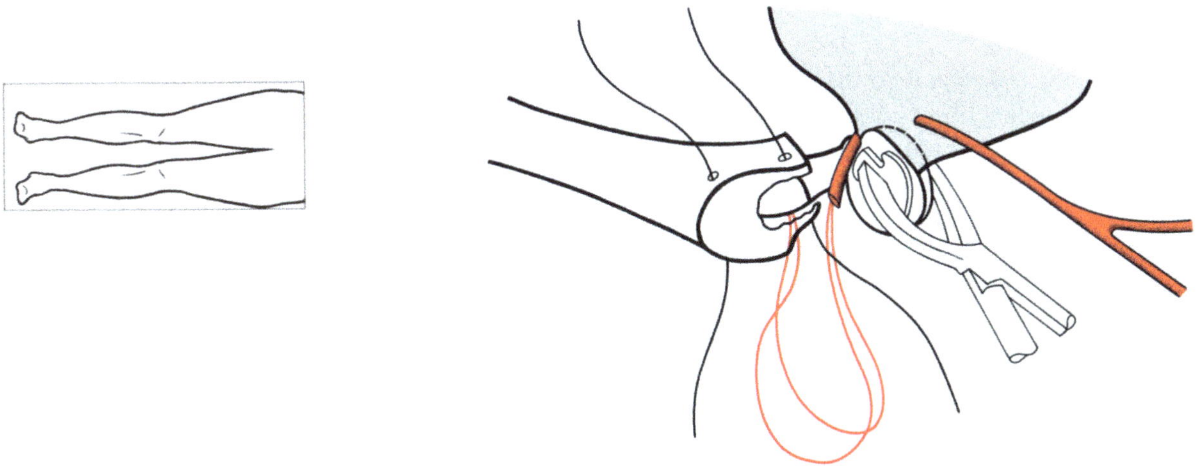

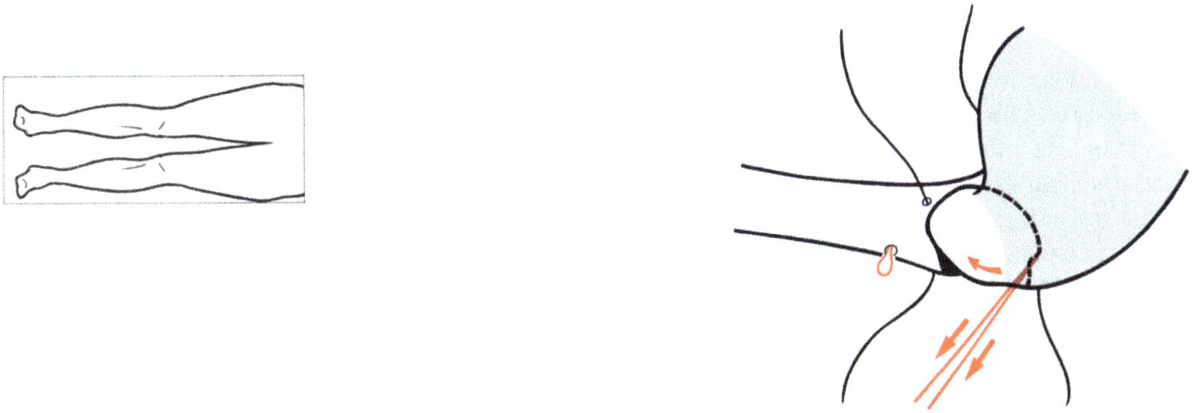

120

Temporary Tacking of Trochanter

This is a most important detail. The awl must have a narrow point, triangular or rectangular in cross-section. [Common surgical awls, with a hole in a flat, diamond-shaped point are useless in this application. On a grinding wheel such a point can be made rectangular in cross-section in a few seconds (Appendix C).] The narrow awl is applied to the trochanter in the centre of the distal end, denoted by the aponeurotic fibres of vastus lateralis still attached. The awl is driven through the thin distal end to project about 0.5 cm from the deep surface.

121

The trochanter is **rotated** so that the aponeurotic fibres lie in line with the corresponding fibres of the vastus lateralis aponeurosis on the femur. The trochanter is pegged in position by driving the awl into the femur with a few blows of the mallet. The **inset diagrams** show that the trochanter can be pegged (*a*) in its original anatomical site or (*b*) projecting beyond the lateral surface of the femur. It is never necessary to project more than 1 cm.

122

Tightening Vertical Double Wire

Turn the loop to lie horizontal. The two ends of the double wire are threaded through the wire loop by passing one end backwards from in front, and the other end forwards from behind. Check at this stage, before attaching the wire-tightener, that the wires are crossing the middle of the trochanter. An error can be that the double wire is too far forwards. If so this may need the double wire being pulled out and passed again further back on the summit of the trochanter. Apply the wire-tightener and tighten.

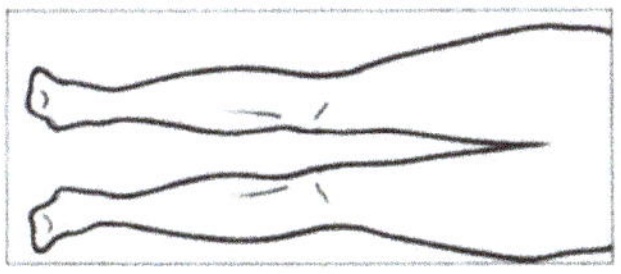

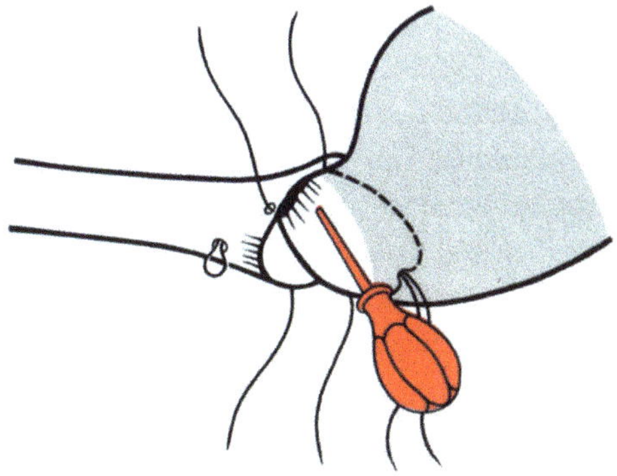

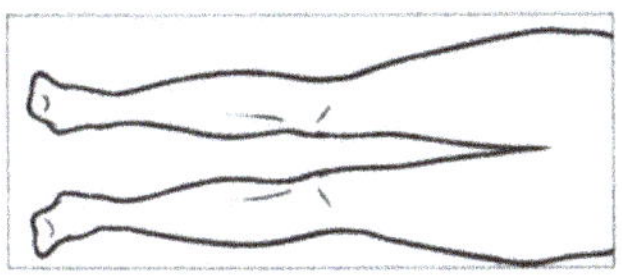

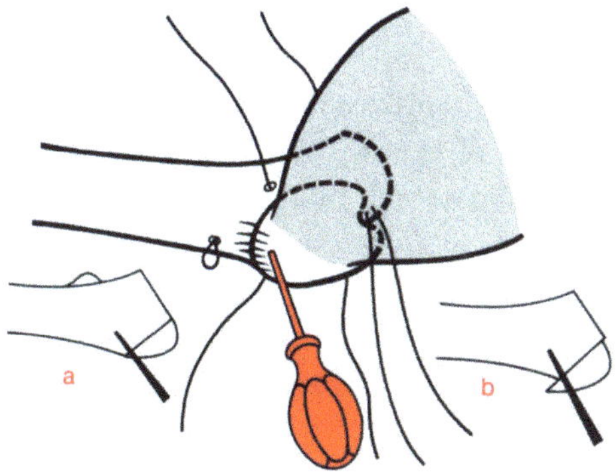
a
b

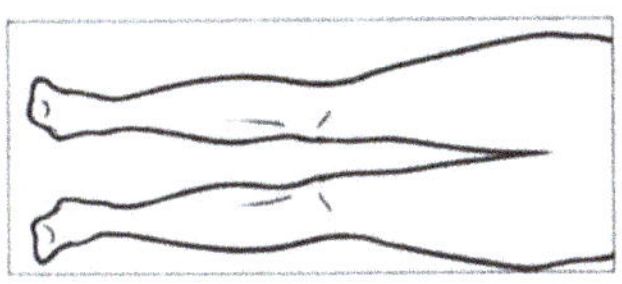

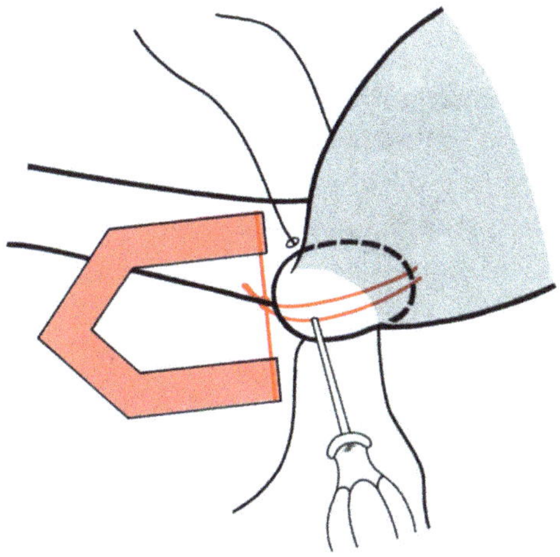

123

Punch to Complete Impaction of Trochanter

Extract the narrow awl. Apply the punch and mallet over the whole visible length of the double wire. This (1) impacts the surfaces of the trochanter and (2) corrects the position of the upper part of the trochanter if it has pulled laterally during tightening to leave a gap underneath it; (3) buries the wire in soft tissues to minimise loosening by necrosis of intervening tissue. Apply the punch to the wire loop. Tighten again; perhaps a quarter of a turn. The amount of tension to apply defies description. There is no point in risking wire breakage or splitting the bone because the cruciate system adds more pressure later.

124

Twisting Wire and Cutting Off

Twisting is preferred to tying knots (Chapt. 12, p. 146). The sequence of steps in the twisting technique using a 'spreader-type' wire-tightener is as follows: (*1*) Pull on the body of the wire-tightener to deflect the wire 0.5 cm from the straight line. (*2*) Maintaining the pull, twist the body of the tightener about 45° in a **clockwise** direction. This will lock the wires by friction. (*3*) Slacken the wire-tightener **at the same time keeping traction on the body of the tightener.** Continue slackening until the wires are nearly at 90° to each other. Twist the body of the tightener **clockwise**. For each clockwise turn of the body of the tightener slacken the tightener screw with one anti-clockwise turn. It is impossible then to brake the wire. Cut off wire and hammer flat against bone with punch.

125

Completion of Vertical Wire

The diagram shows the state at the completion of the vertical double loop. The four wires (two medial and two lateral wires) are now to be made into the cruciate wire system. For clarity of presentation in the subsequent diagrams the completed double vertical wire will be omitted. The cruciate system is applied on top of the vertical double wire.

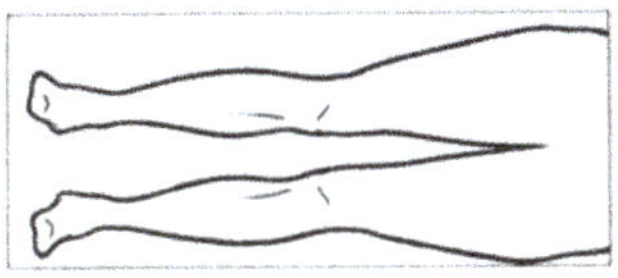

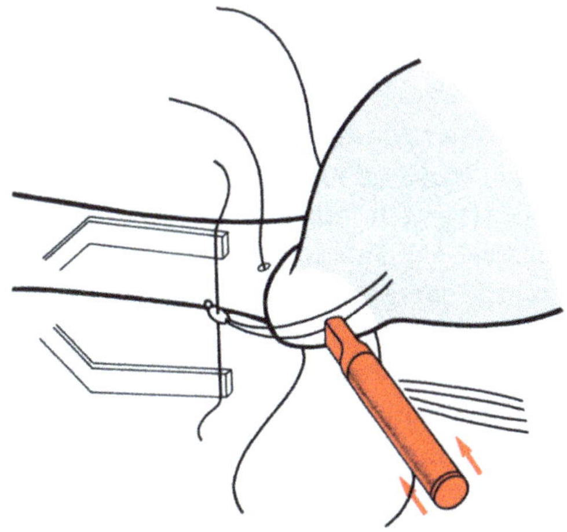

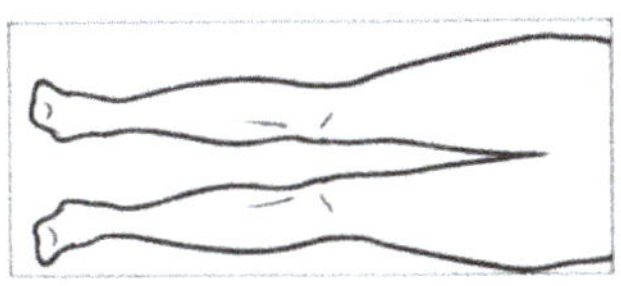

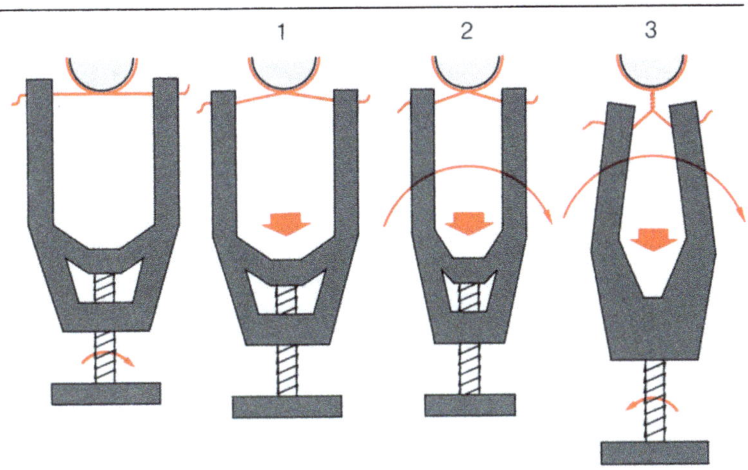
1
2
3

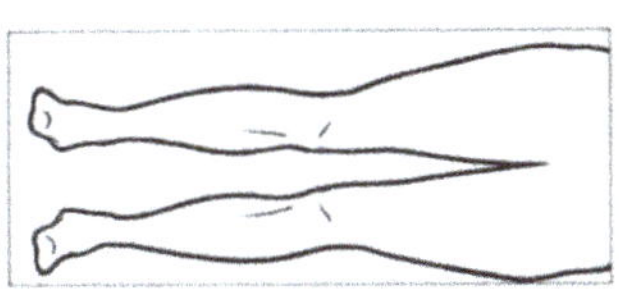

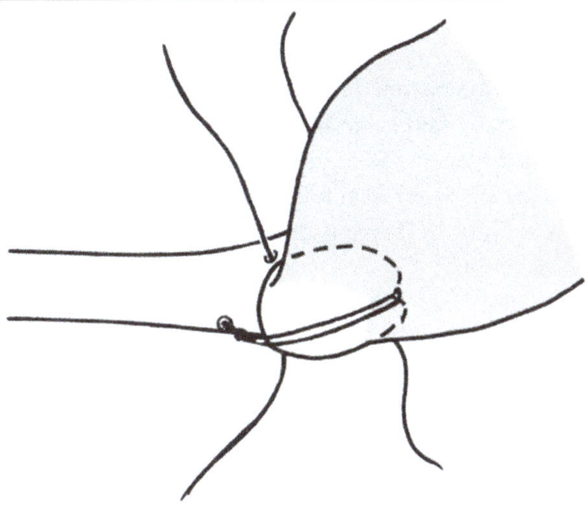

126

Cruciate Wiring Step 1

The anterior end of the medial wire is to be brought out above the trochanter and through the abductor muscles. The wire-passer (quarter-circle) is passed medially and forwards through the track of the double vertical wire to become visible under the anterior edge of the gluteus medius. The anterior end of the medial wire is inserted into the hollow end of the wire-passer. Hold the wire in the forceps with only about 1 cm projecting into the hollow end of the wire-passer. If there is too much wire between the forceps and the wire-passer (say 4 cm) it will bend and fail to push out the wire-passer. Using the forceps, push on the wire in a curved line in continuity with the curve of the wire-passer. The wire-passer is allowed to lie passive and the wire pushes it back and out of the track above the trochanter.

127

Cruciate Wiring Step 2

Reattach the colour-coded wire-forceps and pull out slack from the point of emergence from the neck of the femur. Lay this wire aside by depositing the forceps in an anterior position (*A*). Now take **the posterior end of the medial wire** and bend into a hook (*B*). Take a straight awl with a hole in the tip (Appendix C) and enter this into the same track as the double vertical wire over the tip of the trochanter. Direct the awl posteriorly and medially, in the direction of the point of emergence from the femur of the posterior end of the medial wire. Raise the handle of the awl to vertical; internally rotate the femur; retract tissues posterior to the trochanter till the hole in the awl is visible. Introduce the hook on the posterior end of the medial wire.

128

Cruciate Wiring Step 3

The posterior part of the medial wire has been pulled through the muscle and is laid aside by depositing it in a posterior position (in colour-coded forceps). The posterior end of the lateral wire (henceforth called the PL wire) is now brought forward, to lie between the two medial wires, and its forceps deposited in the direction of the patient's opposite shoulder.

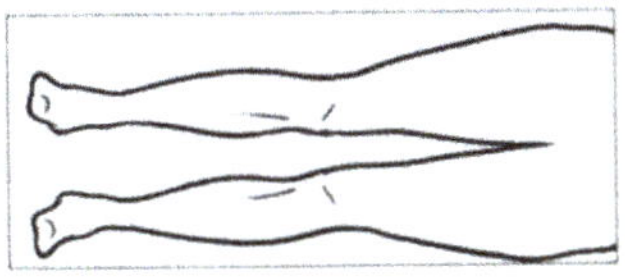

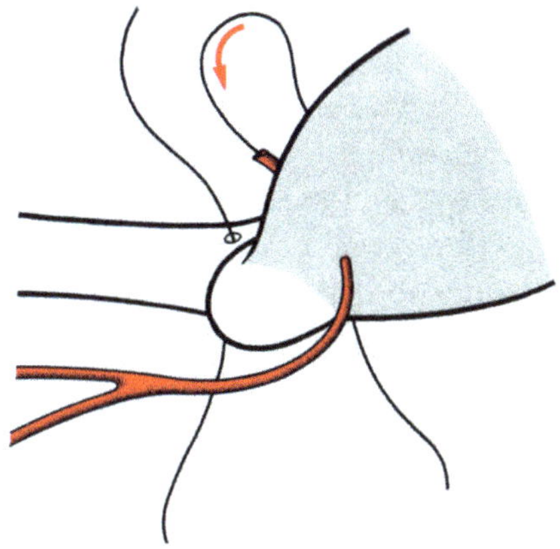

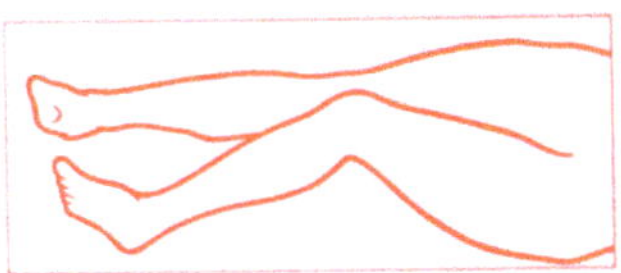

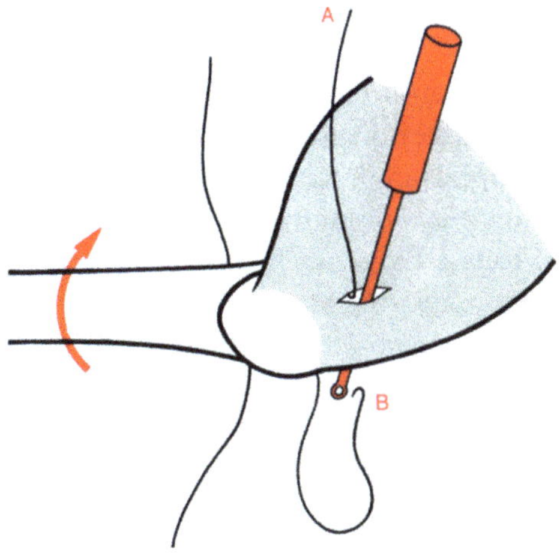
A
B

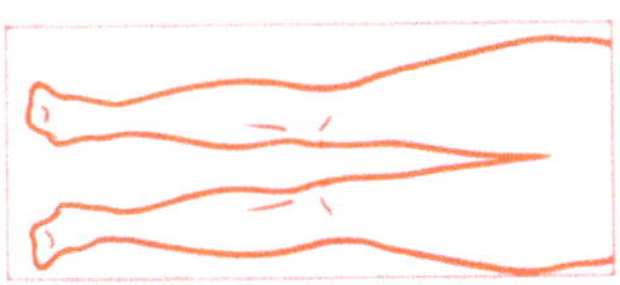

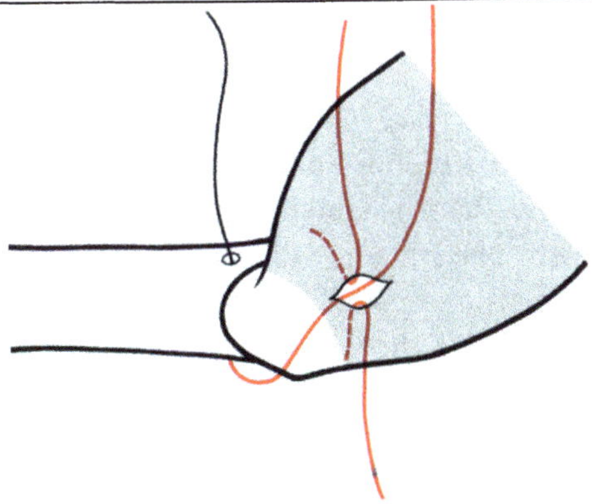

129

Cruciate Wiring Step 4

The PL wire remains untouched. The anterior and posterior ends of the medial wire are crossed over the PL wire by passing the posterior end forwards and the anterior end backwards. Make the cross-over so that it will twist in a clockwise direction. Insert the narrow awl into the trochanter so that the cross-over lies distal to it. (The position of the PL wire in relation to the awl is not important.)

130

Cruciate Wiring Step 5

The awl ensures that the cross-over stays near the centre of the trochanter, and enables the wire to be strongly tightened without the cross-over disappearing proximally into the muscle. To resist strong tightening, the assistant must hold the handle of the awl to prevent its being deflected. On removing the awl the twisted wire tends to slide up into the muscle; but when the PL wire is finally tightened, to act on the pulley made by this cross-over, the planned situation is restored. Tightening of the crossed medial wires ensures that the proximal end of the detached trochanter is compressed against the femur. The crossed wires are twisted and cut off leaving about 1 cm of vertical wire projecting, **for concealment as the last step of the cruciate wiring procedure**.

131

Cruciate Wiring Step 6

The wire-passer is inserted under the anterior edge of the gluteus medius muscle, keeping close to the bone of the trochanter, and is brought out above the trochanter through the same track used for the vertical double wire. The PL wire is inserted into the end of the wire-passer and passed through the muscle to emerge on the deep surface. (Again this is done by pushing the wire-passer back along its own track by the stiff, 18-s.w.g. wire, held by forceps close to the end of the wire-passer.) Note the smooth curve of the PL wire to assist its passage through the muscle.

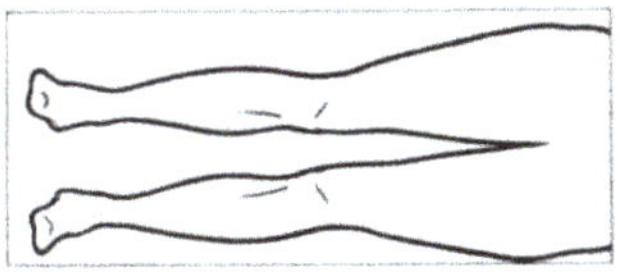

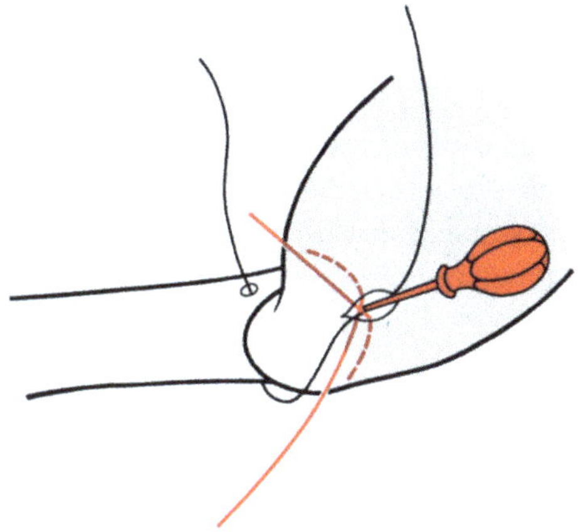

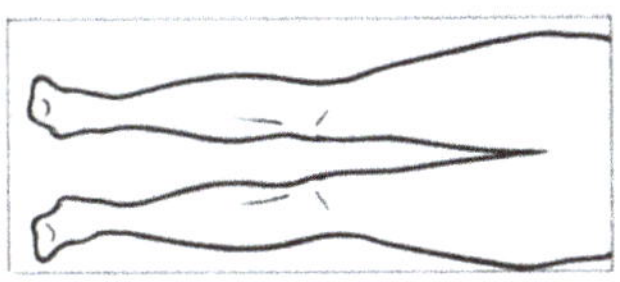

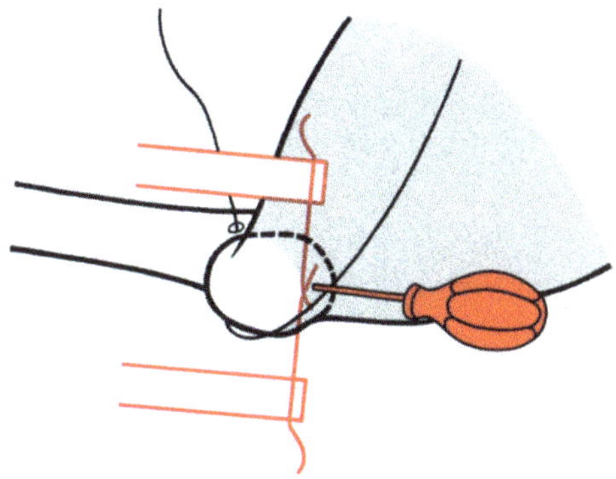

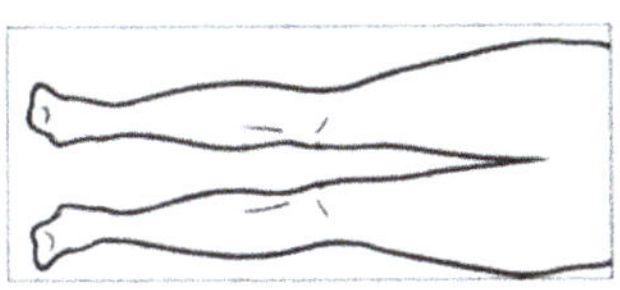

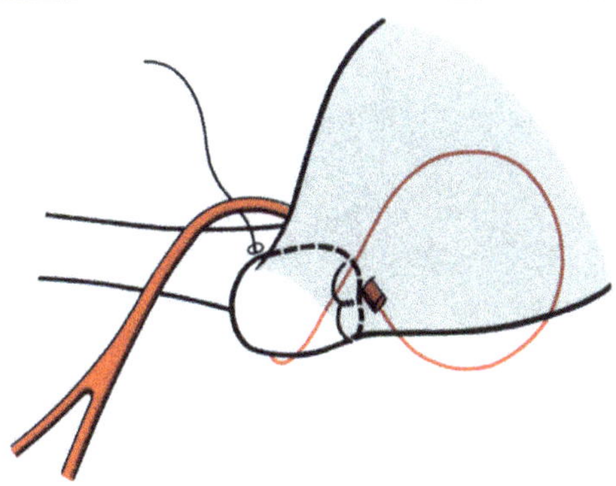

132

Cruciate Wiring
Step 7

The PL wire is brought out from under the anterior edge of the gluteus medius muscle **taking care it runs smoothly from the external loop without kinks**. It is then crossed over the **anterior end of the lateral wire**, the cross-over being for a clockwise twist. The wire-tightener is attached and tightening started.

133

Cruciate Wiring
Step 8

After tightening and twisting (as described in 124) the wire is cut off and the projecting end hammered flat with punch and hammer.

134

Cruciate Wiring
Step 9

This is the final step of removing the projecting, cut end of twisted wire left from step 5 (130). If this is not done the twisted end may project laterally and if seen by the patient in the X-ray the appearance may suggest a cause for pain. The $^{1}/_{4}$-in. (6-mm) awl (Appendix C) is used to make a hole in the lateral cortex of the trochanter close to the base of the twisted and projecting end. This is easily done by rotating the triangular trocar point. The projecting end of wire is then hammered flat to lie across the hole so made. With a narrow punch, having a fish-tail end (Appendix C) the twisted end is punched into the hole. The absence of any projecting wires on the bursal surface of the trochanter at the completion of this technique is very satisfactory.

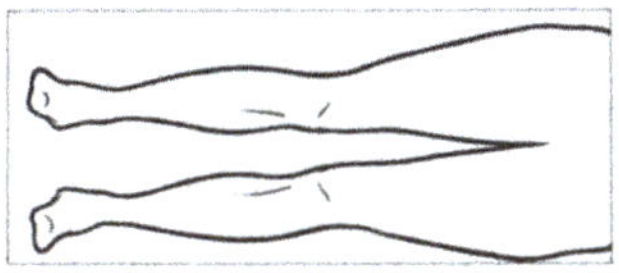

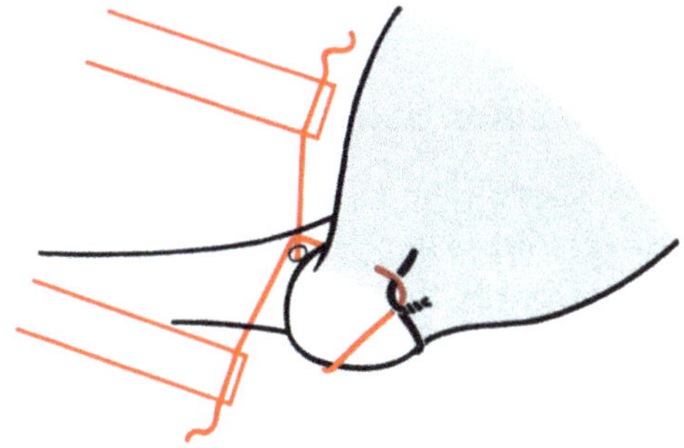

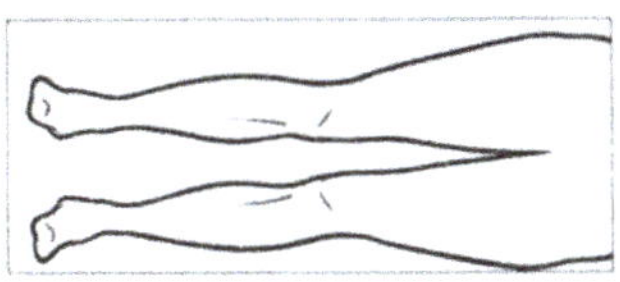

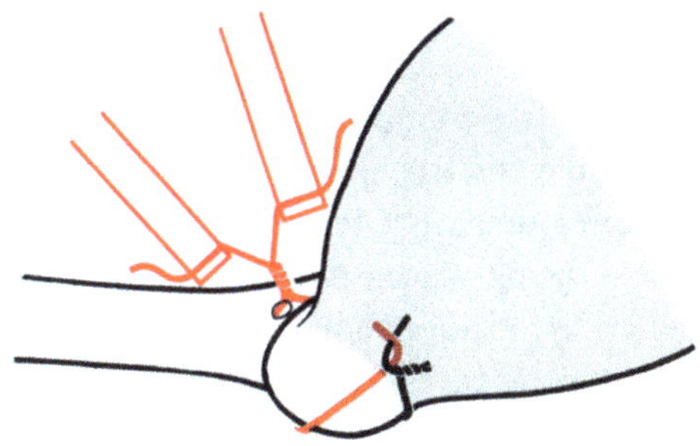

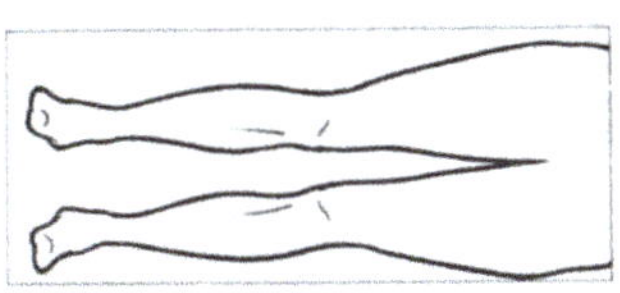

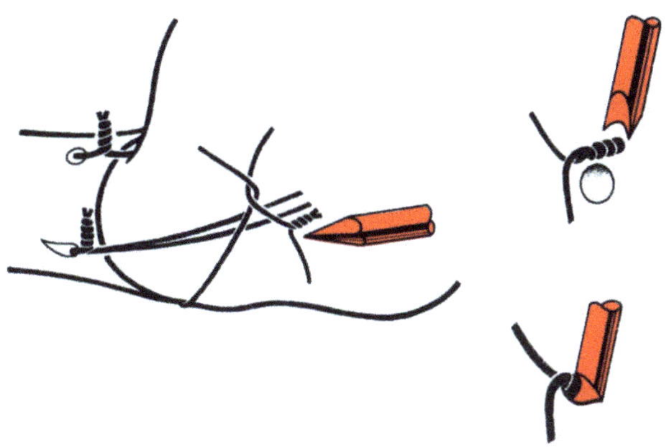

Trochanter Staple-Clamp

The staple-clamp is optional (though considered by the author to be of very great importance) and can be supplementary to any form of wire fixation for the trochanter favoured by the surgeon. When the staple-clamp is to be combined with the cruciate wiring system its insertion is started immediately after 119. The preliminary phases occupy only 3 steps and thereafter the cruciate wiring system proceeds, as already described, from 120 to end at 134. The final steps of the staple-clamp are resumed at 135 to end at 141. The first three steps of the staple-clamp will be designated with the letters A, B and C added to 119.

119 A

Cutting Femur Groove

With a narrow bone rongeur ($^1/_4$-in. or 6-mm-wide jaws) a groove is cut across the trochanteric surface on the femur in a roughly antero-posterior direction. Prominence of the prosthesis may necessitate the groove being placed more laterally than the mid-point. The posterior end of the groove should be as medial as possible, even if this makes the anterior part of the groove incline laterally; this is because prominence of the anterior staple is more easily concealed than prominence of the posterior staple.

119 B

Length-Measuring Gauge

The length-measuring gauge is applied to the groove, as in the diagram, and tightened. The length of rod projecting beyond the sliding component of the gauge will be equal to the length of screw projecting from the nut of the staple-clamp when tightening is complete. The length-measuring gauge is set aside for the later stages.

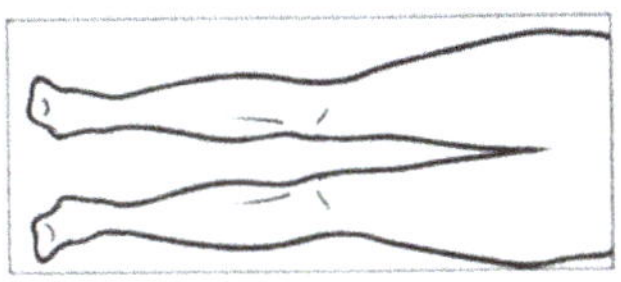

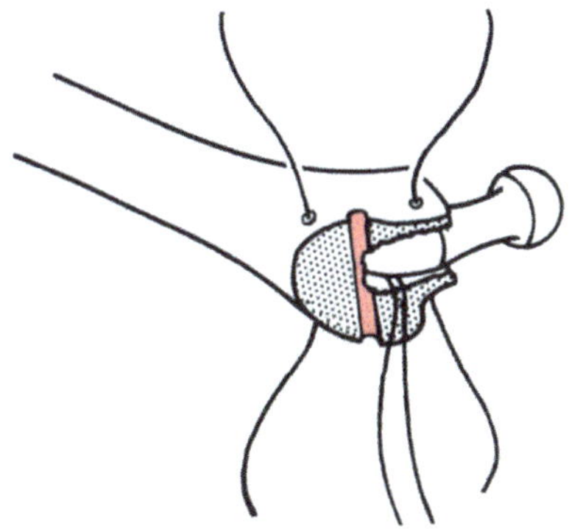

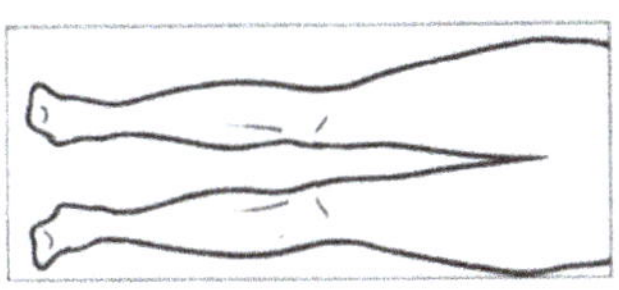

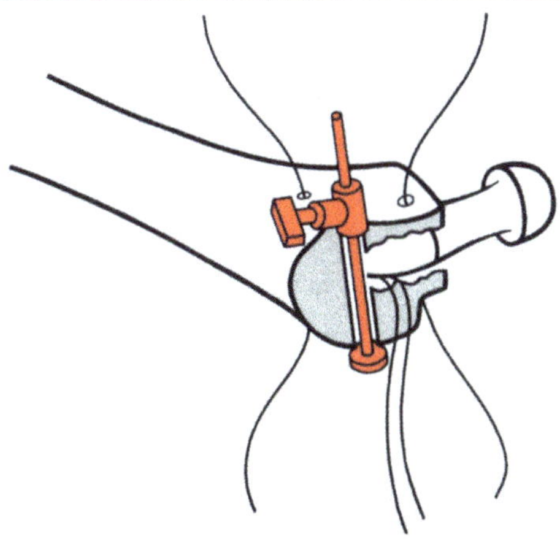

119 C

Application of Staple-Clamp

The nut and the anterior staple are removed from the clamp. The clamp is held by the assistant using (1) a forceps for the posterior staple and (2) a perforated rod for the anterior end (Appendix C). If the screwed rod touches the metal of the prosthesis it should be insulated with the plastic sleeve. **Pinch the plastic sleeve flat** before threading on to the screwed rod, so that it will not slip downwards when the rod is held vertically. The posterior staple should be held 1–2 cm below the level of the femur, so as not to obstruct siting of the trochanter. The assistant presses the staple-clamp into the groove and he remains immobile in this position until the end of the next step, 119 D. The surgeon must thread the vertical double wire and start to tighten it without help from the assistant at this stage.

119 D

Start of Wiring of Trochanter

This stage is stage 120 already described, with the addition of the staple-clamp. From this point the staple-clamp, in situ, is ignored and the cruciate wiring system proceeds till it finishes at 134. Once the tightening of the vertical double wire has been started the assistant can remove the perforated rod holding the anterior end of the staple and ignore the posterior forceps till stage 135 is reached.

This hiatus represents the completing of the cruciate wiring stages **already described and illustrated** as 119–134. The stages in the completion of the trochanter staple-clamp will now be taken up as from 135 onwards.

135

Punch Mark on Staple

Both staples bear punch marks to indicate the end to engage in the detached trochanter. The punch marks are required because, for anatomical reasons, the staples are not symmetrical. Always mount the posterior staple in the forceps with the punch mark towards the handle.

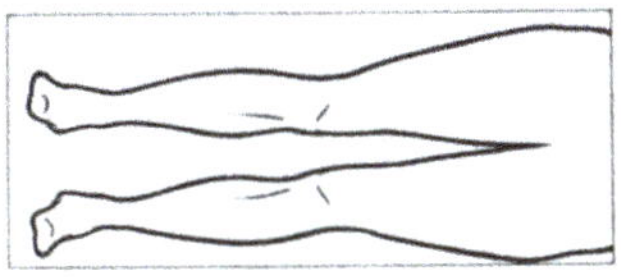

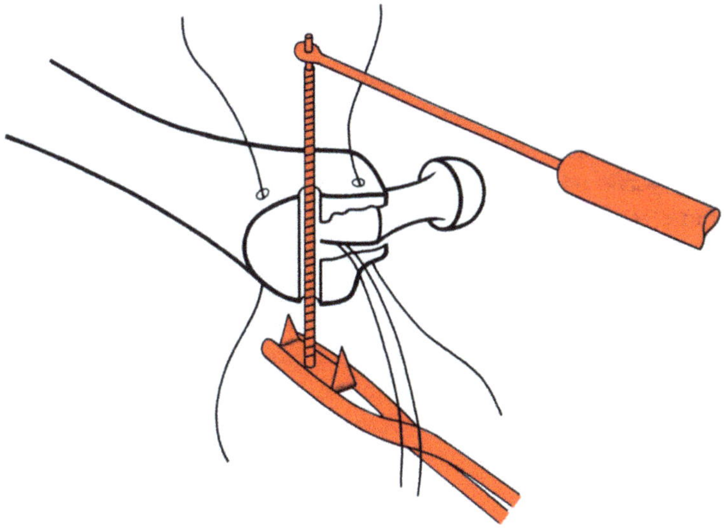

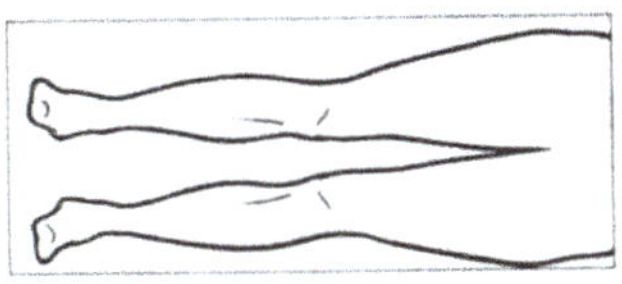

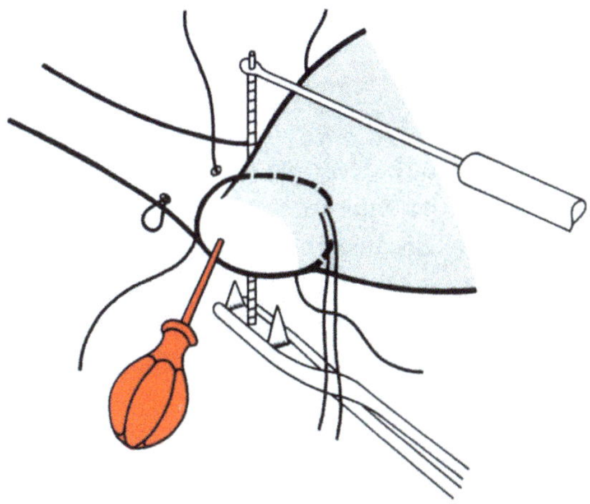

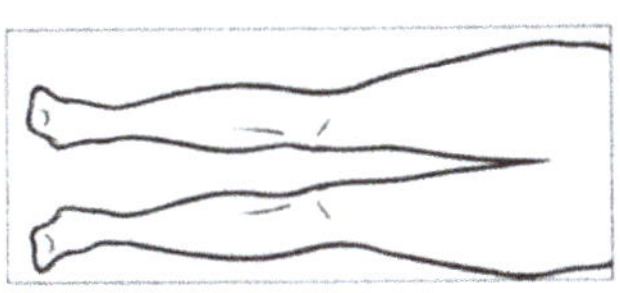

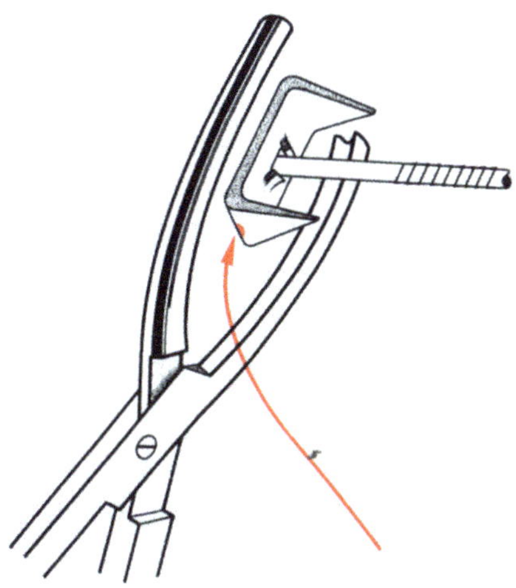

136

Application of Anterior Staple and Nut

The anterior edge of the gluteus medius muscle is retracted, and the anterior staple slipped over the threaded bolt with the punch-mark directed towards the trochanter. The staple should be perpendicular to the line of the osteotomy. The anterior staple should be punched into the bone with hammer and punch used alternately on the two ends. **Note** that the plastic bush in the anterior staple must be inserted by the manufacturer with **the wide flange underneath the staple** (not on top as might be thought best for receiving the pressure of the nut). In the latter case it is impossible to punch the staple into position without the bush being knocked out of the staple. The screw threads will be damaged if the bush does not function properly and the nut will seize on the thread.

137

Tightening the Nut

The nut is slipped over the plain, anterior end of the screwed rod. The hexagonal end of the nut is downwards. A tubular spanner is used to tighten the nut. The posterior staple should be aligned rather more vertically than the anterior staple to make sure it does not project and is not visible. Because the posterior staple is out of sight the line of the forceps gives its direction. Note: The tubular spanner must be in line with the screwed rod to permit tightening of the nut. The curved incision in the deep fascia (4–10) greatly facilitates this and some external rotation of the femur also helps.

138

Final Punch to Anterior Staple

The anterior staple cannot be compressed to its final position by tightening the nut alone. This is because the anterior cortex of the femur is thick and strong while posterior cortices of both femur and trochanter are thin and soft. The posterior staple could sink into the bone while the anterior staple would still be projecting from the surface of the femur. It is most important that the distal spike of the anterior staple (the short spike) should be punched into the cortical bone before final tightening.

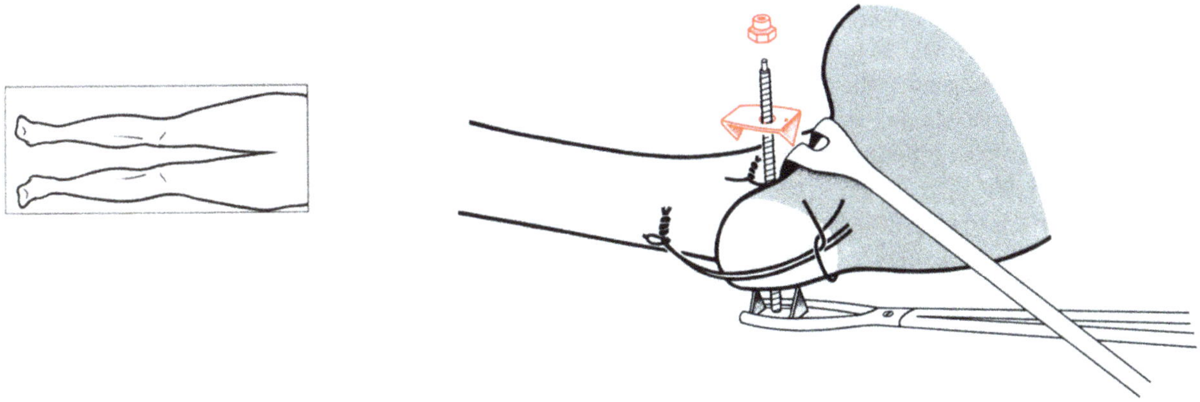

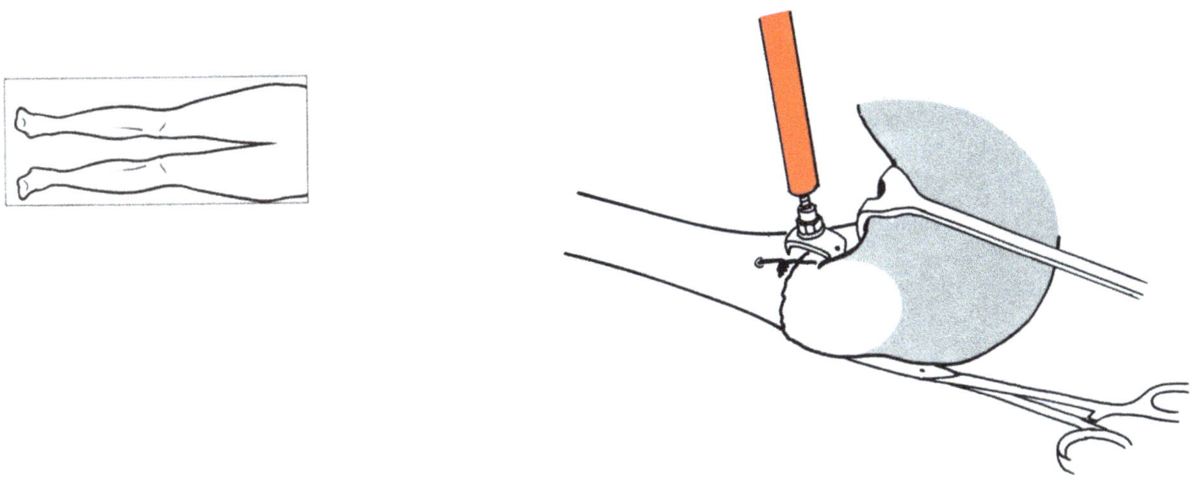

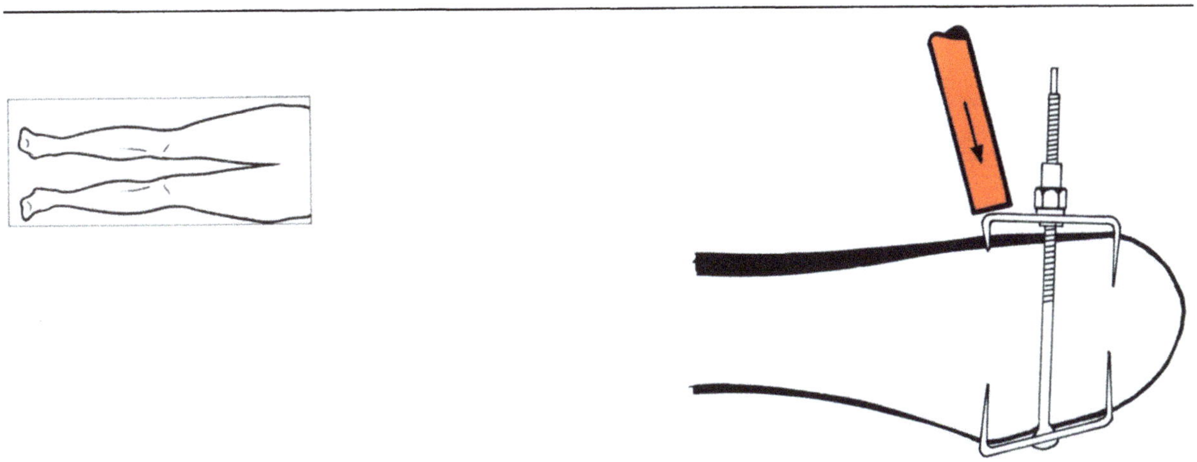

139

Estimating Tightening

The measuring gauge is applied to the projecting screwed rod in the reversed position as shown. When the projecting ends of both the gauge and the screwed rod are equal, tightening is approaching finality. There will be no increased resistance to tightening in osteoporotic bone and the length-gauge alone will indicate the end of tightening. Despite this the staple-clamp is considered to be very important in osteoporotic bone.

140

Cutting Off Screw

A bolt cutter is applied to the nut and both the sleeve of the nut and the screwed rod are cut simultaneously. The crushed sleeve provides a locking mechanism.

141

Filing Cut End of Nut

The bolt cutter leaves two sharp 'ears' which could tear a surgeon's glove when inserting suction drains. A **fine-toothed** file is used to round off the sharp ears. Do not file away too much metal or the locking action will be lost.

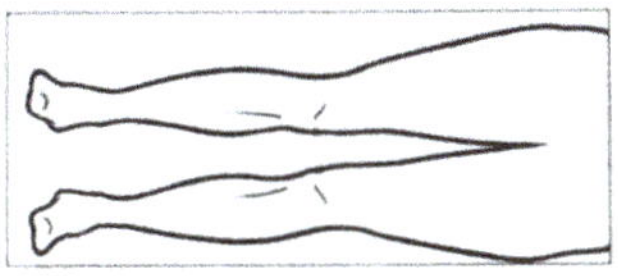

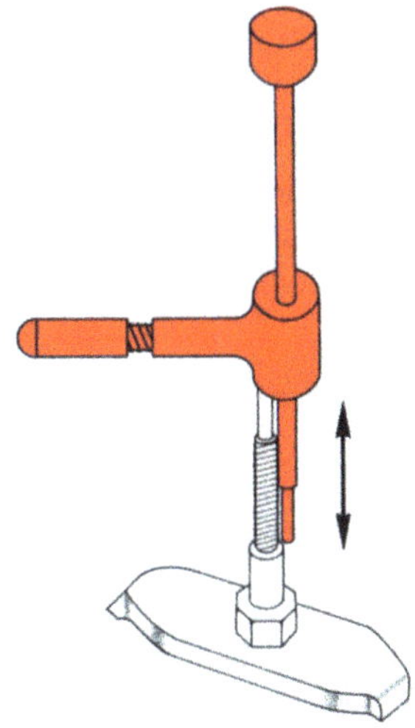

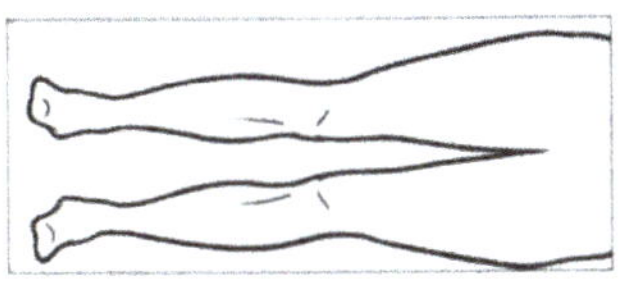

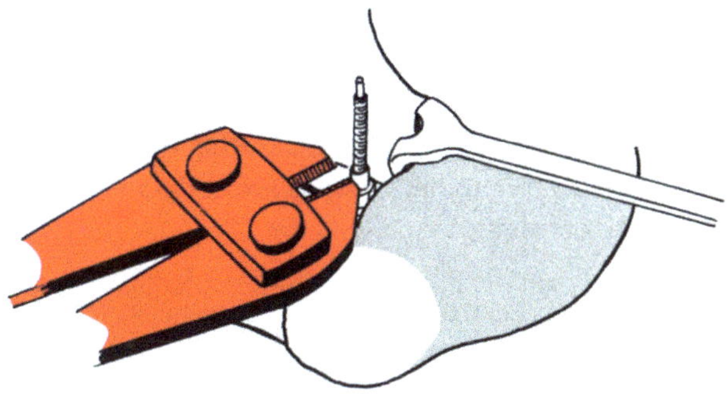

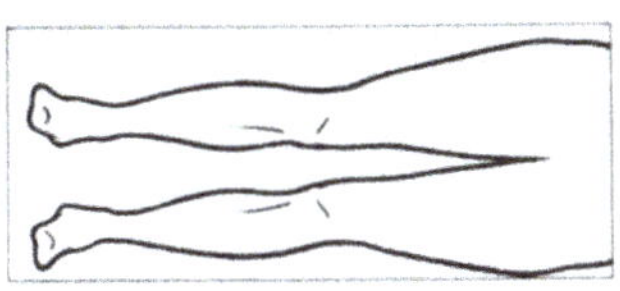

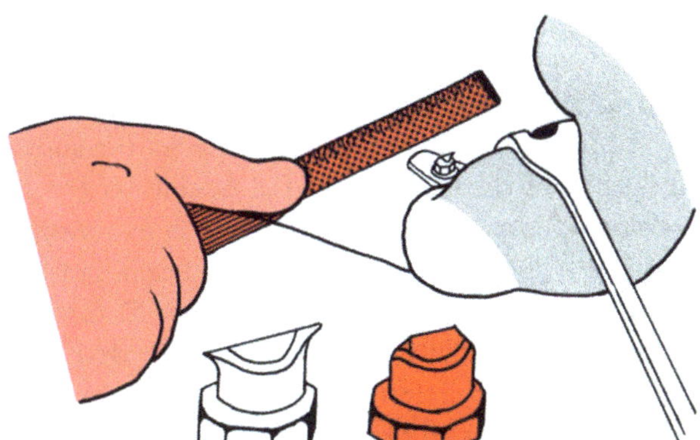

Time: 67 min

142

Suction Drains

Closure of Wound

Two deep suction drains are used. Tubing 3-mm in external diameter is preferred. This type of tube is equivalent to 12 fr stomach tube.

143

Suction Drains

It is preferred that the drains should emerge in a dependent direction to facilitate drainage of the track after the drains have been pulled out. It is quite simple to ensure that the stylets emerge on the postero-lateral aspect of the thigh.

144

Closure of Deep Fascia

Two central sutures are applied first. The diagram shows that when the curved incision in the deep fascia is used the sutures will lie anterior to the site of reattachment of the trochanter (*cross* and *circle*). This is considered important and is effective in avoiding discomfort from mechanical bursitis. Sutures in the deep fascia must never be absorbable. The deep fascia is an important tendon; absorbable sutures are not safe if early, full rehabilitation is to be encouraged. Interrupted, figure-of-eight sutures are preferred. Personal preference is for black silk, which offers high-frictional resistance in knots. Square knots are less likely to slip than are twists made by single-handed ties. The surgeon's square knot (with three throws on the first half-hitch) tied slowly with two hands is the author's preference.

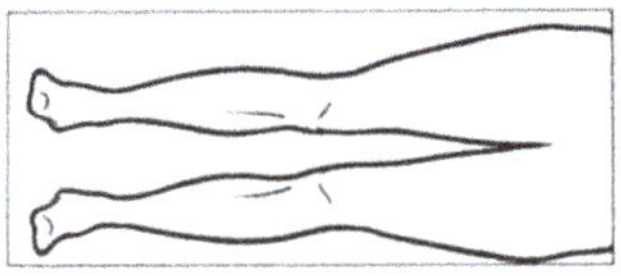

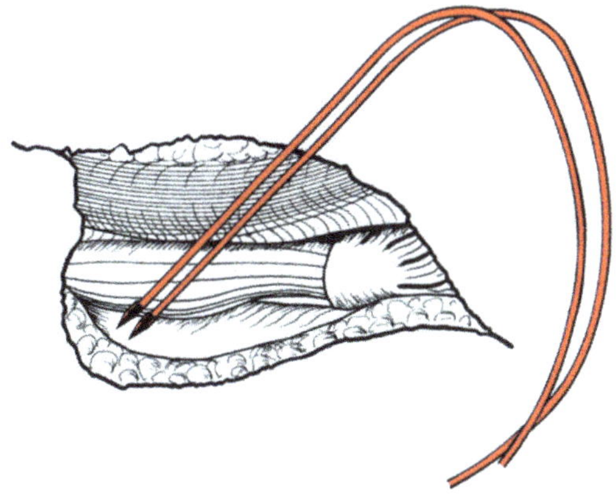

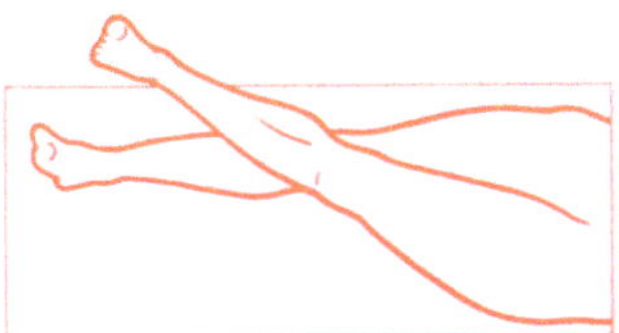

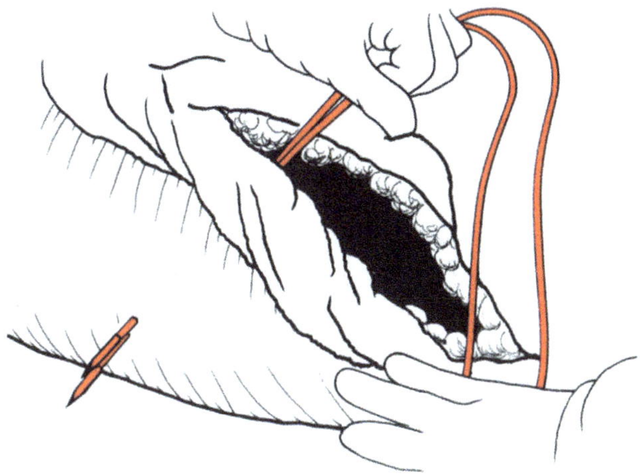

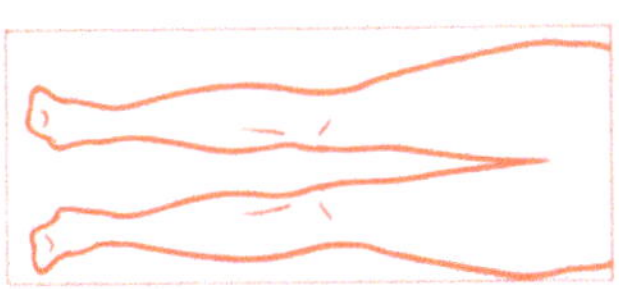

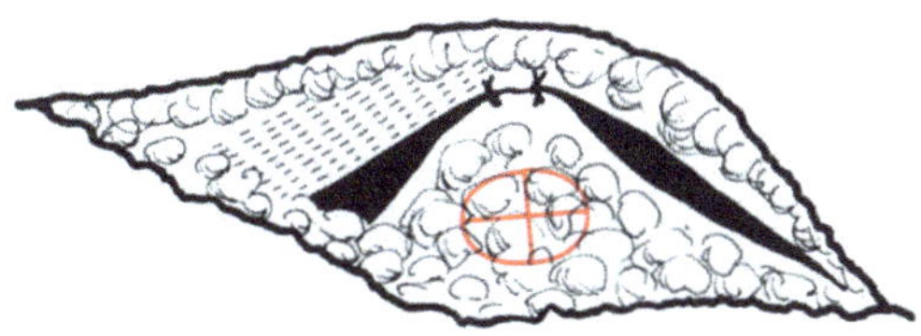

145

Closure of Proximal End of Wound

Closure of the deep fascia in the upper end of the wound is greatly facilitated by flexing and slightly **adducting** the thigh. After the first two stitches in the proximal end of the wound the thigh is **abducted** to slacken the fascia for the remaining stitches.

146

Foam Pressure-Pads Step 1

This technique for preventing subcutaneous haematomata has been in use at Wrightington since 1969: Five sutures are usually adequate. Each suture of monofilament nylon is 14 in. (35 cm) long and armed at each end with curved needles. One needle (the one to be used first) should be round bodied, the other, cutting. The first needle takes a small but effective bite of the deep fascia a few millimetres away from any suture in the deep fascia. The round-bodied needle is used because a cutting needle can cut the figure-of-eight sutures in the fascia without the surgeon knowing.

147

Pressure-Pads Step 2

The anterior needle is brought out through the skin **not more than** 1.5 cm from the cut edge. A common error is to emerge too far from the skin edge and the gentle pressure of the foam pad is then wasted at some distance from the suture line in the deep fascia. The round-bodied needle offers resistance to penetration of skin but if it is held in the needle-holder one-third of its length behind the needle point penetration of the skin then is not difficult.

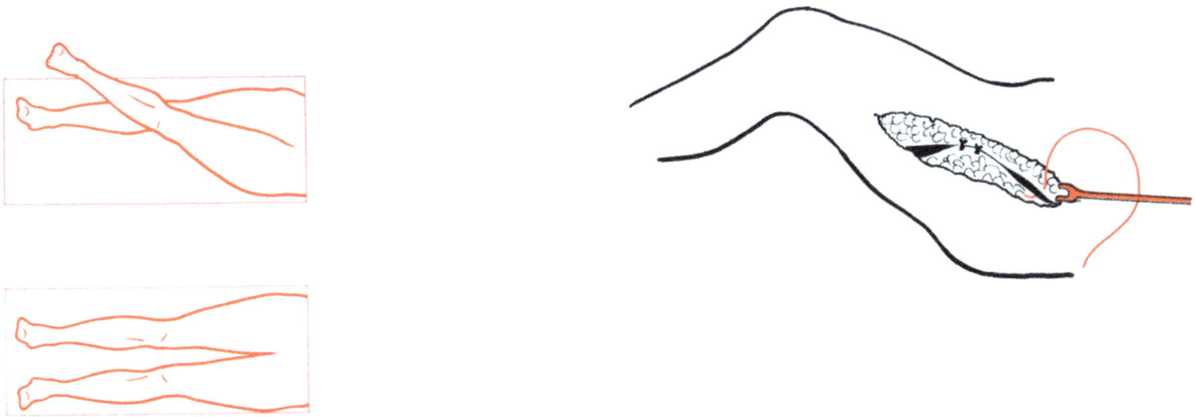

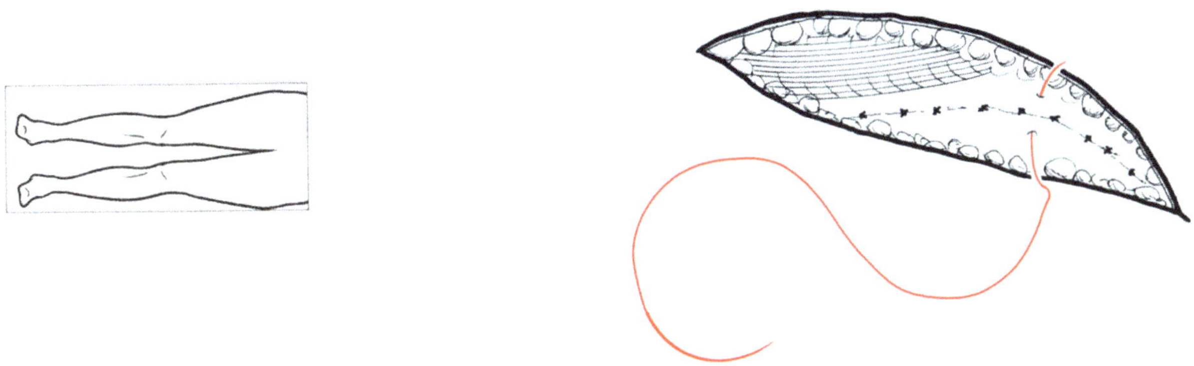

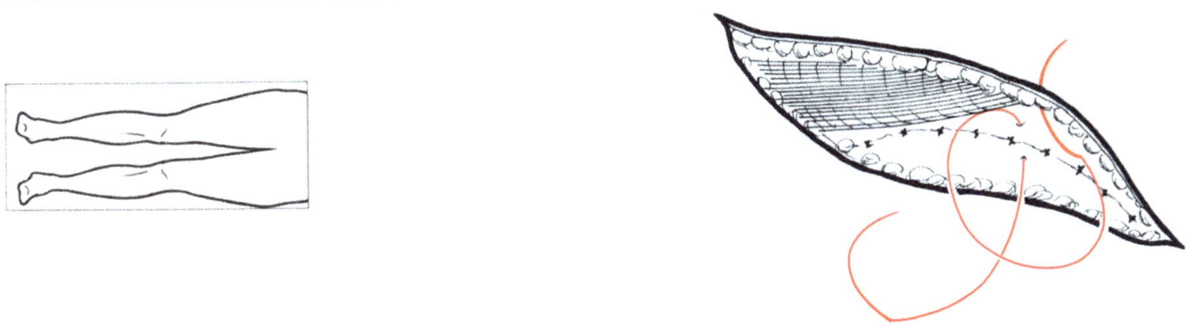

148

Pressure-Pads Step 3

The posterior needle is brought out through the skin, also not more than 1.5 cm from the skin edge. The foam pads are then threaded over the needles.

149

Compressing Pads

Having closed the skin incision the pressure-pads are gently compressed by pulling on one end of the suture and pinching the aluminium buttons. The pads are compressed not more than half their thickness. The pads on opposite sides of the wound should lie in contact in order to exert pressure on the incision. This is preferred to leaving a gap between two rows of pads.

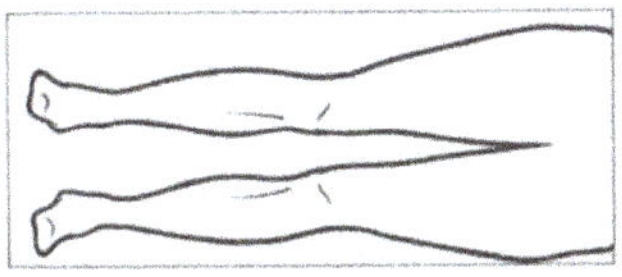

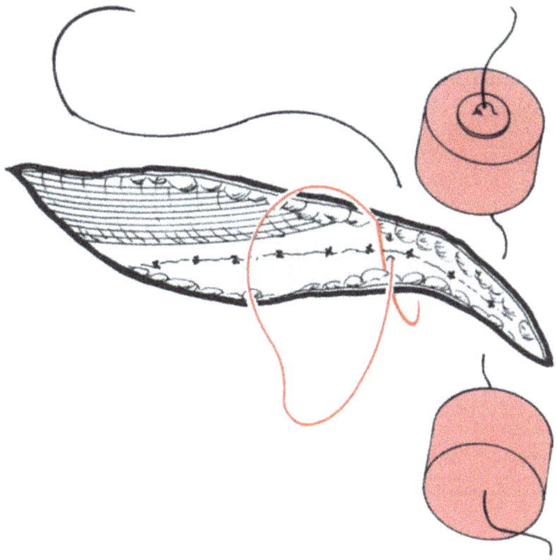

Time: 78 min

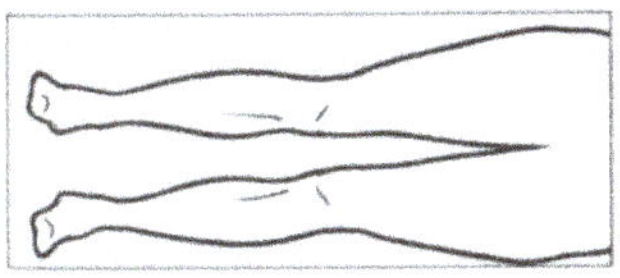

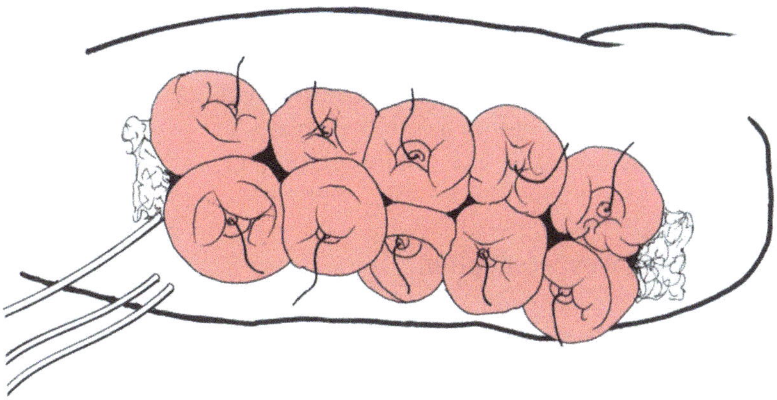

End: 84 min

The time at various stages is the average of five operations and includes use of the neck-length jig (Chap. 16).

Chapter 16

Femoral Neck-Length Jig

In the ordinary method of performing the LFA operation a stage which lacks precision is the 'test reduction'. The 'femoral neck-length jig' has been developed to remedy this and practical experience has shown that it serves several different and important functions. The different functions will be described in the order of their recognition because to present them simultaneously, as happens when the instrument is used, might give an erroneous idea of complexity. When the operator becomes accustomed to it the device not only increases precision but can shorten the total operating time.

Defects of Test Reduction

The main purpose of a test reduction is to assess stability against dislocation before the femoral prosthesis is cemented in position. Stability against dislocation requires that the stump of the neck of the femur should be of such a length that the fascial structures of the thigh will be correctly tensioned. It is undesirable that fascial structures should be over-tensioned, purely to achieve extreme stability, because this can result in the whole extremity being made too long.

In the ordinary operation an element of 'hit and miss' enters at this stage of the test reduction. Most surgeons tend to err on the side of leaving the stump of femoral neck rather longer than is indicated in step 37, and will be ready to shorten this during the test reduction. But when shortening the stump of the neck of the femur it is easy to change a 'snug' reduction into one permitting 2-3-mm distraction of the femoral head from the depth of the socket. Also to correct an excessive degree of anteversion it is difficult to trim the stump of the neck of the femur without at the same time reducing the effective length of the neck, and spoiling what at the first test reduction was a snug fit of the prosthetic head in the socket.

Another source of imprecision concerns changes in the effective length of the femoral prosthesis produced by changes from varus to valgus alignment, when a medullary cavity is very large. When this problem presents, a gauze swab can be packed into the medial part of the medullary cavity to hold the prosthesis in valgus alignment during the test reduction; but the swab may be compressed during the reduction and the final position of the prosthesis, when cemented, may be more valgus than at the test reduction, resulting in the reduction being under tension and the extremity being too long. All these difficulties are rectified by the neck-length jig.

Neck Length

The principle by which stability is achieved by the neck-length jig depends on the fact that all the Charnley prostheses have the same vertical distance between the summit of the head and the level of the notch, where the base of the femoral neck meets the concave medial surface of the stem of the prosthesis. When resecting the femoral head the femoral neck is left longer than will eventually be required and the purpose of the neck-length jig is to transfix the neck, from front to back, with a 3-mm pin at a point which will be the correct site for the notch on the prosthesis (Fig. 16.1). The purpose of the neck-length jig is to locate precisely the placing of this pin. The bone of the stump of the neck lying proximal to the locating pin is then cut away, at a precise angle to the axis of the femur, to leave the correct length of femoral neck for a stable reduction without the limb being made too long.

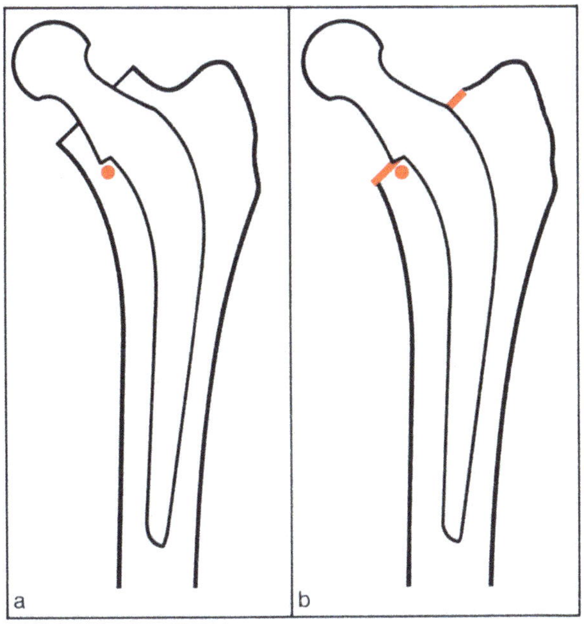

Fig. 16.1. **a** Neck of femur longer than needed in the end-result. Prosthesis superimposed in ideal position: (1) longitudinally; to give correct limb length and correct tissue tension and (2) transversely; to keep axis of stem of prosthesis in axis of femur. The function of the neck-length jig is to place the drill hole in the correct position to coincide with notch on prosthesis. **b** Excess femoral neck resected proximal to pin in the drill hole

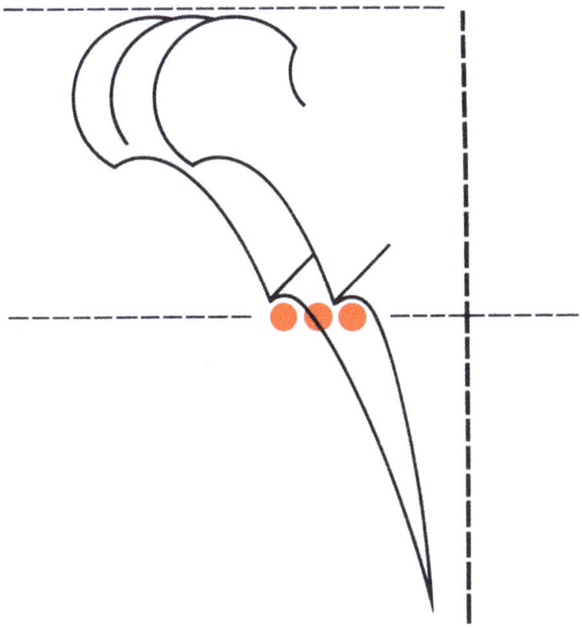

Fig. 16.2. Showing 'nesting' of the bases of the necks of the three offsets of prosthesis: (1) when the axes of the stems are superimposed and (2) when the summits of the heads are all at the same level. The outline of the stem of the 40-mm offset has been excluded for clarity. The three drill holes are separated transversely from each other by 0.5 cm

When the stage of packing the soft cement into the medullary cavity has been completed the pin once again is inserted into its original holes and the femoral prosthesis is then pushed into the cement-filled medullary cavity until the notch of the prosthesis comes to rest on the transfixing pin. Shortly before the final setting of the cement the pin is extracted and local pressure on the cement closes the track left by its withdrawal. In the process of obtaining correct **length**, the transfixing pin is sited in relation to the **longitudinal** co-ordinate of the femur.

Valgus and Varus Alignment

In controlling valgus and varus alignment of the stem of a femoral prosthesis, especially when the medullary cavity of the upper end of the femur is large, the most important element concerns **lateral or medial siting of the base of the prosthetic femoral neck**. The lateral or medial siting of the tip of the stem of the prosthesis in the medullary cavity makes only a small contribution to varus or valgus alignment of the prosthesis.

In the process of controlling **varus or valgus alignment of the prosthesis** the transfixing pin is sited in relation to the **horizontal** or transverse co-ordinate of the femur.

Different Offsets of Prosthesis

The offset of a prosthesis, as already described, is the perpendicular distance between the centre of the head and the axis of the stem. In the Charnley system all the different offsets are obtained with the angle of the femoral neck maintained at a constant angle (50°) to the axis of the stem.

In Fig. 16.2 the three offsets of the Charnley prosthesis are shown with the axes of the three stems superimposed. If the summits of the three femoral heads are arranged to lie on the same transverse line, then the notches of the three prostheses also must lie on a transverse line. If the three stems are superimposed each notch will be separated horizontally from the next by 5 mm (45-, 40- and 35-mm offsets). The neck-length jig therefore is designed to site the transfixing pin in the bone of the femoral neck (a) so that the longitudinal co-ordinate predetermines length and (b) so that three transverse co-ordinates correspond to the three different offsets of prosthesis, so keeping the axis of each prosthesis in the central axis of the femur.

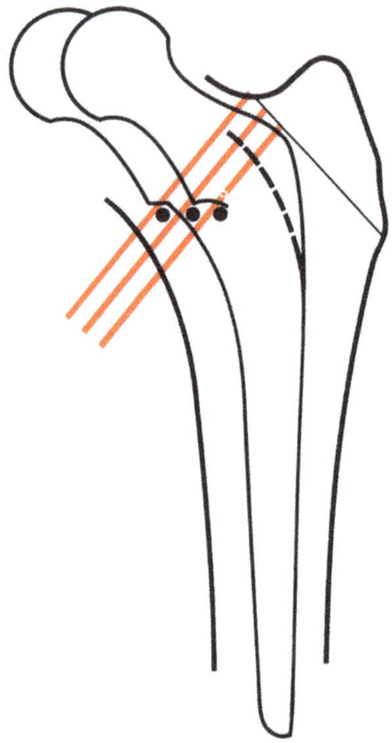

Fig. 16.3

Neutral Axis Alignment

It is the purpose of the neck-length jig always to try to achieve alignment of the prosthetic stem with the central axis of the femur. Only when this can be achieved with consistent success does the availability of different offsets make sense. Without accurate control of alignment a 45-mm-offset prosthesis in valgus could produce less offset **in relation to the axis of the shaft of the femur** than a 35-mm offset in varus.

Level of Section of Stump of Femoral Neck

Because the axis of the femoral neck lies approximately at 45° to the long axis of the femur, changes of length in the axis of the femoral neck will displace the femur equally in longitudinal and medial directions. If for any reason it is desired to keep

Fig. 16.3. As the offset of the prosthesis becomes less, so the length of the neck of the femur must be reduced if we are to keep the axis of the stem aligned with the axis of the shaft of the femur. The three levels for sectioning the femoral neck are demonstrated: the longest femoral neck is for the 45-mm offset; the shortest for the 35-mm. The convex, lateral surface of the 35-mm-offset prosthesis encroaches on the plane of section of the trochanter

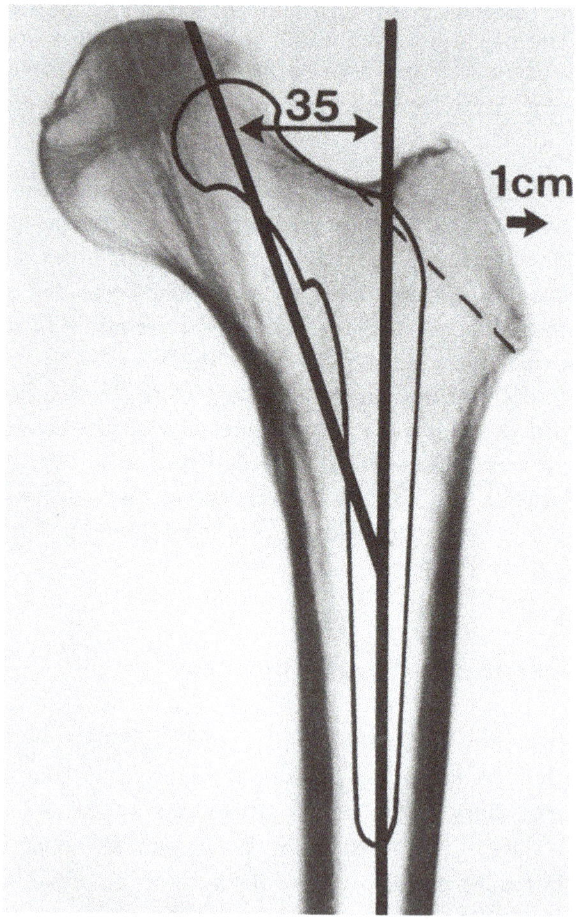

Fig. 16.4. Showing 35-mm offset with projection of lateral ▶ convexity of stem; 1-cm lateral displacement of trochanter avoids the projecting convex surface of the prosthesis

the longitudinal dimension constant but move the shaft of the femur medially (i.e. a reduced offset) the transverse component of the inclined axis of the neck must be shortened without changing the vertical component. This subtlety is explained in Fig. 16.3, showing the 'nesting' of the three parallel planes of section of the neck, corresponding to the three different offsets of prosthesis, when the leg length is kept constant.

When a Charnley design of prosthesis with 35-mm offset is used there is a tendency for the convex lateral surface of the upper end of the stem to project above the plane of the cut surface of the trochanter (Fig. 16.4). This affects only the medial part of the cut trochanteric surface of the femur; it does not impede reattachment of the trochanter, because the trochanter will be reattached more laterally than its original site on the femur when the shaft of the femur is medially displaced.

Anteversion

When the stump of the neck of the femur is transfixed with the locating pin this determines the plane of the section of the neck and ensures that it will correspond to the desired anteversion.

Plane Surface of Section

Because the neck of the femur is sectioned by means of a saw, the plane surface so produced enables a simple pressure injection device to be used (described below) to improve the final step of inserting the soft cement. This is not possible if the cut surface of the femoral neck is irregular as a result of changing anteversion by nibbling 'high spots' with a bone rongeur.

Description of Neck-Length Jig

The full set of instruments (Fig. 16.5) comprise the following parts:

1) **Shaft axis stems** (set of six for different sizes of medullary cavity at the level of the tip of the prosthesis). Each stem is provided with a detachable (screw-on) inserting handle.

2) A **forked plate** used with a mallet is useful for extracting during the process of trial and error to find the stem which best fits the medullary cavity at full depth.

3) **Proximal spacers.** Three sizes of proximal spacer are available for different sizes of medullary cavity in the trumpet-shaped proximal level.

4) An **extractor** is available to help in changing a proximal spacer in case the first to be chosen proves too large or too small. (Fig. 16.6 shows the axis stem and proximal spacer in position.)

5) **Hollow punch** for driving in the proximal spacer.

6) **Drilling jig** with thumb-screw to attach it to head and neck unit, with $^1/_8$-in. (3.2-mm) **drill** (9) for use with jig.

7) **Head and neck unit** with **locking screw** (8) to lock the head and neck unit on to the shaft axis and an **Allan key** to tighten the locking screw.

10) T-shaped **locating pin**.

11) T-shaped **extractor** with screwed end.

Fig. 16.5. Set of instruments for using the neck-length ▶ jig: *1* Six femoral shaft axis stems, each with screw-on heads in position. *2* Forked plate, used with mallet, to extract shaft axis stems during trial and error to find the one which grips best, at desired depth, in medullary cavity. *3* Set of three proximal spacers. These centralize the femoral shaft axis stem in the medullary cavity (as demonstrated in Fig. 16.6). *4* Extractor to engage with bayonet recess on proximal spacers if first spacer (usually middle-size) needs to be changed for one larger or smaller. *5* Hollow punch to drive proximal spacer to full depth. This is essential in ensuring that the shaft axis stem lies truly in the axis of the femur. *7* Head and neck unit (in sequence of use this should have been numbered 6). This is slid over end of shaft axis stem. *8* Allan screwdriver to fix head and neck unit on the end of the shaft axis stem at desired level to achieve perfectly stable reduction without excessively over-lengthening the limb. *6* Drilling jig to be clamped to front of the head and neck unit. *9* Drill, to be passed through appropriate hole in drilling jig, to transfix stump of neck of femur. *10* T-shaped locating pin inserted in hole made by drill; T-handle turned to be transverse to axis of head and neck unit to give correct plane for section of the neck. *11* Extractor to pull out in one piece: shaft axis stem, together with head and neck unit and proximal spacer; at the end of the procedure

Additional tools

The following ordinary tools are required:

1) Mallet
2) Bone rongeur
3) Power operated drill to hold $^1/_8$-in. (3.2-mm) drill
4) Oscillating or reciprocating saw (or handsaw)

Surgical Technique

The medullary cavities of the femoral shaft and the neck of femur are reamed with rotary reamers, the aperture being made large enough to accept the flanged (Cobra) prosthesis. (Later in the procedure shortening of the neck usually requires a second application of the rotary reamer.) It is not necessary to ream the femoral shaft in an exaggerated degree of valgus, but it certainly should reach 5° valgus as judged by alignment with the patient's patella.

Test Prostheses

It will be evident that the neck-length jig renders it unnecessary to have a series of test prostheses. Gauging the size of the reamed medullary cavity is done using the definitive prosthesis in the prosthesis holder.

Conclusion

If a surgeon is prepared to study this technique, so that he can guarantee to achieve a stable reduction of the prosthesis on every occasion and if he masters reattachment of the trochanter by the techniques already described, the author seriously believes that after primary operations the hip can be almost 100% proof against dislocation. This claim covers active rehabilitation with almost no restrictions started 48 h after operation.

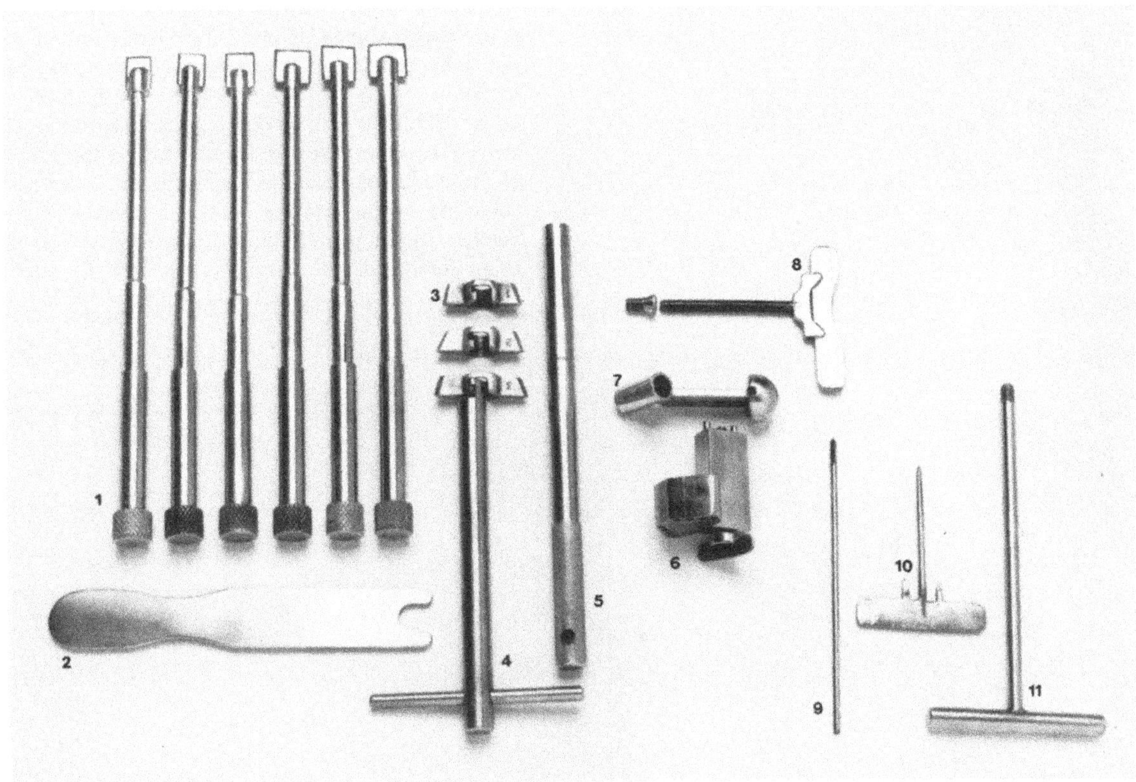

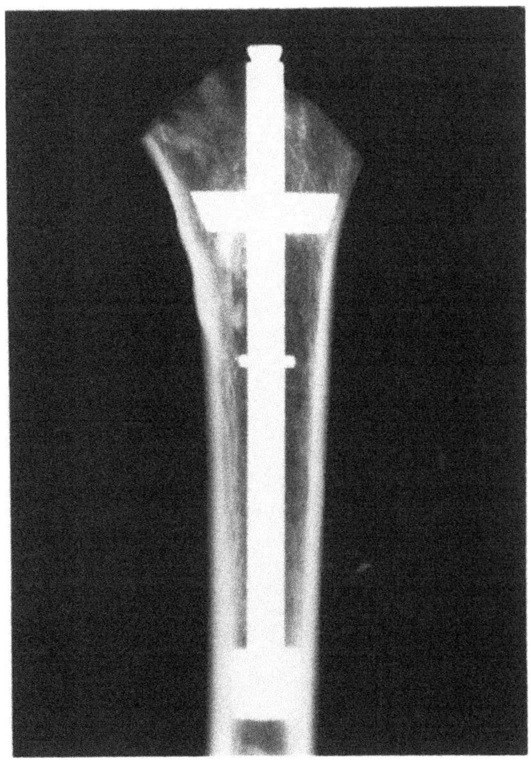

Fig. 16.6. Indicating correct depth of femoral axis stem in femur. Depth controlled by choosing correct size of tip to grip in medullary cavity. Note how proximal spacer controls alignment in axis of femur (unless this is correctly achieved the femoral prosthesis will not be correctly aligned)

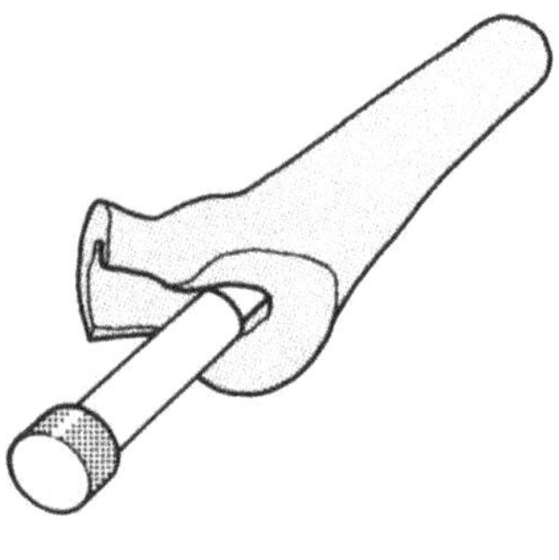

Fig. 16.7 (Stage 1). A **shaft axis stem** is chosen of such a size that it can be driven to full depth without very heavy hammering. Full depth is when the junction of the stem with the screw-on handle is at the level of the cut trochanteric surface of the femur. The tip of the shaft axis stem must take a sufficiently good grip deep in the medullary cavity to resist rotation when at a later stage the locking screw is tightened. Sometimes to achieve a good grip the tip of this device is best placed in an antero-posterior plane

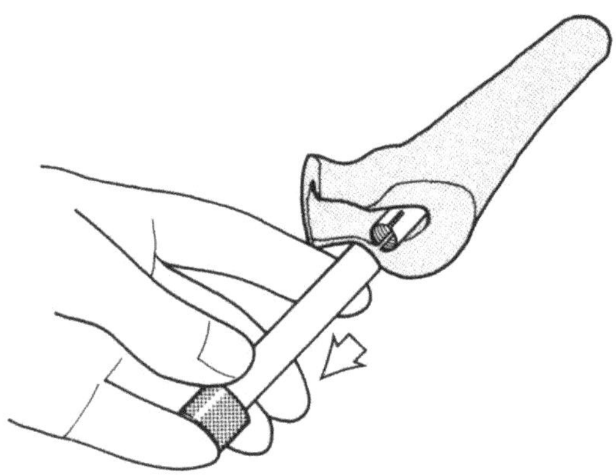

Fig. 16.8 (Stage 2). The screw-on handle is detached

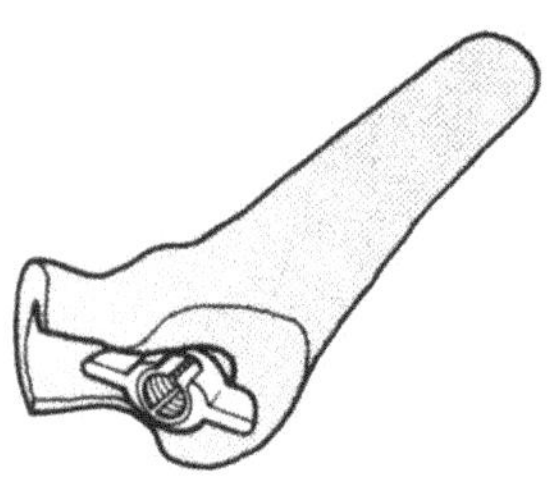

Fig. 16.9 (Stage 3). A **proximal spacer** is chosen appropriate to the size of the proximal medullary cavity. The best routine is to try the middle size (No. 2) first

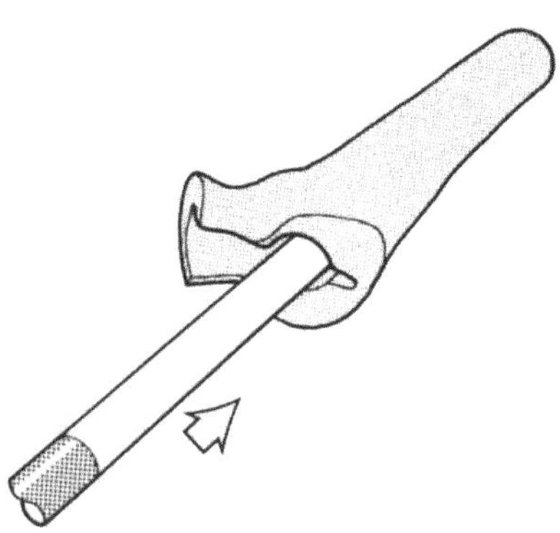

Fig. 16.10 (Stage 4). The **hollow punch** is applied over the shaft axis stem and the proximal spacer is **hammered firmly into position.** It should be noted that the lateral blade of the spacer will reach the endosteal surface of the lateral cortex by cutting its way through the cancellous bone (which it does without destroying much of the area of cancellous bone in the most lateral part of the cut trochanteric surface). Correct use of the proximal spacer locates the axis stem in the neutral position

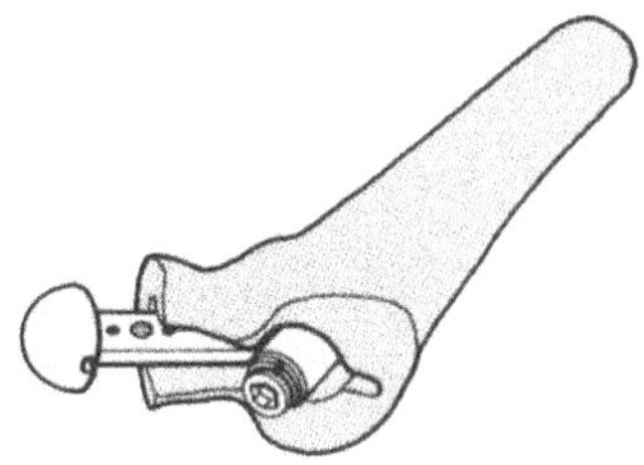

Fig. 16.11 (Stage 5). The **head and neck unit** is slipped on to the shaft axis stem and pushed as far down as seems reasonable. If the head and neck unit will not go sufficiently deep into the cavity of the femur (i.e. if the head and neck unit projects too far to permit an easy test reduction) then the proximal spacer is too large and should be changed for the next smaller size which can be hammered more distally in the medullary cavity. To extract the proximal shaft spacer in order to change it for a different size the tubular extractor (Fig. 16.5.4) is used. To facilitate extraction the shaft spacers should always be inserted with the 'bayonet socket' device uppermost, so that the hook on the extractor also can be inserted uppermost. The **locking screw** is inserted into the end of the stem of the shaft axis and the head and neck unit locked on by tightening with the Allan key. A test reduction is now made and long-axis traction is applied to see whether the test head can be pulled away from the socket. If the test head can be pulled away from the socket the number of millimetres by which this can be done is estimated and recorded. If the head cannot be distracted out of the socket the length of the lower extremity must be estimated to make sure that it has not been made too long. The supine position on the operating table is essential for this. In making this estimate the level of the detached trochanter when it is brought down to the trochanteric surface of the femur is a useful index. To lengthen or to shorten the head and neck unit the hip is dislocated and the locking screw loosened until the head and neck unit can then be pulled out, or pushed in, by the desired amount and the locking screw is re-tightened. A further test reduction can then be made and stability tested in all directions

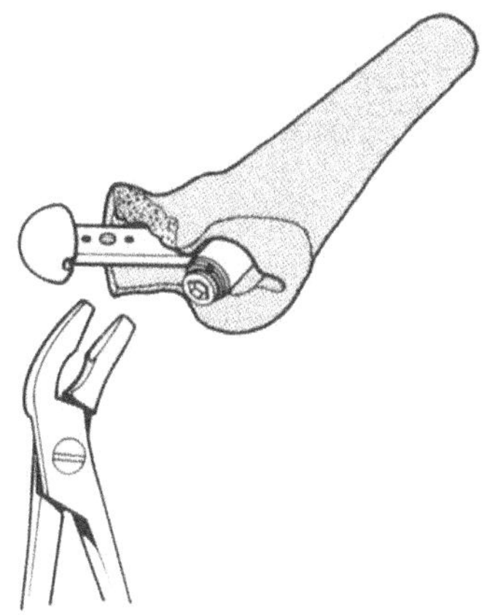

Fig. 16.12 (Stage 6). If the stable position for the head and neck unit is such that the distal holes in the neck are obscured by the anterior cortex of the femoral neck, it is necessary to nibble away bone from the anterior cortex of the neck with rongeur forceps until the drilling jig can be attached and fixed in position with the thumbscrew. An arrow on the drilling jig points distally when it is correctly attached

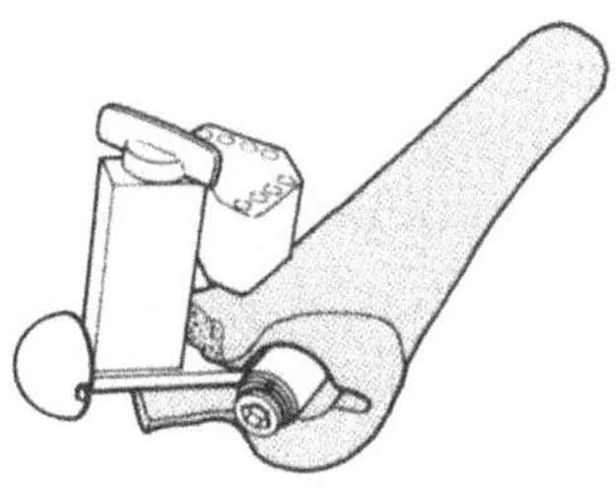

Fig. 16.13 (Stage 7). Because the drilling jig is reversible for left and right hips, it is provided with two sets of three holes, one set for each side. The correct set of holes lies on a line transverse to the long axis of the femur. This illustration shows two sets of four holes (this is incorrect)

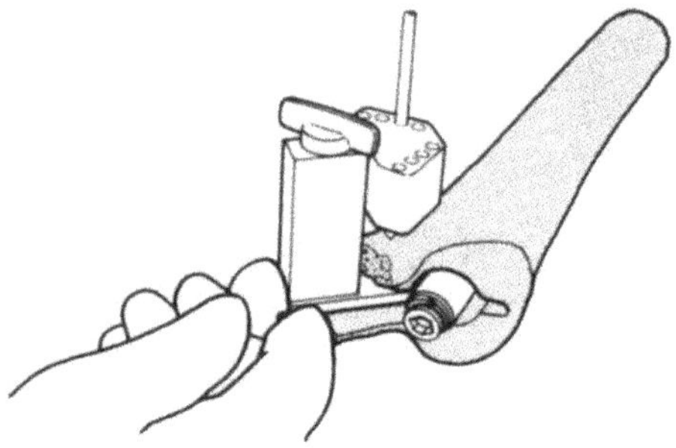

Fig. 16.14 (Stage 8). Choosing the drill hole. Of each set of three holes the most lateral hole (i.e. nearest the axis of the femur) will be for the 35-mm offset; the next will be for the 40-mm offset, and the next again for the 45-mm offset. The $^1/_8$-in. (3.2-mm) drill, mounted in the power drill, is inserted into the appropriate hole of the drilling jig. Before the drill is made to engage the bone, the axis of the head and neck unit is inspected to make sure that it is lying centrally in the reamed medullary cavity of the femoral neck and that this corresponds to an acceptable degree of anteversion (preferably not more than 5° though 10° is permissible). The drill is now passed through both cortices of the femoral neck. The drill is extracted and the drilling jig is detached by undoing the thumbscrew, leaving the head and neck unit in situ

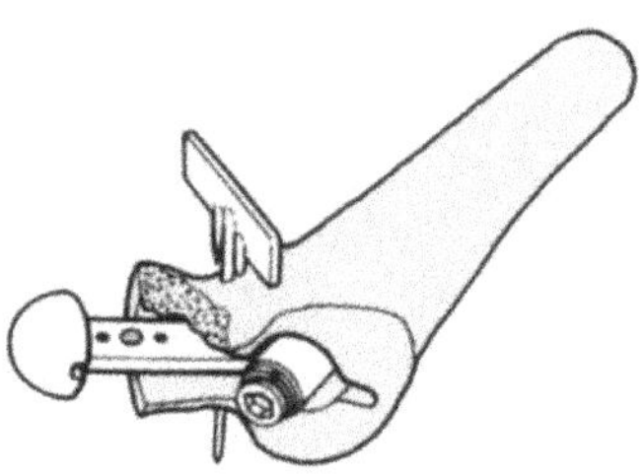

Fig. 16.15 (Stage 9). The **locating pin** is now entered into the hole made by the drill and the plane of the T-shaped handle of the locating pin is turned to lie at right-angles to the axis of the head and neck unit. The locating pin is then gently tapped with the mallet, till one or other of the two spikes engages with the anterior cortex of the femoral neck to prevent the T-shaped handle spinning round and losing its transverse orientation to the axis of the head and neck unit

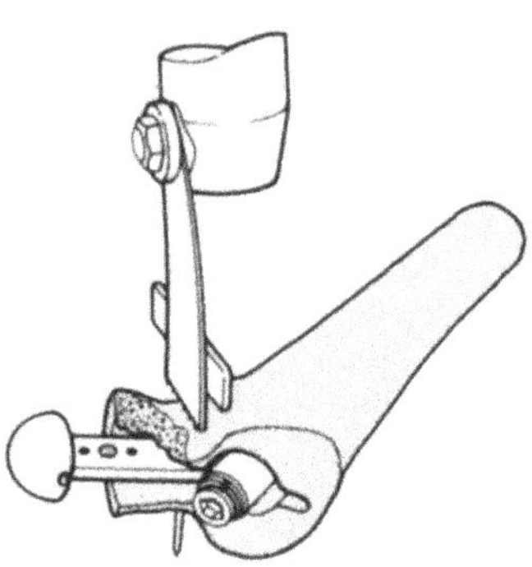

Fig. 16.16 (Stage 10). An oscillating or reciprocating saw is now applied to the anterior cortex of the femoral neck in the plane indicated by the T-shaped handle of the locating pin. The blade of the saw should be kept in contact with the central rod of the locating pin (this is made of very hard steel to resist damage by the saw). The **anterior cortex only** is cut at this stage while the head and neck unit is in situ to determine the angle of the cut

Stage 11. The locating pin is temporarily extracted to permit the assembly to be extracted from the medullary cavity. This can be done in one piece with the T-shaped extractor (Fig. 16.5.11), which is inserted in exchange for the locking screw after extracting the locking screw. A few blows with a mallet on the T-shaped extractor handle may be necessary

Fig. 16.17 (Stage 12). The T-shaped **locating pin is re-inserted** in its original track judging the angle from the saw cut already started. The sawing of the neck is then completed, again keeping the saw blade in contact with the hardened pin. The cut surface of the bone of the femur must be so close to the pin that the pin will be exposed on the cut surface **(Fig. 16.18)**

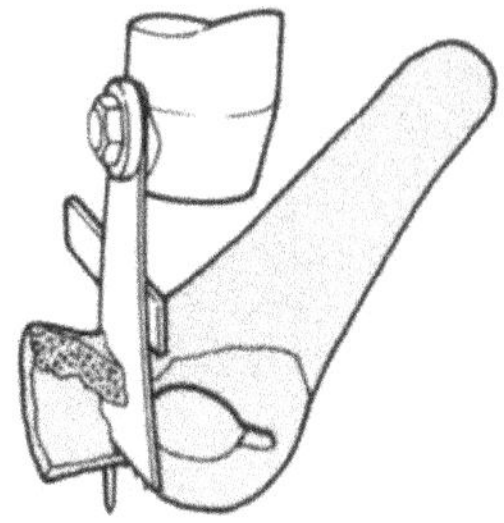

Fig. 16.17

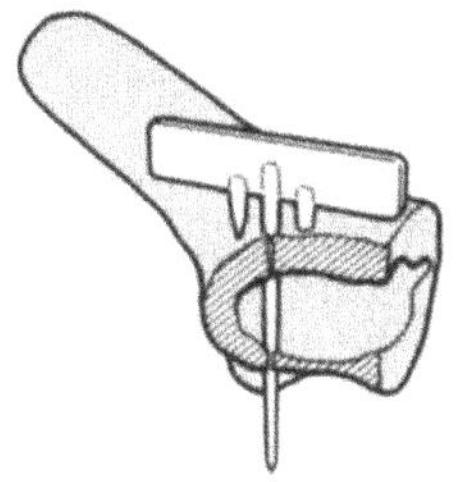

Fig. 16.18

Fig. 16.19 (Stage 13). With the locating pin still in position the chosen prosthesis is tested in the medullary cavity by sliding it into the femur with the medial surface of the stem in contact with the pin. If the flange of the Cobra prosthesis is too wide for the medullary cavity the rotary reamer should be used again

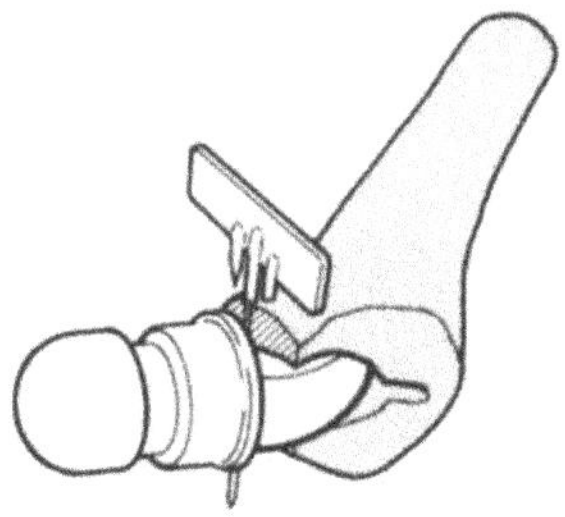

Fig. 16.20 (Stage 14). Keep the rotary reamer in contact with the locating pin so that unnecessary reaming in a lateral direction can be avoided. By keeping the reamer close to the pin the important antero-posterior widening of the cavity can be concentrated at the points related to the widest part of the dorsal flange of the prosthesis

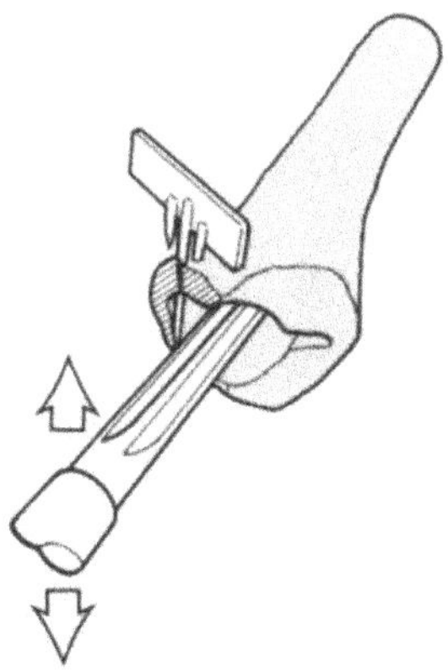

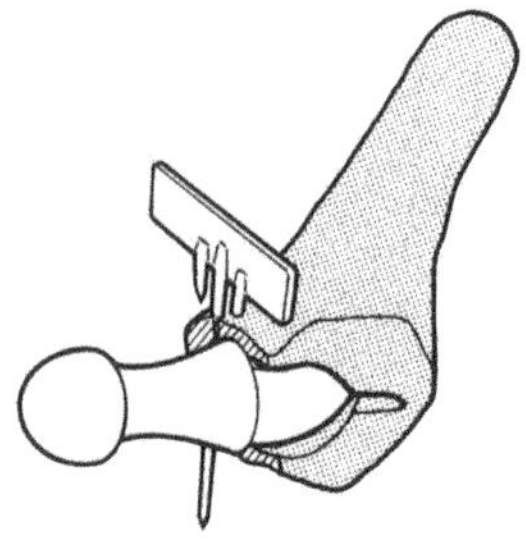

Fig. 16.21

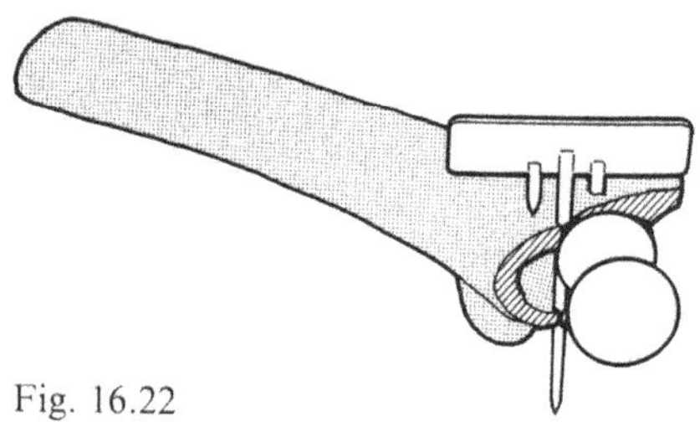

Fig. 16.22

Figs. 16.21 and 16.22 (Stages 15 and 16). Everything is now ready for the insertion of the cement and the prosthesis. A test reduction can be performed if the surgeon wishes; but this is usually unnecessary. The locating pin is extracted and the slits where the drill-holes encroach on the cut surface of the cortex are inspected to make sure they can be identified when the cement is in position. Final curettage and packing of the medullary cavity with dry gauze is completed. The locating pin is placed conveniently at hand **so that it can be found instantly when required** immediately after the last movements of inserting the cement. The **pressure injection cap** (Appendix C 16). This is a device to assist in pressure injection of cement in the region of the medial femoral neck. It replaces the ordinary protective cap (Thackray) but is used to hold the prosthesis in the holder in exactly the same way as the original protective cap. The large-diameter semicircular flange of the injection cap must be orientated in the prosthesis holder so that it lies on the medial aspect of the prosthesis. When testing the prosthesis in position prior to inserting cement the large-diameter flange of the pressure injection cap should automatically make contact with the plane surface of the femoral neck produced by the technique just described. Wires for reattachment of the trochanter should be moved to make sure they are not in the way of this contact.

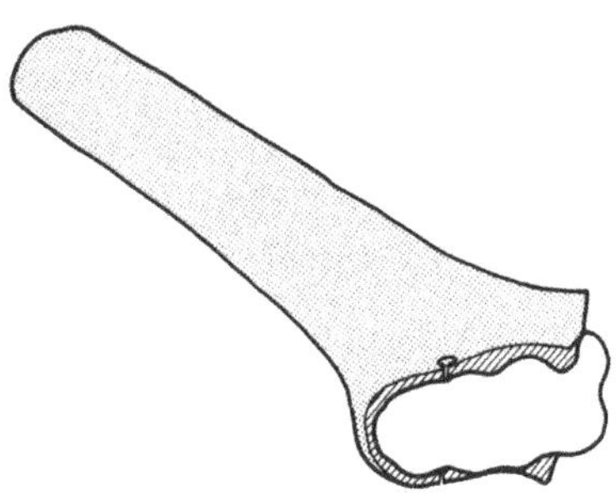

Fig. 16.23 (Stage 17). The cement is inserted into the medullary cavity of the femur. The author prefers to use the two-thumb technique as described (p. 259). When insertion is complete (which need not take longer than a count of 10 s) the surgeon identifies the drill holes encroaching on the cut surface of the femoral neck. This is done by pressing on the cut surface of the bone with the pulp of a thumb to squeeze away the cement and reveal the slots where the holes encroach on the cut surface of the bone

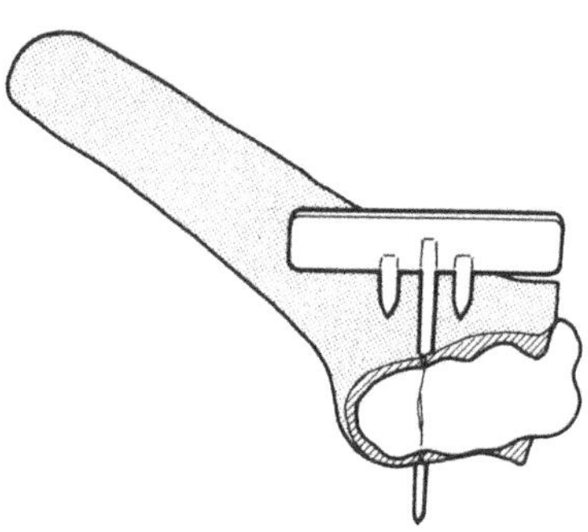

Fig. 16.24 (Stage 18). The locating pin is then slipped into position

Fig. 16.25 (Stage 19). Holding the prosthesis in its holder in one hand, the surgeon applies the thumb of his other hand to the cement bulging from the trochanteric part of the medullary cavity. The tip of the stem of the prosthesis is now inserted into the cement keeping close to the locating pin. As the prosthesis enters the medullary cavity the excess cement extrudes in the region of the locating pin because it is stopped from extruding towards the trochanter by the surgeon's thumb and by the dorsal flange of the Cobra prosthesis

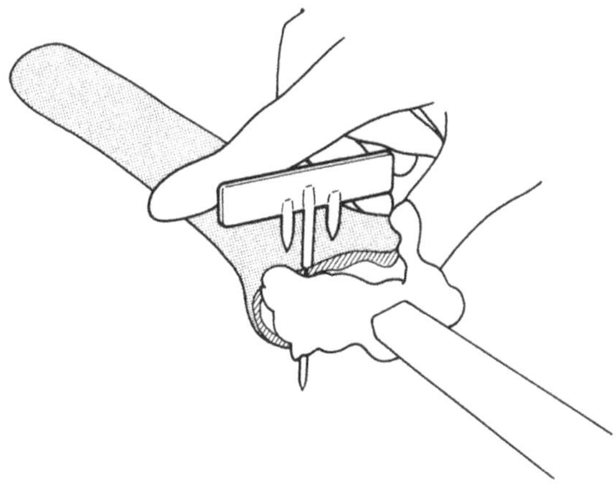

Fig. 16.26 (Stage 20). In the last 5 mm of insertion the large-diameter flange of the injection cap meets the bulging cement and drives it into the medullary cavity of the medial femoral neck. The cement is trapped laterally by the dorsal flange of the prosthesis and medially by the injection flange of the cap

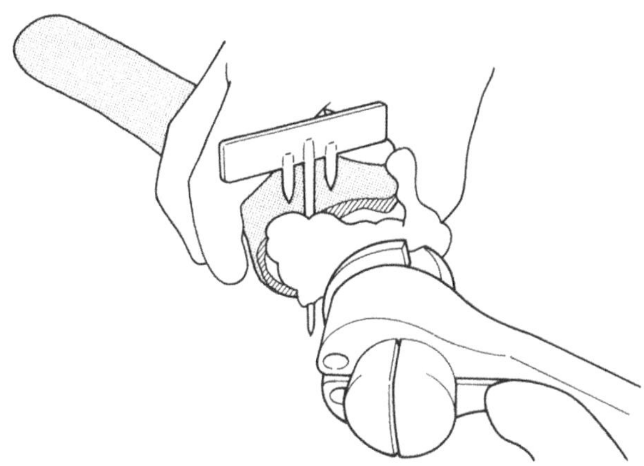

Fig. 16.27 (Stage 21). Hammering on the prosthesis holder ensures that the surface of the injection cap comes into close contact over the whole area of the cut surface of the femur. The medial surface of the prosthesis is still in contact with the locating pin. This position is maintained until the cement is reaching the rubbery stage. There is no danger of accidental movement of the femoral prosthesis while the cement is soft because of contact between the bone and the edges of the dorsal flange and because of contact between the surface of the injection cap and the neck of the femur

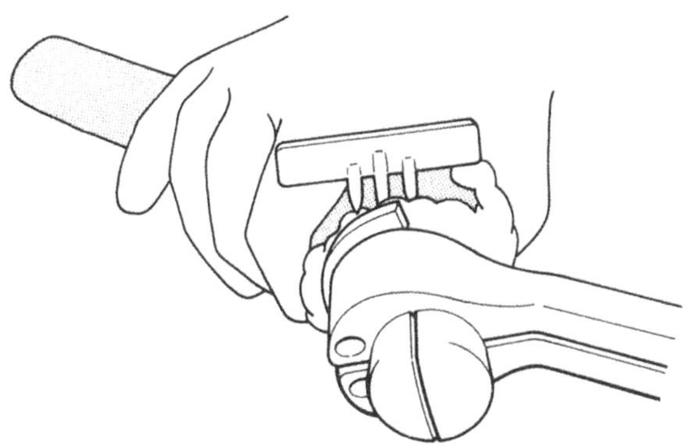

Fig. 16.28 (Stage 22). The prosthesis holder is detached and the two halves of the pressure injection cap removed. The locating pin is extracted and the surgeon applies his thumb to the cement and compresses it to obliterate the cavity in the cement left after withdrawing the locating pin

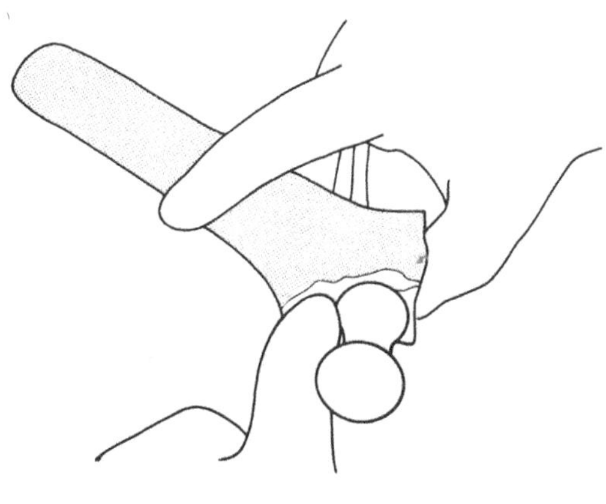

Chapter 17

Post-operative Management

This chapter describes post-operative management leading into rehabilitation. General nursing details, including blood and fluid replacement, are the same as those after all major orthopaedic surgery and need no special comment.

A frequent statement, especially in literature from the United States, is that trochanteric osteotomy is responsible for excessive blood loss. This is not true. The points of arterial bleeding in this operation are only about six in number and are instantly located. When blood loss of any note occurs it is capillary from the whole wound area and commonly is in rheumatoid arthritis. Male patients with osteoarthrosis usually are notably free from haemorrhage, rarely losing more than 250 ml in the operating room though this increases in suction drains in 24 h. The main cause of bleeding during the operation relates to the type of anaesthesia, though it is unnecessary to give hypotensive drugs. In physically fit patients the author would have no hesitation in performing unilateral operation without transfusion though a small transfusion is routinely given. Thrombo-embolic complications after total hip replacement are a special complication of major importance and the prophylaxis of this complication is discussed in Chap. 18.

Two systems of rehabilitation will be described which differ only in the duration of external restraint and the extent to which very vigorous rehabilitation is encouraged. The two systems have been designated (1) the 'original' system; designed to minimise the possibility of non-union of the trochanter and of post-operative subluxation and (2) the 'new' system; used when extreme stability has been obtained by use of the neck-length jig combined with fixation of the trochanter with the cruciate wiring system and staple-clamp.

Leg Bandaging

Bandaging of the legs from the ankles to above the knee (or an elastic stocking) is a logical and worthwhile procedure in the hope of reducing deep venous thrombosis in the calf and popliteal regions. The leg bandages are applied before the patient leaves the operating room. The bandages are of crepe material (i.e. 'Ace' bandages) and are applied using the figure-of-eight method which holds in position longer than simple spiral bandaging because it does not tend to concertina down the leg. The bandages should be reapplied at least every 8 h and be retained day and night until the patient leaves hospital.

Wedge Pillow

The patient returns from the operating room with a special wedge-shaped pillow between the legs (Fig. 17.1). This pillow has an included angle of about 20° and so holds each hip in about 10° of abduction. The pillow is loosely tethered between the patient's ankles by padded ankle straps held together by Velcro. The measurements of the two sizes of wedge pillow are indicated in Fig. 17.1. The pillow should be of firm consistency using an upholsterer's construction and can with advantage be a little heavy. A detachable and washable cover is used. In choosing the size of pillow make sure that too much abduction is not being used because excessive abduction can make the limb roll into external rotation. Even with an ordinary size of wedge pillow excessive abduction can occur if the opposite hip is ankylosed or has limited abduction, the pillow exerting all its action on the operated side. In such a case an ordinary soft pillow may be better than the smallest of the wedge pillows. The purpose of the wedge pillow is merely to ensure that reactionary oedema in the traumatised

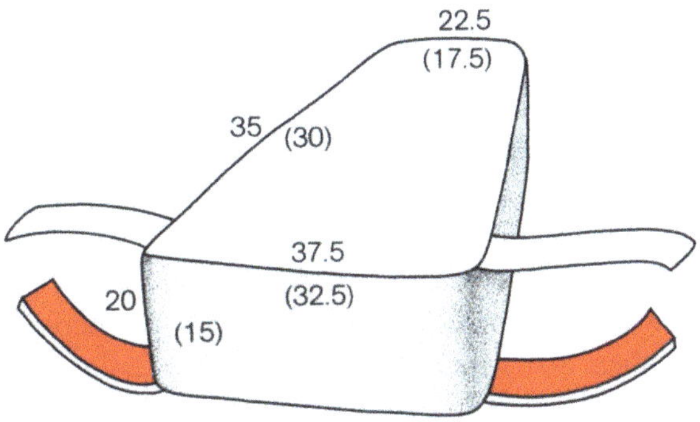

Fig. 17.1. Wedge-shaped pillow with dimensions of small and large size. The ankle straps are held by Velcro

tissues will develop with the hip in a good position. It also helps the nursing staff during the first 2–3 post-operative days when turning the patient for care of pressure points.

Knee Support

The popliteal surfaces of the knees should be supported to hold them comfortably in slight flexion. The 'bean bag' support, using plastic granules (Cubex) has proved noticeably superior to plastic foam pads even when the latter have been sculptured to shape. Prior to adopting the bean bag an incidence of external popliteal palsy of about 2% was encountered.

External Popliteal Nerve Palsy

On the evening ward-round of the day of the operation the patient should be tested for ability to dorsiflex the foot and toes. The negative observation (that **no weakness** exists) should be recorded, because if an external popliteal palsy is discovered 3–4 days after operation it is of the utmost value to know that it was not present immediately after the operation. Pain down the front of the leg radiating into the dorsum of the foot during the first 2–3 post-operative days can precede the appearance of an external popliteal palsy. Any patient who complains in this way should immediately have the head of the fibula inspected for localized tenderness or reddening of the overlying skin caused by external pressure. Failure to attend to this detail can result in a palsy which can take 6 or more months to recover whereas steps to prevent it can take a matter of seconds. During the operation it is important to correct fixed external rotation because a lower extremity which tends to lie persistently in external rotation is prone to develop external popliteal palsy, because it causes the weight of the leg to lie on the head of the fibula.

Heel Pads

Routine inspection of the heels, and maintenance of heel pads disturbed by 'calf pumping' exercises, are routine nursing details.

Posture in Bed

The foot of the bed is elevated for the first 48 h to encourage venous return from the lower extremities. Only one pillow under the head is permitted for the first 4–6 h; thereafter two pillows for the next 48 h. After 48 h a semi-recumbent position is used.

Catheterisation

In men retention of urine is common. After bilateral operations at the same session, a small-calibre indwelling catheter is inserted as a routine prophylactic measure at the end of the operation.

Bed Exercises

Breathing exercises, muscle contractions and the use of elbow crutches are demonstrated to the patient by the physiotherapist before the operation. From the first post-operative day the physiotherapist supervises the patient in the following four exercises which are performed thereafter at regular intervals throughout the day for the duration of the hospital stay.

1) **Dorsiflexion and plantar flexion of the foot and ankle** to encourage venous return from the calf (calf pumping) (10 times every 15 min).

2) **'Bicycling' of the knees.** This consists of moving the knees up and down alternately as though riding a bicycle. The popliteal surface of the knee is lifted from the supporting surface for 2–3 in. (5–7.5 cm) at each movement. On the side where the knee is to be flexed the patient concentrates on attempting to pull the heel a short distance towards the body; on the opposite side the action

is to push the heel towards the foot of the bed. This exercise is encouraged every 15 min while the patient is in bed.

3) **Breathing exercises.**

4) **Gluteal and quadriceps contractions.** These will have been taught by the physiotherapist.

Between exercises and when merely resting in bed patients should be repeatedly reminded that they themselves must control the position of their legs and as far as possible lie with their toes and knee caps pointing to the ceiling.

From the third post-operative day

The following exercises are supervised by the physiotherapist, the wedge pillow having been temporarily removed from between the legs (unless already removed in the new routine).

5) **Abduction exercises.** A polished board using talc on the heels, or skates, is employed.

6) **Combined hip and knee flexion exercises.** These are performed on the polished board with talc.

7) **Quadriceps contractions.** This leads to straight leg raising (SLR) as soon as the patient shows signs of ability to lift the foot from the bed.

Confident SLR should start to be in evidence 6–7 days after the operation but if a patient is slow in this he or she should not be discouraged by criticism. Very occasionally patients will be unable to perform SLR even when ready to return home but all eventually acquire it spontaneously.

8) **'Hip shrugging'.** This is a useful method for encouraging abduction when the operation is unilateral. After unilateral operations patients can dodge true abduction movements of the operated hip by tilting the pelvis and by abducting only the unoperated hip. To perform hip shrugging the patient lies supine in bed, holds the knees in full extension and presses the popliteal surfaces into the bed. The exercise consists of attempting to make the operated limb longer than the other, by pushing one lower extremity towards the foot of the bed, at the same time trying to shorten the other leg by pulling away from the foot of the bed, **all without flexing the knees**.

The exercise is done alternately right and left, but it can be carried out concentrating only on one leg if there is a special need to make this longer, or shorter, than the other.

Standing Out of Bed and Walking

From the morning of the third post-operative day the patient stands out of bed between the physiotherapist and an assistant. Full weight is taken on both legs. Attempts to make walking steps are started, first with the support of the two persons and then with a walking frame. When balance is acquired, and as soon as the general physical condition and age of the patient permits, walking with elbow crutches is encouraged. Quick steps are better than slow steps because the patient spends a shorter load-bearing period on the operated hip and becomes encouraged by speed.

Four-Point Walking

This method of using crutches, or walking-sticks is important in bridging the phase between a walking frame (often needed only for the first post-operative day) and the start of what can be called 'ordinary walking with sticks' (i.e. 'two-point' walking). The special feature of four-point walking is that it minimises (or even eliminates) powerful contraction of the abductor muscles yet it permits the full load of body weight to be placed on the operated hip. Newly cemented implants are stronger than they will ever be at any later stage so that the load of body weight is not important. Attempts to avoid powerful contractions of the abductor muscles is an aid to union of the trochanter.

Axillary crutches are not advised; in the first place because it is not necessary to avoid putting body weight on the hip and in the second place axillary crutches produce a clumsy and abnormal method of walking. Elbow crutches are preferred because they lead naturally to the use of ordinary walking-sticks or canes.

Four-point walking is taught in the following way:

1) Move forward the crutch opposite the operated limb
2) Move forward the foot of the operated limb level with this crutch
3) Move forward the second crutch
4) Move forward the foot of the unoperated limb level with the second crutch, etc., etc.

This sequence progresses naturally to the ordinary two-point gait in which the walking-stick and opposite leg move forwards simultaneously.

The four-point cycle is a sequence of separate quarter-cycles. It demands considerable mental concentration in order to stop the natural tendency for a crutch and foot to move forward together as a half-cycle. Patients usually count to themselves in order not to lose the rhythm which is very easily lost as the speed quickens. It is useful to teach the patient the rhythm before the operation.

Sitting

Sitting is not permitted until the seventh post-operative day. On this day (after removal of the fat sutures and their pressure-pads) the physiotherapist takes the patient to the toilet for the first time instructing how to sit by sliding the operated leg forwards. The patient then sits out of bed in a chair for 0.5–1 h and again in the afternoon. The duration of sitting out of bed is increased daily to a total of about 6 h by the ninth day. When sitting the feet should not hang down for longer than about 1 h; the knees should then be extended and the feet supported on a stool for an equal period. After the mid-day meal all patients are returned to bed for 1–1.5 h.

Height of Chairs and Toilet Seats

Chairs and toilets should be provided with arms to assist the patient in sitting down and getting up. The height of the sitting surfaces should not be less than 20 in. (50 cm) from the floor. Ordinary toilet seats are only about 16 in. (40 cm).

Discarding Crutches

The tenth post-operative day is the usual time to change from elbow crutches to walking sticks (United States: 'canes').

Stairs

Stairs are attempted on the eleventh day. This exercise encourages knee and hip flexion and produces a great increase in confidence.

Ascending and Descending Stairs

The patient holds the bannister with one hand and the stick in the other.

Ascending: Start by placing the **unoperated leg first** on the higher stair. Follow by the stick on to the higher stair. Then bring the operated leg to the same stair.

Descending: First put the stick down to the lower stair. Follow by the operated leg. Unoperated leg last.

For bilateral simultaneous operations the process is the same but the stronger leg is regarded as the unoperated leg.

Returning Home

In the author's practice patients usually return home 14 days after the operation, this being dictated by administrative details, but many patients would be able to return home after 10 days.

Discarding All Walking Aids

Patients return home 14 days after operation using one or two sticks according to their performance. They are instructed to **retain one stick in the hand opposite the operated hip for a further 4 weeks** and they must do this even if able to walk easily without any aid. The first post-operative attendance is 3 months after leaving hospital.

Recovery of Flexion Range

When the hips were very stiff before operation for many years, the recovery of a major range of flexion is possible but it is unpredictable. When hips have been very stiff for many years the muscles may have lost permanently some of their normal range of elasticity; but this is by no means a general rule and reasonable elasticity not infrequently can return spontaneously.

Post-Operative X-Ray

It is important that a good X-ray should be obtained at the time of discharge home because the patient has then been up and about for 2 weeks. This very important film is made for comparison with later films taken at outpatient attendances. The routine post-operative film, if a portable taken when leaving the operating room, is of absolutely no value for comparison with later X-rays.

Prophylaxis Against Thrombo-Embolism

This matter is dealt with in Chap. 18. The patient continues with oral Plaquenil, 400 mg/24 h, for 1 week after returning home.

Speed of Rehabilitation

The difference in duration of the various phases of rehabilitation in the 'original' and the 'new' system of rehabilitation is tabulated:

Days post-op.	**Original method**	**New method** (Neck-length jig and cruciate wiring with staple-clamp)
1st and 2nd	Bed	Bed
3rd–7th	Retain wedge pillow	**Discard** wedge pillow
	Stand and walk morning and afternoon	Stand and walk morning and afternoon
	Return to wedge pillow	**Lie free in bed**
	Caution in flexion exercise	No restriction on movement in any direction. Flexion encouraged
8th–14th	**Discard** wedge pillow but **retain soft pillow between knees**	
	Sleep on back, face up	**Can try to sleep on unoperated side** with pillow between knees
15th day to 2 months	**Sleep on back,** keep pillow between knees	**Sleep on side as soon as desired**

Some of the author's pupils who use the original method of trochanter fixation advise patients to use axillary crutches for up to 6 weeks after the operation. Axillary crutches spare muscular contraction in the abductor muscles more efficiently than do elbow crutches. Nevertheless the most dangerous muscular contractions acting on the trochanter are those which take place when the hip is flexed in the act of sitting down or rising up from the sitting position.

After a unilateral operation a patient with strong arms and a good hip on the other side can sit down, and stand up, without subjecting the operated side to very much muscular action; non-union of the trochanter then is rare. Frail patients (category C) with weak arms, expose the trochanter on the operated side to more stress than do athletic patients. Category C patients therefore should be encouraged to **try** to avoid using the operated side when sitting down and standing up, and encouraged to **try** to use their arms and opposite leg maximally.

Principles Guiding Physiotherapy

The keynotes in rehabilitation are (1) emphasis on learning to walk and (2) encouraging active abduction range.

After returning home emphasis on rehabilitation is still on walking, with rehabilitation by ordinary daily chores (i.e. sitting down and standing up; attempting to put on shoes and socks, etc. all being exercises for increasing hip range). To continue professional physiotherapy after leaving hospital is quite unnecessary in a properly motivated patient.

During the week or two after total hip replacement an important part of the physiotherapist's role is to get acquainted with the patient's psychology. Because the physiotherapist spends more time in close contact with the patient than anyone else in the team, she can discover a patient's secret worries and either communicate them to the surgeon or dispel them herself when she knows how the surgeon likes the common questions to be answered.

General Remarks

In Chapter 12 on reattachment of the trochanter and Chapter 19 on post-operative dislocation it is shown that the original method of rehabilitation following the original surgical technique was associated with a post-operative dislocation rate of only 0.4% and non-union of the trochanter of about 5%. Though these are low rates for mechanical complications the author believes that even these can be almost eliminated (at least after primary interventions) by use of the neck-length jig and reattachment of the trochanter with cruciate wiring and staple-clamp. The increased confidence in pushing the speed of rehabilitation which comes from total confidence in the stability of the hip and the strength of fixation of the trochanter is worth the effort needed to add these advanced techniques. Once the technical details are mastered the author believes that this operation is consistently more successful in avoiding mechanical complications than any method which struggles to avoid detachment of the trochanter.

Chapter 18

Thrombo-embolic Complications

An important function of the two-channel system for recording post-operative complications at Wrightington (Chap. 2) is the monitoring of various forms of prophylaxis against thrombo-embolism (TE). More than 1000 arthroplasties are performed each year at Wrightington, in reasonably controlled circumstances, so that the situation is very favourable for establishing clinical trials of different prophylactic agents.

The background statistics in this chapter are taken from our records of TE complications at Wrightington as studied by Johnson et al.[43, 44, 45].

The possibility of fatal pulmonary embolism (PE) after total hip replacement is a hip surgeon's constant worry. Even so the TE complications of total hip replacement have certain features which appear to make them less serious (with the exception of the absolute catastrophe of death) than those which occur in the course of medical diseases or after some operations in general surgery.

The relatively benign nature of the majority of TE complications after total hip replacement is still not widely appreciated. The facts are (1) that the complications are very rarely recurrent, so that prophylaxis continued for many months after returning home is unnecessary and (2) that the venous obstruction in most cases recovers completely; even after a major PE the patient does not become a pulmonary cripple, nor after deep venous thrombosis (DVT) is leg swelling frequently permanent, except when the patient has had thromboses before the operation. The main concern always is the possibility of a fatal embolism, no matter how rare this might be.

The author makes these sweeping generalisations from a background of considerably more than 7959 total hip operations with 628 cases of non-fatal PE (7.89%) and 83 fatal emboli (1.04%).

Diagnosis of PE

In seeking to prevent PE we are seriously handicapped by the difficulty of diagnosing it by objective tests. Even a research based on pulmonary arteriography might not be conclusive, because it might not be reasonable to use it in the least serious and numerically most common cases.

Research into the prophylaxis of PE has tended therefore to be indirect, based on the idea that anything which reduces the incidence of DVT must 'pay off' in a reduced rate of PE. Because it is now accepted that some degree of symptomless DVT in the calf veins occurs in more than 50% of patients after total hip replacement, it is clearly possible (by clot-seeking radio-active isotopes) to make statistically significant tests of anticoagulant procedures in a few hundred post-operative observations. On the other hand we must not ignore a theoretical possibility that radio-active tests might be too sensitive for total hip work: if a prophylactic agent were to be so effective that it completely suppressed clot formation in the calf, it might interfere with the beneficial aspects of the clotting mechanism so necessary inside the operated hip.

The incidence of clot formation in the deep femoral and iliac veins is much more important than the incidence in calf veins, as a parameter for studying the prevention of major grades of PE; but routine venography is impossible in a unit performing over 1000 total hip operations a year.

Clinical Diagnosis of PE

At Wrightington we have studied the effects of different prophylactic agents on PE diagnosed by simple clinical methods. We realize that this is scientifically unacceptable but in support of the clinical diagnosis of PE are the following matters:

1) There does not exist a non-symptomatic PE, or one which can be overlooked in the way that 30%–40% of DVT in the lower extremities can be overlooked.

2) Errors will be positive from accepting as PE a few cardiac or pulmonary complications of another type.

3) In arriving at the diagnosis of PE the clinical picture is checked and rechecked over several days, and the diagnosis is made retrospectively.

4) The clinician's judgement is enhanced when working in a unit where total hip replacement is highly concentrated. PE after total hip replacement follows recognisable patterns, 45% occurring in the second and 30% in the third post-operative week.

Background of Present Policy of PE Prophylaxis

From proformata at Wrightington designed to record PE complications prospectively, data were analysed from the study of 7959 total hip replacements from the end of 1962 to the end of 1973. During this 12-year period a number of different forms of prophylaxis were used. Over this 12-year period Johnson[43] was able to extract 1174 operations where no prophylaxis of any kind had been used and these showed 2.3% of fatal PE and 15.2% of non-fatal. This is an important statistic because all methods of prophylaxis are better than none and therefore it is no longer justifiable to use an untreated series as a control.

The various methods of prophylaxis in relation to the incidence of fatal and non-fatal PE are tabulated:

Year	Method of prophylaxis	No. of operations	Fatal PE	%	Non-fatal PE	%
1966	Dindevan	450	3	0.8	29	6.5
1970	Heparin (intravenous)	138	1	0.7	13	9.5
1971	Heparin (subcutaneous)	47	3	6.4	3	6.4
1970–1973	Macrodex	4096	46	1.1	339	8.2

Anticoagulant Prophylaxis

The trial of Dindevan (Phenindione) in 450 patients undergoing total hip replacement was against a controlled group of 450 patients having the same operation without prophylaxis (Crawford et al.[46]). Fatal emboli were reduced from 1.8% in the control group to 0.8% in the Dindevan group, but the benefit was neutralised by three deaths from bleeding (0.7%) attributable to the anticoagulant.

Intravenous Heparin

Intravenous heparin was administered as a continuous infusion for 2 days, at a rate of 5000 units 8-hourly (15,000 units per 24 h) for a total dose of 30,000 units. In 138 cases there was 1 fatal embolus (0.72%) and 13 (9.5%) non-fatal emboli.

Low-Dosage Subcutaneous Heparin

Our short and unfortunate experience with low-dose subcutaneous heparin is included for general interest and because of the important lesson that it should never be combined with dextran prophylaxis. The method was that of Sharnoff and DeBlasio[47]. An initial dose of 5000 units of heparin was given subcutaneously at 6.00 a.m. on the morning of the operation followed by 2500 units 6-hourly, until the patient was fully mobile, which is usually 10–14 days post-operatively. The method had to be abandoned after 47 cases because of the high complication rate (Charnley[48]). The subcutaneous heparin was an addition to the routine current at that time of giving 1 unit of dextran 70 immediately after the operation followed by another 24 h later. There were three fatal emboli (6.4%) and three non-fatal emboli (6.4%). The total fatality rate in this very small sample of low-dose subcutaneous heparin prophylaxis was 8.5%, because one patient with haemoptysis could not be controlled with full doses of vitamin K.

There are reports in the literature of ineffectiveness of heparin in total hip replacement (Harris et al.[49]) but our specially bad experience would seem to be the result of combining it with dextran.

High-Molecular-Weight Dextran

In this study 4096 patients were given intravenous dextran 70 which became the standard method of prophylaxis for 3 years. The routine dosage consisted of 500 ml Macrodex 70 on the day of operation followed by 500 ml Macrodex 40 on the following day. Dextran was not started until the end of the operation because of increased capillary bleeding from the open wound. The rate of fatal PE with dextran was 1.1% and non-fatal, 8.2%.

Hydroxychloroquine (Plaquenil)

The action of Plaquenil (hydroxychloroquine sulphate, Winthrop) as an anti-thrombotic agent is attributed to its ability to prevent platelet adhesiveness and to a lesser degree the aggregation which follows adherence of platelets to damaged endothelium (Carter and Eban, 1974[50]).

Carter and Eban (1974)[50] compared the incidence of DVT in 107 general surgical patients on Plaquenil with 97 controls, using radioactively tagged fibrinogen and venography for diagnosis. The incidence was reduced from 16% to 5%. Chrisman et al. (1976)[51] using the same drug in 100 patients undergoing orthopaedic surgery between the knee and pelvis, reduced the frequency of TE complications from 8 out of 50 (including 4 instances of PE) to 1 out of 50 without a pulmonary embolus.

Between April 1974 and April 1976, 2144 total hip replacements were performed at Wrightington with Plaquenil 200 mg administered orally 6- or 8-hourly. The drug was started on the morning prior to surgery and continued until the patient was fully mobile, usually between 10 and 14 days. This usually involved a total dose of 8–10 g, which is well within the acceptable limits of 80–100 g, above which irreversible damage to the retina may occur. Of these patients, 1300 also received dextran 70 500 ml, starting at the completion of surgery and continuing slowly by intravenous infusion over several hours.

The standard post-operative regime consisted of the patient standing out of bed for a few minutes after 48 h, with mobilisation increasing daily until discharge from hospital usually between 2 and 3 weeks. A minority of patients were kept in bed longer than 2 days if technical or medical problems were encountered. All cases of fatal emboli were confirmed by post-mortem.

Results

The results evaluated for the efficacy of Plaquenil as a prophylactic against embolism, with and without dextran, are shown in the following table:

Emboli	Plaquenil alone	Plaquenil plus dextran
No. of cases	844	1300
Fatal	1 (0.1%)	5 (0.4%)
Non-fatal	29 (3.4%)	60 (4.6%)

The difference with or without dextran is not statistically significant, but taken together 2144 operations using Plaquenil, with 6 (0.28%) fatal emboli and 89 (4.15%) non-fatal emboli, is significant.

Bilateral Simultaneous Operations

A statistic which came out of the Wrightington study of 7959 LFA operations under different forms of prophylaxis and with no prophylaxis, was a higher rate of PE (fatal and non-fatal) following bilateral LFAs performed at the same operation (so-called simultaneous) compared with unilateral operations. The incidence of PE for the whole series of 7959 cases was 1.04% fatal PE and 7.89% non-fatal, and out of 243 bilateral simultaneous LFAs there was an incidence of 1.65% fatal PE and 12.8% non-fatal.

It is natural to interpret a higher rate of PE after bilateral simultaneous operations to an increased metabolic load on the patient, but the suggestion was advanced that purely from chance any patient having two total hip operations would face double the ordinary risk of having one pulmonary embolism even when the operations were at two different sessions. The Wrightington statistics were therefore re-examined to see whether the bilateral simultaneous operation carried a total risk of embolus of twice that of the single operation and this was found not to be the case, as shown in the following table:

	PE	Total no. of operations	% Incidence PE
Bilateral simultaneous	35	243	14.4%
Unilateral	676	7716	8.76%
	711	7959	

The observed bilateral rate, 14.4%, is certainly less than twice the observed unilateral rate, 8.76%.

Additional Personal Experience

The author's personal experience of PE on 760 total hip operations performed between December 1969 and November 1977 in a hospital quite separate from Wrightington (King Edward VII Hospital, Midhurst, Sussex) is of interest in relation to the optimal dosage of Plaquenil and is shown in the following table:

Prophylaxis	Single LFA	Bilateral simultaneous LFA	Total
Dextran	308 35 emboli (1 fatal) 11.4%	36 6 emboli (0 fatal) 16.7%	12%
Dextran plus Plaquenil 800 mg/24 h	115 7 emboli (0 fatal) 6%	18 0 0%	5.3
Dextran plus Plaquenil 1200 mg/24 h	259 0 emboli 0%	26 1 embolus (fatal) 4%	0.35%

From these figures Plaquenil in the dose of 1200 mg/24 h is favoured and we have had no increase in complications compared with 800 mg/24 h.

Complications

Plaquenil caused allergic rashes in 18 cases, temporary blurring of vision in 6 cases and bleeding from the genito-urinary tract in 5 cases. Vomiting and temporary gastric dilation occurred in 7 cases but these are complications of total hip replacement even in the absence of special drugs. All these adverse effects subsided when the drug was stopped.

Total Results

After the various forms of prophylaxis of PE used at Wrightington between 1966 and 1973 (excluding the 47 patients with the unfortunate combination of subcutaneous heparin and dextran) there were 4684 total hip operations with a total of 53 fatal pulmonary emboli (1.13%) and 381 non-fatal emboli (8.13%). The incidence of fatal emboli ranged from 0.7% to 1.1% and non-fatal from 6.5% to 9.5%. In 2144 patients treated with prophylactic Plaquenil there were 6 fatal emboli (0.28%) and 89 non-fatal (4.15%).

In a separate series of the author's, in a different hospital, with prophylactic dextran, in 344 total hip operations there was 1 fatal embolus (0.29%) and 40 non-fatal emboli (11.6%). Using Plaquenil in 418 similar operations there was 1 fatal embolus (0.23%) and 7 non-fatal emboli (1.7%).

Plaquenil therefore is significantly better than anything in the author's previous experience when using clinical criteria to diagnose PE.

Further Observations on PE After LFA

Arising out of the statistics relating to 711 emboli in 7959 LFA operations at Wrightington the following items have been selected from the papers of Johnson et al.[43, 44, 45] because of their special relevance to practical problems after this type of surgery.

PE After Second Side Without PE After First

There were 1140 patients who had a total hip replacement on the second hip without having had a PE after the first operation and the incidence of PE in this group has been examined.

	No.	Fatal	%	Non-fatal	%
Same hospital stay	252	0	–	5	1.98
Within 1 year	487	2	0.41	10	2.05
Later than 1 year	401	0	–	13	3.24

Grouping fatal and non-fatal emboli together there was no significant difference between the three different periods: $p > 0.2$.

PE After Second Operation Following PE After First

Sixty-one patients had total hip replacement on the second hip following a PE on the first side. These were divided into three groups as above.

	No.	PE	%
Same hospital stay	5	3	60
Within 1 year	25	3	12
Later than 1 year	31	1	3.2

Grouping the within-1-year figures together resulted in a highly significant difference compared with later than 1 year: $p < 0.001$. Therefore to operate on the second side following embolism on the first side, and especially within the same period of hospitalisation, very significantly increases the risk of a second embolism. The risk becomes significantly less the longer the period between operations.

Treatment of Established PE

Johnson[44] examined the results of different regimes instituted after the diagnosis of PE in 603 patients at Wrightington between 1962 and 1973. For details readers are referred to the original paper.

The methods used were:

1) Intravenous heparin 123 cases
2) Warfarin 82 cases
3) Heparin and warfarin 90 cases

Judged by recurrent embolism and DVT developing later, the worst results were with heparin alone. Heparin with warfarin was not as good as warfarin alone. The results of no treatment were only marginally worse than the best, i.e. warfarin alone. The figures are tabulated:

Method	No. of cases	Recurrent emboli	DVT later
Heparin alone	123	25 (20.3%)	3 (2.4%)
Warfarin alone	82	2 (2.4%)	0
Heparin and warfarin	90	11 (12.2%)	2 (2.2%)
Total with anticoagulants	295	38 (13.0%)	5 (1.7%)
No anticoagulants	308	10 (3.2%)	3 (1.0%)

In the total series of 603 pulmonary emboli there was only one that heralded a second embolus which proved fatal. This patient had been treated with heparin as soon as the first embolus was diagnosed. It is considered therefore that if it is felt necessary to start active treatment after a PE it should be with warfarin alone and not with heparin as a method of speeding up anticoagulation before warfarin comes into action. There is a good case for no treatment at all and no case for prolonged anticoagulation after return home.

Streptokinase Therapy

Only two patients were treated with streptokinase in the whole series and both had disastrous consequences. In one the embolism occurred 8 days after the operation and the wound started to ooze while streptokinase was being administered and was clearly infected by the 12th post-operative day. In due course the prosthesis had to be removed. In the other case the embolism occurred on the 13th post-operative day and a haematoma occurred which had to be evacuated on the 29th day. A deep infection developed and the prosthesis was later removed. Streptokinase was given here on emotional grounds and we feel that both patients, having already survived several days after a massive embolism, were (in our experience) past the worst and most unlikely to succumb thereafter.

Final Remarks

It is emphasized that in the prophylaxis of PE the diagnosis throughout this study has been purely clinical without confirmation by objective tests such as pulmonary scanning and pulmonary angiography. From out total clinical experience with different methods of TE prophylaxis we are satisfied that hydroxychloroquine has shown itself the most satisfactory and with the least serious side-effects of anything we have yet tried.

A clinical observation not capable of statistical analysis, is the reduction in frequency of TE complications after the patient has returned home when Plaquenil has been used. This used to be a source of great worry in the past because telephone calls and letters from patients and family practitioners had a particularly aggrieved tone. This aspect of the problem has been notably changed by the use of Plaquenil.

It is accepted that the experience reported here can only be regarded as impressions because of the absence of controls. Whether we should still find a rate of embolism of 2.3% fatal and 15% non-fatal if we were to use no form of prophylaxis no-one will ever know. Also it is not impossible that improved surgical technique over the last 5 years (especially related to better methods of fixing the trochanter) as a result of a better quality of early function, might have helped to reduce PE.

Despite our satisfaction with Plaquenil our overall results are still not as good as those claimed by Jennings et al.[52] for aspirin and Coventry et al.[53] for the delayed administration of warfarin, as shown in the table presented below.

In a study of the effect of aspirin on post-operative DVT in patients undergoing total hip replacement, Stamatakis, Kakkar et al.[54] used the ^{125}-I fibrinogen uptake test with ascending venography between the 14th and 16th day, unless a thrombosis was indicated by ^{125}-I when the venography was carried out immediately. Aspirin (600 mg twice daily) was given by mouth starting the day before operation. DVT was demonstrated by venography in 24 cases (80%). The clot was in the operated limb in 11; contralateral limb, 4; both limbs, 9. Clots were in the femoral vein in 13 and extensive in 4.

Method	Hospital	No of cases	Fatal	Non-fatal
Plaquenil	Wrightington	2144	0.28%	4.15%
Plaquenil	Author's personal: King Edward VII hospital Midhurst Sussex	762	0.26%	5.5%
Aspirin	Harris	528	0	1.3%
Warfarin	Coventry et al.	2012	0.05%	2.0%

The whole subject is therefore still wide open from the scientific point of view and surgeons can do no more than follow whatever prophylactic method appears to have given the best results when balancing complications against success. It is not impossible that empirical trials in the prophylaxis of embolism may lead to a solution before the scientific approach through investigating the clotting mechanisms responsible for producing DVT. This is because the factor which causes clots to detach is, in some ways, more important than the clots themselves. Even if an accurate study by venography of the effectiveness of Plaquenil were to prove it ineffective in preventing DVT, as with aspirin, the author will continue to put his first trust in Plaquenil to reduce the incidence of **embolisation** until some better regime is available.

Summary of Dosage

Hydroxychloroquine sulphate by mouth in 200-mg capsules; 1200 mg/24 h starting 24 h before operation and continued for 2 weeks. Then reduced to 400 mg/24 h for 1 week.

Chapter 19

Post-operative Dislocation

Fear of dislocation is one of the reasons why the very small prosthetic femoral head (22.25-mm diameter) has not become universally popular. But our dislocation rate at Wrightington even prior to 1966 did not average more than about 1% whereas a dislocation rate of 5% with a 41-mm-diameter head was reported by McKee and Chen[55] in their first 100 cases. Dislocation of Thompson and Moore prostheses of large diameter are also not uncommon. Therefore the size of a femoral head in itself is not the essential factor in susceptibility to dislocation.

Our low rate of dislocation in the early days was attributed to a combination of a number of different factors, notably: correct alignment of the implants; avoidance of excision of the capsule; correct reattachment of the trochanter; the use of an abduction pillow for 1 week, etc. By 1970 it was realized that dislocation might be associated with a tendency for the socket to be placed too high in the acetabulum, the centre of rotation thus being higher than the anatomical level and Shenton's line not being completely restored. This sometimes explained the persistence of shortening of a lower extremity after the operation. A high position of the socket (Fig. 19.1a, b) was sometimes the result of deepening the acetabulum in a headward direction as a result of directing the reamers more than the 20° towards the head which was the standard teaching at that time.

The rationale of increasing stability against dislocation by restoring full length to the leg has an important analogy in the case of arthroplasty of the knee. It is now universally agreed that in 'unconstrained' arthroplasty of the knee-joint an unstable knee can be made stable by restoring correct tension to the ligaments and capsular structures merely by inserting implants of a thickness appropriate to the amount of bone lost by disease.

In arthroplasty of the hip the total length of the lower extremity appears to be governed by the length of the fascial structures in the thigh. These fascial structures comprise the fascia lata, the three intermuscular septa of the thigh and the ilio-tibial band. In different positions of the thigh different aspects of this complex of fascial structures control leg length: the medial structures are tight in abduction, and the lateral structures in adduction, etc.

From November 1970 a policy of keeping the centre of the socket low in the acetabulum (but not lower than the anatomical level) was started

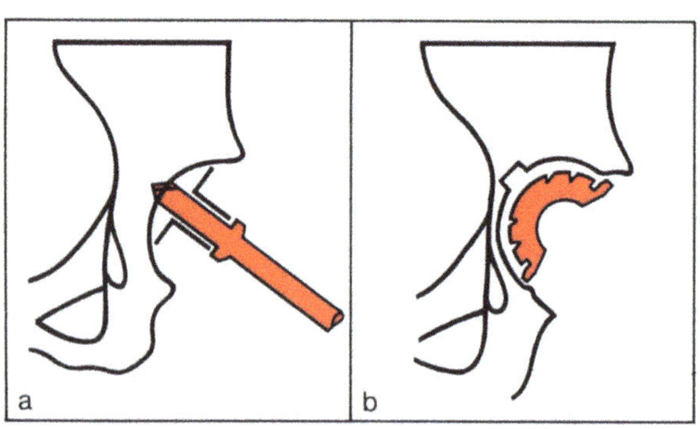

Fig. 19.1. a Deepening acetabulum in a headward direction giving **b** high position of socket

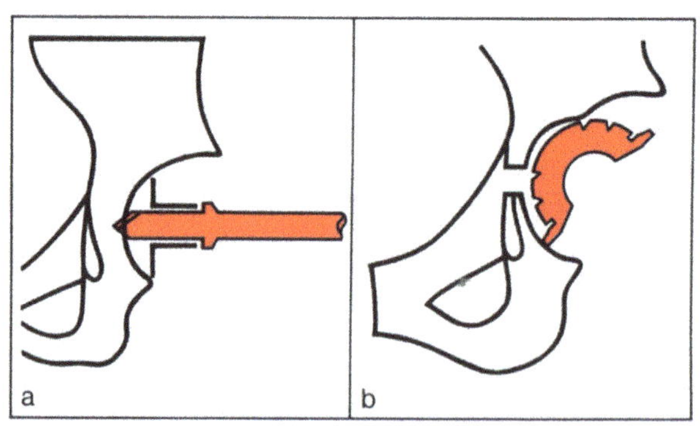

Fig. 19.2. a Deepening acetabulum transversely giving **b** low, or anatomical level of socket

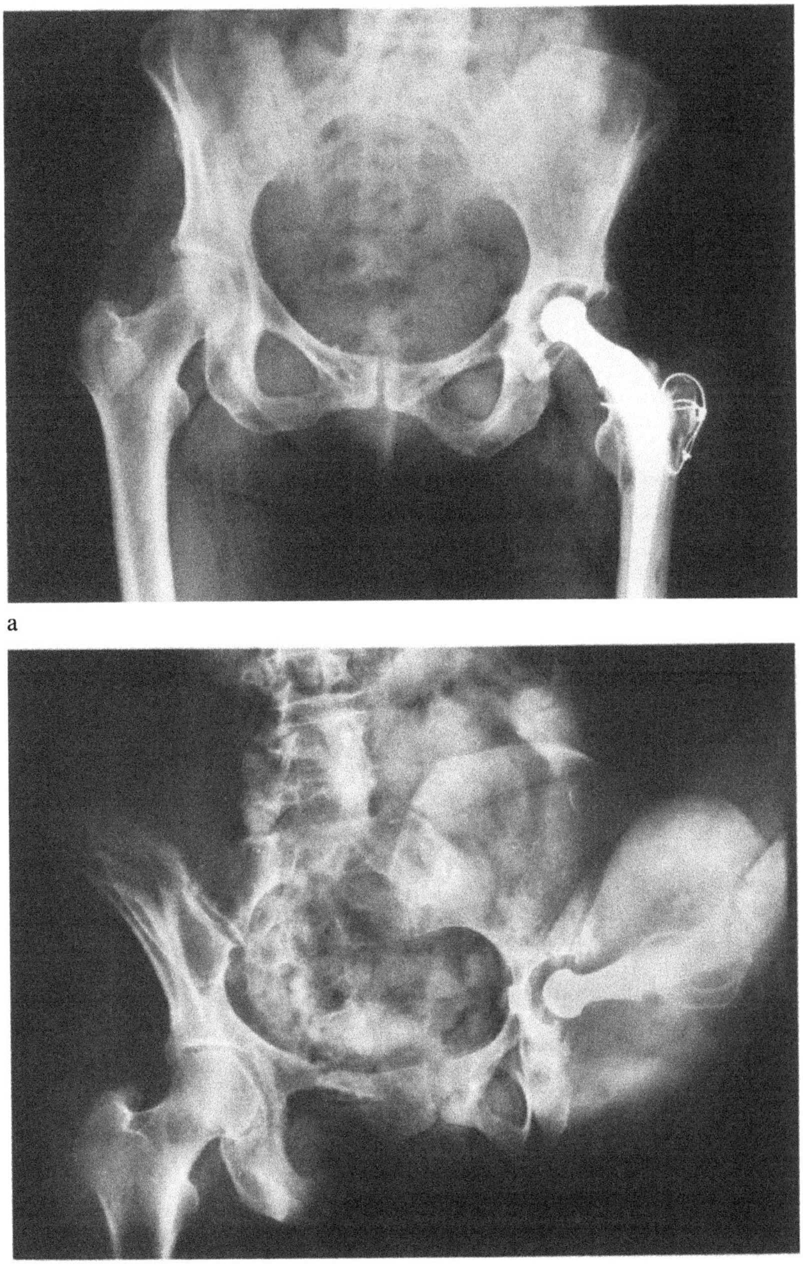

a

b

Fig. 19.3. a Extended position of hip. **b** Hip in 110° of flexion showing femoral head well located in socket and no subluxation despite fact that neck of prosthesis must be in contact with inner lip of plastic socket

by directing the pilot drill and reamers at 90° (transversely) to the long axis of the body rather than inclined 20° headwards (Fig. 19.2a, b).

In May 1972 a new design of hip socket was introduced to offer special resistance to posterior dislocation. In this new design the posterior wall was longer than the anterior wall (long posterior wall, or LPW socket.) The rationale of the LPW design of socket is to achieve increased stability against posterior dislocation. The first act in dislocation is for the femoral head to cross the 'watershed' of the posterior rim of the socket and the LPW design gives more latitude before the watershed is reached (Fig. 7.11, p. 100). When using LPW sockets anteversion should be avoided because this will exaggerate the projection of the

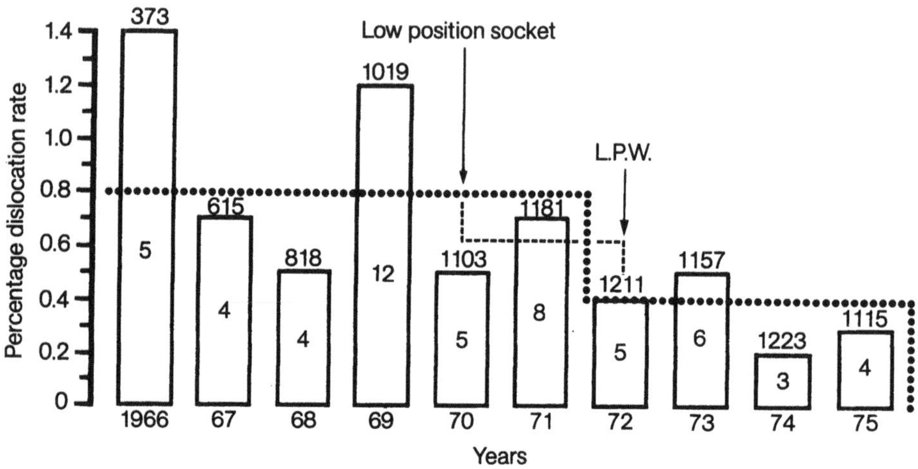

Fig. 19.4. Dislocation by years. See text

posterior wall with the possibility of impingement with the femoral neck in the extended position of the hip.

It is unnecessary to antevert plastics sockets to avoid impingement of the femoral neck. When the socket is not anteverted full flexion is obtained by slight abduction and external rotation even though impingement between femoral neck and rim may occur at 90° of flexion (Fig. 19.3a, b). In long-term post-mortem specimens impingement can sometimes be seen to have accommodated itself to the situation by the sharp internal lip of the central cavity of the socket having received a rounded impression in the superior and lateral quadrant.

The 'low' position of the socket and the LPW design were not both routinely put into action until after May 1972 and the individual contribution of each innovation therefore cannot be isolated in the total statistics. During 1971 the transverse direction of reaming was not employed in all cases. For this reason dislocation rates are compared before 1970 and after 1971. The statistics in the following study are taken from the study by Etienne and Cupic (1978)[56].

In Fig. 19.4 the percentage dislocation rate per year is represented by the height of each column in the histogram. The number of operations performed per year is recorded above the column and the number of dislocations within the column. It will be seen that during the years 1966–1969 (inclusive) the annual dislocation rate ranged from 1.4% to 0.5%. During this period of 4 years 2825 arthroplasties were performed with an average dislocation rate of 0.9% but there was no progressive control of dislocation because of the rise to 1.2% in 1969.

In May 1972 the LPW socket was added to the low socket position and by the end of December 1975 a further 4706 arthroplasties had been performed with an average dislocation rate of 0.4%. The annual rate of dislocation during this second period was more consistent and during these 4 years ranged from 0.5% to 0.2% as shown in Fig. 19.4.

Other Factors Accompanying Dislocation

Position of Pilot Hole

The position of the metal wire-mesh cement restrictor, visible in the X-ray, indicates whether a socket was deepened transversely or in a slightly upward direction. Figure 19.5 shows that before 1971 68% of the dislocations (38) had a high pilot hole but only 11% of the dislocations (18) after 1971.

Shortening of the Limb

Figure 19.5 shows that shortening of the limb closely followed the position of the pilot hole. Before 1971, 50% of the dislocations occurred with persistent shortening but after 1971, only 16%.

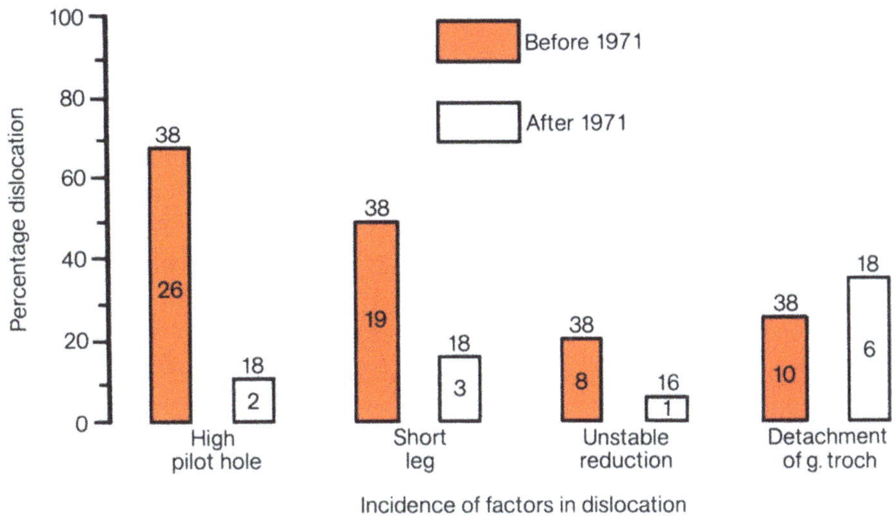

Fig. 19.5. Dislocation in relation to: transverse deepening of socket; shortening of limb; instability while under anaesthetic; and non-union with complete detachment of trochanter

Instability at End of Operation

Figure 19.5 demonstrates that before 1971, eight cases of instability out of the 38 dislocations (21%) were recorded while the patient was still under anaesthesia at the end of the operation. After 1971 there were three cases of instability out of 18 dislocations (16%) but two of these were explained by the fact that they were particularly difficult secondary operations (one a conversion after a Ring arthroplasty, and the other replacing a very deeply sited, loose socket).

Detachment of Great Trochanter

Figure 19.5 shows that before 1971, 10 of the 38 dislocations were associated with non-union of the great trochanter (26%) and after 1971, 6 out of 18 dislocations were associated with detachments (33%). Of the 10 dislocations associated with non-union of the great trochanter before 1971, 7 also had a high position of the socket in the acetabulum; but after 1971 the 6 dislocations with detachment of the trochanter all had correct siting of the socket. Therefore non-union of the trochanter would appear to be an important factor in rendering the arthroplasty susceptible to dislocation. In 6 cases of dislocation where the great trochanter was reattached dislocation did not recur.

In accordance with previous teaching these sockets are implanted without anteversion to maximise the effective length of the anterior wall of the socket and, when combined with the intact and re-tensioned anterior capsule of the joint, make it difficult for anterior dislocation to occur in external rotation (Fig. 19.6). With conventional sockets the common practice is to antevert the socket to increase the effective length of the posterior wall to prevent posterior dislocation, and also with the idea of encouraging flexion range, but anteversion reduces stability against dislocation in external rotation especially when the anterior capsule has been excised.

Recurrent Subluxation

Though not studied statistically there was, prior to the details introduced in 1972, a small incidence of patients reporting that their hips would 'click' in certain positions. In a few cases it was possible to demonstrate laxity of the articulation by applying traction under the image intensifier. On two occasions the head of the femur could be distracted from the socket by about 0.5 cm. The same has been observed with the large-diameter McKee–Farrar implant, indicating that this is a matter of the length of fascial structures and nothing to do with the diameter of the head. Since insisting on restoration of full length, and employing the LPW design of socket, this complaint is now very rarely heard.

Over-Lengthening of the Lower Extremity

It is possible that parallel with the complaint of 'clicking' of the hip no longer being heard there

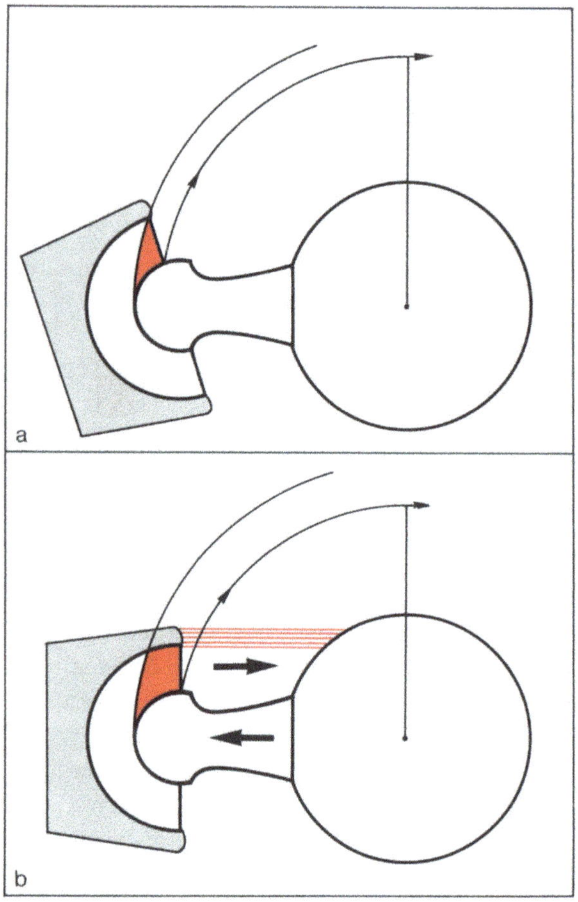

Fig. 19.6. a Anterior capsule excised with socket anteverted. Low resistance to dislocation in external rotation. **b** Preservation of anterior capsule with avoidance of anteversion of socket. Interaction of these two factors produces high resistance to dislocation in external rotation

may now sometimes be a complaint in the early post-operative period that the leg 'feels too long'. There is no need ever to incur gross over-lengthening of the leg (such as by 2.5 cm) in the interests of avoiding subluxation, but occasionally to err on the side of being up to 1 cm over-length can be justified, and most certainly after difficult secondary interventions.

Over-lengthening of up to 1 cm can be justified because (1) the stability which is assured permits active rehabilitation almost without any restrictions whatsoever and this is good for the prevention of PE, and (2) patients very soon become adjusted to 1 cm of over-lengthening. A complaint of feeling that the leg is over-length in the early weeks after the operation usually is the result of some fixed abduction still being present which will disappear in a few weeks.

If patients do not become completely adjusted to a slight increase in length then a small raise to the opposite heel (0.5 cm) is no hardship in comparison with the boon conferred by absolute stability. A patient can be justifiably disappointed if shortening, especially if not originally present, is incurred and slightly less so if previous shortening is not fully corrected; but since men nowadays wear raised shoes for cosmesis, slight lengthening is less important. The author usually, but not always, prefers not to adjust the height of a heel for 6 months to give the patient time to settle in.

Summary

This study shows that combining the 'low' position of the socket (by which is meant the anatomical level of the centre of rotation) with the LPW configuration of socket, reduced the total dislocation rate by 50% (0.9% to 0.4%). This improvement is even more striking when one considers the consistency of behaviour in the later years compared with the earlier years.

Non-union of the great trochanter is an important factor in precipitating dislocation, emphasized by the fact that after 1971, when the rate of dislocation was at its lowest (0.4%), non-union of the great trochanter accompanied 33% of the dislocations.

Final Remarks

The foregoing chapter is based on the study (Etienne and Cupic)[56] of dislocation as it was experienced at Wrightington up to the end of 1975. Since 1975 two technical advances in the author's own practice have contributed towards almost eliminating dislocation entirely. These are: improved method of reattachment of the trochanter (Chap. 12); and the new technique of the neck-length jig (Chap. 16). By this latter technique it can almost be guaranteed that it will be impossible to distract the femoral head out of the socket at the test reduction and before the trochanter is reattached, and to do this with safeguards against the lower extremity being made significantly too long. With the addition of these two new details of surgical technique the author believes that this operation might provide the most stable early post-operative result of any current method and permit even earlier unrestricted rehabilitation than when the trochanter is not detached.

Finally the point must be made that an occasional post-operative dislocation, in the week or two after leaving hospital, is no disgrace. Patients can sometimes be quite irresponsible and unreasonable during this period. If the implants are correctly orientated and the reduction was adequately stable on the operating table, one can confidently look forward to a permanently successful result after reduction. It is only in **recurrent** subluxation or dislocation that the surgeon might have to hold himself responsible for a technical error of orientation or of lack of tissue tension.

Chapter 20

Wear of Hip Sockets

If total hip replacement is to be undertaken in vigorous male patients above the age of 45 we must have some definite information regarding the wear of hip sockets if we are to extrapolate, from our present knowledge of 10 years, to 25 years. Three radiological studies of wear in vivo have been undertaken at Wrightington, covering periods averaging 8–10 years after the operation, and these studies are reviewed in this chapter.

1) Cupic, 1973[15]

This was primarily a general study of long-term clinical results but it included our first study of wear in vivo and related to 72 patients measured between 9 and 10 years after the operation. All these patients were derived from the first year's work of the prospective series between November 1962 and December 1963, when 185 low-friction arthroplasties using cemented HMWP sockets were performed in 170 patients. The first 14 patients had sockets without a circumferential wire marker, and only 72 of the cemented sockets from the first year were available for wear measurement 9–10 years later.

The average wear for the whole series in this study was considered to be 0.12 mm/year: 86% (62 hips) wore on average 0.10 mm/year; 14% (10 hips) wore on average 0.30 mm/year. The accuracy of the method used for measuring wear by clinical radiology in this study (for which the author accepts responsibility) has been criticised and will be discussed later in the chapter.

2) Halley, 1975[57]

This study was devoted entirely to radiological estimates of wear and it re-examined the same group of 72 patients measured by Cupic but using an improved method of measurement. In this technique of measurement the thickness of HMWP in the region of wear was measured on each film and corrected for the individual radiographic magnification of each film. Wear was the difference between the thickness of plastic in the early postoperative film and the most recent film. The validity of this technique is discussed later in the chapter. The average wear for the whole series after 10 years was 0.15 mm/year.

The results were divided into a **low-wear** group and a **high-wear** group. The **low-wear** group comprised patients with total wear up to and including 1.5 mm in 10 years. This comprised 68% of the whole series of 72 patients. The **high-wear** group comprised patients wearing more than 1.5 mm after 10 years. This comprised 32% of the series.

An extremely important part of this paper was an investigation to determine whether the rate of wear changed with the passage of time. The average wear for the whole series year by year was plotted against time and is shown in Fig. 20.1. Each annual point represents the average wear of the same 72 hips measured each year. It will be seen that after the first 5 years the rate of wear diminished.

For the series as a whole the wear rate fell by 44.4% in the last 4 years compared with the wear in the first 5 years (i.e. 0.18 mm/year for the first 5 years and 0.10 mm/year for the last 4 years). In the **low-wear** group (Fig. 20.2) there was a reduction of 58.3% in the rate of wear in the last 4 years. In the **above-average wear** group (Fig. 20.3) there was a reduction of 38.7% in the last 4 years.

All attempts to predict ultimate wear from early behaviour failed. The best that could be attempted was totally unhelpful: if zero wear persisted during the first 3 years there was a 50% chance that wear

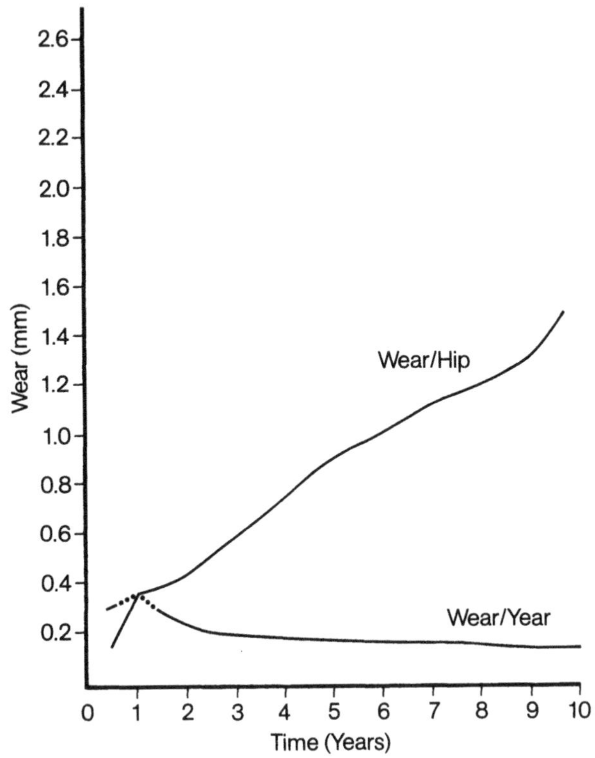

Fig. 20.1. Average wear for 72 patients plotted year by year (Halley)

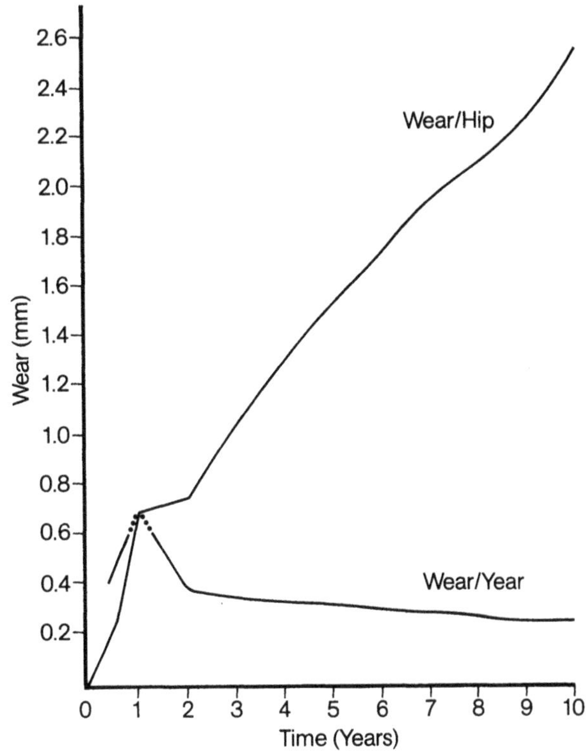

Fig. 20.3. High-wear group (more than 1.5 mm after 10 years)

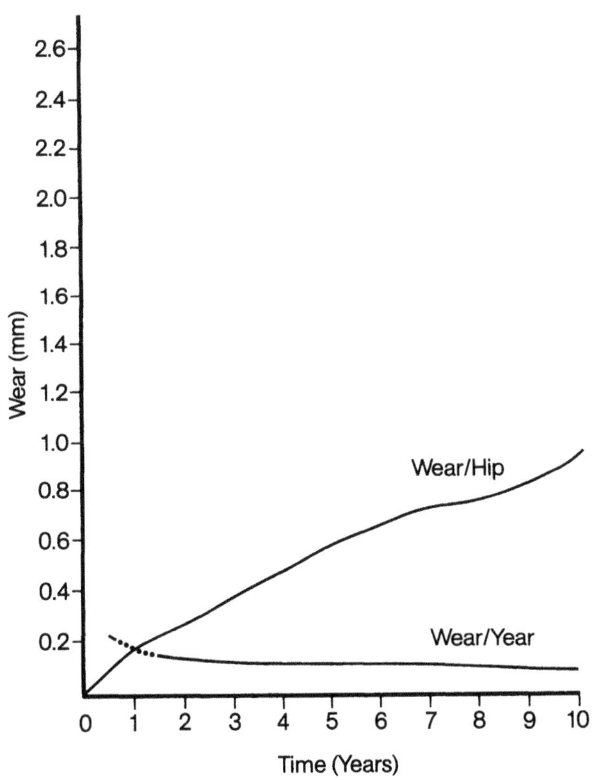

Fig. 20.2. Low-wear group (up to 1.5 mm after 10 years)

would not exceed 1 mm after 9–10 years. Prediction in the high-wear group also was quite impossible: many hips showed rapid wear in the first 3 years (i.e. 0.5–1.00 mm) but this would slow down to stay within the medium range and not wear more than 2.5 mm after the total 9–10 years.

Weight and Wear

The weights of the 72 patients in this series ranged from 100 to 180 lb (45–81 kg) representing nearly a 100% difference. Nevertheless this did not appear to affect the rate of wear.

In order to examine the **simultaneous action of the two factors** most likely to affect wear, i.e. physical activity combined with weight, two separate plots were made showing the distribution of wear in relation to weight in (1) patients exposing the hip to low functional activity (category C patients) (Fig. 20.4) and the distribution of wear in relation to weight in (2) patients considered to have normal functional activity for their age (category B patients) (Fig. 20.5). Category A patients were too few to be considered.

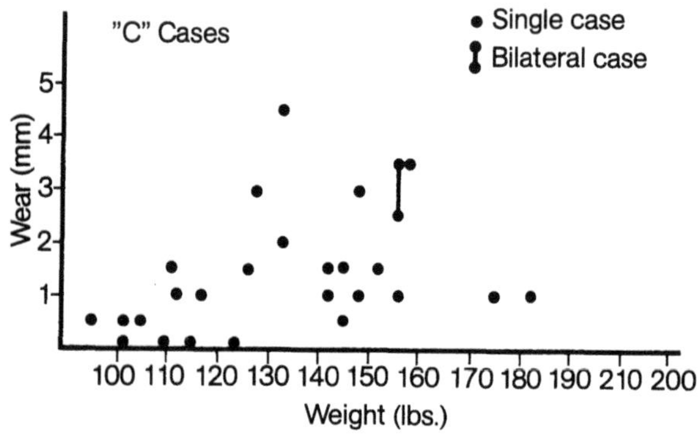

Fig. 20.4. Weight plotted against wear. Category C patients

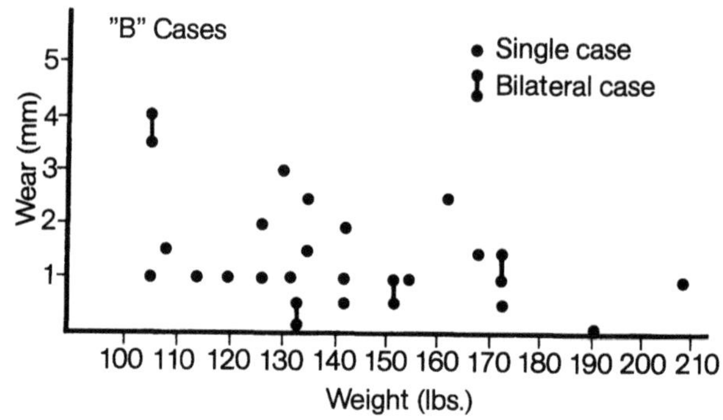

Fig. 20.5. Weight plotted against wear. Category B patients

It is interesting to see that the two plots of wear against weight showed the same distribution in the disabled (category C) patients and in the category B patients. There was no preponderance of heavy wear in patients weighing more than the median weight (140 lb or 63 kg) nor a preponderance of low wear below this level. In the centre of the range of wear the rate of wear covered the whole gamut from high to low wear.

This lack of correlation between weight and physical activity in governing the rate of wear was emphasized by the difference in the numerical grading representing the average post-operative functional activity. The average figure for post-operative function in category B was 5.8, which is very close to the figure of 6.0, which represents normal function. The average post-operative function in the category C group was only 3.5, which implies that the patients still had a very considerable restriction of walking activity. This makes it all the more surprising that the pattern and amount of wear in the two plots were the same.

Wear in Patients Under 30 Years of Age

Halley[57] measured the wear of sockets in patients under 30 years of age at the time of the operation. This group comprised 33 patients with 59 sockets (26 being bilateral). All were extremely disabled before operation as a result of: rheumatoid arthritis, late effects of Still's disease, and congenital dislocation of the hip after previous surgery. It was because of the widespread nature of their disability (category C) that they were accepted for surgery at less than 30 years of age in accordance with the criterion of 'built-in restraint' taught by the author when selecting very young patients for total hip replacement.

Built-in restraint means that the pre-operative disability is such that even after two successful total hip replacements the general physical activity of the patient still would not compete with that of a **normal** person of 30 years of age even though the operation would have totally changed the quality of the young person's life.

Though this section of Halley's paper is of great interest it is difficult to draw firm conclusions because of wide variations in rate of wear and because of the miscellaneous combinations of stiff and deformed hips in this group. Moreover the average follow-up was only 38.4 months ranging from 6 months to 8 years. Halley's conclusions were that after rapid wear in the first 2 years the rate of wear settled '... to a figure not very different from the 9–10 year series', i.e. about 0.18 mm/year. But even so the heaviest rate of wear we have ever encountered in any of our wear studies (0.6 mm/year) was in this series. This was a patient with ankylosing spondylitis only 20 years of age at the time of the operation and observed for 5 years after the operation; moreover this patient had a similar arthroplasty on the opposite hip wearing at the same rate (0.6 mm/year) though at that time observed for only 1.5 years.

This study of wear in very young patients is the only one so far undertaken in this unit. It is the author's opinion that very great caution must be observed for a number of years yet in patients below 30–35 years of age. In these young patients rapid wear not infrequently is associated with considerable radiological demarcation of the socket, though the clinical result may be perfect and it is almost certain that failure will result from loosening of the socket long before total wear-out of the HMWP socket (Figs. 22.2c and 22.3c).

Wear in Patients Under 50 Years of Age

Halley measured wear in four male patients, all category A, with average age of 38.5 years and average weight of 168.5 lb (75.8 kg) followed up for an average period of 5 years. The average wear, surprisingly, was only 0.1 mm/year. As a further check on this important group of vigorous category A males (i.e. single-sided arthroplasties) the author, at the end of 1977 traced nine male, category A, patients (including the previous four) all now averaging 8 years since operation (7–9 years). The average age was 42.9 years (27–52 at the time of operation) and average weight, 173 lb (87 kg). With the exception of two showing heavy wear, the remaining seven averaged only 0.054 mm/year, which is the lowest rate of wear in a series we have yet encountered.

One of the two patients with very heavy wear (0.44 mm/year at 7.25 years) was a teacher of ballroom dancing. For the first 5 years after the operation he worked long hours but in the last 2 years he has been only working 2 hours per evening though not because of any defect in the hip (the rest of the time he administers his two dancing schools). His weight was 189 lb (85 kg) at the operation but had fallen to 175 lb (79 kg). As is not uncommon in very vigorous, relatively young patients showing socket wear there has been some migration of this socket. The result was excellent and graded A. 6.6.6.

The small number of young active males in category A available for this study reflects the cautious selection in force up to 1969.

Direction of Wear

It is fundamental to understanding how wear can be measured radiologically in vivo to appreciate that a small-diameter prosthetic femoral head bores into the material of the socket to produce a cylindrical wear track terminating in a hemispherical surface. This observation was made very early in our experience as a result of the gross amount of wear which occurred with Teflon (PTFE) sockets (Fig. 1.6, p. 7). The very-small-diameter prosthetic head does not wear erratically to produce an enlarged basin-like socket in which the metal ball is lying loose.

It was a surprising fact in Halley's study that in 59 patients (64.4%) the wear took place in an upward and outward direction (i.e. in the plane of the face of the socket). Vertical wear was present in 32.2% (19 patients). Only 3.4% showed wear with a medial inclination (i.e. in the direction one would expect from the direction of the joint force). It is difficult, even impossible, to study the direction of wear unless a marked degree of wear is present; if no more than about 2 mm present, any estimate of the direction can often be only an impression.

The predominance of wear with a lateral component (i.e. in the face of the socket) probably explains why the 'uni-radiographic' method of measuring wear used by Cupic gave an average result not grossly different from the more precise 'duo-radiographic' technique. The uni-radiographic method of estimating wear consists of measuring the narrowest radial distance between the head and the semicircular wear marker and subtracting this from the widest radial distance at the lowest part of the head. The difference is then divided by 2 to give the wear. There is no need to correct for magnification and the estimate can be made on a single film without the need for an early post-operative film to compare. The uni-radiographic technique still can be useful in making a fair estimate of wear, bearing in mind that if wear is vertical it can underestimate wear by about 20% (0.12 compared with 0.15) but it should never be used in a serious scientific study of wear.

Summary

Grade A men under 50 years
6 patients average rate 0.054 mm/year
2 patients average rate 0.38 mm/year

3) Griffith, Seidenstein and Williams, 1978[58]

This is the most recent study of socket wear from this unit and presents a number of important features. The author is particularly grateful to Mr. Maldwyn Griffith who undertook the laboratory assessment of the accuracy of methods of measurements while his associates worked with him on the clinical measurements.

The study includes a reassessment of the accuracy of clinical radiographic measurements in view of the opinion expressed by Clarke, Black, Rennie and Amstutz (1976)[59] that there are so many variables in clinical radiography that it is impossible to make valid wear measurements in vivo. Griffith et al. believe that the variables which made accurate measurements impossible for Clarke et al. probably resulted from: (1) their use of routine anteversion of the socket, (2) the absence of radio-opaque cement to provide a check on coronal alignment of the socket and (3) the design of their experimental model.

Radio-opaque cement makes it possible to check whether the semicircular wire marker was in the coronal plane originally and whether in subsequent years it might have tilted out of the coronal plane. If the socket is implanted more than 10° from the coronal plane a radiolucent crescent becomes visible between the radio-opaque cement and the semicircular wire (Fig. 20.6). Even if this happens it is still possible to **estimate** the thickness of the plastic socket using the outline of the radiolucent crescent rather than the wire marker.

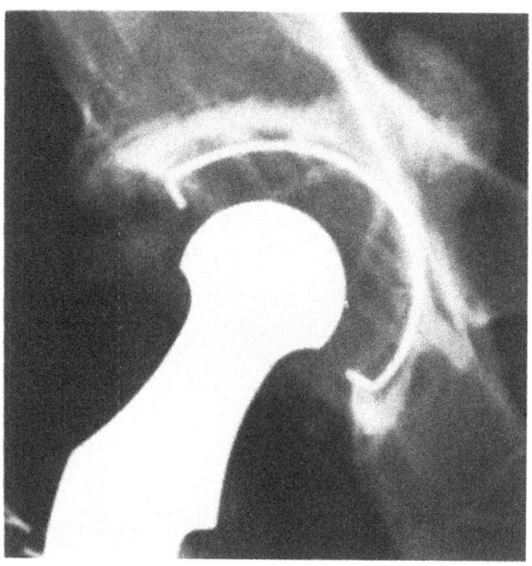

Fig. 20.6. Radiolucent crescent of HMWP visible outside semicircular wire marker when socket is tilted out of coronal plane and visible only when radio-opaque cement is used

The laboratory model used by Clarke et al. to simulate radiographic measurements is criticised because in attempting to show how anteversion and retroversion can falsify the measurement of wear, the direction of the wear-track was given a posterior component when the socket was anteverted and an anterior component when retroverted. The model would be valid only in the unlikely circumstance of the prosthetic femoral head always wearing in the plane of the semicircular wire marker irrespective of the orientation of the socket. There are no grounds for doubting that the direction of a wear track always lies in the coronal plane of the pelvis irrespective of the orientation of the socket. For further details the reader is referred to the original paper.

Clinical Radiological Method of Measuring Wear

Working in this unit Halley was able to get consistent wear measurements taken to the nearest 0.5 mm which had been made in X-rays at yearly intervals over a period of 10 years for 72 different patients (i.e. over 700 films). This would have been impossible if the method was essentially erratic and sensitive to slight variations in alignment of the X-ray tube produced by the numerous radiographers employed during 10 years. In view of the doubt thrown on the validity of clinical radiographic measurements of socket wear, we have repeated and extended experimental observations on a model (Fig. 20.7) originally designed and constructed in this unit by Christensen in 1968.

1) **Effect of variations in centring the X-ray tube.** It is our normal practice always to X-ray both hips on a 17 × 14 in. (42.5 × 35 cm) film and to centre the X-ray over the symphysis pubis (in order that the film should include the lower limits of a femoral prosthesis). The model was therefore radiographed first with the X-ray tube centred 4.5 in. medial to the prosthesis, to represent centring on the symphysis pubis, and then centred on

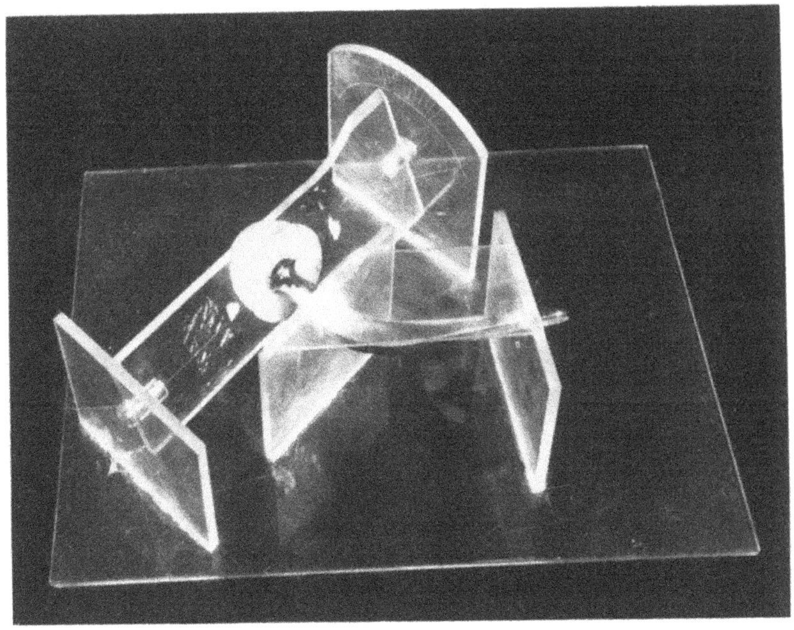

Fig. 20.7. Model for simulating clinical conditions in vitro (C.M. Christensen)

the head of the femoral prosthesis itself. Also, the X-ray tube was centred on high and low positions consistent with possible errors in clinical practice. The model reproduced the average height of the centre of the hip joint above the top of the X-ray table and the level of the film below the table top was at the normal level used in clinical practice. The X-ray tube-to-plate distance was 40 in. (100 cm), the minimum distance likely to be used in clinical practice, and tests at 75 in. (187.5 cm) showed no significant change in proportions. These variations in position of the X-ray tube made differences of only about ± 0.2 mm to measurements of the thickness of the socket provided the wire marker was in the coronal plane.

2) **Orientation of socket.** Our model allowed rotation about a horizontal axis across the centre of the face of the socket to represent anteversion (or 'anterior cup opening') and about an axis at right angles to this to represent 'polar' rotation. Malorientation of the socket in this way results in the wire marker appearing to lie closer to the femoral head in certain zones and so to simulate wear. When radio-opaque cement is used malorientation is revealed by a translucent ellipse of polyethylene appearing between the outer margin of the wire marker and the cement.

The error associated with malorientation of the socket in theory is proportional to the cosine of the angle of inclination of the wire marker from the coronal plane. The inaccuracies increase with the angle of tilt. The first 10° of anteversion causes only little difference to the measured thickness but each succeeding 10° causes an increasing error. This is shown diagrammatically in Fig. 20.8. Thus 10° of deviation from the coronal plane of the pelvis cup will only result in up to 1.5% underestimate of the radius of the socket or a 3.3% underestimate of the socket thickness; 20° malorientation may result in a 14% underestimate of thickness.

The actual radius of the socket as measured to the inside of the wire marker is 20 mm. The thickness of the socket is 9.0 mm. If the cup is rotated 10° from the coronal plane then the smallest apparent radius is $20 \times$ cosine $10° = 20 \times 0.985 = 19.7$ mm. This apparent diminution in the thickness of the cup is 0.3 mm or $0.3/9 \times 100 = 3.3\%$. Similarly with the cup malrotated 20° the maximal apparent diminution in the thickness of the cup is

$$\frac{20-(20 \times 0.94)}{9} \times 100 = 13.3\%,$$ for 30° malrotation is

$$\frac{20-(20 \times 0.866)}{9} \times 100 = 29.8\%,$$ and for 40° malrotation is

$$\frac{20-(20 \times 0.766)}{9} \times 100 = 52.0\%$$

Differences in radius

10° = 1.5%	30° = 13.4%
20° = 6.0%	40° = 23.4%

These theoretical considerations were substantiated by direct measurement of the radiographs of the specimen in varying degrees of anteversion.

Thus errors of up to 10° in orientating the cup will at most cause only 0.3 mm difference in the

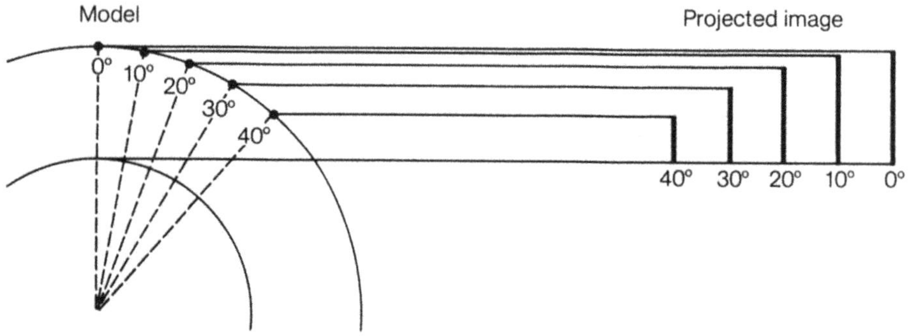

Fig. 20.8. Showing how errors of projected image increase beyond 10° of anteversion

Degrees of anterior cup opening	0°	10°	20°	30°
'Thickness' of the cup (mm) measured on X-rays on model	9.0	8.8	7.7	6.5
Theoretical 'thickness' (mm) of the cup (calculated from angles)	9.0	8.7	7.8	6.3

Fig. 20.9. Results of observations of effect of socket positions on a model compared with calculations

apparent thickness of the cup when the position of the X-ray beam is constant (Fig. 20.9).

3) **Malorientation of socket plus variation in positioning the X-ray tube.** When the radiographic marker does not lie in the coronal plane the separation of its image from the image of the femoral head will become sensitive to varying positions of the X-ray beam, as indicated diagrammatically in Fig. 20.10. This was tested practically in the following way. The socket was rotated on the model to represent degrees of anteversion and/or polar rotation varying from 0° to 30° and each example of malrotation of the socket was then radiographed with the tube centred in the four ways previously described (medial to hip, over hip, high and low) in order to represent maximal variation in radiographic technique. The results are shown in Fig. 20.11. Varying positions of X-ray tube, as previously described, did not alter the measurements of the cup by more than 0.3 mm when the cup was rotated up to 10° from the coronal plane.

When there is 20° or more rotation of the cup from the coronal plane then variation in centring the X-ray tube considerably alters the measured thickness of the socket. In the important superior segment, where wear is to be expected, the maximum errors in the thickness of the cup occur when the X-ray tube changes from being high to low relative to the socket. Changes in centring of the tube in a medial to lateral direction, (i.e. centred over the prosthesis or over the symphysis pubis) made much less difference to the measured thickness in the important superior segment of the malorientated socket.

These experiments show that if the wire marker lies within 10° of the coronal plane of the body radiological measurements of the thickness of the cup are not seriously affected by variation in radiological centring well within the range of clinical practice. If, however, the socket is rotated by more than 10° from the coronal plane, measurements will be unreliable. When radio-opaque cement has been used malorientated sockets can be identified by the translucent ellipse of polyethylene between the wire marker and the cement. In this case films that show an ellipse between bone and cement are unsuitable for wear measurements unless exactly the same appearance is present in both films, but in some cases when the interface between polyethylene and cement is clearly defined this can be used as the point of reference instead of the wire marker.

Griffith et al. checked the accuracy of the duoradiographic technique in 14 patients by comparing clinical radiographic measurements with direct measurements when the socket was later available as a result of revision or post-mortem. Direct measurements of wear were made from acrylic casts of the cavity of the socket using an optical profile instrument. With the exception of one case (where there was an unexplained minus error of 0.5 mm) the wear of the remaining 13 specimens as measured on clinical radiographs agreed with the actual wear measured on socket replicas within plus or minus 0.20 mm (Fig. 20.12).

An important detail which emerged from this study was that observer errors (three different observers measuring the same X-ray) most often were traced to variations in the particular radius chosen by different observers to represent the direction of maximum wear. It was possible to achieve errors in the final calculation of more than 100% by different observers choosing different radii but when the direction of the radius was agreed differences could be ignored.

Clinical Measurement of Wear

In the study of socket wear by Griffith et al.[58] a new group of patients was chosen rather than the original prospective group operated on before 1965, which had been measured on the two previous occasions already reported. The patients in this new group had been operated on in 1967 and 1968. For this study 351 patients were X-rayed and there were also 196 patients who had been examined within the current year with X-rays suitable for measurement. There were thus 491 hips suitable for measurement with a mean follow-up period of 8.3 years (range 7–9 years) (Fig. 20.13).

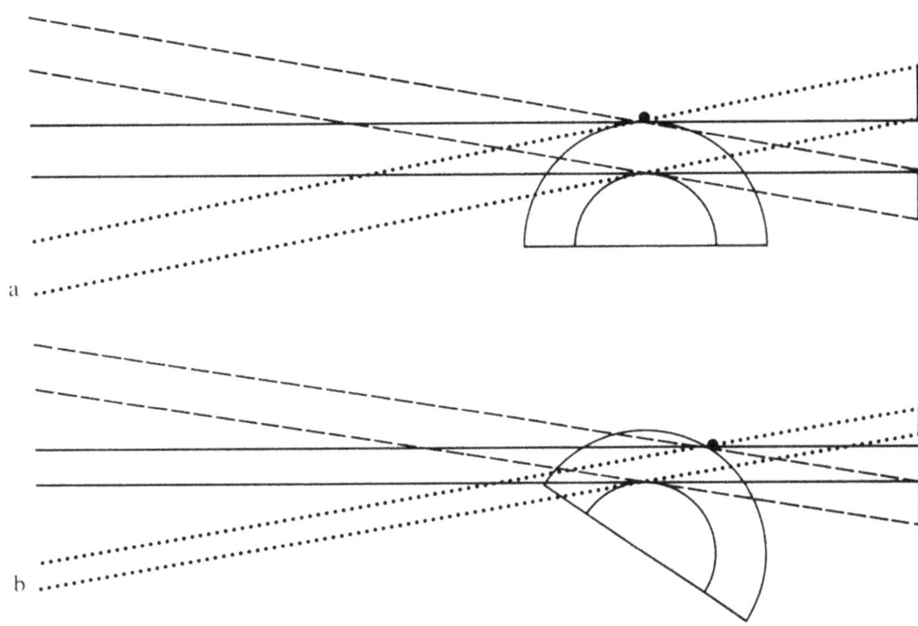

Fig. 20.10a, b. Showing how variations in direction of X-ray beam will distort wear measurements (**b**) if wire marker is not in coronal plane. Not so (**a**) if wire marker is in coronal plane

Anterior cup opening	No polar rotation				10° Polar rotation				20° Polar rotation			
	0°	10°	20°	30°	0°	10°	20°	30°	0°	10°	20°	30°
Location of cup on film												
Central high	8.9	8.7	8.3	7.8	8.6	8.2	7.6	6.8	8.2	7.6	6.7	5.9
Central low	9.0	8.9	8.6	8.2	8.9	8.6	8.0	7.4	8.6	8.1	7.5	6.7
$4^1/_2''$ Lateral high	8.8	8.6	8.1	7.7	8.6	8.2	7.5	6.7	8.0	7.4	6.8	5.8
$4^1/_2''$ Lateral low	8.9	8.9	8.7	8.3	8.8	8.5	8.1	7.3	8.4	8.1	7.3	6.6

Fig. 20.11. Socket thickness measured on model with 0°–30° of anteversion and polar rotation, and with four positions of X-ray tube

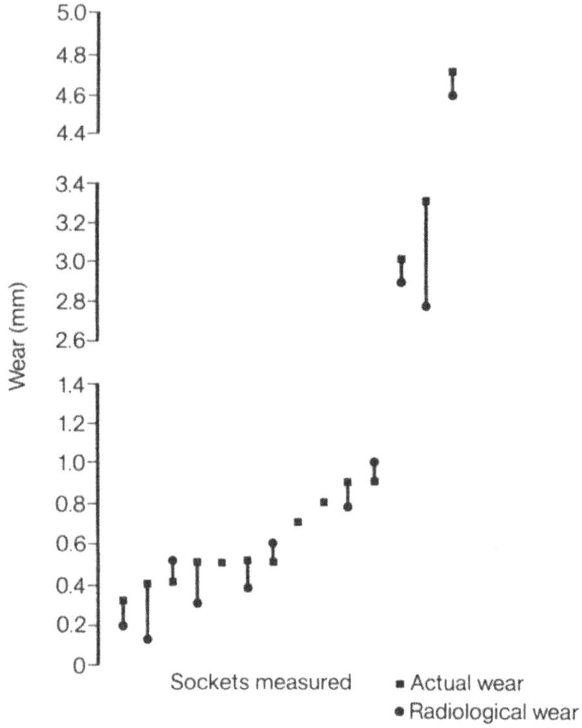

Fig. 20.12. Clinical radiographic estimates of wear on last available film compared with direct measurement of removed socket

The average rate of wear for the whole series of 491 sockets was 0.07 mm/year. This, rather surprisingly, is one-half the previous average figure of 0.15 mm/year for the patients of the prospective study from November 1962 to December 1965. In this most recent study 63.5% (312 hips) showed less than 0.5 mm wear in the total period of study (0.06 mm/year). Only 20 sockets (4%) had worn between 1.5 and 2.8 mm (average 1.9 mm), corresponding to an average for high wear of 0.24 mm/year. These results were examined for factors which might explain differences in rates of wear.

Sex. Of the sockets with more than 0.18 mm/year rate of wear 70% were in males; yet the males formed only 23% of the whole series. On these figures males seemed to be more at risk, except for the remarkable results for category A patients averaging 43 years of age (p. 323).

Age. Heavy wear was commoner in young patients than in old (Fig. 20.14).

Weight. There was no correlation with weight. In the minimum wear group the average weight was 67 kg (147 lb) ranging widely from 38 to 110 kg (84–244 lb). In the group with heav-

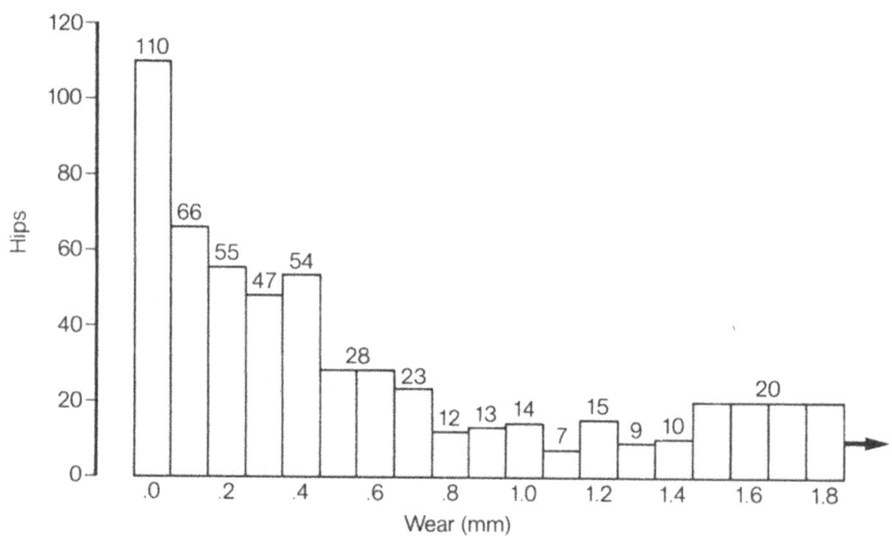

Fig. 20.13. Wear of sockets measured by duo-radiographic technique in 1967–1968 series averaging 8.3 years after operation

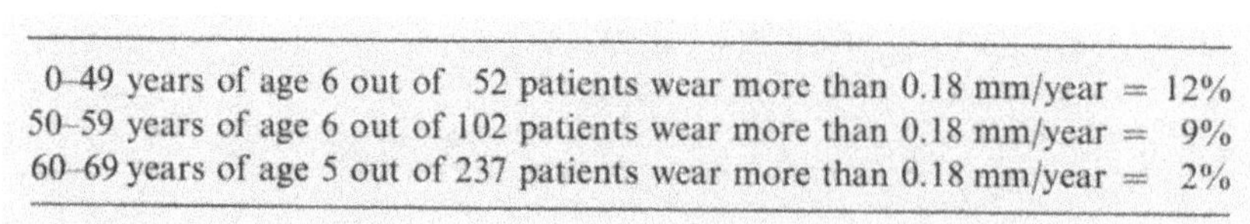

0–49 years of age 6 out of 52 patients wear more than 0.18 mm/year =	12%
50–59 years of age 6 out of 102 patients wear more than 0.18 mm/year =	9%
60–69 years of age 5 out of 237 patients wear more than 0.18 mm/year =	2%

Fig. 20.14. Age of patients related to socket wear

Grade of function	0.06 mm/year total wear	0.06–0.18 mm/year total wear	0.19 mm/year total wear
1	4 (1.3%)	1 (0.6%)	0 –
2	25 (8.0%)	8 (5.0%)	2 (10%)
3	42 (13.5%)	19 (12.0%)	0 –
4	47 (15.0%)	16 (10.1%)	4 (20%)
5	49 (15.7%)	29 (18.2%)	0 –
6	145 (46.5%)	86 (54.1%)	14 (70%)
	312	159	20

Fig. 20.15. Functional grade of patient related to socket wear

iest wear the average weight was 70 kg (154 lb) ranging from 41 to 85 kg (91–187 lb).

Post-operative function. In Fig. 20.15 the functional grades of the patients are plotted against wear in three groups. It will be seen that of 245 patients in function grade 6 (normal) only 14 patients (5.7%) wore more than 0.19 mm/year over 8.3 years. Combining these with grade 5 function there are still only 14 patients wearing more than 0.19 mm/year in 323 patients = 4.9%.

The 50% improvement in average wear resistance of HMWP in this study of patients operated on in 1967 and 1968, compared with those operated on in 1963 to 1965, is of great interest. As in the previous study there was the same tendency for something over 60% to show average wear less than the average for the whole series, but in this study a smaller percentage (4%) showed wear more than three times the average. In this series the percentage rated as three times the average was one-quarter of that in the previous study.

Summary of Wear

	Halley, 1963–1965	Griffith et al., 1967–1968.
Average wear for the whole series	0.15 mm/year	0.07 mm/year
Average wear and under	68%	63.5%
Three times average wear	15%	4%

Grade A men under 50 years of age

6 patients, average rate 0.054 mm/year
2 patients, average rate 0.38 mm/year

Direction of Wear and Anteversion

Though a purely theoretical matter, the author believes that anteversion of a hip socket may, over a period of many years, lead to wear of the socket taking place in a forward direction. The theory is explained in Fig. 20.16 where two hips are com-

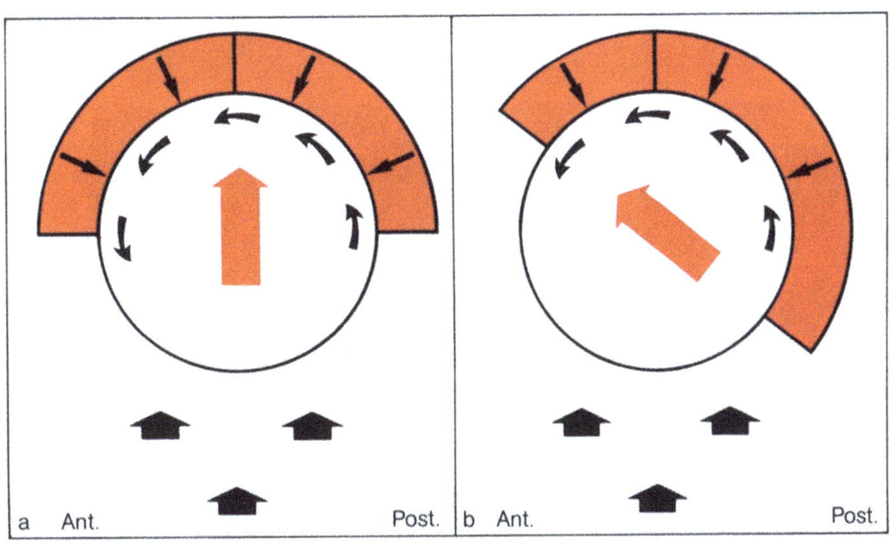

Fig. 20.16a, b. Theoretical possibility of anteversion of a socket favouring forward migration of the head as wear progresses. Lateral views of socket. **a** Equal area of plastic front and back to resist wear. **b** Less plastic in front to resist wear in forward direction

pared in lateral view. Wear in general will take place in an upward direction because of the vertical load, but as regards the sagittal plane because of the 'principle of symmetry', the direction of wear must have an anterior component in case B because the area of socket presented to resist wear is less in front than behind.

Conclusions

From the new study of the 1967 and 1968 patients it is encouraging to find that the rate of wear in vivo was significantly less than the 0.15 mm/year found in the prospective study, though as yet we cannot explain this.

The rate of wear of HMWP would now seem to be one of the less important matters in total hip replacement and certainly not as important as the search for a method of making a perfect bond between acrylic cement and the acetabulum. We have not yet had to replace a worn socket without the cement-bone bond already having loosened. The operation of changing a socket for loosening of the cement-bone junction always presents a more unpredictable future than a primary implantation on a bed of fresh cancellous bone.

There still remains the question of the effects of abraded particles of HMWP draining into iliac and aortic lymph nodes. Particles of HMWP can be seen in these glands under polarised light

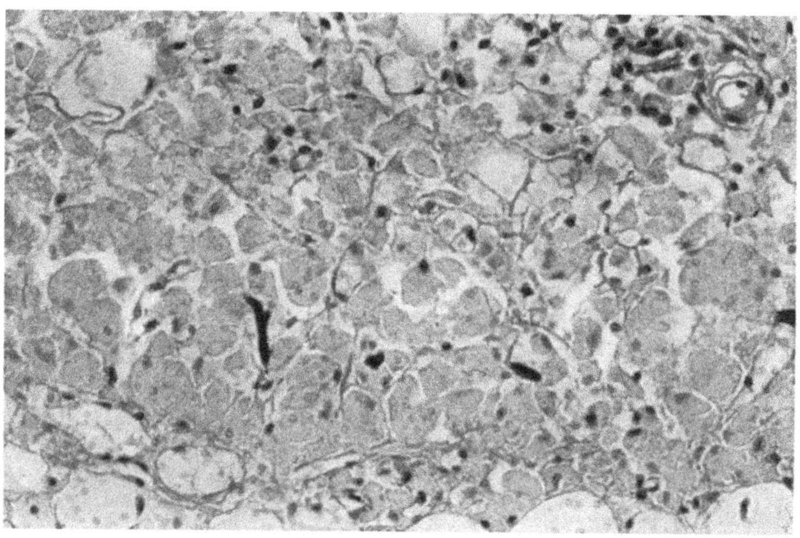

a

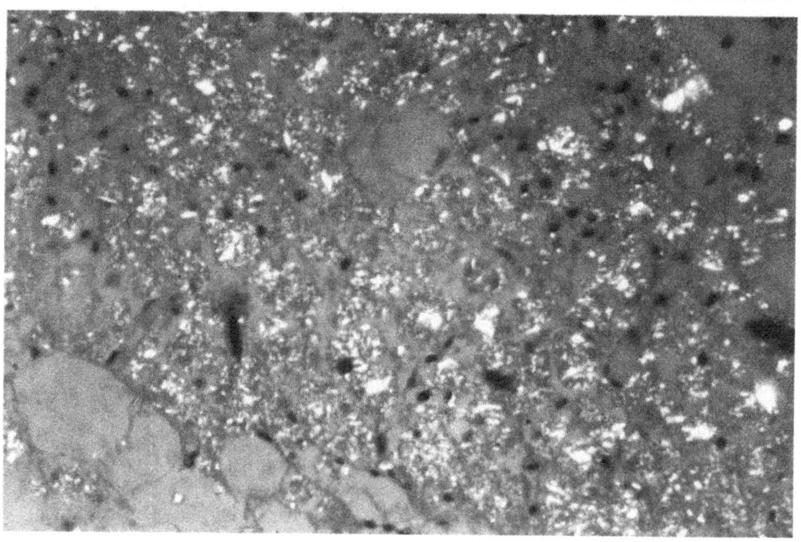

b

Fig. 20.17. a Iliac lymph node replaced by histiocytes (H.E). **b** Same section under polarised light. Histiocytes full of small, brightly birefringent particles of HMWP

(Fig. 20.17) contained inside sheets of histiocytes which are replacing lymphoid tissue. Macroscopically the glands were not enlarged nor were they palpable and indeed they were not at all easily found at post-mortem examination. This is quite different from the effects of particles of PTFE in the solitary post-mortem specimen which was available; here there was considerable enlargement, with palpable induration (this specimen is in the Wrightington museum).

Considerations such as these contribute to the author's reluctance to perform total hip replacement in very young patients even though there is much to indicate that these very small particles may be clinically innocuous. Emphasis here is on the small size of particles because large particles of HMWP produce a giant-cell reaction with the production of foreign-body granulomata with caseation and the production of sterile 'pus'. Therefore research into the wear of HMWP must not be confined merely to the amount of wear but must look into the factors which control the size of the abraded particles. The author's impression is that particles of HMWP from 'unconstrained' knee joints are significantly larger than those he has seen with the small, 22.25-mm-diameter, femoral head prosthesis and he suggests that the high loading on the small diameter femoral head may 'burnish' particles into the surface and minimise the 'third body wear' mechanism possible under low loading. Also small-diameter prosthetic femoral heads can be fabricated, relatively cheaply, at very high degrees of sphericity. Surface polish is not expensive to achieve but to maintain a very high degree of sphericity on a large-diameter sphere and at the same time superimpose a high polish introduces serious technical complications and will escalate manufacturing costs.

Chapter 21

Biomechanics

In this chapter an attempt is made to explain an approach to the analysis of forces acting on the hip which was not evident when Pauwels (1935[60]) first taught orthopaedic surgeons the meaning of the 'moment of a force' as applied to the hip 40 years ago.

The author is indebted to his engineering colleague, Dr. R.D. McLeish[61] for help with a large part of the substance of this chapter. He attempts to interpret some of the work of McLeish and his colleagues on the analysis of one-legged stance and strain-gauge studies on femoral prostheses cemented into cadaveric and artificial femora.

The subject is of immense complexity because of the wide range of variables which can operate simultaneously and it is specially difficult for surgeons because graduate engineers often fail to appreciate the abysmal ignorance of mathematics which hampers surgeons in this field.

Moments of Forces About the Hip Joint

The simple theory of moments of forces, first applied to the hip by Pauwels, was the basis of the author's early enthusiasm for the lateral approach to the hip joint, which facilitated lateral transplantation of the great trochanter and medial displacement of the centre of rotation of the hip joint. By changing the proportions of the lengths of the lever arms, the force transmitted through an artificial joint could be raised or lowered and to achieve a minimum value is obviously desirable when seeking to ensure the longest possible life for an implant in the human body.

To emphasize this approach the author often used to refer to his operation as total hip **reconstruction** to distinguish it from total hip **replacement,** because the latter could signify merely the implantation of a replica of a normal hip joint without making any advantageous changes by engineering design.

Figure 21.1 reminds the reader of the principle of the moment of a force and how, by shifting the fulcrum of a lever, one can change the total load on the fulcrum. For an easily readable exposition of these principles the surgical reader is referred to the paper by Denham[62]. The essence of the mechanics of the hip is that the total load on the hip joint is created more by the abductor muscles than by the mere weight of the body. If a change in ratio of the levers puts the abductor muscles at an increased mechanical disadvantage

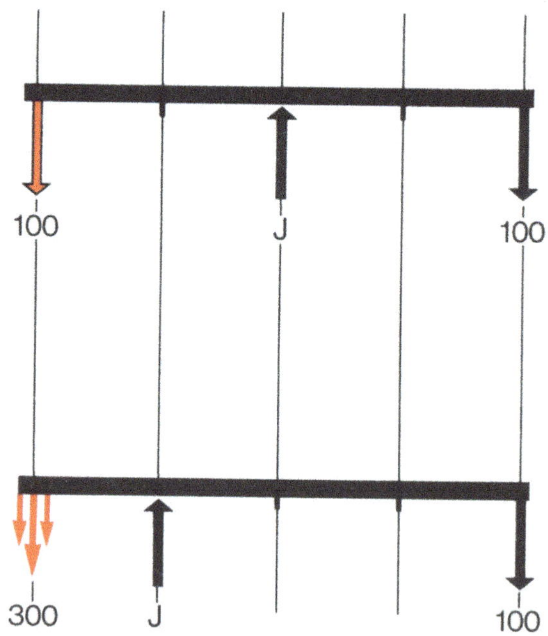

Fig. 21.1. Simple principle of moments of a force. The body weight is constant at 100. The site of the fulcrum changes from a ratio 1:1 to 1:3. Abductor force has to rise to maintain equilibrium. Load on fulcrum also rises

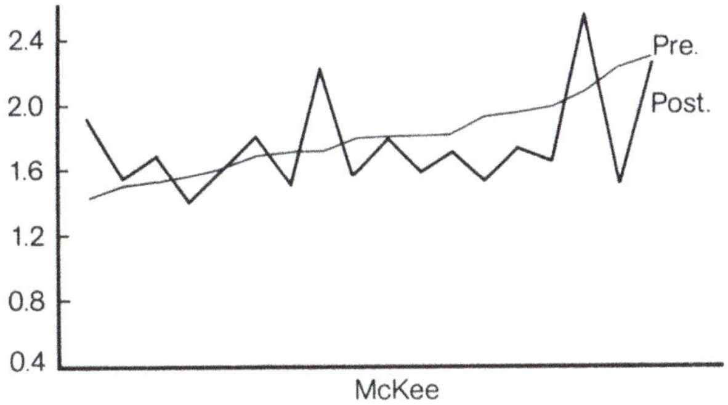

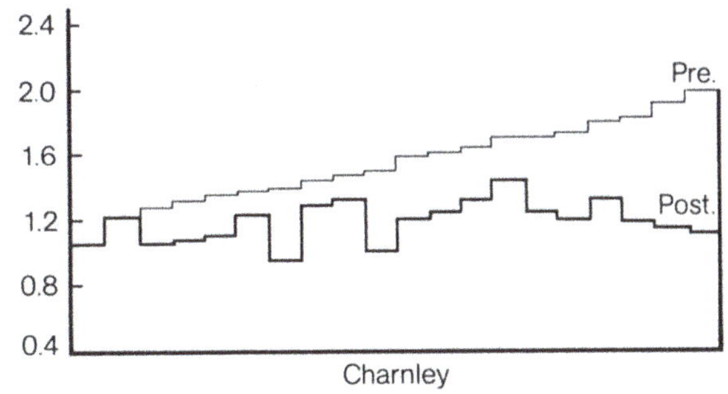

Fig. 21.2. Ratios are: lengths of body weight levers to lengths of abductor muscle levers, measured as in Fig. 21.1. Data arranged in ascending order. McKee cases, without transferring trochanter, show erratic changes in ratios post-operatively. Charnley cases, with transfer of trochanter and deepening of acetabulum, show more consistent improvement in ratios

the muscle force necessary to maintain the pelvis in equilibrium must increase.

Applying the elementary theory of moments to 18 McKee-Farrar operations (all of the original design with the large-diameter 41-mm prosthetic head) Dall[63] by measuring X-rays found that the ratio of body-weight levers to abductor muscle levers averaged about 1.74:1 **before** and 1.65:1 **after** the operation. This corresponded to a reduction in load on the hip of about 3%. On the other hand measuring 20 Charnley arthroplasties with transplantation of the trochanter and medial displacement of the centre of the femoral head the ratios averaged 1.54:1 **before** and 1.19:1 **after** the operation. This meant a reduction in load on the joint of about 13%.

The erratic effect of the McKee-Farrar operation, sometimes resulting in a higher load on the joint after the operation than before, is seen in Fig. 21.2, whereas a consistent improvement, though variable in amount, is seen with the Charnley reconstruction.

Tracings of superimposed X-rays before and after operation are seen in Fig. 21.3a, b.

The foregoing estimates are of course very crude but the order of magnitude of the difference is probably not far off the mark as far as **load on the socket is concerned.** It is the purpose of the rest of this chapter to show that the mere magnitude of the load on a socket is not in itself sufficient to assess the forces acting on the stem of a prosthesis (or on the cement in the region of the medial femoral neck). It is necessary to know the **direction** of the joint force.

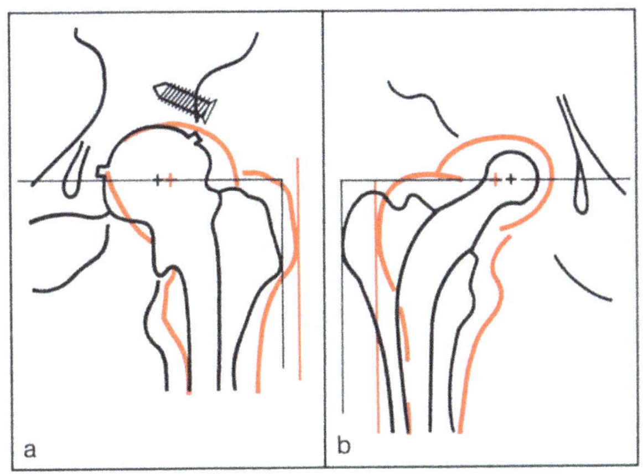

Fig. 21.3. a Pre-operative profile in **red.** Slight medial displacement of centre of rotation of head post-operatively. Lateral projection of trochanter reduced post-operatively. **b** Greater medial displacement of centre of prosthetic head than before operation, compared with **a**, and trochanter projects further laterally

Vector Forces in the Hip

In Fig. 21.1 the forces of body weight and the abductor muscles were drawn as acting vertically and therefore the resultant force on the hip joint will be vertical; but it has long been known that the force passing from the acetabulum to the head of the femur does not act vertically but has a lateral component in its direction.

The architecture of the neck of the femur has always been the most perfect example of Wolff's Law in connecting bone structure with function. Dixon (1910)[67] comments: '... much doubt exists as to whether the disposition of the stronger system of lamellae is to be regarded as associated with direction of pressure, or strain, due to

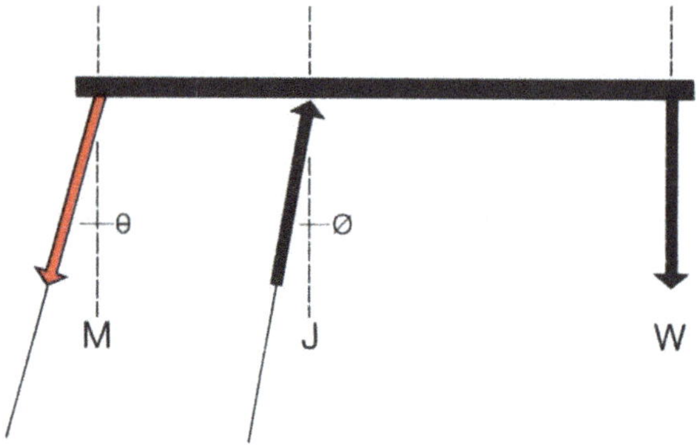

Fig. 21.4. Abductor muscle pull inclined laterally by angle θ. This causes joint force J to incline laterally (though to a lesser degree)

the weight of the body in the erect position ... **or as due to the direction of pull of the muscles which hold the bones in contact at the hip joint**' (Author's boldface).

The lateral component of the resultant force (J) on the hip joint is produced by the direction of the abductor muscle force. We therefore have to redraw our simple diagram as in Fig. 21.4.

Direction of the Abductor Force M

When estimating joint force in the hip the problem is how to determine the angle of the abductor muscle force in relation to the vertical, generally denoted θ. It is sufficient for this account to take the findings of McLeish[61] who estimated the direction of the abductor force for different inclinations of the pelvis by combining data from anatomical dissection with antero-posterior X-rays of subjects in one-legged stance.

In a cadaveric dissection the four abductor muscles (gluteus medius, gluteus minimus, tensor face femoris, and the anterior fibres of gluteus maximus) were identified and a Kirchner wire was threaded longitudinally in each muscle mass to represent the central axis of each muscle. The specimen was X-rayed and the direction of the resultant force, M, of the four muscles was calculated from their relative strengths, which was assumed to be in the order of their relative weights, given by Inman[65] for the first three muscles as 4:2:1 in the order enumerated above.

Magnitude of Abductor Force M

The magnitude of the abductor force, M, is derived by the principle of moments but because the direction of the abductor force is inclined at an angle ($\theta°$) to the vertical it is necessary to measure the length of the abductor moment arm in a direction perpendicular to the line of the abductor muscle force (Fig. 21.5).

Direction of the Joint Force J

The direction of the joint force, J, will depend on whether it is taken in relation to the pelvis or in relation to the vertical (the two coinciding when the pelvis is level). The **direction** of the joint force can be derived graphically or by calculation. The graphical method is instructive.

The theorem of the Triangle of Forces states that 'if three forces acting on a body are in equilibrium they can be represented **in magnitude** and **in direction** by the sides of a triangle taken in rotation (i.e. with the directions following round in the same sense)'.

If we are to construct a triangle of forces for the lever system in Fig. 21.5 where the abductor muscle force of magnitude M is inclined at $\theta°$ to the vertical, **we first establish a linear scale to represent units of force** and the triangle of forces is constructed as follows (Fig. 21.6):

Draw a vertical line of scale length to represent the body weight, W. From the lower end of this vertical line set off a line at $\theta°$ to the vertical and mark off on it the scale length representing the abductor muscle force M (calculated from body weight and the ratio of the abductor and body weight lever arms). The direction and magnitude of the joint force (Φ and J) will then be represented by the line joining the top of line W to the bottom of line M. This line is now transferred, in length and direction, to the hip joint.

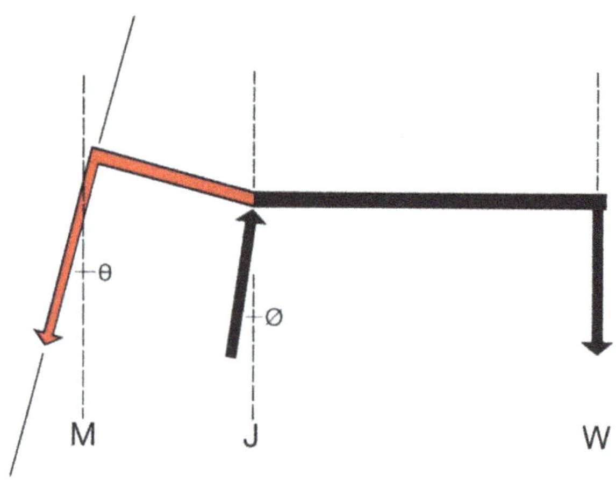

Fig. 21.5. The length of abductor moment arm is measured perpendicular to the direction of the force; abductor lever therefore visualized as inclined (also at $\theta°$) to the body weight lever

It will be seen that the direction of the joint force will always be more vertical than the direction of the muscle force.

Direction of Joint Force in Relation to Femur

The angle of the joint force in relation to the axis of the femur is constantly changing as the posture of the body changes, becoming smaller (i.e. more vertical and more nearly parallel to the axis of the femur) as the free side of the pelvis is elevated, and vice versa. These variations in the direction of the joint force are illustrated in Figs. 21.7, 21.8 and 21.9 taken from the paper by McLeish. Note how the gravity line of the body changes position with the tilt of the pelvis in relation to the hip joint, and how the direction of the joint force changes in relation to the vertical and the axis of the shaft of the femur. If the pelvis were to be elevated 15° the angle of the joint force to the axis of the femur would be about 10° and if the pelvis sagged 15° it would increase to about 35°.

Figure 21.10 shows an X-ray of a femur and how a line through the centre of the head of the

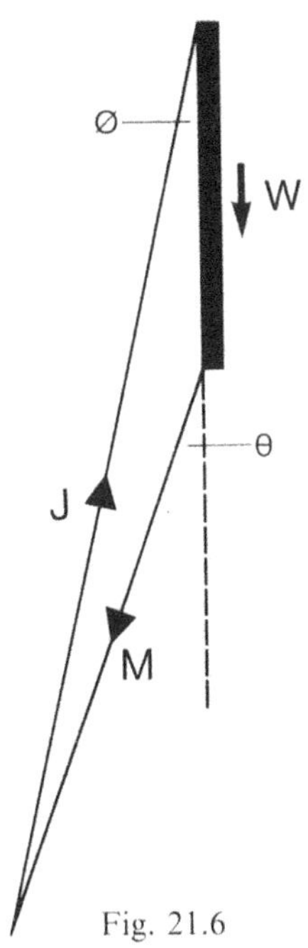

Fig. 21.6

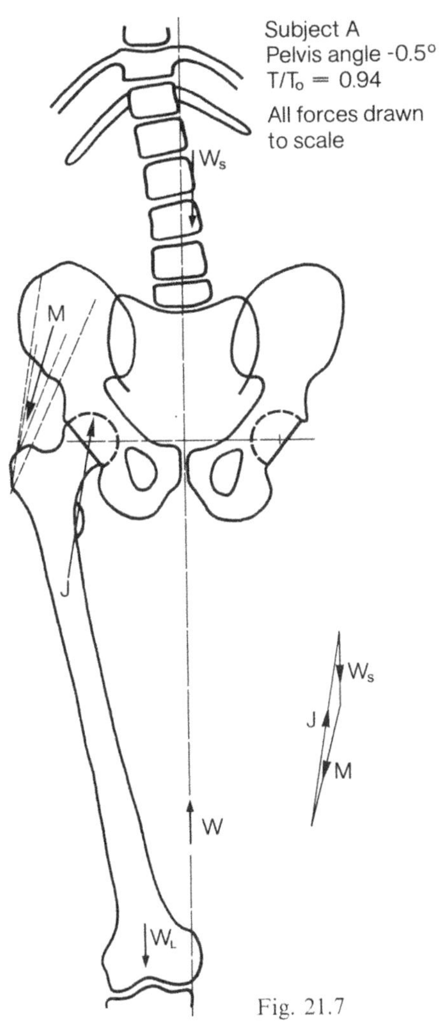

Fig. 21.7

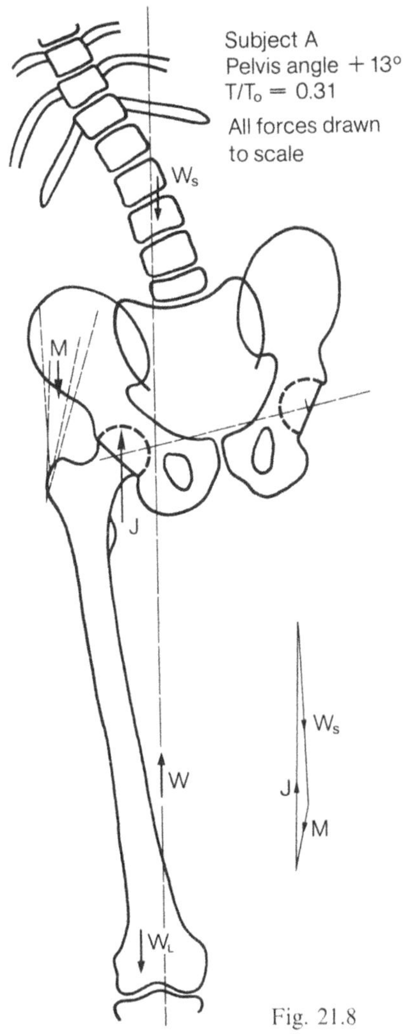

Fig. 21.8

Fig. 21.6. Triangle of forces. Length of M on same scale as W. J therefore represents magnitude and direction of the joint force

Fig. 21.7. Alignment of forces in frontal plane; in vivo studies of one-legged stance (McLeish[61]). With pelvis almost horizontal

Fig. 21.8. Same as Fig. 21.7, with pelvis elevated 13° (Duchenne position with centre of gravity of body nearly above the hip joint)

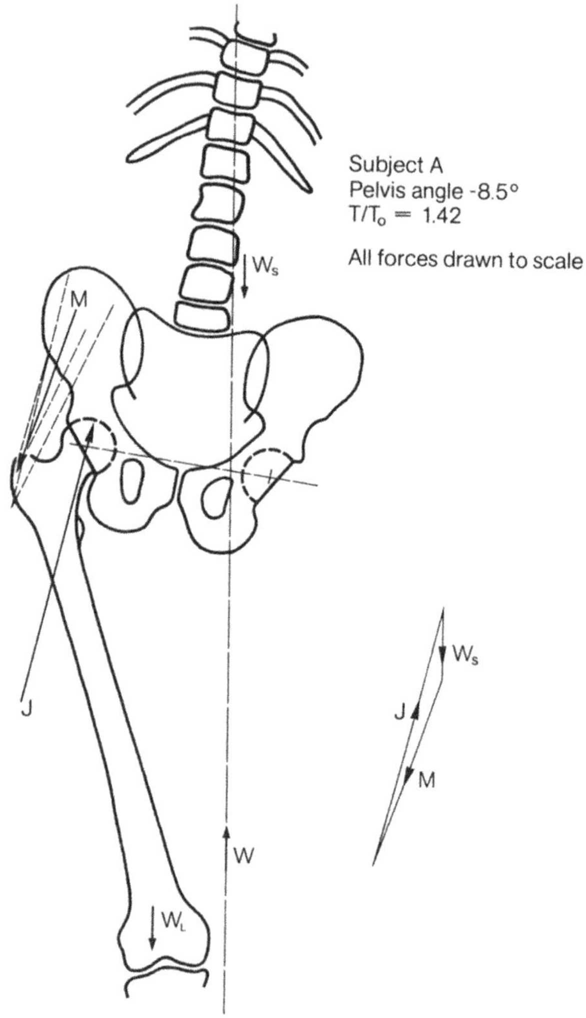

Fig. 21.9. Same as Figs. 21.7 and 21.8, with pelvis sagging 8.5° (Trendelenburg position)

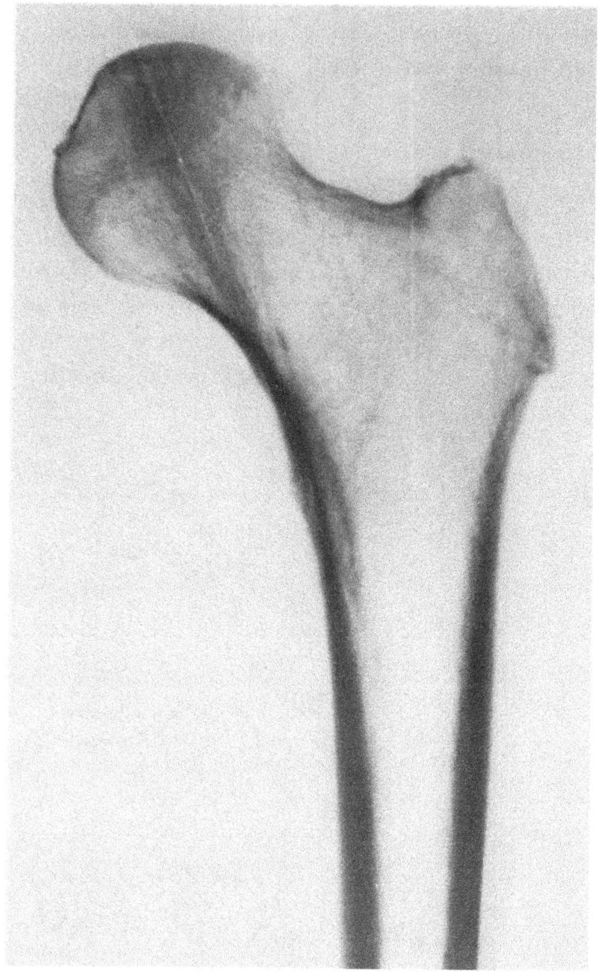

Fig. 21.10. a Normal femur showing load-bearing (compression) trajectories in cancellous bone of medial femoral neck

femur and through the centre line of the trajectories of cancellous bone condensing on to the calcar femoris, meets the axis of the femur at an angle of about 20°. According to Wolff's Law this implies that the angle of the joint force to the axis of the femur **in daily activities** averages about 20°. The 'ideal position' for the stem of a femoral prosthesis therefore would be for it to replace the medial femoral cortex where it would be in pure compression without any bending moment acting on it; for obvious reasons we are forced to use a more lateral, endosteal, position and so expose it to bending moments.

Offset of the Normal Femur

The X-ray of Fig. 21.11 shows the offset of the centre of a normal femoral head in relation to the axis of the femur; 45 mm in this case. This offset was accepted by the author in 1958 as normal for an average adult femur. Therefore a prosthesis with an offset of 45 mm, with its stem in the central axis of the femur, will have the centre of its head coinciding with the anatomical centre of the femoral head. In recent years the author thinks that the 45-mm estimate was too great and that 40 mm is better.

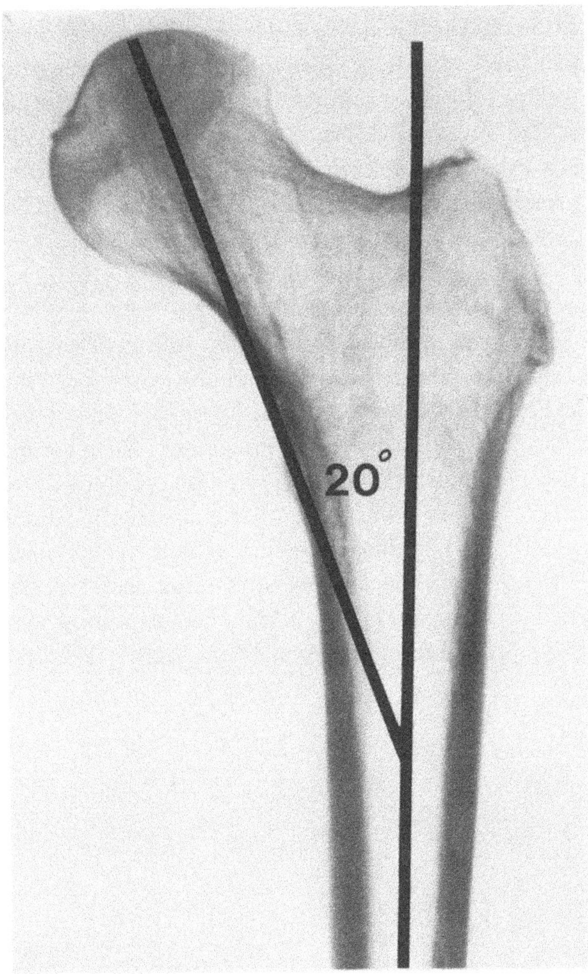

Fig. 21.10. b General direction of cancellous trajectories at 20° to long axis of femur

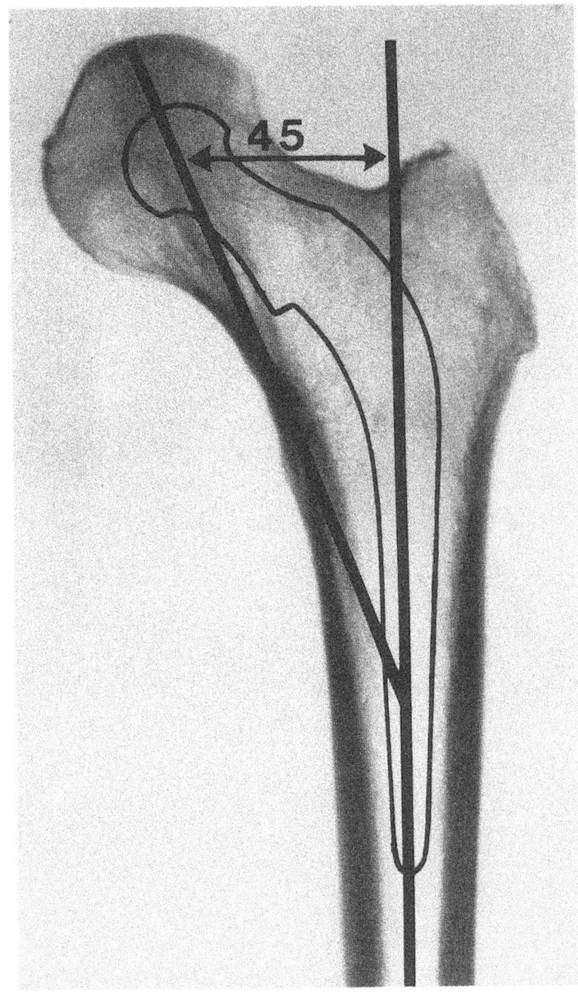

Fig. 21.11. 45-mm-offset prosthesis with stem in axis of femur showing joint force (through centre of head) in physiological direction. Note that later experience indicates 45-mm offset a little too great for average European patients

In the early days of developing this arthroplasty the author was always worried that too short an offset might lead to instability and subluxation of the hip, especially when combined with a deep-set socket. To counteract the potential weakness of a prosthesis with a long offset it was hoped to support it by retaining a long stump of femoral neck. In that era other femoral prostheses required resection of the femoral neck almost to the lesser trochanter (as in the Thompson and Austin-Moore femoral head prostheses and the McKee and Muller total hips) (Fig. 21.12).

The possibility of using prostheses with offsets shorter than anatomical followed from experiences when the femoral prostheses had been implanted in exaggerated valgus alignment. Valgus alignment displaces the centre of the prosthetic head laterally and in effect reduces offset. An exaggerated example of valgus alignment of a 45-mm prosthesis is shown in Fig. 21.13 where a vertical through the head of the prosthesis touches the medial edge of the cut femoral neck. We found no tendency to dislocation even with this very short offset.

An example of modest valgus alignment of a 45-mm prosthesis is shown in Fig. 21.14 and for many years we regarded this alignment as admirable because it so clearly avoided the varus alignment. Nevertheless a prosthesis with a shorter off-

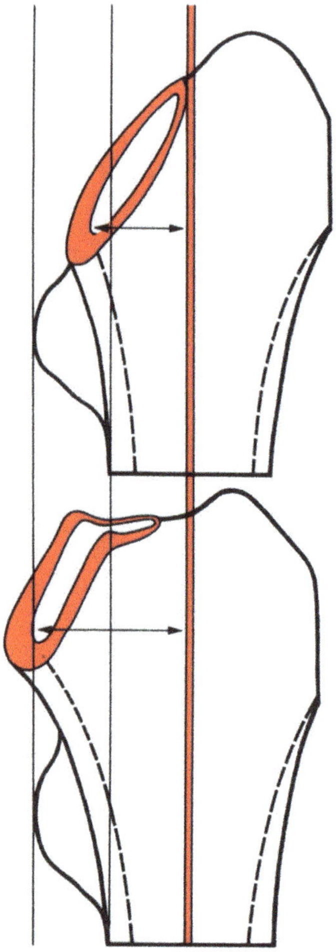

Fig. 21.12. *Upper diagram* illustrates resection of neck almost to level of lesser trochanter as practised for Thompson and Moore prostheses. Note shortness of moment arm to resist rotation of prosthetic stem inside medullary cavity. *Lower diagram* illustrates long stump of medial femoral neck in Charnley design of prosthesis. Originally thought to support extra offset of prosthesis and to resist rotation of stem in axis of femur

set and no valgus would be better (Fig. 21.15) because this would bring the stem of the prosthesis into the neutral axis of the femur while retaining the same offset of the femoral head in relation to the femur. Reducing the offset will increase the strength and stiffness of the prosthesis.

If the 'average' direction of the joint force lies at 20° to the axis of the femur the effect of different offsets is shown, diagrammatically, in Fig. 21.16a, b, c. Because the line of the joint force can be taken as passing through the centre of the prosthetic head it will be seen that if the offset is 'physiological' the direction of the joint force will pass through the medial femoral cortex, Fig. 21.16b. If the offset of the prosthesis is less than physiological the line of the joint force well fall lateral to the medial femoral cortex and nearer to the stem of the prosthesis (Fig. 21.16c) and this will be advantageous in reducing the bending moment on prosthesis and cement. The worst thing would be to have an offset greater than physiological, Fig. 21.16a, because this would increase the bending moment on prosthesis and cement.

The magnitude of the bending moment on the stem of a prosthesis will of course vary with the level in the femur under consideration. This is because the length of the moment arm is measured as a perpendicular from the line of the joint force to the point in the stem of the prosthesis about which the bending moment is being calculated. The taper of the stem provides more metal at the higher levels where the moment arm is long and therefore bending moments are high, and less

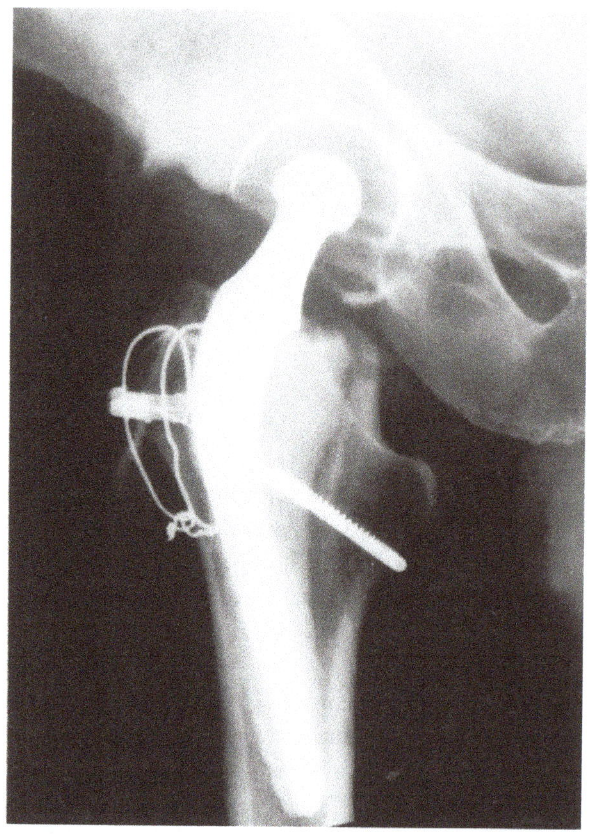

Fig. 21.13. Example of gross valgus alignment. Experiences such as this showed that a short offset of prosthetic head **in relation to axis of femur** did not cause dislocation or subluxation

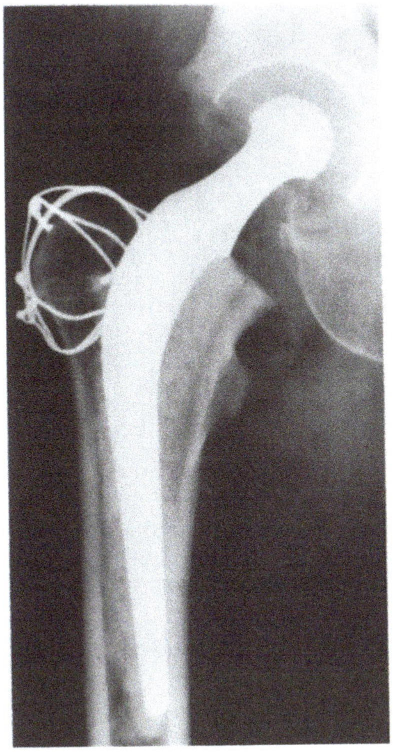

Fig. 21.14. Modest valgus alignment of 45-mm-offset prosthesis considered in 1970 ideal situation. Now considered unnecessary and better to use a straighter (and therefore more rigid) prosthesis

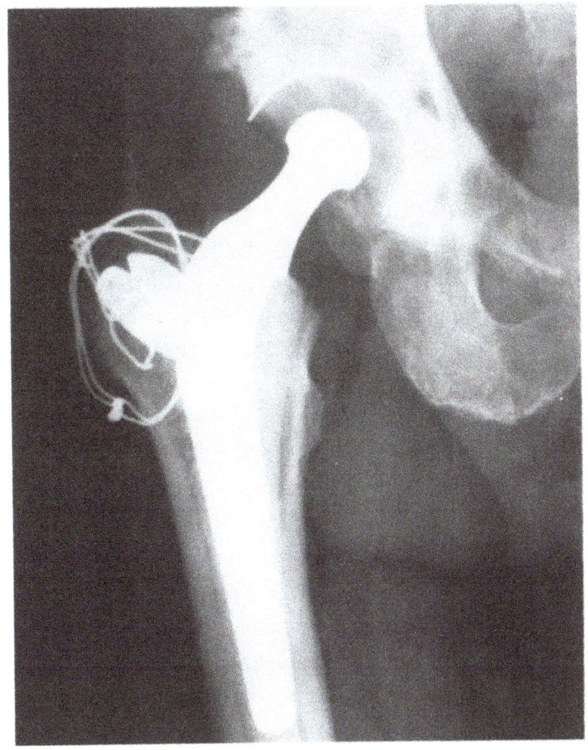

Fig. 21.15. Ideal situation: 40-mm-offset prosthesis with stem in central axis of femur. Prosthesis stiffer and stronger in this arrangement than in Fig. 21.14

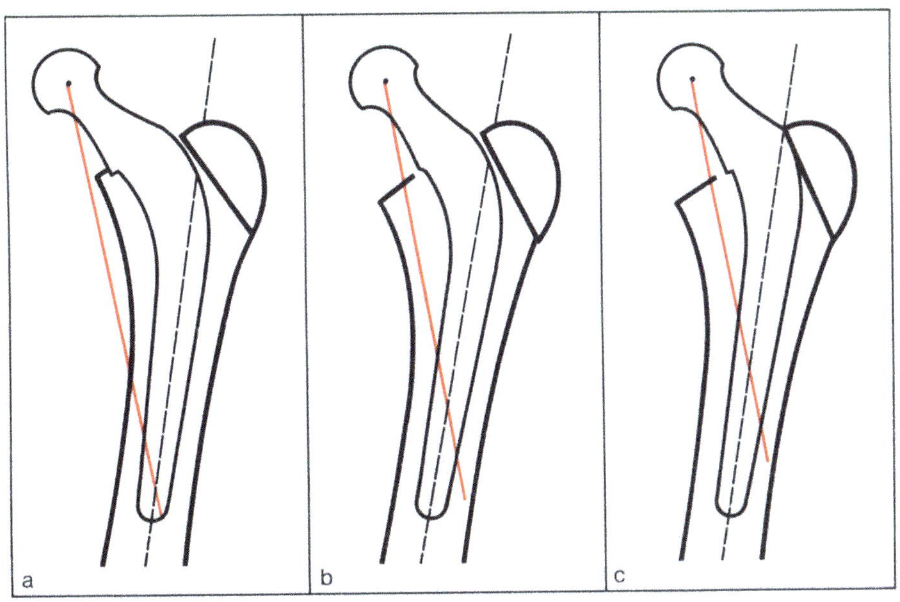

Fig. 21.16a–c. Line of joint force, J (assumed to act at 20° to midline of femur in all cases) in relation to bone of medial femoral neck as result of different offsets of prosthesis. **a** Large offset: line of joint force passes medial to femur. Heavy stress on cement: high bending moment on prosthesis. **b** Anatomical offset (in relation to size of bones). Line of joint force physiological direction. **c** Short offset; less than physiological. Line of joint force lateral to medial femoral neck. Low stresses on cement; reduced bending moments on prosthesis. Best effect obtained only if trochanter displaced laterally to maintain length of abductor lever and angle, θ, of abductor force

metal lower down where the moment arm is short and therefore bending moments are low.

Penalties of Excessively Short Offsets

A prosthesis with a short offset produces medial displacement of the shaft of the femur, and if the great trochanter moves medially with the femur there will be two disadvantageous consequences:

1) The **length of the abductor lever will be reduced** and so a more powerful abductor force will be required. This will increase the joint force and so impair the benefit of the short offset in reducing bending moment on the prosthesis.

2) The **angle θ will be reduced** and the direction of the abductor force will therefore become more vertical. Consequently the joint force will become more vertical. The more the direction of the joint force tends towards becoming parallel with the axis of the femur, the higher the bending moment on the stem of a femoral prosthesis. Both these factors combine to increase the bending moment on a prosthesis.

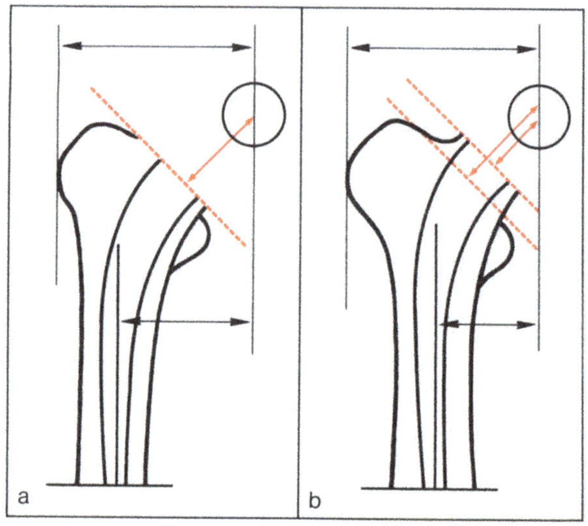

Fig. 21.17. a L-shaped upper end of femur; long prosthetic neck without transference of trochanter. **b** T-shaped reconstruction of upper end of femur; relatively short prosthetic neck with transfer of trochanter. Length of abductor levers same in both cases. T-shaped femur = bovine, heavy-load-bearing design

Lateral Transplantation of the Trochanter

It is therefore logical to transplant the trochanter laterally, in relation to the femur, in order to maintain the normal length of the abductor lever and the normal inclination, θ, of the pull of the abductor muscles. This is essential if one is to achieve the maximum benefit in reduction of bending moment when using a short offset prosthesis. This principle, maintaining the length of the abductor lever and reducing the bending moment on the femur, has long been taught by the author using the analogy that the anatomy of the upper end of the femur should be changed from the L-shape of the normal human femur to the T-shape of the femora of quadrupeds (Fig. 21.17).

It must be emphasized that we are attempting to retain the trochanter at its anatomical distance from the mid-line of the body and not attempting a 'super-human' lateral siting. There are surgical limitations to the amount of lateral displacement of the trochanter which is feasible. In order to obtain rapid union in the presence of full activity,

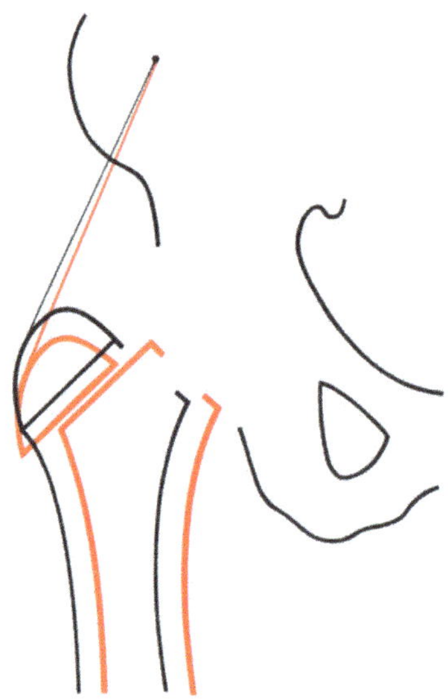

Fig. 21.18. Lateral displacement of trochanter to maintain length of abductor lever and abductor force angle θ, when shaft of femur is slightly displaced medially by short offset prosthesis. No need to increase lateral projection of trochanter beyond physiological distance from centre of body

the maximum lateral displacement possible without reducing too much the area of bone contact is not more than 1 cm. But, because of the geometry of the situation (Fig. 21.18) 1-cm lateral displacement of the trochanter in relation to the cut surface of the femur does not increase the length of the abductor moment arm by more than about 0.5 cm. Nevertheless quite small movements of the trochanter produce valuable contributions to the mechanics of the situation because the abductor forces are very high, being in the region of 1.5–2.0 times greater than body weight.

If one wishes to increase lateral displacement of the trochanter more significantly, it would be necessary to insert a bone graft between the trochanter and femur as has been advocated by English[66], but there could be disadvantages to such a radical step and especially one which is not absolutely necessary.

Deepening of the Acetabulum

This is the aspect of hip reconstruction on which discussions with Dr. McLeish have modified one of the author's concepts based on the simple teaching of Pauwels.

Because the abductor muscles involve forces considerably greater than body weight the abductor lever is more sensitive to changes in length than the body weight lever. Thus in terms of mere magnitude of force we could say that 0.5 cm of abductor lever is equivalent to about 1.0 cm (or even more) of body weight lever. To keep the angle of the abductor muscle (θ) normal (and prevent the joint force J from acting vertically on the head of the prosthesis) we must maintain the normal projection of the trochanter. **If a short offset prosthesis is used the normal projection of the trochanter could be lost by too much deepening of the acetabulum.**

But there are surgical considerations in any policy of minimum deepening of the acetabulum. It is a sound surgical principle always to deepen sufficiently to contain the socket under the roof of the acetabulum. In the average patient the acetabulum is not deepened more than 0.5 cm because there is not sufficient bone in the floor of the acetabulum to permit more than this.

Where deliberate conservation of deepening is important is in large men with very large acetabula; in these patients it is possible to deepen 1 cm and sometimes as much as 1.5 cm. But even here in recent years surgical facts have been leading us away from gross deepening, because in these cases to deepen to the full depth can produce excessive projection of the rim of the acetabulum and particularly so if projection of the rim is already increased by osteophytic outgrowths.

Quantitative Effects of Surgical Variables

In reconstruction of the hip three basic dimensions can be modified by the surgeon:

1) Length of the body weight lever (distance of the centre of rotation from the midline of the body)
2) Offset of the prosthesis (perpendicular distance of centre of prosthetic head from axis of femur)
3) Length of the abductor lever (distance of trochanter from centre of prosthetic head, approximately)

A fourth variable, varus or valgus alignment of the prosthesis in the femur, can have important effects on stresses in the stem of the prosthesis but for the purposes of simplicity the author excludes this because (a) the object of Chapter 16 is to describe a technique whereby the axis of the prosthesis can be made to coincide with the axis of the shaft of the femur so that the chosen offset of the prosthesis will be the actual offset in the patient, and (b) because varus and valgus siting of the prosthesis displaces the femoral head in relation to the axis of the femur in the same way as different offsets of prosthesis.

In order to give some idea of the effects of changing the three surgical variables, in numerical values, the author is indebted to Dr. McLeish for processing, through his own computer programme, data prepared by the author by graphical construction. A solution by computer was necessary because the second stage of the graphical method (i.e. finding the angle of the joint force) was found not to be sufficiently accurate, compounding as it did any errors of drawing in the first stage (and by this illustrating how sensitive the geometry is to small changes in dimensions, especially angles). It is emphasized that Dr. McLeish cannot be held responsible for the exact figures presented below because these are derived from theoretical data of the author's. In McLeish's own computer programme the input data are derived from actual measurements of stresses in strain-gauged prostheses in cadaveric femora with load angles derived from studies of stance in human subjects, but his work is too complex for an elementary presentation such as the author is attempting here. It is hoped that this chapter may help in the understanding of the work of McLeish and his colleagues when eventually it is published.

Data

The theoretical or artificial data presented for the computer analysis were derived from the tracing of an X-ray with a 45-mm prosthesis in situ as indicated in Fig. 21.19.

The length of the body weight lever (*l*) is taken as the horizontal distance from the centre of the femoral head prosthesis to the *mid-line* of the body. This is quite unrealistic as regards equilibrium in one-legged stance because, as already mentioned, the gravity line of the body changes grossly in relation to the hip according to the posture of the body. Nevertheless the gravity line crosses the mid-line during each half-cycle when walking and therefore the mid-line site could be justified as an instantaneous position of the gravity line at some point in the walking cycle.

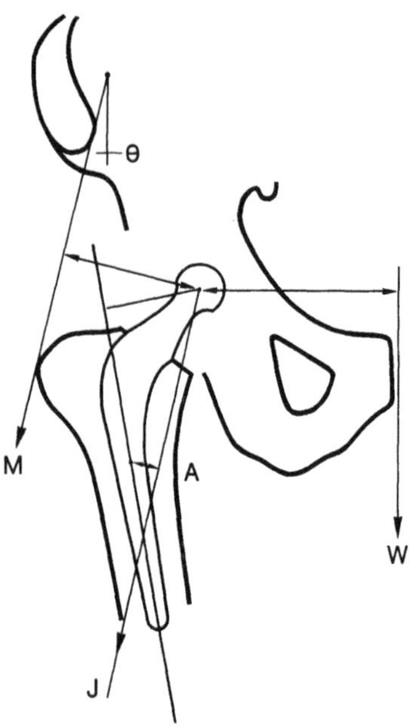

Fig. 21.19. Data traced from X-ray with 45-mm-offset prosthesis in situ. *A*, length of the moment arm concerned in bending prosthesis at a point 8 cm above tip of prosthesis. See text for point of origin of abductor force on ilium

The angle of the axis of the femur to the vertical was fixed arbitrarily at 10°. The author has no data to judge how far this fails to represent the situation in slow walking, when the gravity line of the body is crossing the mid-line of the body, but 10° would seem to be a not unreasonable estimate.

The pelvis is assumed to remain horizontal. The point on the ilium from which a line should be drawn to the lateral outline of the trochanter, to represent the direction of the abductor force, presents a problem. For the purpose of this demonstration the author, from McLeish's diagrams (Fig. 21.7) has taken a point 2.5 cm medial and 2.5 cm above the antero-superior iliac spine as seen in the antero-posterior projection. This corresponded to a point (measured directly on the X-ray at 1.2 times magnification) 15.65 cm lateral to the mid-line, and 11 cm above the level of the centre of the prosthetic femoral head.

The length of the abductor lever (d) is the perpendicular distance from the centre of the prosthetic femoral head to the line of the abductor force, M.

The bending moment exerted by the joint force on the stem of the femoral prosthesis is critically dependent on the level in the stem from which the perpendicular is drawn to the line of the joint force. The author has assumed a fixed point, 8 cm above the tip of the prosthesis, because this represents the average level of fatigue fractures. The length of this moment arm is denoted A, so that the bending moment is JA.

Graphical constructions were made for **three offsets of prosthesis (45 mm, 40 mm and 35 mm)** with **two positions of the centre of the hip joint** (the normal centre, and deepened 1 cm medially) and with **three positions of the trochanter** (the normal site and displaced 0.5 cm and 1.0 cm) (Fig. 21.20). Data from 1-cm lateral displacement of the trochanter was not used because, due to the inclination of the line of the osteotomy, maximum lateral shift in relation to the femur in practice produces the equivalent of only about 0.5 cm shift as regards the improved leverage.

The information required by the computer from these graphical constructions was: the ratio d/2

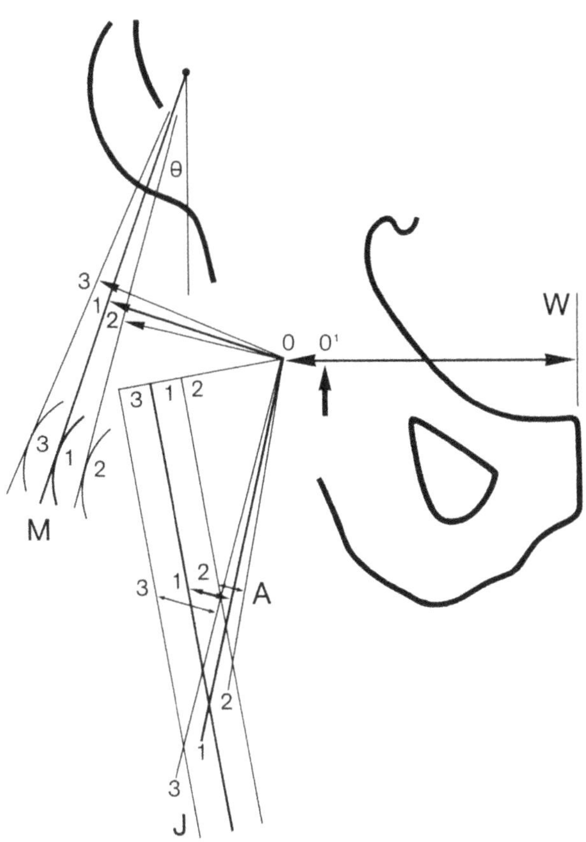

Fig. 21.20. Data supplied to computer for: three offsets of femoral prosthesis; three positions of trochanter; two sites for centre of rotation of femoral head (O, normal; O^1, deepened 1 cm).

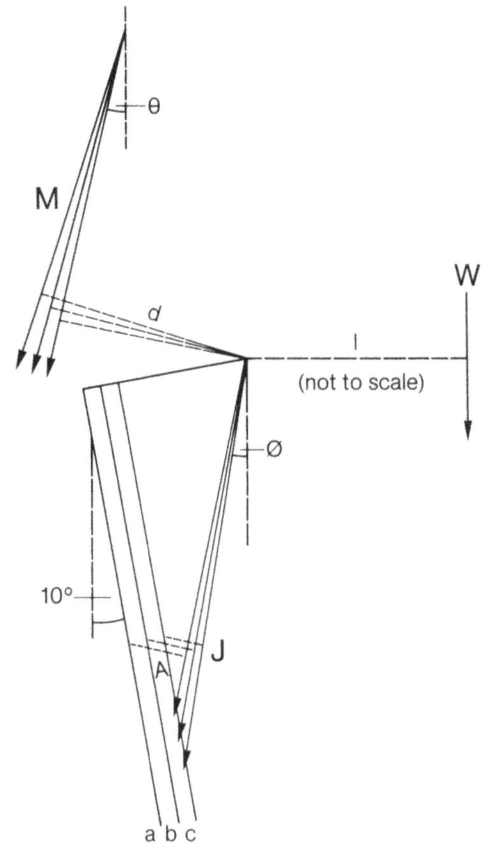

Fig. 21.21. Trace of computer print-out. *l*, body weight lever; *d*, abductor muscle lever; axis of femur in all cases 10° to vertical; bending moment, *JA*, in all cases at 8 cm above tip of prosthesis

(the ratio giving the magnitude of the joint force from body weight) and the angle of the abductor force (θ). The output of the computer used in this presentation concerns the ratio J/W, JA and A. Figure 21.21 is traced from one of the computer print-outs and shows the effects of the three different prosthesis offsets.

To compare the combined effects of these variables the **45-mm-offset** prosthesis, with **trochanter in normal position,** and **without deepening** the acetabulum, is taken as the **standard 100%**. Comparisons with the 100% standard are made as + or − percentages. Four combinations of socket position and trochanter position have been studied for each of the three different prosthesis offsets of 45 mm, 40 mm and 35 mm.

The four combinations are:

1) Normal socket centre; normal trochanter position
2) Socket deepened 1 cm; normal trochanter position
3) Normal socket centre; trochanter displaced laterally 0.5 cm on femur
4) Socket deepened 1 cm; trochanter displaced laterally 0.5 cm on femur

(Note: trochanter displaced **laterally** 0.5 cm means displaced 1 cm distally and laterally as in Fig. 21.18).

The results are shown in the table on p.344. J/W is the ratio of joint force to body weight and is a measure of the joint force. JA/Std is the ratio of the bending moment in the stem of the test prosthesis 8 cm above the tip, to the bending moment in the standard.

45-mm-Offset Prosthesis

Deepening the socket 1 cm produces a 10% reduction in joint force but it increases the bending moment on the prosthesis by nearly 20%. Transferring the trochanter 0.5 cm reduces the harmful effect of deepening the socket on the bending moment; but still leaves the bending moment 5% greater than in the standard.

The best situation for the 45-mm prosthesis is with 0.5-cm lateral movement of the trochanter without deepening the acetabulum. In this case the bending moment on the femoral prosthesis is reduced by more than 10% and the joint force not significantly changed from the standard position. This situation would increase the projection of the trochanter more than the physiological amount and might be cosmetically objectionable or even cause trochanteric bursitis.

1) Normal socket			3) Normal socket	
	Normal trochanter		Trochanter 0.5 cm lateral	
	J/W	JA/Std	J/W	JA/Std
45	100%	100%	−3.0%	−12.5%
40	+4.3%	−13.6%	+0.5%	−28%
35	+8.5%	−30.9%	+3.8%	−47%

2) Socket deepened 1 cm			4) Socket deepened 1.0 cm	
	Normal trochanter		Trochanter 0.5 cm lateral	
	J/W	JA/Std	J/W	JA/Std
45	−10%	+17.8%	−12.8%	+5%
40	−6.6%	+5.0%	−10%	−0.6%
35	−2.9%	−9.2%	−6.6%	−23.7%

40-mm-Offset Prosthesis

Deepening of the socket here is also bad as regards increasing the bending moment on the prosthesis. A reduction in bending moment of 13% when the prosthesis was inserted without any other change of variables, was changed to an increase of 5% when the socket is deepened. Lateral transplantation of the trochanter neutralises the ill effects of deepening the socket.

The best situation for the 40-mm prosthesis is with lateral transplantation of the trochanter without deepening of the socket. This reduces bending moments by nearly 30% without significantly altering the joint force. This combination will not cause abnormal projection of the trochanter.

35-mm-Offset Prosthesis

The most marked improvements are seen in certain combinations with the 35-mm-offset prosthesis but this prosthesis as yet is not commonly used in primary operations in a femur with normal anatomy. It is not easy to place a 35-mm-offset prosthesis in correct alignment without the neck-length jig and **a varus position will reduce the estimates for reduction of bending moments.** Transferring the trochanter is essential with this small offset. When the stem is in neutral alignment the following data will be applicable:

With the trochanter laterally displaced 0.5 cm and socket in normal position, bending moment on the prosthesis will be reduced by 47% of the standard, for a rise in joint force of only 3.8% over the standard.

With the trochanter transferred laterally 0.5 cm and the socket deepened 1.0 cm the bending moment on the prosthesis will be reduced by 23.7% of the standard and the joint force reduced by 6.6%.

Conclusions

It is emphasized that this is purely a theoretical exercise to give some idea of the order of magnitude of changes in joint force, and in bending moment on the stem of the prosthesis, which can be produced by small variations in the disposition of those components of an arthroplasty which are under the surgeon's control. It is emphasized that despite the mathematical disadvantage of deepening of the acetabulum, a hip socket must at all times be fully contained under the roof of the acetabulum. In the average case 0.5 cm of deepening is usually sufficient to achieve this. It is only in men with large bones, where even 1.5 cm of deepening would be easily possible, that mathematical theory advises restraint in this direction.

Chapter 22

Selection of Patients

To try to enunciate golden rules to guide the choice of patients for total hip replacement is an impossible task. The following paragraphs are offered merely to establish certain perspectives rather than give help in specific, and always difficult, cases.

Age Groups

When total hip replacement becomes a true science, as the author believes some day it will, there ought to be no need for a chapter on how to select patients, because then perhaps all hip disorders will be treated by total replacement. This happy situation in fact has already been achieved for patients **over 65 years of age**. Between **45 and 65 years of age** the surgeon must exercise sensitive and informed judgement in selecting and rejecting patients. For operation on patients in this group high-precision technology is essential and this is the group to which this book is dedicated. **Below 45 years of age** we are still only at the beginning of our experience. A few guide-lines for positive acceptance can be indicated and some guide-lines for methods of organizing delaying tactics. The chapter ends with the **15–25-year age group** and highlights the problem of the acetabulum in young people and attempts to point to certain lines of research for the future.

Alternatives to Total Hip Replacement

In the treatment of **osteoarthrosis** of the hip alternative procedures to total hip replacement are being performed less and less commonly and the author is firmly of the opinion that osteotomy no longer has any place. Osteotomy is tempting as a means of bridging 10 years in patients in the 45-year age group, but a previous operation can prejudice subsequent total hip replacement by raising the risks of post-operative infection two to four times. Osteotomy has no scientific basis. One sometimes wonders whether the most successful results of osteotomy might not be those that never needed the operation; because the rate of evolution of osteoarthrosis is unpredictable and remarkably variable. The X-ray when the patient is first seen gives no clue to the rate of future deterioration.

Until quite recently the surgeon's problem was complicated by the dogma that unless osteotomy is performed early in the course of the disease, it had no chance of 'reversing' the pathological process. Therefore so that the surgeon should not be accused of leaving the operation too late, it was often performed with the idea that even if not very successful 'it could do no harm'. But this frequently proved not to be true. Experienced hip surgeons have all seen the case of a patient between 45 and 50 years of age, still just able to manage a round of golf, who after osteotomy has never played golf again and moreover has never been able to get away from dependence on a cane which he did not originally use. Examples as bad as this perhaps are not very common but **they are always possible**; they are very damaging to a surgeon's reputation and nowadays even more so when all patients know the quality of results after total hip replacement.

When patients with osteoarthrosis seek a consultation for the first time they are usually about 45–50 years of age. The surgeon should ask 'Is your pain so bad **at the present moment** that you cannot continue to tolerate it?' 'If I were to reassure you that your pain and disability are unlikely to get much worse during the next few years, would you be prepared to put up with it if I advise this as the best course of action?' These patients often in the past have been athletic and it is their intolerance of minor impairment of physical prowess, and fear of even worse future disablement, more than present disability, which usually urges them to submit to surgery. Usually the reply will be quite emphatic, 'If it does not get any worse than this I can easily put up with it **but are you sure I dare risk it?'** 'Would it not be better for me to have something done now before it is too late and not to take any risks?' If patients in this age group accept to have nothing done and if they continue to try to play golf (even with a restricted number of holes) and if they have physiotherapeutic or osteopathic treatment, what does in fact happen to them? The answer is that if they are seen every year it will be found that more than 50% will go 5 years or more before true disability demands treatment. By this delaying tactic, based on informed reassurance, the patient will be able to get into an age and disability bracket where total hip replacement is the method of choice and in this way the number of years they have delayed will then be in hand at the other end.

It is not adequately appreciated that in the pathology of the early phases of osteoarthrosis biological attempts to restore lubrication go side by side with deterioration. The process is not simply one of relentless mechanical abrasion as goes on in the unlubricated bearings of an engine. It is everyday experience that there is no correlation between the radiological appearances of an osteoarthrosic hip and the amount of pain. Patients can present for the first time with total absence of joint space and advanced osteophytosis and still with reasonable function, so that in these cases some kind of lubrication must still be present. Patients given to assiduous home exercises and to osteopathic treatment with its associated psychological encouragement, quite frequently not only retain a remarkable range of movement but also experience discomfort which is tolerable even in the presence of advanced radiological changes. One sometimes wonders whether the periodic variations in the amount of pain and function which are common in osteoarthrosis may not depend merely on variations in the amount of synovial fluid available to lubricate the eburnated bone surfaces, more than any change in the rubbing surfaces themselves.

On the other hand, though two or three out of every four patients applying for advice for the first time in the 45–50 age group may last 5 years without significant deterioration after a regime based on reassurance has been planned for them, about one in four will proceed to deteriorate within weeks of the consultation and within a year in such a case the head of the femur may have totally disintegrated. Such a case originally was indistinguishable radiologically from the others. Ischaemic necrosis may be the underlying process causing this rapid loss of the femoral head, but in the type of case the author has in mind the degeneration involves the acetabulum from the very beginning. This condition therefore is different from idiopathic ischaemic necrosis, which is confined to the head for several years before the acetabulum is finally involved.

The point of this brief account is that, had osteotomy been performed on all of these patients when seen at the first consultation between 45 and 50 years of age, the slowly evolving cases would have been recorded as successful results of osteotomy and the rapidly evolving case would have produced one of the very sad failures of osteotomy we have all encountered. The failures of osteotomy associated with progressive, unarrested destruction of the femoral head can be as tragic as the failures of total hip replacement because the patient is much worse than before operation and the treatment was proposed as a prophylactic measure. This would still be true if we did not have total hip replacement to salvage these failures.

Over Age of 68

Over the age of about 68, and certainly over the age of 70, osteotomy for osteoarthrosis does a patient disservice. This is the age-group where total hip replacement is one of the greatest boons to mankind. To submit a patient to osteotomy at the age of 70 is nowadays inhumane.

Age and Disability

In deciding to recommend total hip replacement in osteoarthrosis of the hip there are interesting clinical combinations of age and disability to be considered. Though it is an over-simplification, let us take the age of 65 as a dividing line in this exercise.

Over 65 there are no problems of mechanical failure in the future by wearing out of the socket nor need there now be problems (so the author believes!) of loosening of the implants. These patients always must be made to understand that it is a major operation and carries certain, rare risks to survival. The patient must be informed of the risk of being made worse by infection. If the patient fully realizes these matters then almost any patient over the age of 65 can be accepted for total hip replacement **on grounds of pain alone**. To emphasize this point one can almost accept this type of patient by telephone without examination! An X-ray is required, but this is merely to establish the diagnosis and so exclude unsuspected and more serious lesions, and a medical assessment is needed merely for their physical fitness for anaesthesia and surgery rather than for the state of the hip.

Above 65 years of age the X-ray is not required to establish the **extent** of the arthrosic disease. The X-ray does not influence the surgeon's decision whether or not to operate. At this age the decision to perform total hip replacement depends solely on the patient's statement about the pain and what effect it is having on daily life and happiness. In other words in this age bracket the patient is accepted for total hip replacement on their subjective sensations and the objective scrutiny of the surgeon relates mainly to the patient's psychological state (i.e. their motivation, their personality and their mental health).

Below Age of 65

Below the age of 65 the situation is very different. The younger the patient the more the surgeon must guard against allowing the patient's subjective symptoms to influence his judgement. The decision to operate should be made almost entirely on the surgeon's objective assessment. He must turn deaf ears to exaggerated adjectives used to describe the intolerable quality of the pain. Objective assessment relates to: the use of a walking aid; the gait without a walking aid; the range of movement in the hip; the range of separation of the ankles; and, most important, any **spasm** on forcing the hip to the extreme of any range. Spasm is noticed by flinching of the patient's face and **never** by the surgeon asking, 'Does that hurt?'

Below 65 years of age the X-rays of the hip are of very great importance. The X-ray will show how much of Nature's articular cartilage is still available for lubrication and therefore if it is going to be reasonable to recommend delaying tactics. Finally one will ascertain the nature of the patient's work; whether still working; whether the patient could go back to work if the operation were performed.

It is not possible to be more specific than this in emphasizing how physical signs must take precedence over subjective sensations when accepting the younger patients for total hip replacement. It is of paramount importance to emphasize that total hip replacement must never be performed as a 'prophylactic' against the possibility of severe disability at some indefinite time in the future. No arthrosic hip can get too bad to be salvaged by total hip replacement when the time comes. Early operation does not give better results than late; in fact the opposite can sometimes be the case, because operation demanded when the disease is radiologically and clinically early may be more a measure of a patient's low threshold for pain than the degree of disability itself. In these cases there might also be pain after the operation (tenderness over the trochanter) but no sweeping statements can be made and this is a field for an acute clinical sense.

Technique of Delaying Operation

Obviously not many patients between 35 and 45 years of age will accept the advice to delay surgery for a more or less indefinite period of years (say 5 years) unless the method of presenting this advice is adjusted to their particular psychology. A good way of doing this is never to accept for operation **at the first consultation** very young patients with only moderate physical signs. It is essential to see the patient several times; at first perhaps at 6-

month intervals. At each attendance (and especially at the first attendance) a very careful clinical record should be made and the state carefully quantitated by measurements. At subsequent attendances the fact that no deterioration—assessed objectively—has taken place can be proved to the patient by comparing records and their interest can thereby be held. The use of the visual display of ranges of movement on the type of record card illustrated in Fig. 3.2, p. 21, can be easily understood by the patient and, even more important, a series of cards visually demonstrating no deterioration can be more easily understood than mere lists of measured angles.

Several consultations suitably spaced after the first interview will benefit both patient and surgeon in their attempts to understand each other's point of view, and not infrequently the surgeon will learn more from repeated consultations than the patient.

25–45 Years of Age

In this age group the conditions for which total hip replacement can be confidently recommended are: rheumatoid polyarthritis and ankylosing spondylitis. In this age group we look for factors which offer a 'built-in restraint' which will continue after the operation, such as defective knees or ankles, and impose some general physical limitations on the patient. Built-in restraint is **any factor which will persist, after total hip replacement, to hold back physical activity below that expected of a normal subject of the same age**. This is still compatible with offering the type of patient one has in mind a very great boon and a new start in life.

Another method of assessing very young patients is by the 'pseudarthrosis test' though it is only rarely helpful in difficult situations. In this test one asks oneself whether the present state of the patient would be improved by resection of the head and neck of the femur. If the answer is an emphatic 'no' then total hip replacement must be considered with the greatest reluctance. If the answer is 'yes' then one can be confident that if the operation were to fail the young patient's lot would not be worsened. Young patients who could be helped by a primary pseudarthrosis are rare because they would have to combine at one and the same time most of the following factors: (1) severe pain as the main feature, (2) spasm when the hip is moved passively, (3) fixed deformity, (4) 2–3 in. (10–12.5 cm) of shortening and (5) severe dependence on crutches or two canes. It will be recognized that this is not a very common picture and therefore the pseudarthrosis test only rarely helps in a positive way but when it is applicable it is very reassuring.

In the young age group the commonest hip conditions, and the most difficult, are the result of congenital dislocation and fractures of the acetabulum resulting from traffic accidents. These are usually in patients who are of athletic fitness except for the one hip. They are therefore totally without built-in restraint. Regrettably very little can be said to help in laying general rules other than to discuss arguments to uphold delaying tactics.

In **congenital subluxation in young women** currently in their 16th or 17th years old, surgeons must remind the younger generations of surgeons that before total hip replacement became an everyday subject for conversation (which is less than 10 years ago) young women with congenital dislocation almost always had reached 35 or 45 years of age before pain reached a point when the idea of surgery had to be seriously considered. These young women by then were usually married and often had children. In the modern world unfortunately the mere rumour of a new treatment makes it imperative that it should be employed with minimum delay! Modern ideas on sex and marriageability, combined with the worries of these young patients' mothers on this score, all must be seen against the history of the untreated condition. Anything that can be done to get these patients to postpone total hip replacement will be to their ultimate advantage. There is still a lot of research needing to be done in this field.

When it is considered that decisions to perform total hip replacement in these young women must be seen against the background of the next 50 years, patients can be very foolish not to try to adapt themselves to the surgeon's informed advice and opinion. If they force the surgeon's hand one wonders whether they have only themselves to blame.

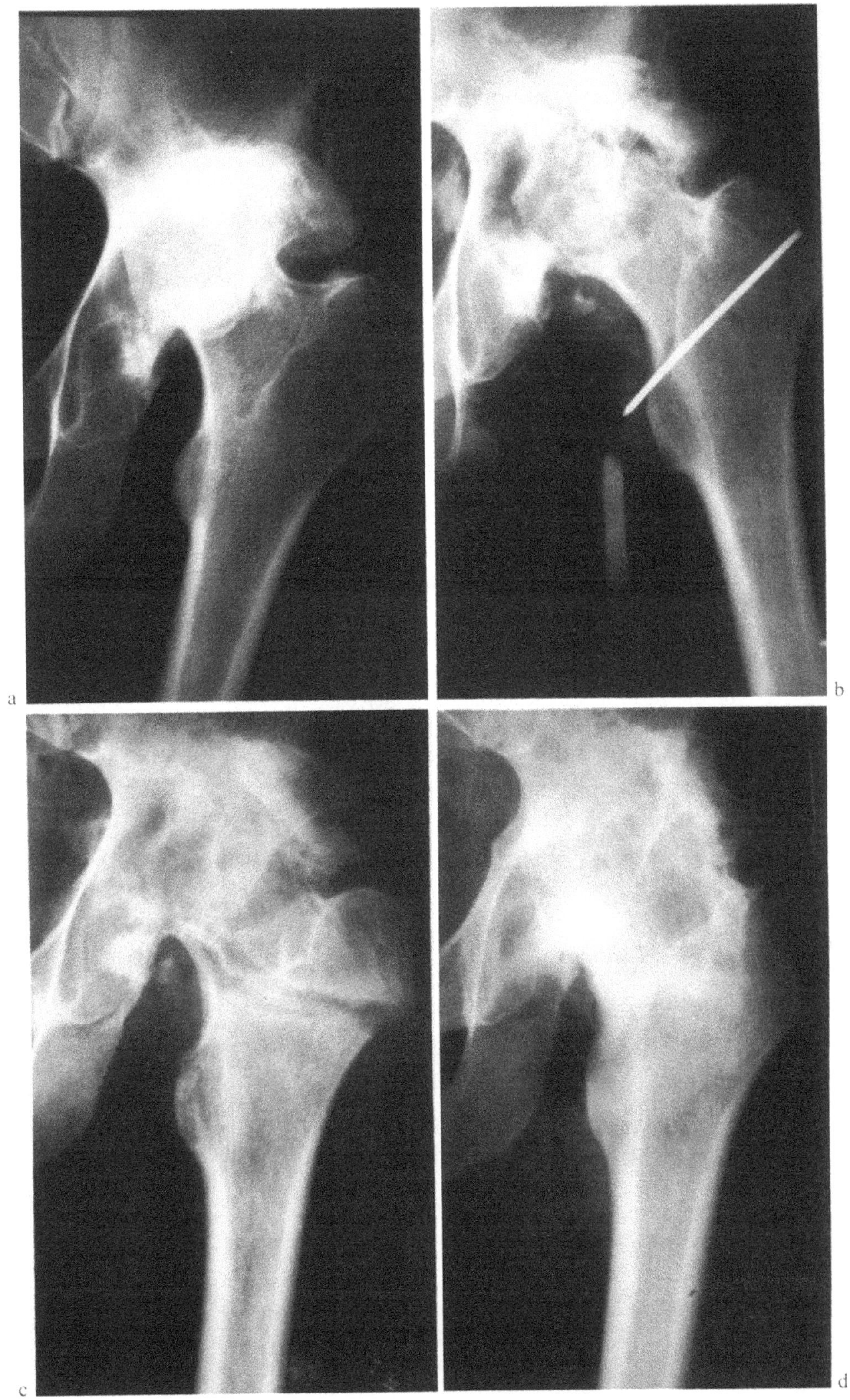

Fig. 22.1 a–d. Arthrodesis of the hip in a male patient 22 years old. **a** Pre-op. state of fracture dislocation of the hip. **b** Post-op.; after first stage. **c** Post-op.; after second stage 4 weeks later. **d** End result at 18 months post-op.

Traumatic Conditions of the Acetabulum in Young Men

In young men the role of arthrodesis must not be overlooked even when they do not earn their livelihood with heavy physical exertion. There is a tendency nowadays to forget what splendid results can be obtained by arthrodesis in young patients **when the opposite hip and both knees are normal**. Patients are naturally repelled by the idea of having a hip 'stiffened' but they do not realize that if they have a mobile spine, two good knees, and a good opposite hip they will hardly notice an arthrodesed hip. The only handicap not encountered very much in the past is the tendency for young people nowadays to be very much taller than they were 20 years ago and, unlike short patients, a very tall man is handicapped by an arthrodesed hip.

After 20–30 years with an arthrodesed hip a patient is in a perfect situation for conversion to a total hip replacement possibly with no further operation for the rest of his life. After arthrodesis the state of the bone in the acetabulum is perfect for a long-lasting implant. It is a pity that young women with unilateral CDH and the grossly defective acetabulum which is usually present can no longer be expected to undergo 20 years with an arthrodesis because this is the ideal way of reconstructing an acetabulum to receive a total hip socket. It must be emphasized that a happy married life, with children and with good athletic performance is possible even in a woman with an arthrodesis in good position, because in CDH the spine and knees are perfect.

Figure 22.1 shows a hip arthrodesis, performed April 1975, in a man of 22 years of age with the idea of converting to a total hip 20 years hence. A two-stage operation was used so as to (1) guarantee quick osseous union and (2) have no 'hardware' in situ when the time comes for the total hip replacement.

The 'two-stage' arthrodesis is essentially 'abduction-osteotomy' arthrodesis. The author uses his 'central dislocation arthrodesis' tools. The femur is approached by elevating the trochanter. The tip of the head of the femur is reamed into a conical shape **taking away minimal bone**. The floor of the acetabulum is pierced with conical reamers and enlarged only sufficiently for the **tip** of the conical femoral head to engage in the reamed hole, so as not to lose length by penetrating unnecessarily deep into the pelvis. The thigh is positioned at any alignment which achieves the best lie of the head in the hole in the floor of the acetabulum; this is usually about 20° abduction and 10° internal rotation. Considerable stability is achieved when the head penetrates about 1 cm in the acetabular hole and the limb is held in the appropriate attitude. The detached trochanter is laid in position and anchored with one wire or even a stitch. A **single-sided** hip spica cast is applied from chest to foot. The cast is retained for about 4 weeks during which time the patient can ambulate. After 4–6 weeks a high intertrochanteric osteotomy is performed under X-ray control to bring the

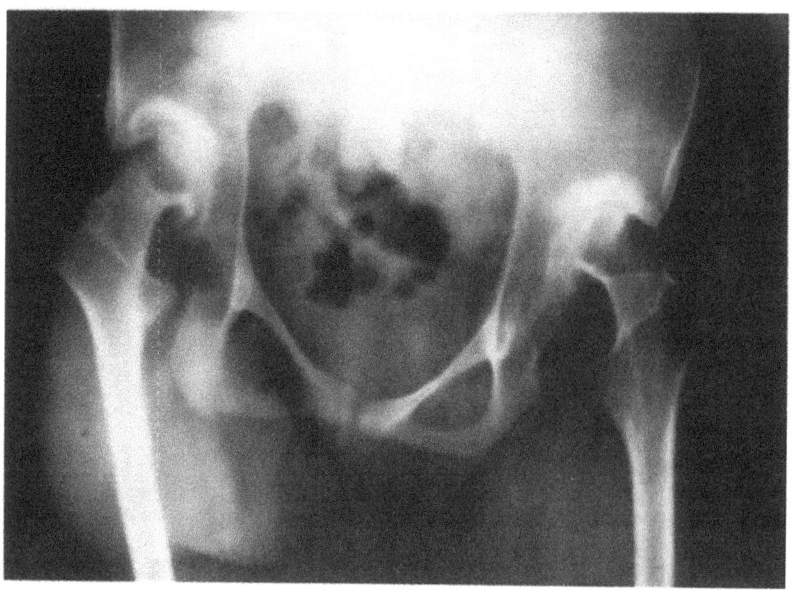

Fig. 22.2. a 17-year-old girl with defective result of bilateral Chiari procedures for CDH.
b Post-op. result March 1971
c Appearance 7 years post-op. Note good hypertrophy of femoral cortices but demarcation of left socket cement

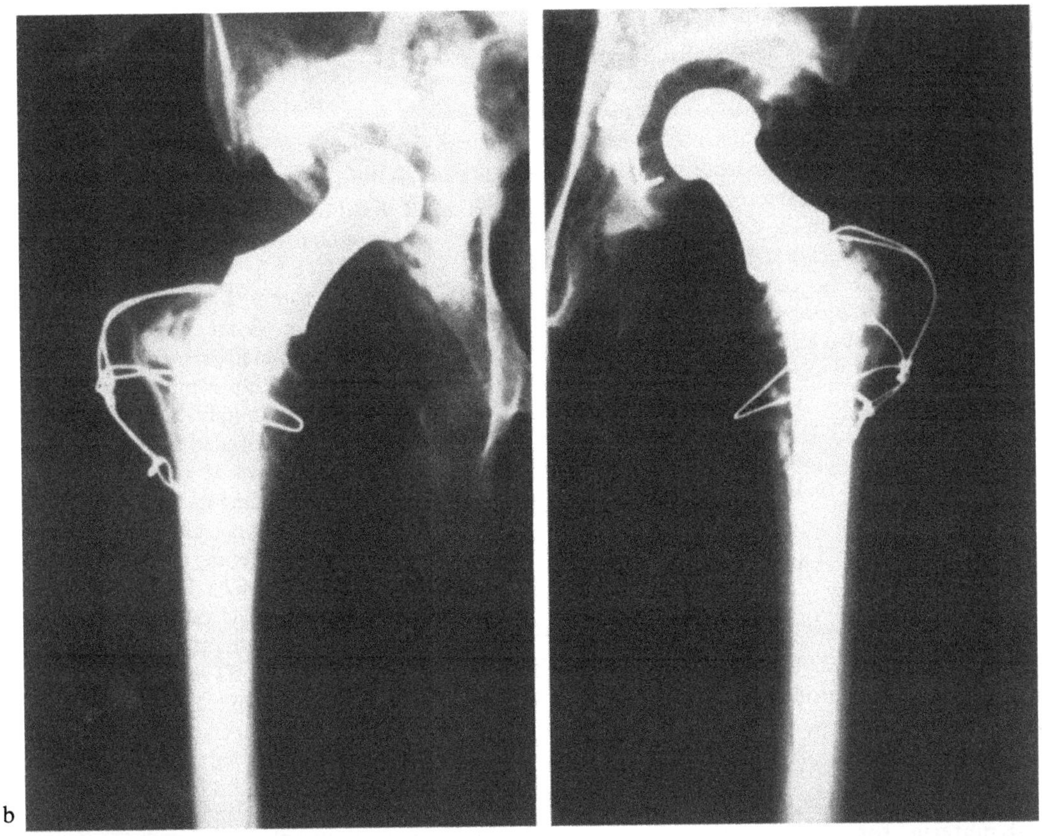

b

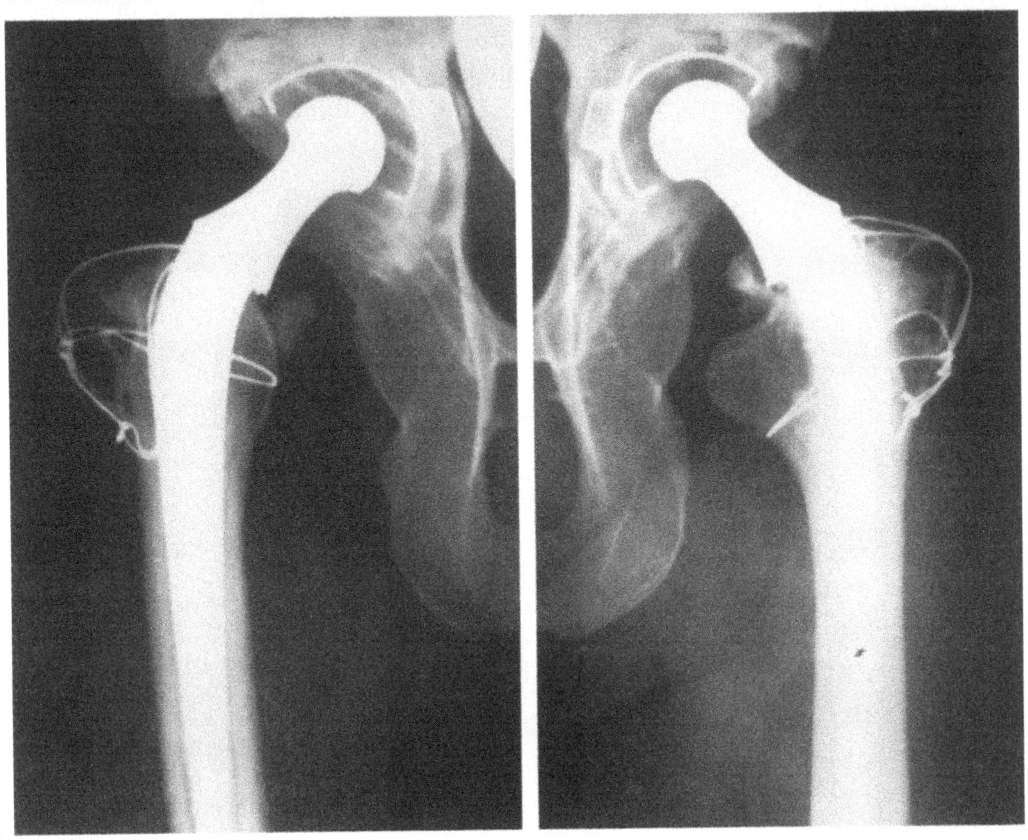

c

femur into correct alignment (neutral abduction and rotation, with not more than 5°–10° flexion) and a new **single-sided long hip spica** cast is applied. Because the osteotomy is performed through hyperaemic bone, osseous union is rapid. Also the thickened periosteal tissues from the previous operation prevent the osteotomy being freely mobile and becoming spontaneously displaced; it is only necessary to 'bend' the osteotomy 10°–20° in the direction of adduction and 10° in the direction of external rotation. The osteotomy is best not fixed with screws and plate because a defunctioning element is necessary to precipitate rapid union in the acetabulum.

After another 4 weeks (8 weeks so far) the single-sided cast is changed for a short, above-knee, single-sided cast and these young patients can ambulate within a day of the application of this last cast. Clinical union should be present in a total period of 12 weeks and full knee movement will have returned in 6 months.

15–25 Years of Age

Hip replacement under 20 years of age occasionally has to be performed even by the most conservative of surgeons. In emotional terms the results are dramatic not only in quality but in the speed of returning to full activity in comparison with the very much older patients who constitute the normal material for this operation. This should not blind surgeon and patient to the possibility of gross disability 25–30 years later with an acetabulum beyond all hope of further replacement.

Two brief clinical histories are presented to demonstrate the problems which will face such patients in the future and to suggest lines on which future research might be pursued.

A.D. 32673. 17-year-old girl; bilateral CDH treated by very imperfect Chiari operations (Fig. 22.2a). There was 80° fixed flexion deformity in both hips and before operation separation of ankles was only 8 in. (20 cm). No pain. B. R6.2.2 L6.2.2. Bilateral LFA operations performed within a month of each other March 1971. Post-operative result Fig. 22.2b. X-ray at 7 years (Fig. 22.2c); note hypertrophy of cortices of both femoral shafts. Patient's life completely changed and very happy though still has an ugly, rolling gait without sticks (which she rarely uses). Graded B. R6.5.5 L6.5.5. Note demarcation of left socket which will certainly require further surgery at some time in the future.

J.S. 29025. 18-year-old girl with juvenile rheumatoid arthritis and moderate involvement of knees and hands (Fig. 22.3a) C. R4.2.1 L3.2.1. Bilateral LFA operations performed within 1 month of each other March 1970 (Fig. 22.3b). Very happy and now married. State of hips after 7.5 years Fig. 22.3c. Note excellence of femoral cortices. C. R6.5.5. L6.5.5. Note wear of sockets. Note demarcation of left acetabular cement and less so in right. Future surgery will be necessary.

There can be no doubt that the decision to perform arthroplasties in these two young patients was correct. The effect on these two young people's lives has been truly miraculous. What do we learn from these cases?

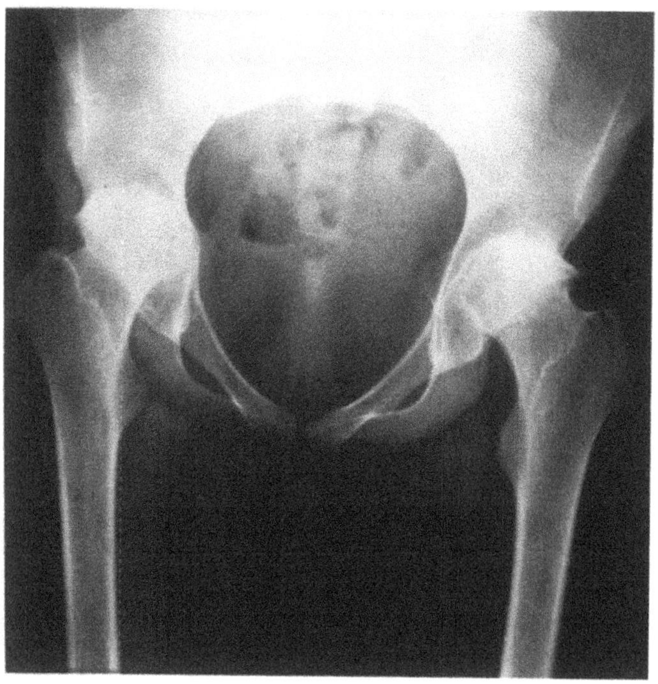

a

Fig. 22.3. **a** 18-year-old girl with rheumatoid arthritis. **b** Early post-op. result March 1970. **c** State 6.5 years post-op. Note excellence of femoral cortices but wear and demarcation of sockets

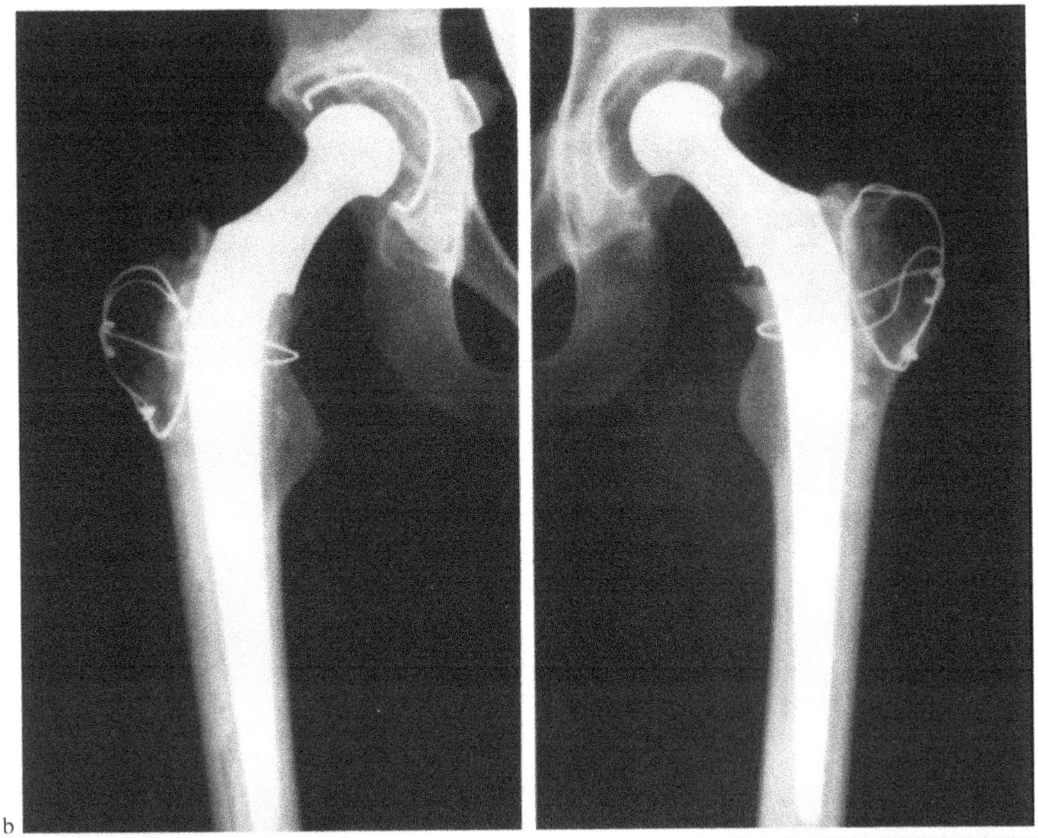

b

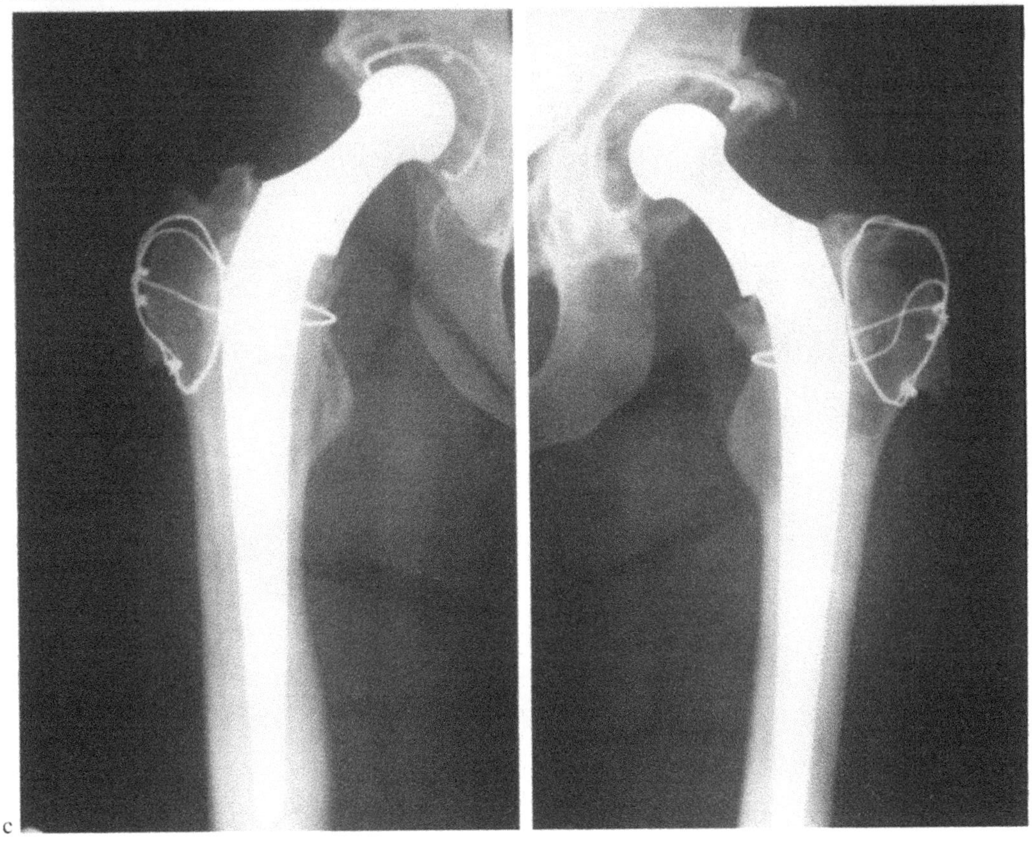

c

The acceptance of the cemented prostheses in the femora again is established as sound treatment. The tendency to resorption of the medial femoral neck may be a relatively unimportant side-issue because the 12–15-year follow-up suggests that calcar resorption becomes arrested.

Clearly it is the future of the cemented sockets which is at stake. In these very young patients the essential problem for cement in the acetabulum might be the greater flexibility of the bones of the pelvis compared with older patients. This is likely to cause an even more abrupt transition between the elastic modulus of the pelvis and the cement than in the adult so that at every load-bearing step the acetabulum must distort significantly round the cement. The risks of a foreign-body histiocyte reaction with increased resorption of the bone of the acetabulum is therefore very high. In this type of patient it is possible that a socket using the 'expanded surface' technique with perhaps **6 months** of avoidance of load-bearing might be the solution.

Appendix A

Ectopic Ossification After LFA of the Hip

DeLee and Ferrari[67] studied ectopic bone formation in 2173 hips over an average period of 1.8 years (1–5 years) after the LFA operation. They made a classification of the site and amount of ossification.

There were 318 cases of ectopic bone formation (14.6%) but if the least significant grade was excluded (ectopic bone extending **less than** 50% of the distance between femur and pelvis at any site) the incidence was 10%. The ectopic bone stabilized in amount by 12 months. Males developed new bone more commonly than females in the proportion of 26% to 8.5%. Osteoarthrosic patients were at greatest risk of producing new bone (16.6%) with congenital subluxation or dislocation (12.3%) and rheumatoid arthritis (11%) not a great deal less. The tendency to form ectopic bone seemed to be a systemic characteristic of the patient. There was a 90% chance of forming ectopic bone in the second hip if ectopic bone had occurred after operation on the first hip. Also if previous failed surgery of any kind on a hip had produced ectopic bone there was a 100% probability that a subsequent total hip replacement would show ectopic bone.

In the very rare instances of very severe ectopic bone formation after the LFA operation, with more or less complete ankylosis of the hip, the few attempts which have been made to resect the bone have been total failures. Total replacement after failed surgery did not have a high risk of producing new bone if the previous operation had not done so.

The patients who developed the greatest amount of bone were those with most restriction of movement before operation.

The commonest site for ectopic bone was lateral to the neck of the prosthesis as seen in the antero-posterior X-ray (i.e. the abductor region) and nearer the femur than the pelvis (54%). This obviously might be related to detachment of the trochanter. Of special interest was how infrequently new bone occurred medial to the prosthesis. Bone arising from the lower lip of the rim of the acetabulum is the region where osteophytes are most frequently resected and it is encouraging to find that this was the most rare of all sites (1%) for ectopic bone.

Nature of Ectopic Bone Formation

It is quite certain that after total hip replacement new bone formation is only very rarely the result of myositis ossificans. The author has encountered this disorder only two or three times after this operation and the clinical pattern was characteristic: in the first 3 post-operative months there was **unexplained pain and limitation of movement with 10°–15° of fixed flexion.** A cloud of new bone was detected only when X-rayed 3–6 months post-operatively. In the early post-operative period the picture led to suspicion of deep infection but the limitation of movement and the pain was greater than in an infection.

The common form of ectopic bone is associated with a more or less normal range of movement in the hip and the bone appears to form as a plaque, or plaques, lying behind and above the neck of the femur. The bony plaque is slightly mobile in relation to the femur which may explain why it interferes so little with the range of movement of the hip.

The common site of new bone is compatible with the deposition of bone debris in the bottom of the wound during the operation. It is possible that bone marrow from the reaming of the medullary cavity of the femur might be a more active producer of new bone than bone dust from the acetabulum. Since taking precautions to isolate the stump of the neck of the femur with gauze swabs before starting to ream the medullary cavity of the femur and carefully collecting all the marrow paste, the author has the impression that new bone formation is less common.

Conclusion

Ectopic bone formation after total hip replacement is more of a radiological incident than a serious clinical problem.

Appendix B

Re-surfacing Arthroplasty of the Hip

A new approach to total hip replacement is currently attracting attention, the idea being to 're-surface' the head of the femur with a hollow metal cap, thereby avoiding a femoral endoprosthesis. The principle of re-surfacing is commonly used in arthroplasty of the knee, though even in the knee some surgeons believe that better fixation of implants is obtained if an intramedullary extension is used.

Because in 'double-cup' arthroplasty of the hip one must sacrifice as little of the femoral head as possible, the hollow metal ball has a large external diameter and consequently the socket a large internal diameter. This leaves no alternative but for the plastic socket to have a relatively thin wall and be anchored in the acetabulum with a thin layer of cement.

The desire to avoid a femoral endoprosthesis seems to spring from bad results experienced with cement in the medullary cavity of the femur, and also from the belief that by this technique it will be possible to encourage hip replacement in young patients, leaving an intramedullary prosthesis for a secondary procedure many years later.

The author's experience of the 12–15-year results of the LFA operation lead him to an almost diametrically opposite point of view. Experience with the femoral endoprosthesis suggests that this is the site where almost 100% success with cement might very well be possible, if one considers the success already obtained with the original, unsophisticated technique and the greatly improved technologies which are now available. On the other hand the 12–15-year results lead the author to identify the socket as the most likely cause of long-term failures. Even with the low frictional torque principle there was a 25% incidence of sockets showing severe demarcation or migration. A thin-walled socket of large external diameter makes it impossible to use any shape other than a simple hemisphere and this makes it impossible to incorporate any features of design which could enhance the suitability of the socket for use with cement, as with the socket described in this book.

But the most serious criticism of all, in the author's opinion, is the idea that after the double-cup procedure it will be an easy matter to change the socket if the operation is encouraged in a young patient. It is a central theme of the present book that when using cement, the first time is the best time; secondary operations in the acetabulum encounter a bone surface which is never ideally suited to accepting cement. After second operations it is unlikely that the socket will remain successful, clinically and radiologically, for as long as it did after the first operation; and success after the third time will be of shorter duration even than after the second time.

In favour of the double-cup concept is the avoidance of the bending moments on the metal implant which lead to fatigue fractures of endoprostheses in heavy patients. Time alone will show whether cement failures of the femoral component are less with this new technique than the intramedullary procedure. On the other hand with the knowledge of the causes of fatigue fracture of femoral prostheses, which is only just becoming finalized, it is almost certain that a solution to this problem has already been found, though it will still take a number of years more to prove.

As regards surgical technique it would seem unlikely that the double-cup operation will prove any easier to perform for surgeons who have had difficulty with conventional methods. To facilitate work on the femoral head a very wide exposure might damage an essential blood supply to the bone inside the hollow metal cap. Detachment of the trochanter to facilitate the exposure also might damage the blood-supply to the femoral neck and lead to fracture (Freeman[68]).

The technique of re-surfacing the femoral head is not universally applicable and is feasible only where the hip joint has a reasonable anatomical shape. It is not attractive in congenital subluxation. It will always be necessary for surgeons who specialize in total hip replacement to be skilled in the use of the femoral endoprosthesis.

The author attributes much of the long-term success of his own operation to what he calls the 'safety valve' of the arthroplasty (p. 13). This is the ability of the prosthetic femoral head to escape, momentarily, from the acetabulum when the joint is traumatically forced beyond its designed range as for instance when a patient falls. The larger the diameter of the femoral head the greater will be the force needed to stretch the capsule when the neck of the femur acts as a lever with the edge of the acetabulum as a fulcrum. High-intensity, short-duration stressing of this kind could react on the fixation of the hollow metal ball and on the stump of the femoral neck.

A large-diameter socket will always offer problems of being contained completely inside the acetabulum. If a thin-walled socket projects beyond the rim of the acetabulum the unsupported part will not be in a good position for taking load.

Possible problems in the use of a thin-walled socket have been discussed at the end of Chap. 1 as a result of photo-elastic studies.

Appendix C

Special Instruments

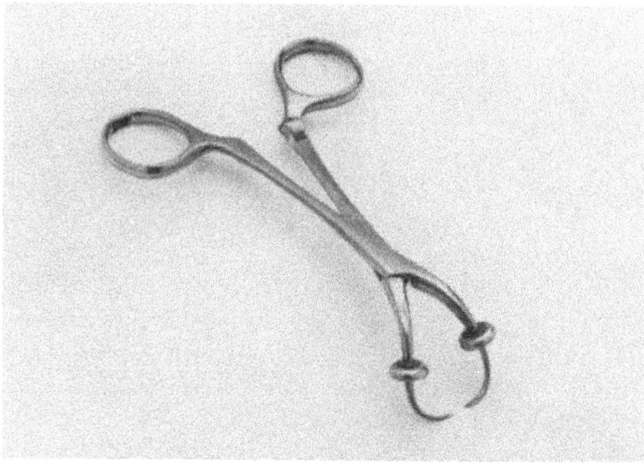

Fig. C 1. Mayo Towel Clips with Ball-Guarded Points
These can be made very easily from ordinary towel clips by brazing on small discs, appropriately drilled, as in the illustration. This detail greatly improves the precision of closing the skin-edge towels at the top and bottom of the wound. Can be used with advantage for all drapes

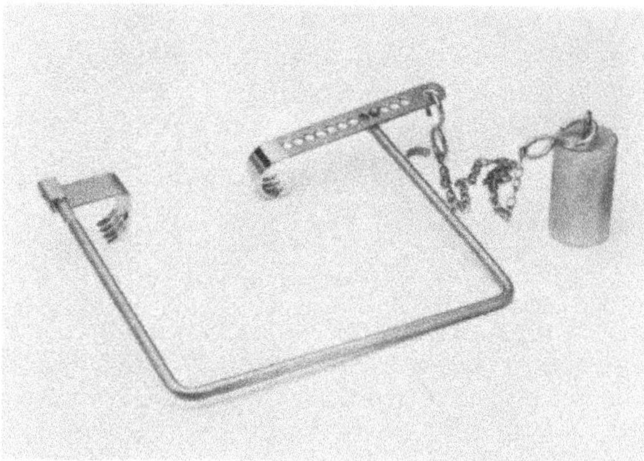

Fig. C 2. Initial Wound Retractor

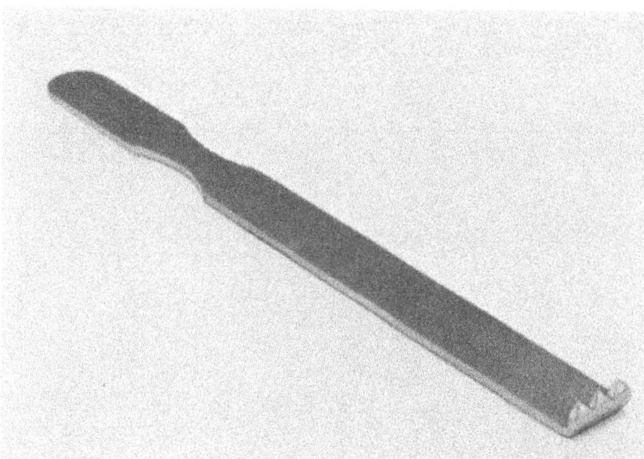

Fig. C 3. Angulated and Serrated Femur Lever
This is used extensively in the operation:
1) To expose the femoral head when resecting (step 33)
2) When reaming the medulla of the femur (step 86)
3) When drilling the femur and passing the medial and lateral wires (step 100)

It enters on tray 2 and is retained till the end of wiring the trochanter. It is about 12 in. (30 cm) long and 1 in. (2.5 cm) wide

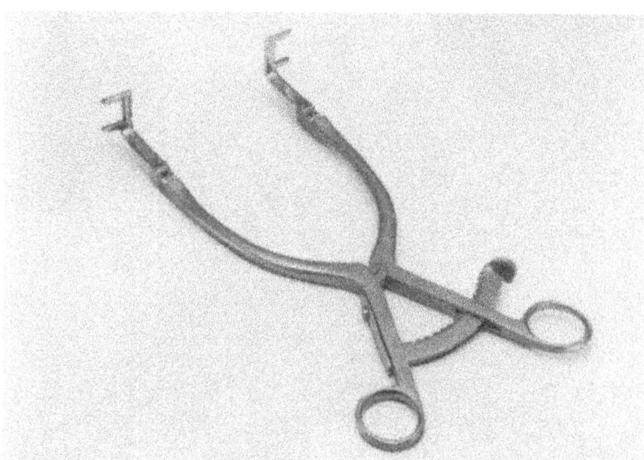

Fig. C 4. Horizontal Retractor
The special details are:
1) It is of heavy calibre
2) The jaws are specially shaped for this purpose

Fig. C 5. Screw-Jack
This is of paramount importance for use with (4). The screw thread is quick-acting. It is operated with a Kocher's forceps inserted, closed, as a lever into the holes of the turnbuckle. Each movement of the lever is through 90°. Remember to add a few additional turns before inserting the cement into the acetabulum in order to achieve optimum exposure at that moment. It is very important for good exposure of the acetabulum when the stump of the neck of femur is left rather long

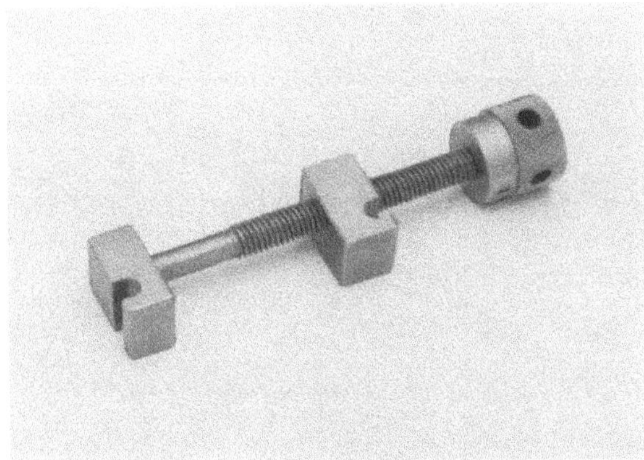

Fig. C 6. Nail Retractor and Handle
These nails tend to bend during use and afterwards must be hammered straight again (it is important that they should not be of such hard metal that they might break in situ). Take care not to blunt the teeth of the expanding reamer by siting the nail so that it enters the cavity of the acetabulum. The pilot hole or starting drill also can be blunted, when making the superior cement hole, if it is directed towards the nail. Two nails can be used if desired

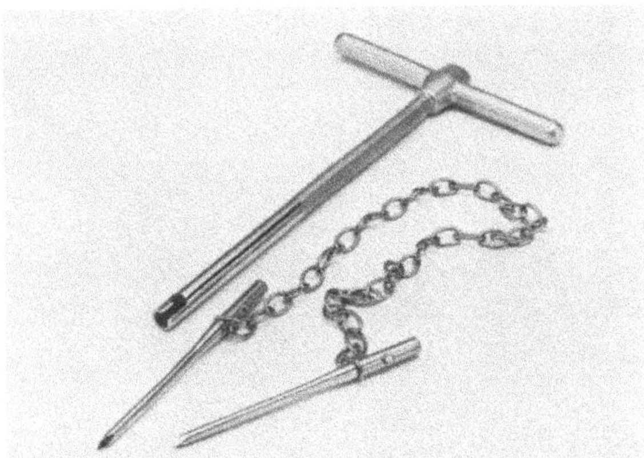

Fig. C 7. Angulated Hohman Retractor
This is used to reveal the anterior margin of the acetabulum and the bend keeps the handle out of the surgeon's way

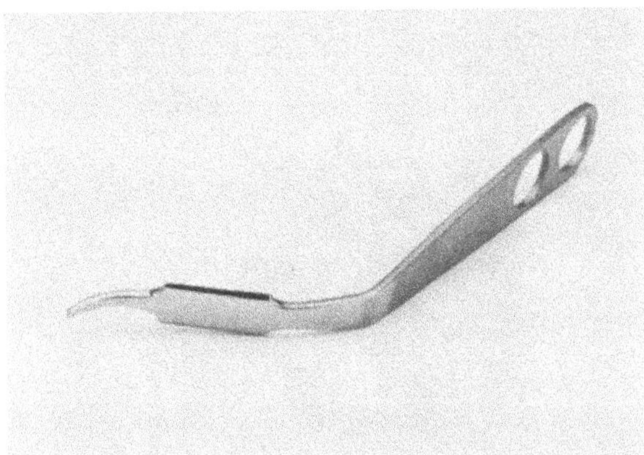

Fig. C 8. Double-Handed Curettes
The small curette will enter the 0.5-in. (12.5-mm) hole made by the centring or pilot drill. These curettes should be **kept very sharp** by rubbing the **exterior** on a small oilstone. These instruments are about 13.5 in. (34 cm) long. The T-handle lies in the same plane as the mouth of the curette

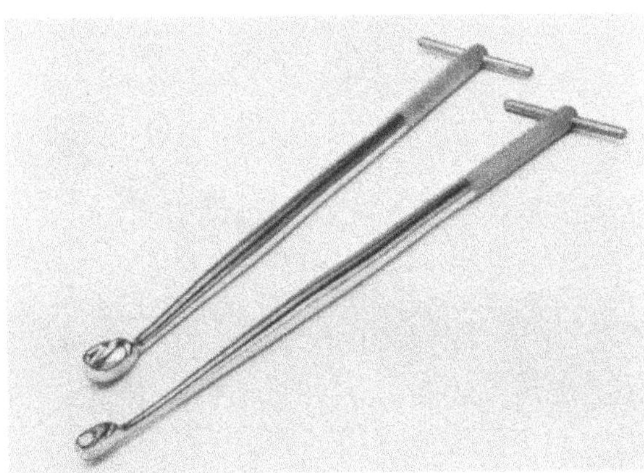

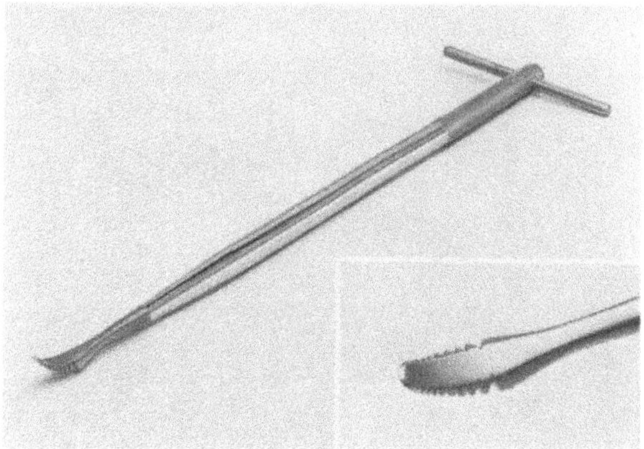

Fig. C 9. Ring Curette
The sharp teeth on this double-handed curette are invaluable for roughening the surface of eburnated bone or removing remains of cartilage

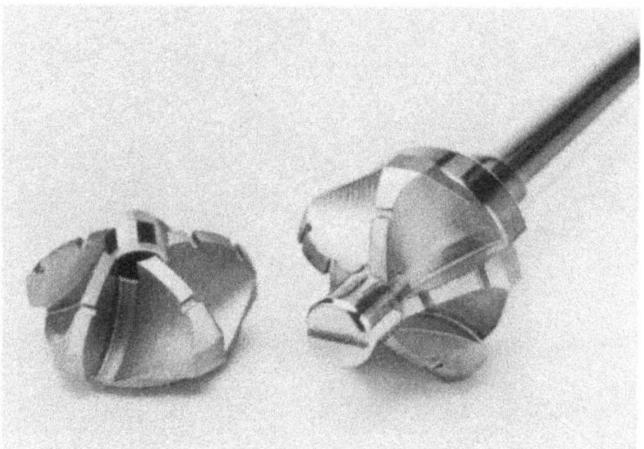

Fig. C 10. Deepening Reamer
The cutters can be changed for sharpening. The spigots on this and on the expanding reamer are an essential detail in this operation. Only by the spigot and the pilot hole is it possible to locate precisely the centre of the deepened and reamed area of bone. Without a spigot the reamers can wander and 'shy away from' hard eburnated bone by cutting towards the least resistant quadrants of the acetabulum

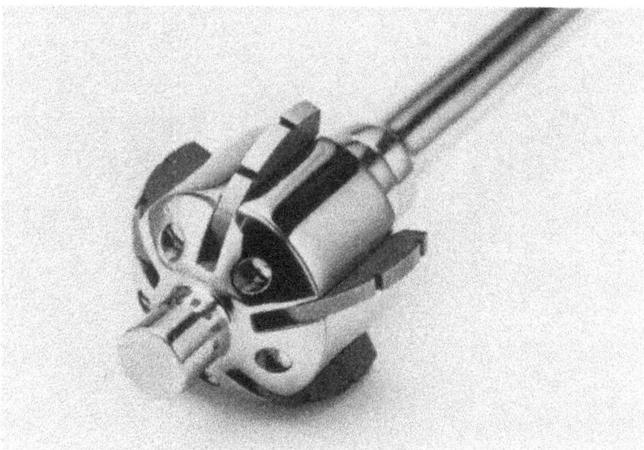

Fig. C 11. Expanding Reamer
Both these reamers cut easily (if kept with sharp blades) in the large brace with a 5-in. (12.5-cm) throw. They should not be used with a power source except at slow speeds (not more than about 150 r.p.m.)

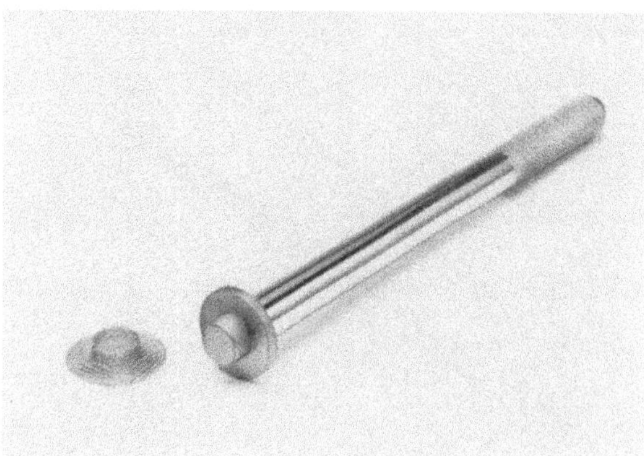

Fig. C 12. Cement Restrictor and Holder
The flange on the holder enables it to be used as a punch, with a hammer, to drive the 'turned-over' edge of the cement restrictor into the cancellous bone. This prevents the rough edges of the wire mesh catching on gauze swabs and so being pulled out, at the critical moment, just before inserting the cement

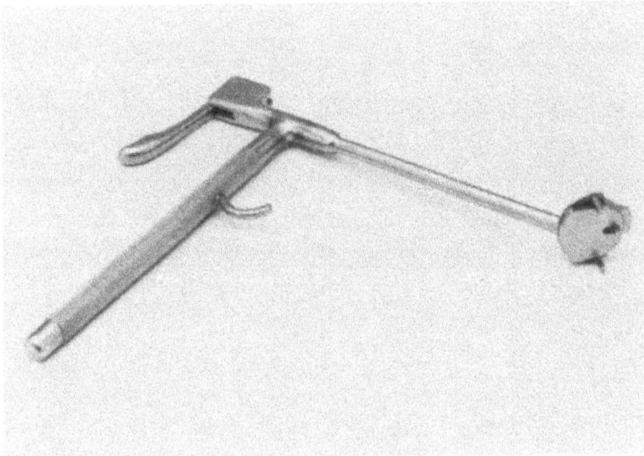

Fig. C 13. Self-Ejecting Socket-Holder
An essential tool. The length of the transverse limb is such that the index finger of the hand holding it, when extended, will just reach the edge of the wound to act as a 'steady'. When used with PIJ sockets the stability of the socket depends on contact between the rim and the acetabulum **under pressure from the pusher.** The surgeon can thus relax his hold on the socket-holder

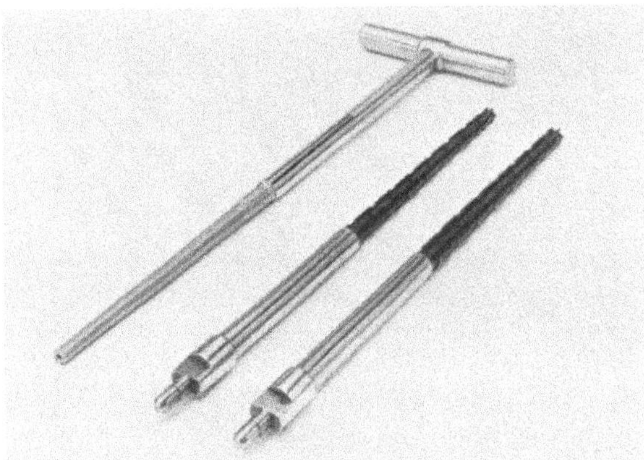

Fig. C 14. Hand-Operated Taper Reamer
The tip of the reamer is $^3/_8$ in. (9 mm) in diameter. Important for finding the direction of the medullary cavity of the femur.

Rotary Reamers
Used in the large hand brace with 5-in. (12.5-cm) throw. These have completely supplanted the use of broaching tools and mallet. Rotary reamers are an essential part of using large-calibre femoral prostheses to avoid fatigue fracture. Can only be used after detachment of the trochanter. Encroachment into the cut surface from which the trochanter was removed is not important if the cruciate wiring system is used to reattach the trochanter

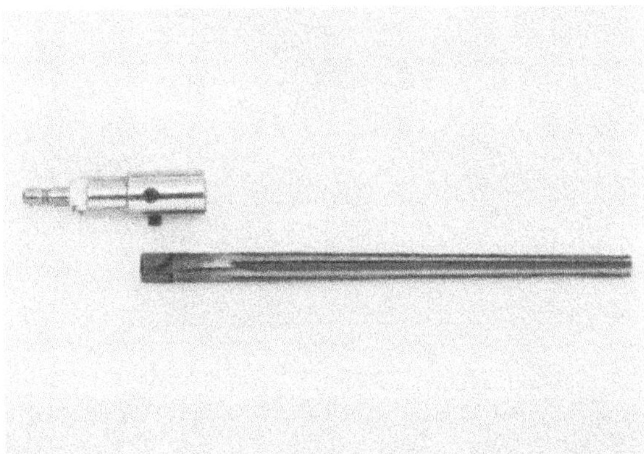

Fig. C 15. Specially Sharp Rotary Reamer
This reamer is of paramount importance for cutting dense bone (or cutting cement). **It is not used routinely but only when specially needed,** in order to keep it sharp. The cutting blade is an engineer's 'taper pin reamer' $^3/_8$-in. (approx. 9-mm) diameter at the tip and $^1/_2$ in. (12.5 mm) at the widest part. It is not stainless steel and will rust if not looked after. It is almost razor sharp when new. Because it is relatively cheap it can be discarded when it becomes blunt. Different countries (U.K., U.S.A., Germany, etc.) have different sizes so that the holder to fit the brace must be made locally. Messrs. Chas. Thackray Ltd. will provide blank adaptors to fit the heavy brace and the hole can be made larger to receive whatever size of taper pin reamer is locally available

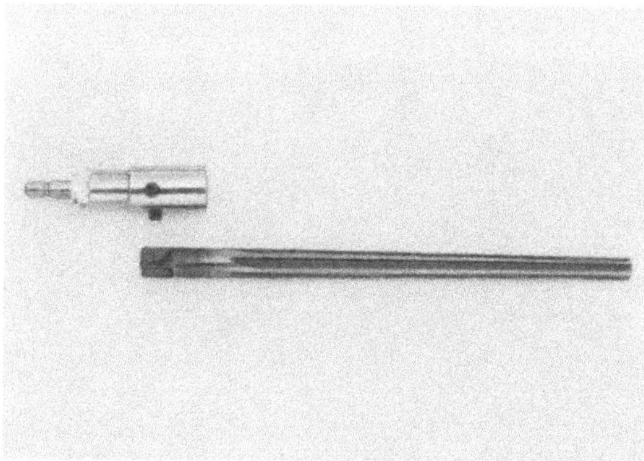

Fig. C 16. Prosthesis-Holder with Cement Injection Cap
All Charnley prostheses are protected with a polypropylene cap by which they are held in the prosthesis-holder so that the precision-finished head does not need to be exposed until the moment comes for reducing into the acetabulum after the hardening of the cement. When gripped in the holder it is unnecessary for the grip to be totally rigid against rotation, provided it is not loose. The 'pressure injection' cap replaces the medial half of the regular protective cap and is mounted in the holder so that it faces the medial femoral neck. These caps cannot be sterilized by dry heat but only by autoclaving

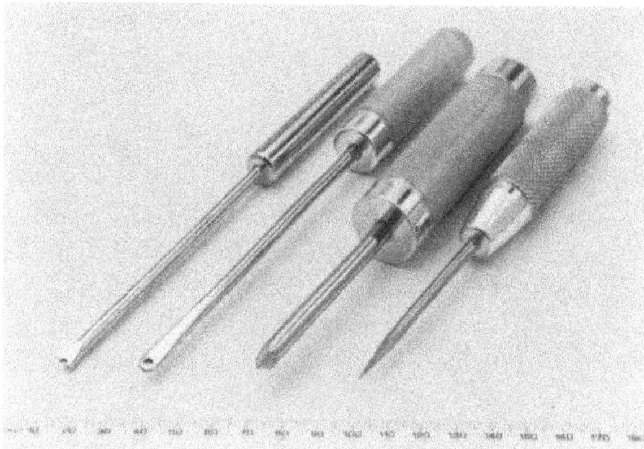

Fig. C 17. Set of Trochanter Tools
The large awl, with trocar point, is $^1/_4$ in. (6.25 mm) in diameter. It is used (1) to pass the double wire over the summit of the trochanter at the same time making the 'notch' in the bone, (stage 116) and (2) to bury under the surface of the trochanter the last cut and twisted end of wire at the completion of the wire fixation (step 134).
The small awl is used (1) to 'tack' the lateral end of the trochanter temporarily in position while starting to fix the trochanter (stage 120) and (2) to present a fixed point in the centre of the trochanter, when tightening the wires in the making of the pulley, so that the cross-over does not slide upwards into the abductor muscles (step 129)
The perforated awl is used (1) for the assistant to use to hold the anterior end of the staple-clamp while the surgeon is starting the wiring of the trochanter (stage 119c) and (2) to pull back through the abductor muscle the posterior end of medial wire after fashioning the end into a hook (step 127).
The fish-tail awl is used (1) to push into the medullary cavity the loop of the medial wire as it crosses the medullary cavity lateral to the prosthesis: if lying on the cut surface of the trochanter this loop would interfere when making the groove for the staple bolt, (stage 102) and (2) to drive the last cut and twisted end of wire under the surface of the trochanter, into the hole made for it by the large awl, as the final step in the wiring (stage 134).
These four instruments can easily be made by the surgeon himself and together with the punch are favourite early exercises for postgraduates under instruction in the biomechanical machine shop

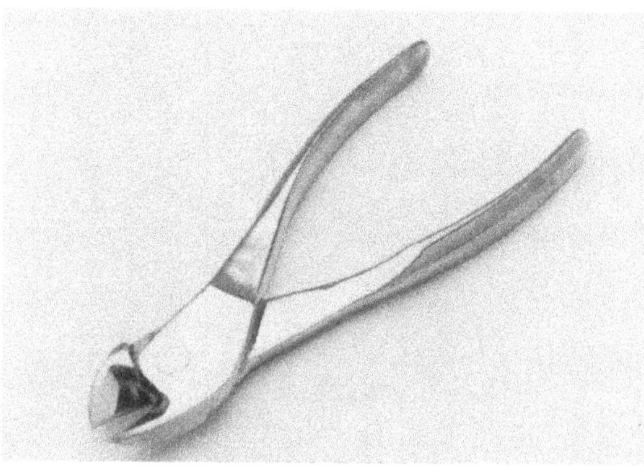

Fig. C 18. Wire-Cutter
This wire-cutter cuts 'on the flat' and is more convenient than 'end cutting' patterns though these often have a double-acting hinge. It should be about 8 in. (20 cm) long if it is to cut 18 s.w.g. wire (doubled) easily and without a double-acting mechanism. Non-stainless engineer's cutter can be used for this purpose ("8-in. diagonal cutting nippers")

Fig. C 19. Punch
This punch is important (1) for impacting the trochanter on to its bed on the femur, before finally tightening the vertical double wire (stage 123) (2) for punching in the anterior staple of the staple-clamp (stage 136) and (3) for punching in the three cut and twisted ends of wire (stages 124, 132, 134)

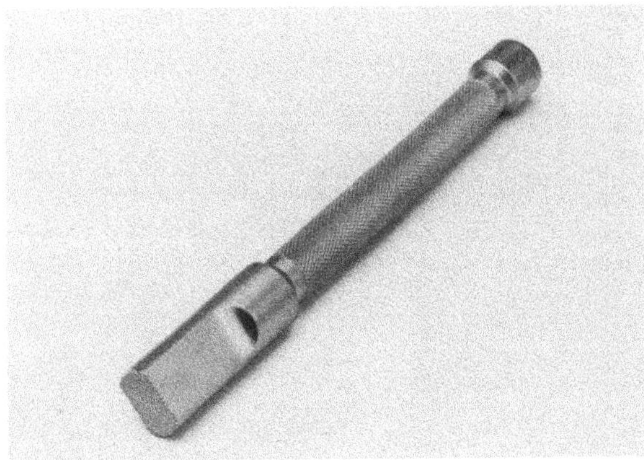

Fig. C 20. Bolt Cutter for Staple-Clamp
This duty can be performed by an engineer's (non-stainless) 12-in. bolt cropper

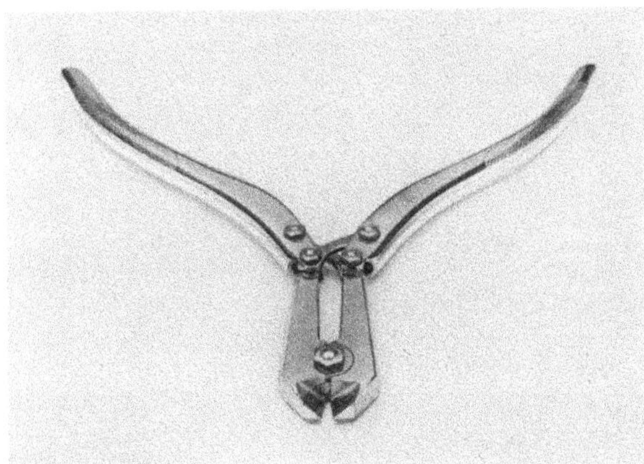

Fig. C 21. Gouges with Concave Bevels
These gouges are important in surgery on a difficult acetabulum. They do not 'shy away from' the bone in the way that gouges bevelled on the convex surface tend to do. They are very useful in a congenital subluxation and dislocation to prepare the way for the deepening reamer

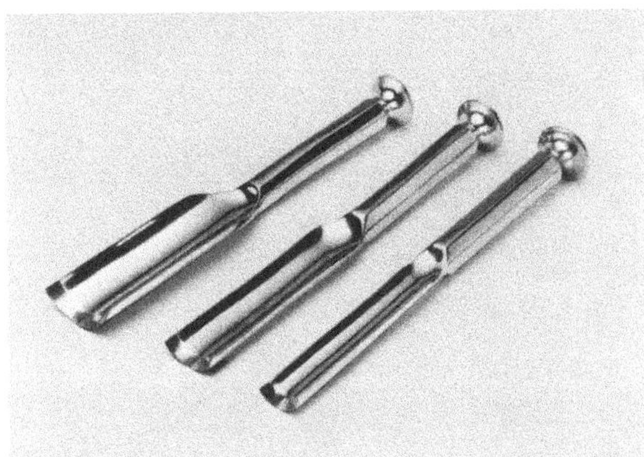

Fig. C 22. Length-Measuring Gauge
The use of this instrument is described in stages 119 B and 139. In size it is equal in dimensions to a staple-clamp

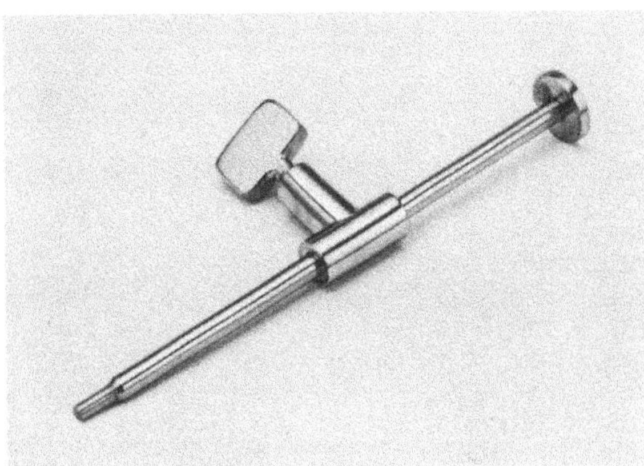

References

Chapter 1

1) Charnley, J. (1961): Arthroplasty of the Hip. A New Operation. Lancet **1**, 1129
2) MacConnaill, M.A. (1950): Movement of Bones and Joints. 3. Synovial Fluid and its Assistants. J. Bone Joint Surg. **32** B, 244
3) Jones, E.S. (1936): Joint Lubrication. Lancet **1**, 1043
4) Elson, R.A., Charnley, J. (1968): The Direction of the Resultant Force in Total Prosthetic Replacement of the Hip Joint. Med. & Biol. Engineering, Vol. 6, pp. 19–27. Pergamon Press
5) Simon, S.R., Radin, E.L. (1973): Lubrication and Wear of the Charnley, Charnley-Muller, and McKee-Farrar prostheses with Special Regard to their Clinical Behaviour. The Hip Society, Proceedings 1973. Saint Louis: Mosby
6) Dowson, D., Wright, V. (1977): Evaluation of Artificial Joints, p. 19. Biological Engineering Society, Department of Engineering, University of Leeds, England.
7) Andersson, G.B.J., Freeman, M.A.R., Swanson, S.A.V. (1972): Loosening of the Cemented Acetabular Cup in Total Hip Replacement. J. Bone Joint Surg. **54** B, 590

Chapter 2

8) Wiltse, L.L., Hall, R.H., Stenehjem, D.D.S. (1957): Experimental Studies Regarding the Possible Use of Self-curing Acrylic in Orthopaedic Surgery. J. Bone Joint Surg. **39** A, 961

Chapter 3

9) d'Aubigné, M.R., Postel, M. (1954): Functional Results of Hip Arthroplasty with Acrylic Prostheses. J. Bone Joint Surg. **36** A, 451

Chapter 4

10) Charnley, J. (1970): The Reaction of Bone to Self-Curing Acrylic Cement. A Long-Term Histological Study in Man. J. Bone Joint Surg. **52** B, 340
11) Charnley, J. (1970): Acrylic Cement in Orthopaedic Surgery Edinburgh, London: Livingstone
12) Willert, H.G., Semlitsch, M. (1976): Tissue Reactions to Plastic and Metallic Wear Products of Joint Endoprostheses. In: Total Hip Prosthesis. Gschwend, N., Debrunner, H.U. (eds.) Bern, Stuttgart, Vienna: Huber
13) Vernon-Roberts, B., Freeman, M.A.R. (1977): The Tissue Response to Total Joint Replacement Prostheses. In: The Scientific Basis of Joint Replacement; Pitman Medical p. 86

Chapter 5

14) Eftekhar, N. (1971): Charnley Low Friction Torque Arthroplasty. A Study of Long-Term Results. Clin. Orthop. **81**, 93
15) Charnley, J., Cupic, Z. (1973): Results of Low Friction Arthroplasty of the Hip. Clin. Orthop. **95**, 9
16) Charnley, J. (1972): The Long-Term Results of Low-Friction Arthroplasty of the Hip Performed as a Primary Intervention. J. Bone Joint Surg. **54** B, 61
17) Griffith, M.J., Seidenstein, M., Williams, D., Charnley, J. (1978): 8 Year Results of Charnley Arthroplasty of the Hip with Special Reference to the Behaviour of Cement. Clin. Orthop. (in press)
18) Muller, M.E. (1975): Total Hip Replacement: Planning, Technique and Complications. In: Surgical Management of Degenerative Arthritis of the Lower Limb, p. 91.: Lea & Febiger
19) Stuhmer, G. (1976): Loosening of Prostheses. In: Total Hip Prostheses. Gschwend, N., Debrunner, H.U. (eds.) p. 125. Bern, Stuttgart, Vienna: Huber

Chapter 6

20) Weber F.A., Charnley, J. (1975): A Radiological Study of Fractures of Acrylic Cement in Relation to the Stem of a Femoral Head Prosthesis. J. Bone Joint Surg. **57** B, 297
21) DeLee, J., Charnley, J. (1976): Radiological Demarcation of Cemented Sockets in Total Hip Replacement. Clin. Orthop. **121**, 20
22) Evans, E.M., Freeman, M.A.R., Miller, A.J., Vernon-Roberts, B. (1974): Metal Sensitivity as a Cause of Bone Necrosis and Loosening of the Prosthesis in Total Joint Replacement. J. Bone Joint Surg. **56** B, 626

23) Miller, A.J. (1972): Late Fractures of the Acetabulum after Total Hip Replacement. J. Bone Joint Surg. **54** B, 600
24) Follacci, F.M., Hammond, B.T., Charnley, J. (1968): The Long-Term Reaction of Bone to Self-Curing Acrylic Cement. J. Bone Joint Surg. **50** B, 822
25) Blacker, G., Charnley, J. (1978): Long-Term Study of Changes in the Upper Femur after Low Friction Arthroplasty. Clin. Orthop. (in press)
26) Bocco, F., Langan, P., Charnley, J. (1977): Changes in the Calcar Femoris in Relation to Cement Technology in Total Hip Replacement. Clin. Orthop. **128**, 287
27) Al-Habboobys, S., McLeish, R.D. (1969): A Study of the Load Transfer from Prosthesis to Femur. Dissertation for M.Sc. in Victoria University of Manchester, Manchester Institute of Science & Technology
28) Harris, W.H., Schiller, A.L., Scholler, J., Freiberg, R.A., Scott, R. (1976): Extensive Localized Bone Resorption in the Femur Following Total Hip Replacement. J. Bone Joint Surg. **58**A, 612

Chapter 9

29) Charnley, J. (1975): Fracture of Femoral Prostheses in Total Hip Replacement. A Clinical Study. Clin. Orthop. **111**, 105
30) Wroblewski, B.M. (1978): Mechanics of Fracture of Femoral Prostheses in Total Hip Replacement. Int. Orthop. (in press)

Chapter 12

31) Boardman, K.P., Bocco, F., Charnley, J. (1978): An Evaluation of a Method of Trochanteric Fixation Using Three Wires in the Charnley Low Friction Arthroplasty. Clin. Orthop. (N°132)
32) Brady, L.P. (1976): Lateral Oblique Incision for the Charnley Low Friction Arthroplasty. Clin. Orthop. **118**, 7

Chapter 13

33) Charnley, J. (1972): Post-operative Infection after Total Hip Replacement with Special Reference to Air Contamination in the Operating Room. Clin. Orthop. **87**, 167
34) McLauchlan, J., Logie, J.R.C., Smylie, H.G., Smith, G. (1976): A Study of the Wound Environment during Total Hip Arthroplasty Postgrad. Med. J. **52**, 550
35) Franco, J.A., Baer, H., Enneking, W.F. (1977): Airborne Contamination in Orthopaedic Surgery. Clin. Orthop. **122**, 231
36) Davidson, A.I.G., Smylie, H.G. Macdonald, A., Smith, G. (1971): Ward Design in Relation to Postoperative Wound Infection: Part II Br. Med. J. 72
37) Charnley, J., Eftekhar, N. (1969): Penetration of Gown Material by Organisms from the Surgeon's Body. Lancet 172
38) Van Niekerk, G.A., Charnley, J. (1977): Post-Operative Infection after Charnley Low Friction Arthroplasty of the Hip. Internal Publication No. 68, Centre for Hip Surgery, Wrightington Hospital
39) Fitzgerald, R.H., Lowell, F., Peterson, A., Washington, J.A., Van Scoy, R.E., Coventry, M.B. (1973): Bacterial Colonization of Wounds and Sepsis in Total Hip Arthroplasty. J. Bone Joint Surg. **55**A, 1242
40) Cruess, R.L., Bickel, W.S., Van Kessler, K.L.C. (1975): Infections in Total Hip Replacement Secondary to a Primary Source Elsewhere. Clin. Orthop. **106**, 99
41) Del Sel, H., Charnley, J.: Total Hip Replacement Following infection in the Opposite Hip. Clin. Orthop. (in press)
41a) Charnley, J. (1976): Letter to Lancet **1**, Vol. 2, pp. 1557–1558
42) Hamilton, H.W., Booth, A.D., Lone, F.J., Clark, N. (1978): Penetration fo Gown Materials by Organisms from the Surgeon's Body. Clin. Orthop., submitted August 1978

Chapter 18

43) Johnson, R., Green, J.A., Charnley, J. (1977): Pulmonary Embolism Following the Charnley Total Hip Replacement and its Prophylaxis. Clin. Orthop. **127**, 123
44) Johnson, R., Charnley, J. (1977): Treatment of Pulmonary Embolism in Total Hip Replacement. Clin. Orthop. **124**, 149
45) Johnson, R., Charnley, J. (1977): Hydroxychloroquine in Prophylaxis of Pulmonary Embolism Following Hip Arthroplasty. Internal Publication No. 74, Centre for Hip Surgery, Wrightington Hospital
46) Crawford, W.J., Hillman, F., Charnley, J. (1968): A Clinical Trial of Prophylactic Anticoagulant Therapy in Elective Hip Surgery. Internal Publication No. 14, Centre for Hip Surgery, Wrightington Hospital
47) Sharnhoff, J.G., DeBlasio, G. (1970): Prevention of Fatal Post-operative Thromboembolism by Heparin Prophylaxis. Lancet **2**, 1006
48) Charnley, J. (1972): Letter to Lancet Vol. 2, p. 134.
49) Harris, W.H., Salzman, E.W., Athanasoulis, C., Waltman, A.C., Baum, S., De Saudis, R.W. (1974): Comparison of Warfarin, Low-Molecular-Weight Dextran, Aspirin and Subcutaneous Heparin in Prevention of Venous Thromboembolism following Total Hip Replacement. J. Bone Joint Surg. **56**A, 1552
50) Carter, A.E., Eban, R. (1974): Prevention of Postoperative Deep Venous Thrombosis in Legs by Orally Administered Hydroxychloroquine Sulphate. Br. Med. J. **3**, 94

51) Chrisman, O.D., Snook, G.A., Wilson, T.C., Short, J.Y. (1976): Prevention of Venous Thrombosis by Administration of Hydroxychloroquine. J. Bone Joint Surg. **58**A, 918
52) Jennings, J.J., Harris, W.R., Sarmiento, A. (1976): A Clinical Evaluation of Aspirin Prophylaxis of Thromboembolic Disease after Total Hip Replacement. J. Bone Joint Surg. **58**A, 926
53) Coventry, M.B., Nolan, D.R., Beckenbaugh, R.D. (1973): "Delayed" Prophylactic Anticoagulants: A Study of Results and Complications in 2012 Total Hip Arthroplasties. J. Bone Joint Surg. **55**A, 1487
54) Stamatakis, J.D., Kakkar, V.V., Lawrence, D., Bentley, P.G., Nairn, D., Ward, V. (1978): Failure of Aspirin to Prevent Post-operative Deep Vein Thrombosis in Patients Undergoing Total Hip Replacement. Br. Med. J. **1**, 1031

Chapter 19

55) McKee, G.K., Chen, S.C. (1973): The Statistics of the McKee-Farrar Method of Total Hip Replacement. Clin. Orthop. **95**, 26
56) Etienne, A., Cupic, Z. (1978): Post-Operative Dislocation After Charnley Low Friction Arthroplasty. Clin. Orthop. **133** (in press)

Chapter 20

57) Halley, D.K., Charnley, J. (1975): Rate of Wear in Total Hip Replacement. Clin. Orthop. **112**, 170
58) Griffith, M.J., Seidenstein, M., Williams, D., Charnley, J. (1978): Socket Wear in Charnley Low Friction Arthoplasty of the Hip. Clin. Orthop. (in press)
59) Clarke, I.C., Black, K., Rennie, C., Amstutz, H.C. (1976): Can Wear in Total Hip Arthoplasty be Assessed from Radiographs? Clin. Orthop. **121**, 126

Chapter 21

60) Pauwels, F. (1935): Der Schenkelhalsbruch, ein mechanisches Problem. Stuttgart: Enke
61) McLeish, R.D., Charnley, J. (1970): Abduction Forces in the One-Legged Stance. J. Biomech. **3**, 191
62) Denham, R.A. (1959): Hip Mechanics. J. Bone Joint Surg. **41** B, 550
63) Dall, D., Charnley, J. (1971: Comparison of the Lever System in the Low Friction Arthroplasty and the McKee-Farrar Arthroplasty. Internal Publication No. 34, Centre for Hip Surgery, Wrightington Hospital
64) Dixon, A.F. (1910): J. Anat. Physiol. **44**, 15
65) Inman, V.T. (1947): Functional Aspects of the Abductor Muscles of the Hip. J. Bone Joint Surg. **29**, 614
66) English, T.A. (1975): The Troachanteric Approach to the Hip for Prosthetic Replacement. J. Bone Joint Surg. **57**A, 1128

Appendix A

67) DeLee J., Ferrari, A. (1976): Ectopic Bone Formation after Low Friction Arthoplasty of the Hip. Clin. Orthop. **121**, 53

Appendix B

68) Freeman, M.A.R.: Personal Communication.

Patents Details

Protective Clothing Patents

(Body Exhaust System)

	Patent Number		Patent Number
Australia	448393	South Africa	69/5091
Canada	928451	Sweden	323942
France	6927285	Switzerland	505576
Great Britain	1208284	U.S.A.	3529594
Great Britain	1239492	U.S.A.	3625206
Italy	885216		

Acetabular Prosthesis Patents

(Flanged, PIJ, Prosthesis)

	Application Number		Application Number
Australia	36061/78	Japan	53-64853
Canada	303223	South Africa	78/2844
France	7816950	Sweden	7805244-6
Germany	P2823306.9	Switzerland	599784
Great Britain	30385/76	U.S.A.	904752
Ireland	927/78		

Long Posterior Wall Hip Socket Patent

	Patent Number		Patent Number
Australia	471468	Sweden	72-017676
France	72-3934	U.S.A.	3722002
Great Britain	1296162		

Femoral Prosthesis Patents

(Flanged Prosthesis)

	Patent Number		Patent Number
Australia	83938/75	Ireland	1756/75
Canada	234136	Japan	104454/75
France	7526569	South Africa	75/5186
Germany	P2537807.8	Sweden	7509285.8
Great Britain	37732/74	Switzerland	11167/75
Great Britain	38965/74 (Cognate)	U.S.A.	604608

Index

www.ingramcontent.com/pod-product-compliance
Ingram Content Group UK Ltd.
Pitfield, Milton Keynes, MK11 3LW, UK
UKHW051004220926
475831UK00003B/109

9783642670152